Twin and Higher-order Pregnancies

Springer Nature More Media App

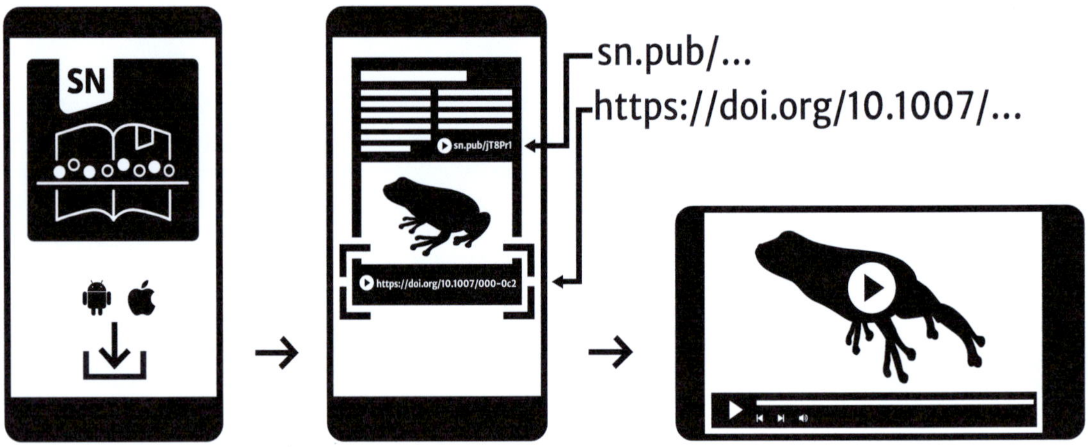

1. Download → **2. Scan Link** → **3. Enjoy Video**

Support: customerservice@springernature.com

Asma Khalil • Liesbeth Lewi • Enrico Lopriore
Editors

Twin and Higher-order Pregnancies

Springer

Editors
Asma Khalil
Fetal Medicine Unit
St George's University Hospitals
NHS Foundation Trust
London, UK

Vascular Biology Research Centre,
Molecular and Clinical Sciences
Research Institute
St George's University of London
London, UK

Liesbeth Lewi
Department of Obstetrics &
Gynaecology
University Hospitals Leuven
Leuven, Belgium

Department of Development and
Regeneration, Biomedical Sciences
KU Leuven
Leuven, Belgium

Enrico Lopriore
Division of Neonatology,
Department of Pediatrics
Leiden University Medical Center
Leiden, The Netherlands

Head of the Neonatal Intensive
Care Unit
Leiden University Medical Centre
Leiden, The Netherlands

This work contains media enhancements, which are displayed with a "play" icon. Material in the print book can be viewed on a mobile device by downloading the Springer Nature "More Media" app available in the major app stores. The media enhancements in the online version of the work can be accessed directly by authorized users.

ISBN 978-3-030-47651-9 ISBN 978-3-030-47652-6 (eBook)
https://doi.org/10.1007/978-3-030-47652-6

This Springer imprint is published by the registered company Springer Nature Switzerland AG
The registered company address is: Gewerbestrasse 11, 6330 Cham, Switzerland

Foreword

This textbook, written by leading international experts, constitutes essential reading for all healthcare professionals involved in the care of multiple pregnancies with the ultimate goal to improve their outcomes. The book provides a detailed account on the management of multiple pregnancies before, during, and after birth. Also, the book incorporates the patient's perspective in testimonials and experience of twin advocacy groups. The reader will gain a clear understanding of the biology, the complications, and the recommended care of multiple pregnancies, and there is special attention to parental well-being and childhood development. The textbook offers a practical guide with a wealth of illustrations, figures, and videos. Each chapter also contains multiple-choice questions to challenge the reader's knowledge.

Kypros Nicolaides
Professor of Fetal Medicine
Harris Birthright Centre
King's College London
London, UK

Contents

VI Postnatal Care

VII Childhood Development

VIII Research, Registries and Parent Views

Contributors

Laoreti Arianna Fetal Therapy Unit "U. Nicolini", Department of Obstetrics and Gynecology, "Vittore Buzzi" Children's Hospital, University of Milan, Milan, Italy

Amir Aviram Sunnybrook Health Sciences Centre, Department of Obstetrics and Gynecology, Division of Maternal-Fetal Medicine, University of Toronto, Toronto, ON, Canada
amir.aviram@sunnybrook.ca

Christian Bamberg Department of Obstetrics and Fetal Medicine, University Medical Center Hamburg-Eppendorf, Hamburg, Germany
c.bamberg@uke.de

Jon F. R. Barrett Sunnybrook Health Sciences Centre, Department of Obstetrics and Gynecology, Division of Maternal-Fetal Medicine, University of Toronto, Toronto, ON, Canada
jon.barrett@sunnybrook.ca

Jeffrey J. Beck Avera Institute for Human Genetics, Avera McKennan Hospital and University Health Center, Sioux Falls, SD, USA
jeffrey.beck@avera.org

Vincenzo Berghella Maternal Fetal Medicine Division, Obstetrics and Gynecology Department, Sidney Kimmel Medical College at Thomas Jefferson University, Philadelphia, PA, USA
vincenzo.berghella@jefferson.edu

Isaac Blickstein Department of Obstetrics and Gynecology, Kaplan Medical Center, Rehovot, and the Hadassah-Hebrew University School of Medicine, Jerusalem, Israel†
blick@netvision.net.il
liesbeth.lewi@uzleuven.be

Dorret I. Boomsma Avera Institute for Human Genetics, Avera McKennan Hospital and University Health Center, Sioux Falls, SD, USA

Netherlands Twin Register, Department of Biological Psychology, Behavioral and Movement Sciences, Vrije Universiteit Amsterdam, Amsterdam, The Netherlands
di.boomsma@vu.nl

Clifton Brock Department of Obstetrics, Gynecology and Reproductive Sciences, University of Texas Health Science Center at Houston, Houston, TX, USA
Clifton.O.Brock@uth.tmc.edu

Susanne Bruins Netherlands Twin Register, Department of Biological Psychology, Behavioral and Movement Sciences, Vrije Universiteit Amsterdam, Amsterdam, The Netherlands
s3.bruins@student.vu.nl

Alyson Chorley Twins Trust, Aldershot, Hampshire, UK
AlysonChorley@twinstrust.org

M. A. Clayton Department of Anaesthesia, Northwick Park Hospital, London, UK

Gareth E. Davies Avera Institute for Human Genetics, Avera McKennan Hospital and University Health Center, Sioux Falls, SD, USA

Netherlands Twin Register, Department of Biological Psychology, Behavioral and Movement Sciences, Vrije Universiteit Amsterdam, Amsterdam, The Netherlands
gareth.davies@avera.org

Eco de Geus Department of Biological Psychology, Vrije Universiteit Amsterdam, Amsterdam, The Netherlands
j.c.n.de.geus@vu.nl

Natasha Fenwick Twins Trust, Aldershot, Hampshire, UK
NatashaFenwick@twinstrust.org

J. L. Gibson Ian Donald Fetal Medicine Centre, Queen Elizabeth University Hospital, Glasgow, UK
janice.gibson@ggc.scot.nhs.uk

Noa Gilad Fetal Medicine Unit, Department of Obstetrics and Gynaecology, Mount Sinai Hospital and University of Toronto, Toronto, ON, Canada

Ontario Fetal Centre, Toronto, ON, Canada

L. R. I. Gurney West Midlands Fetal Medicine Centre, Birmingham Women's and Children's NHS Foundation Trust, Birmingham, UK
leo.gurney@doctors.org.uk

Guillermo Gurza Maternal Fetal Medicine Division, Obstetrics and Gynecology Department, Sidney Kimmel Medical College at Thomas Jefferson University, Philadelphia, PA, USA

Kurt Hecher Department of Obstetrics and Fetal Medicine, University Medical Center Hamburg-Eppendorf, Hamburg, Germany
khecher@uke.uni-hamburg.de

Titia Hompes Department of Neuroscience, Department of Adult Psychiatry, KU Leuven – University Psychiatric Center KU Leuven, Leuven, Belgium
titia.hompes@upckuleuven.be

Anthony Johnson The Fetal Center at Children's Memorial Hermann Hospital, Houston, TX, USA
anthony.johnson@uth.tmc.edu

Johannes Keunen Fetal Medicine Unit, Department of Obstetrics and Gynaecology, Mount Sinai Hospital and University of Toronto, Toronto, ON, Canada

Ontario Fetal Centre, Toronto, ON, Canada
johannes.keunen@sinaihealth.ca

Asma Khalil Fetal Medicine Unit, St George's University Hospitals NHS Foundation Trust, London, UK

Vascular Biology Research Centre, Molecular and Clinical Sciences Research Institute, St George's University of London, London, UK
akhalil@sgul.ac.uk

M. D. Kilby West Midlands Fetal Medicine Centre, Birmingham Women's and Children's NHS Foundation Trust, Birmingham, UK

Centre for Women's and Children Health, Institute of Metabolism and Systems Research, University of Birmingham, Birmingham, UK
m.d.kilby@bham.ac.uk

Janine R. Lam Twins Research Australia, The University of Melbourne, Melbourne, Australia

Ann Langedock Department of Obstetrics & Gynaecology, University Hospitals Leuven, Leuven, Belgium
ann.langedock@uzleuven.be
Ann.Langedock@yperman.net

Liesbeth Lewi Department of Obstetrics & Gynaecology, University Hospitals Leuven, Leuven, Belgium

Department of Development and Regeneration, Biomedical Sciences, KU Leuven, Leuven, Belgium
liesbeth.lewi@uzleuven.be

Becky Liu Fetal Maternal Medicine Unit, St George's University Hospitals, London, UK
Bexliu@doctors.org.uk

Enrico Lopriore Division of Neonatology, Department of Pediatrics, Leiden University Medical Center, Leiden, The Netherlands

Head of the Neonatal Intensive Care Unit, Leiden University Medical Centre, Leiden, The Netherlands
E.Lopriore@lumc.nl

D. N. Lucas Department of Anaesthesia, Northwick Park Hospital, London, UK
nuala@tuesday5.co.uk
nuala.lucas@nhs.net

Pierre Macé Service de Gynécologie-Obstétrique, Hôpital Necker-Enfants Malades, Assistance Publique – Hôpitaux de Paris (AP-HP), Université Paris Descartes, Paris, France

Miguel Macedo University Hospital of S. João, Porto, Portugal

Houman Mahallati Department of Radiology, University of Calgary, Calgary, AB, Canada

Lanna Mariano Fetal Therapy Unit "U. Nicolini", Department of Obstetrics and Gynecology, "Vittore Buzzi" Children's Hospital, University of Milan, Milan, Italy
mariano.lanna@asst-fbf-sacco.it

Alexandra Matias Department of Obstetrics and Gynecology, Faculty of Medicine, University Hospital of S. João, Porto, Portugal

R. L. May Department of Anaesthesia, Northwick Park Hospital, London, UK
rosiemay@nhs.net

Hamdi Mbarek Netherlands Twin Register, Department of Biological Psychology, Behavioral and Movement Sciences, Vrije Universiteit Amsterdam, Amsterdam, The Netherlands
h.mbarek@vu.nl

Elad Mei-Dan Department of Obstetrics and Gynecology, North York General Hospital, University of Toronto, Toronto, ON, Canada

Nir Melamed Sunnybrook Health Sciences Centre, Department of Obstetrics and Gynecology, Division of Maternal-Fetal Medicine, University of Toronto, Toronto, ON, Canada
nir.melamed@sunnybrook.ca

R. K. Morris West Midlands Fetal Medicine Centre, Birmingham Women's and Children's NHS Foundation Trust, Birmingham, UK
Centre for Women's and Children Health, Institute of Metabolism and Systems Research, University of Birmingham, Birmingham, UK
r.k.morris@bham.ac.uk

Kate Murphy Twins Research Australia, The University of Melbourne, Melbourne, Australia
murphyks@unimelb.edu.au

Veronika Odintsova Department of Biological Psychology, Vrije Universiteit Amsterdam, Amsterdam, The Netherlands
Kulakov National Medical Research Center for Obstetrics, Gynecology and Perinatology, Moscow, Russia
v.v.odintsova@vu.nl

Vagisha Pruthi Fetal Medicine Unit, Department of Obstetrics and Gynaecology, Mount Sinai Hospital and University of Toronto, Toronto, ON, Canada
Ontario Fetal Centre, Toronto, ON, Canada
vagisha.pruthi@sinaihealth.ca

Alexandra Ramirez Maternal Fetal Medicine Division, Obstetrics and Gynecology Department, Sidney Kimmel Medical College at Thomas Jefferson University, Philadelphia, PA, USA

Paul Ian Ramler Department of Obstetrics, Leiden University Medical Center, Leiden, The Netherlands
p.i.ramler@lumc.nl

Amanda Roman Maternal Fetal Medicine Division, Obstetrics and Gynecology Department, Sidney Kimmel Medical College at Thomas Jefferson University, Philadelphia, PA, USA
amanda.roman@jefferson.edu

Neal Russell Paediatric Infectious Disease Research Group, St Georges University, London, UK
nrussell@sgul.ac.uk

Sophie Russell Women's Health, Lewisham and Greenwich NHS Trust, London, UK
Sophie.russell7@nhs.net

Greg Ryan Fetal Medicine Unit, Department of Obstetrics and Gynaecology, Mount Sinai Hospital and University of Toronto, Toronto, ON, Canada

Ontario Fetal Centre, Toronto, ON, Canada
greg.ryan@sinaihealth.ca

Laurent J. Salomon Service de Gynécologie-Obstétrique, Hôpital Necker-Enfants Malades, Assistance Publique – Hôpitaux de Paris (AP-HP), Université Paris Descartes, Paris, France

Mercede Sebghati Fetal Medicine Unit, St George's University, London, UK
Mercedesebghati@doctors.org.uk

Shiri Shinar Fetal Medicine Unit, Department of Obstetrics and Gynaecology, Mount Sinai Hospital and University of Toronto, Toronto, ON, Canada

Ontario Fetal Centre, Toronto, ON, Canada
shiri.Shinar@sinaihealth.ca

M. S. Spruijt Division of Neonatology, Department of Pediatrics, Leiden University Medical Center, Leiden, The Netherlands
m.s.spruijt@lumc.nl

Faiola Stefano Fetal Therapy Unit "U. Nicolini", Department of Obstetrics and Gynecology, "Vittore Buzzi" Children's Hospital, University of Milan, Milan, Italy
Stefano.faiola@asst-fbf-sacco.it

Beatriz Teixeira Department of Obstetrics and Gynecology, Faculty of Medicine, University Hospital of S. João, Porto, Portugal

L. S. A. Tollenaar Department of Obstetrics, Division of Fetal Therapy, Leiden University Medical Center, Leiden, The Netherlands
l.s.a.tollenaar@lumc.nl

Thomas van den Akker Department of Obstetrics, Leiden University Medical Center, Leiden, The Netherlands

Athena Institute, Faculty of Science, VU University, Amsterdam, The Netherlands
t.h.van_den_akker@lumc.nl

J. M. M. van Klink Division of Pediatric Psychology, Department of Pediatrics, Leiden University Medical Center, Leiden, The Netherlands
j.m.m.van_klink@lumc.nl

Tim Van Mieghem Fetal Medicine Unit, Department of Obstetrics and Gynaecology, Mount Sinai Hospital and University of Toronto, Toronto, ON, Canada

Ontario Fetal Centre, Toronto, ON, Canada
tim.vanmieghem@sinaihealth.ca

Mieke Vanoppen Department of Obstetrics & Gynaecology, University Hospitals Leuven, Leuven, Belgium
Mieke.vanoppen@uzleuven.be
mieke.vanoppen@jessazh.be

Femke Vanwetswinkel Department of Adult Psychiatry, University Psychiatric Center KU Leuven, Leuven, Belgium
femke.vanwetswinkel@upckuleuven.be

Gonneke Willemsen Department of Biological Psychology, Vrije Universiteit Amsterdam, Amsterdam, The Netherlands
a.h.m.willemsen@vu.nl

Biology

Contents

The Vanishing Twin Syndrome

Isaac Blickstein†

Contents

Electronic Supplementary Material The online version of this chapter (https://doi.org/10.1007/978-3-030-47652-6_1) contains supplementary material, which is available to authorized users. The videos can be accessed by scanning the related images with the SN More Media App.

A. Khalil et al. (eds.), *Twin and Higher-order Pregnancies*,
https://doi.org/10.1007/978-3-030-47652-6_1

1

Trailer

The vanishing twin syndrome (VTS) is used to describe the spontaneous loss of one developing embryo early in a multiple pregnancy. The incidence of the VTS in spontaneous pregnancies is largely unknown, whereas the incidence in pregnancies following assisted reproduction is estimated to be 3–10%. Regardless of chorionicity, the VTS has been associated with adverse outcomes, especially related to cerebral palsy and premature births. The retained products of the vanished twin may lead to errors in risk estimation using biochemical markers as well as with more advanced techniques such as cell-free DNA in maternal blood. While the VTS is mainly diagnosed during the late first trimester, the advent of early sonography, especially following ART, will soon allow an earlier diagnosis.

Definitions

Vanishing twin syndrome: Loss of one developing embryo early in a multiple pregnancy.

Learning Objectives

- To understand the biology of the VTS
- To acknowledge the adverse outcomes attributed to the VTS
- To identify errors in risk estimation of prenatal diagnosis resulting from the VTS

1.1 Introduction

The vanishing twin syndrome (VTS) is used to describe the spontaneous loss of one developing embryo early in a multiple pregnancy. Although suspected for many years, it is a relatively new diagnosis that emerged only after the implementation of ultrasonography in early gestation. In the beginning, this finding was met with skepticism; however, careful examination of the placenta revealed in 1986 the histological evidence that confirmed the validity of VTS, consisting of a chorion-lined sac containing amorphous material [1]. The incidence of the VTS in spontaneous pregnancies is largely unknown because the vast majority of women are not scanned in early pregnancy, and many cases of VTS are thus unnoticed. The best estimate comes from pregnancies following assisted reproduction technologies (ART). Pinborg and her coworkers observed that 1 in 10 ART singletons originated from a twin gestation in early pregnancy [2]. A more recent approximation lacks data about VTS in as many as 1:8 pregnancies, and therefore, the quoted 3% appears to be an underestimate [3].

Birth certificates are also to no avail. Despite a constantly increasing clinical interest, VTS is rarely, if ever, recorded in birth certificates. Pharoah [4] opined that whereas it is a legal requirement of parents to register a fetal death (a dead fetus born after 24 weeks' gestation), there is worldwide confusion regarding fetal death before 24 weeks. Hence, a legal definition for the registration of embryonic/fetal death, including the VTS, requires international agreement and application [4].

The VTS can be considered as a natural equivalent of multifetal pregnancy reduction (MFPR) performed to reduce the number of fetuses in a high-order multiple gestation. However, the main difference between MFPR and VTS is that in the former, the final number of remaining embryos is usually (but not exclusively) two, whereas the VTS is usually (but not exclusively) referring to a singleton survivor after a twin pregnancy. Hence, it is basically incorrect to compare outcomes of MFPR and VTS.

With these caveats in mind, this chapter will discuss several clinical issues related to the VTS.

1.2 Embryonic Loss After ART

Every conception has its own risk of loss. Thus, it is conceivable that each twin has, potentially, an equal chance for survival or loss. It has been repeatedly shown that following ART, the chance of early loss of the entire singleton pregnancy is significantly (2 to 5 times) higher than the entire early loss of a twin pregnancy [5]. This observation suggests that the intuitive view about the gloomy outcome of early twin gestations should be reappraised [6]. Although most data point to better implantation rates as a feasible explanation of better twin survival, it is unknown why in some early pregnancies this presumable advantage of twins is partially lost and results in VTS [6]. Put differently, if indeed ART represents an advantage for early twin gestations, than the VTS or entire early loss of the twin set might represent an effect of an unspecified hostile uterine environment. More importantly, it is unknown if the situation following ART is equivalent to spontaneous pregnancies. Some idea comes from Márton et al. [7] that the incidence of VTS was significantly higher after natural than after ART conceptions. However, a clear explanation for this observation remains elusive.

Pereira and co-workers [8] looked at the VTS by day of embryo transfer and showed that cleavage- and blastocyst-stage embryo transfers were associated with early VTS in 11.6 and 6.32% patients, respectively, which represented 0.5 times lower odds, albeit not significant, of early VTS in the blastocyst-stage group compared to the cleavage-stage group.

1.3 Types of VTS

In principle, four types of VTS may exist. The first is the unknown case of the VTS, namely a singleton is seen by sonography, and there is no clue that a co-twin existed. These may present with a hint of an ill-defined gestational sac or with a hematoma formation adjacent to the other sac that contains an embryo. The second is the VTS with an empty sac ("blighted ovum"), namely a singleton is seen by sonography along with a blighted ovum (◘ Fig. 1.1). The third is the clear-cut VTS with two embryos—one alive and the other dead—which is easily diagnosed during the first trimester (◘ Fig. 1.2). It is unknown if there is a difference in the VTS between the presence of an empty sac and the presence of a "missed" twin in terms of outcome. Finally, all the above may occur in high-order multiple gestations affecting one or more of the multiples.

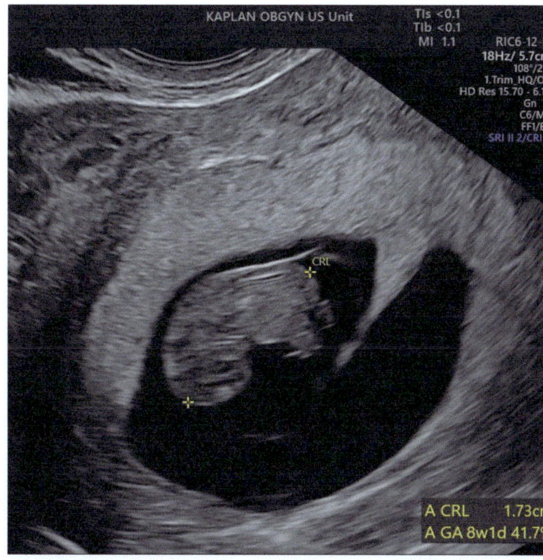

◘ **Fig. 1.1** Empty sac along a gestational sac containing an 8+ weeks' embryo in dichorionic pregnancy. (Image courtesy Dr. Y. Chazan)

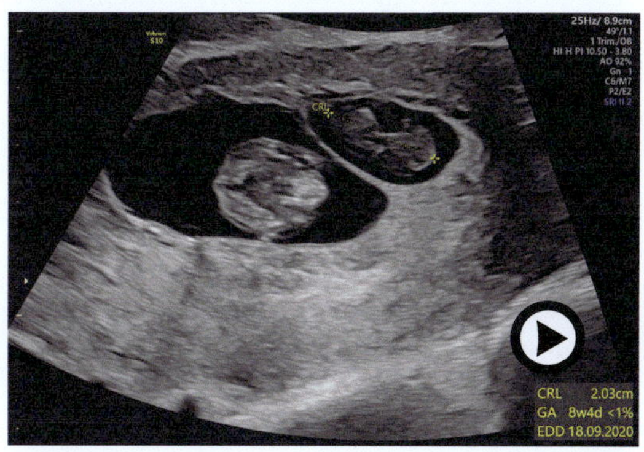

◘ **Fig. 1.2** Vanishing twin with crown-rump length of 8+ weeks in a dichorionic twin pregnancy at 12 weeks) (https://doi.org/10.1007/000-2sw)

1.4 VTS and Cerebral Palsy

Regardless of the etiology, most studies on the VTS show an increased incidence of perinatal complications [2, 7]. For the death of one twin to cause damage to the survivor, one may assume a vascular connection between the two twins. This is the case in monochorionic (MC) twins where the inter-twin anastomoses are invariably present. Following single fetal death, blood is shunted to the low resistance circulation of the demised twin, and depending on the magnitude of this shunt, the survivor twin may die, may become handicapped, or may have an intact survival [9]. Early cases of twin-twin transfusion syndrome (TTTS) in the first trimester were observed, but as stated above, even in the case of diagnosed twins, in the vast majority of the VTS we are blind to placental signs of chorionicity. Based on the idea that numerous singletons exist that are, actually, survivors of the VTS, Pharoah and Cooke [10] further hypothesized that the VTS might explain cases of brain damage in singletons following a normal pregnancy and birth, just because nobody knows that this singleton was a survivor of the VTS. This attractive hypothesis was criticized because most documented cases, especially after ART, were dichorionic twins who lack inter-twin anastomoses [10]. Given that our knowledge on inter-twin anastomoses comes from second- and third-trimester specimen, it is unknown if the early first-trimester dichorionic placenta does or does not have anastomoses. Thus, we are blind to the possibility of inter-twin anastomoses in early first trimester dichorionic twins. Conceivably, such anastomoses and the placenta vanish together with the vanishing twin, just after causing a significant shunt and brain damage [11].

Speculations aside, Pinborg and her colleagues [2] did not find an excess risk of neurological sequelae in survivors of a VTS compared to a singleton cohort, but pointed out the almost double odds cerebral palsy (1.9, 95% CI 0.7–5.2). Two years later, Anand et al. [12] tested the hypothesis that the VTS may be associated with an increased risk of cerebral impairment in the survivor. Among pregnancies classified as first-trimester VTS ("definite" and "probable"), the development and neurological function of surviving infants were assessed at 1 year of age. Although the numbers were extremely small, there was a significant difference between the vanishing twin and singleton group (RR 6.1; 95% CI 1.5–8.3) [12]. Subsequently, the same authors [13] found that the sub- and general quotient scores in singletons and surviving co-twins of a vanishing twin did not differ significantly.

One of the greatest arguments against a cause-and-effect relation between the VTS and brain damage comes from MFPR. This frequent procedure is performed since the 1980s mainly in high-order multiples, but also in twins. Being a common practice, one should anticipate that adverse outcomes such cerebral palsy would be observed. To date, there is no evidence that MFPR is related to cerebral palsy. For example, MFPR in triplets [14] showed that the cerebral palsy prevalence was similar in trichorionic triplets who had or did not have a MFPR.

1.5 VTS and Prenatal Diagnosis

The retained products of the vanished twin may lead to errors in risk estimation using biochemical markers. Spencer et al. [15] made the distinction between the VTS (second gestational sac containing a dead fetus with a measurable crown-rump length) and cases with a presumable VTS (second empty gestational sac). The VTS caused an increase in PAPP-A, which was related to a fall from 85 to 75% in the detection rate for trisomy 21. In contrast, Gjerris et al. [16] assessed the impact of a VTS on first-trimester combined biochemical and ultrasound screening after ART and first-trimester biochemical screening markers in women pregnant after ART and observed that VTS diagnosed at early ultrasound do not differ from those of other ART singleton pregnancies. However, when VTS was diagnosed at the time of the nuchal translucency scan, the serum risk assessment might not be as precise as it is in singleton ART pregnancies. The same authors [17] published in 2012 an extensive literature review and concluded that in VTS pregnancies (second sac with a dead fetus), first trimester screening should be based exclusively on the maternal age and the nuchal translucency scan as the tested biomarkers were found to be significantly altered.

It appears that the more advanced non-invasive prenatal testing (NIPT, cell-free DNA testing) also exhibits diagnostic errors between fetal screening and postnatal phenotype [18, 19]. In such cases, such as discordant sex and RhD typing, the VTS might be a plausible explanation for the discrepant genetics of the survivor. It has been suggested that cases of the VTS result in as much as 42.1%

of confirmed false-positive NIPT results [20]. However, the interval between the diagnosis of the VTS and the presence of a false-positive NIPT is unknown. In one case [20], the persistence of cell-free fetal DNA from the vanished twin for at least 15 weeks was documented. Given these observations, both patients and laboratories should be advised about this potential limitation of the NIPT in cases of the VTS.

1.6 VTS and Perinatal Outcomes

There is little doubt that singletons are doing better than twins in terms of perinatal outcomes. Thus, the early demise of one twin may improve, worsen, or do not change perinatal outcomes in the survivor. Several studies in the last couple of years looked specifically into this question. Evron et al. [21] used multivariable logistic regression models and found that VTS (as compared with singletons) was an independent risk factor for adverse outcomes including gestational diabetes, growth restriction, very low birth weight infants, low Apgar scores, and perinatal mortality. A 2017 meta-analysis [22] identified two case-control studies and three cohort studies for the final analysis. The pooled mean gestational age and preterm delivery rate were not increased in the VTS group; however, the prevalence of extremely preterm delivery rate was higher in the VTS group (pooled risk ratio 3.5, 95% CI 1.7, 7.1). No difference was found in low birth weight rate, very low birth weight rate, and rate of small for gestational age. Magnus et al. [23] looked at the Norwegian ART database and found a reduction in birth weight and increased risk of small for gestational age ART singletons with VTS. This group proposed the presence of harmful intrauterine factors with long-term health impact. Similarly, Kamath et al. [24] used a 20-year database of the United Kingdom Human Fertilization and Embryology Authority. The data suggest that the VTS is associated with an increased risk of preterm birth and low birth weight. One should mention that this was not the case in the study of Romanski et al. [25] who found that if the survivor of the VTS made it past 24 weeks of gestation, the VTS survivor and singleton pregnancies had similar perinatal and peripartum outcomes.

As is the case with MFPR, it is well established that the uterus "remembers" the initial number of implantation, whereby twins reduced from triplets do much better than twins reduced from quadruplets or more. Thus, the lower gestational age and birth weight associated with the VTS appear to follow the same rule. What is more important from the perinatal point of view is the risk of preterm births rather than a lower gestational age and the risk of low birth weight rather than the risk of lower birth weight. To this point, the data are, at best, inconclusive. Indeed, many confounders may significantly affect these outcomes, such as smoking, past obstetric history, obesity, and maternal comorbidity [24].

One of the neglected areas of research concerning the survivor of the VTS is the psychological health of these children. De Pascalis et al. [26] evaluated the attitude of ART parents towards the survivors of the VTS. Using sophisticated psychological assessment, the authors observed that despite the perceived motor difficulties and the difficulties in the process of individuation-separation that appear at the beginning of the educational circumstances, parents of singletons following the VTS perceive their children as "invincible" (as compared to the vanished twin) and thus less vulnerable compared to singletons without the VTS.

1.7 Epilogue

One way to look at the current complexity of the VTS is by referring to the seminal monograph of Landy and Keith [27] some two decades ago, which was the basis of their later detailed contribution [28]. At these points in time, the VTS was some kind of curios of Nature, which cited "The main complication associated with vanishing embryos is vaginal bleeding." In the meantime, the VTS was better defined and related to outcomes.

At present, it appears that the death of the vanished twin affects, directly or indirectly, and in whatever way, the well-being of the survivor of the VTS. The extent of this consequence also varies depending on different determinants such as maternal characteristics as well as by the twining process in terms of chorionicity and timing of the embryonic demise.

While the VTS is mainly diagnosed during the late first trimester, the advent of early sonography, especially following ART, will soon allow an earlier diagnosis. This might lead to the disambiguation of this exciting period of human development.

1.7.1 Review Questions

? 1. How does the vanishing twin syndrome influence screening for Down's syndrome?

? 2. How does the vanishing twin syndrome influence perinatal outcomes?

1.7.2 Multiple-Choice Questions

? 1. The following statement about vanishing twin syndrome is correct:
   (a) Screening for aneuploidy is not possible and an invasive test should be offered.
   (b) In the screening for aneuploidy, PAPP-A is decreased as compared to singleton pregnancies.
   (c) Screening for aneuploidy is best based on maternal age and the nuchal translucency scan.
   (d) In the screening for aneuploidy, the non-invasive prenatal test is as precise as in singleton pregnancies.

✓ Answer: (c)

? 2. Vanishing twin syndrome commonly causes:
   (a) Cerebral palsy in the surviving co-twin.
   (b) False-positive results of the non-invasive prenatal test.
   (c) Psychological vulnerability in the surviving co-twin.
   (d) Macrosomia in the surviving co-twin.

✓ Answer: (b)

References

1. Sulak LE, Dodson MG. The vanishing twin: pathologic confirmation of an ultrasonographic phenomenon. Obstet Gynecol. 1986;68:811–5.
2. Pinborg A, Lidegaard O, la Cour Freiesleben N, Andersen AN. Consequences of vanishing twins in IVF/ICSI pregnancies. Hum Reprod. 2005;20:2821–9.
3. Magnus MC, Ghaderi S, Morken NH, Magnus P, Bente Romundstad L, Skjærven R, Wilcox AJ, Eldevik Håberg S. Vanishing twin syndrome among ART singletons and pregnancy outcomes. Hum Reprod. 2017;32:2298–304.
4. Pharoah PO. Fetal death registration in multiple births: anomalies and clinical significance. Twin Res Hum Genet. 2006;9:587–90.
5. Matias A, La Sala GB, Blickstein I. Early loss rates of entire pregnancies after assisted reproduction are lower in twin than in singleton pregnancies. Fertil Steril. 2007;88:1452–4.
6. La Sala GB, Nucera G, Gallinelli A, Nicoli A, Villani MT, Blickstein I. Lower embryonic loss rates among twin gestations following assisted reproduction. J Assist Reprod Genet. 2005;22:181–4.
7. Márton V, Zádori J, Kozinszky Z, Keresztúri A. Prevalences and pregnancy outcome of vanishing twin pregnancies achieved by in vitro fertilization versus natural conception. Fertil Steril. 2016;106:1399–406.
8. Pereira N, Pryor KP, Petrini AC, Lekovich JP, Stahl J, Elias RT, Spandorfer SD. Perinatal risks associated with early vanishing twin syndrome following transfer of cleavage- or blastocyst-stage embryos. J Pregnancy. 2016;2016:1245210.

9. Blickstein I, Perlman S. Single fetal death in twin gestations. J Perinat Med. 2013;41:65–9.
10. Pharoah PO, Cooke RW. A hypothesis for the aetiology of spastic cerebral palsy- the vanishing twin. Dev Med Child Neurol. 1997;39:292–6.
11. Blickstein I. Reflections on the hypothesis for the etiology of spastic cerebral palsy caused by the "vanishing twin" syndrome. Dev Med Child Neurol. 1998;40:358.
12. Anand D, Platt MJ, Pharoah PO. Vanishing twin: a possible cause of cerebral impairment. Twin Res Hum Genet. 2007;10:202–9.
13. Anand D, Platt MJ, Pharoah PO. Comparative development of surviving co-twins of vanishing twin conceptions, twins and singletons. Twin Res Hum Genet. 2007;10:210–5.
14. Dimitriou G, Pharoah PO, Nicolaides KH, Greenough A. Cerebral palsy in triplet pregnancies with and without iatrogenic reduction. Eur J Pediatr. 2004;163:449–51.
15. Spencer K, Staboulidou I, Nicolaides KH. First trimester aneuploidy screening in the presence of a vanishing twin: implications for maternal serum markers. Prenat Diagn. 2010;30:235–40.
16. Gjerris AC, Loft A, Pinborg A, Christiansen M, Tabor A. The effect of a 'vanishing twin' on biochemical and ultrasound first trimester screening markers for Down's syndrome in pregnancies conceived by assisted reproductive technology. Hum Reprod. 2009;24:55–62.
17. Gjerris AC, Tabor A, Loft A, Christiansen M, Pinborg A. First trimester prenatal screening among women pregnant after IVF/ICSI. Hum Reprod Update. 2012;18:350–9.
18. Thurik FF, Ait Soussan A, Bossers B, Woortmeijer H, Veldhuisen B, Page-Christiaens GC, de Haas M, van der Schoot CE. Analysis of false-positive results of fetal RHD typing in a national screening program reveals vanishing twins as potential cause for discrepancy. Prenat Diagn. 2015;35:754–60.
19. Masala M, Saba L, Zoppi MA, Puddu R, Picciau A, Capponi V, Iuculano A, Monni G, Rosatelli MC. Pitfalls in noninvasive fetal RhD and sex determination due to a vanishing twin. Prenat Diagn. 2015;35:506–8.
20. Niles KM, Murji A, Chitayat D. Prolonged duration of persistent cell-free fetal DNA from vanishing twin. Ultrasound Obstet Gynecol. 2018;52:547–8.
21. Evron E, Sheiner E, Friger M, Sergienko R, Harlev A. Vanishing twin syndrome: is it associated with adverse perinatal outcome? Fertil Steril. 2015;103:1209–14.
22. Sun L, Jiang LX, Chen HZ. Obstetric outcome of vanishing twins syndrome: a systematic review and meta-analysis. Arch Gynecol Obstet. 2017;295:559–67.
23. Magnus MC, Ghaderi S, Morken NH, Magnus P, Bente Romundstad L, Skjærven R, Wilcox AJ, Eldevik Håberg S. Vanishing twin syndrome among ART singletons and pregnancy outcomes. Hum Reprod. 2017;32:2298–304.
24. Kamath MS, Antonisamy B, Selliah HY, Sunkara SK. Perinatal outcomes of singleton live births with and without vanishing twin following transfer of multiple embryos: analysis of 113 784 singleton live births. Hum Reprod. 2018;33:2018–22.
25. Romanski PA, Carusi DA, Farland LV, Missmer SA, Kaser DJ, Walsh BW, Racowsky C, Brady PC. Perinatal and peripartum outcomes in vanishing twin pregnancies achieved by in vitro fertilization. Obstet Gynecol. 2018;131:1011–20.
26. De Pascalis L, Monti F, Agostini F, Fagandini P, La Sala GB, Blickstein I. Psychological vulnerability of singleton children after the 'vanishing' of a co-twin following assisted reproduction. Twin Res Hum Genet. 2008;11:93–8.
27. Landy HJ, Keith LG. The vanishing twin: a review. Hum Reprod Update. 1998;4:177–83.
28. Landy HJ, Keith LG. The vanishing fetus. In: Blickstein I, Keith LG, editors. Multiple pregnancy: epidemiology, gestation, and prenatal outcome. London: Taylor and Francis Group; 2005. Chapter 17.

Key Reading

Chaveeva P, Wright A, Syngelaki A, Konstantinidou L, Wright D, Nicolaides KH. First-trimester screening for trisomies in pregnancies with vanishing twin. Ultrasound Obstet Gynecol. 2020;55:326–31. (this reference replaces the older reference 10 in the chapter)

Kamath MS, Antonisamy B, Selliah HY, Sunkara SK. Perinatal outcomes of singleton live births with and without vanishing twin following transfer of multiple embryos: analysis of 113,784 singleton live births. Hum Reprod. 2018;33:2018–22.

Niles KM, Murji A, Chitayat D. Prolonged duration of persistent cell-free fetal DNA from vanishing twin. Ultrasound Obstet Gynecol. 2018;52:547–8.

Romanski PA, Carusi DA, Farland LV, Missmer SA, Kaser DJ, Walsh BW, Racowsky C, Brady PC. Perinatal and peripartum outcomes in vanishing twin pregnancies achieved by in vitro fertilization. Obstet Gynecol. 2018;131:1011–20.

Placentation in Multiple Pregnancy

Enrico Lopriore and Liesbeth Lewi

Contents

Electronic Supplementary Material The online version of this chapter (https://doi.org/10.1007/978-3-030-47652-6_2) contains supplementary material, which is available to authorized users. The videos can be accessed by scanning the related images with the SN More Media App.

A. Khalil et al. (eds.), *Twin and Higher-order Pregnancies*,
https://doi.org/10.1007/978-3-030-47652-6_2

Trailer

Twins face higher risks during their intrauterine journey, and the placenta often provides clues that explain problems such as growth restriction and ascending infection. Especially, the pattern of anastomoses and degree of placental sharing explain the typical monochorionic complications. In this chapter, we explain how to examine the placenta after birth to confirm the chorionicity, the typical twin-related placental problems, how to document the anastomoses with color dye injection and their role in the monochorionic twin-specific complications, and finally the possible cord complications in twin pregnancies.

Definitions

TTTS = Twin-twin transfusion syndrome

TAPS = Twin anemia-polycythemia sequence

sFGR = Selective fetal growth restriction

Learning Objectives

- To learn how to confirm the chorionicity after birth
- To know the placental and cord abnormalities that are more common in twin pregnancies
- To know how to document the vascular anastomoses in monochorionic twin pregnancies and their importance in monochorionic twin complications

2.1 Introduction

Twins are born earlier and more often smaller than singletons, because they share the same womb. About 20% of twins also share the same placenta (monochorionic) and placental vascular anastomoses connect the circulations of both twins. These anastomoses may cause transfusion imbalances and make their well-being interrelated. The placenta is the black box of their intrauterine journey. In this chapter, we explain how to examine the placenta after birth to confirm chorionicity; we address some twin-specific placental problems, the typical placenta and anastomoses in complicated monochorionic twin pregnancies, and twin-related cord abnormalities.

2.2 Monochorionic Versus Dichorionic Placentas: Macroscopy and Histology

2.2.1 Macroscopic Chorionicity Determination After Birth

In a dichorionic pregnancy, each twin has its separate placenta. Nevertheless, in about 50%, these separate placentas fuse and thus appear as one placental mass at the time of birth [1]. On the other hand, the monochorionic placenta can consist of two separate lobes, the so-called bipartite or bilobar placenta [2], which implies that chorionicity cannot be determined just by counting the number of placental masses. Moreover, although most monochorionic placentas have anastomoses, their absence does not exclude monochorionicity. As such, chorionicity determination at birth requires the careful inspection of the intertwin membrane. In dichorionic placentas, the intertwin membrane is thicker and opaque (◘ Fig. 2.1a) and consists of two layers of amnion separated by one or two layers of chorion. The chorionic membrane is firmly attached to the chorionic surface, forming a ridge that cannot be removed. Therefore, in a dichorionic placenta, one can remove the amniotic membrane on either side of the opaque chorionic layer, thereby reproducing the first-trimester ultrasound image of a dichorionic twin pregnancy (amnion-chorion-amnion) (◘ Fig. 2.1b) (▶ Chap. 6). In contrast, the monochorionic diamniotic intertwin membrane is thinner and transparent (◘ Fig. 2.2a). It consists of only two layers of amnion and is only loosely attached to the chorionic plate without forming a ridge. We can easily separate the amniotic membranes from each other, recreating the first-trimester ultrasound image of a monochorionic-diamniotic twin pregnancy (amnion-amnion) (◘ Fig. 2.2b). In contrast to dichorionic placentas, we can also completely remove

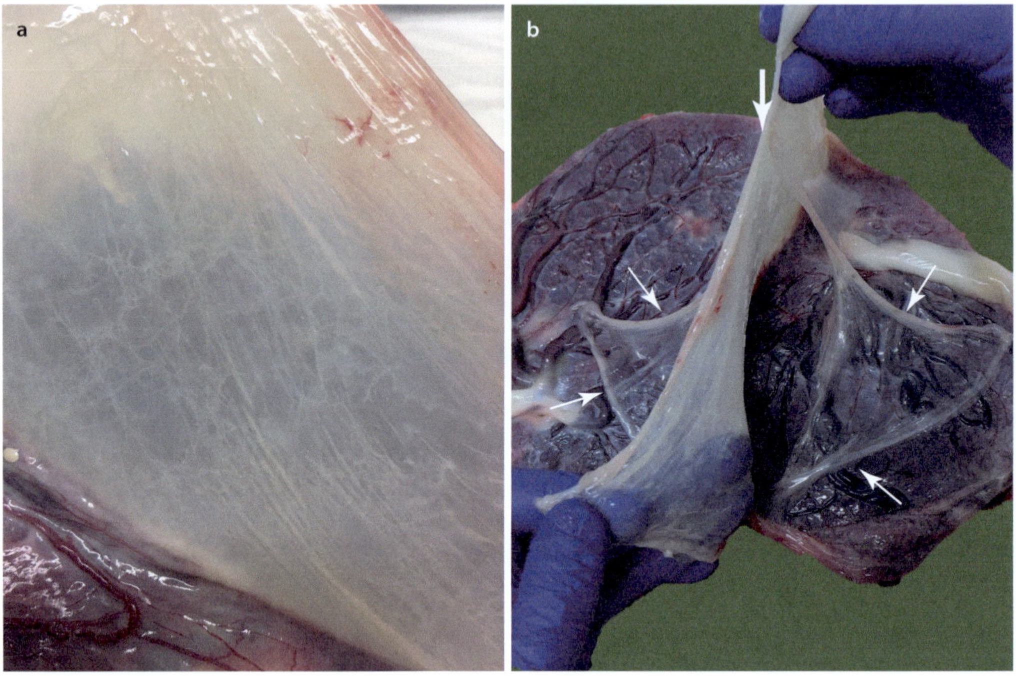

Fig. 2.1 **a** Details of the septum of a dichorionic twin placenta. The septum is thick and opaque. **b** Image of the septum of a dichorionic twin placenta after the removal of the amniotic membranes (thin arrows) from the chorionic layer (thick arrow), recreating the image on the first-trimester ultrasound scan (amnion-chorion-amnion). The chorionic part cannot be removed

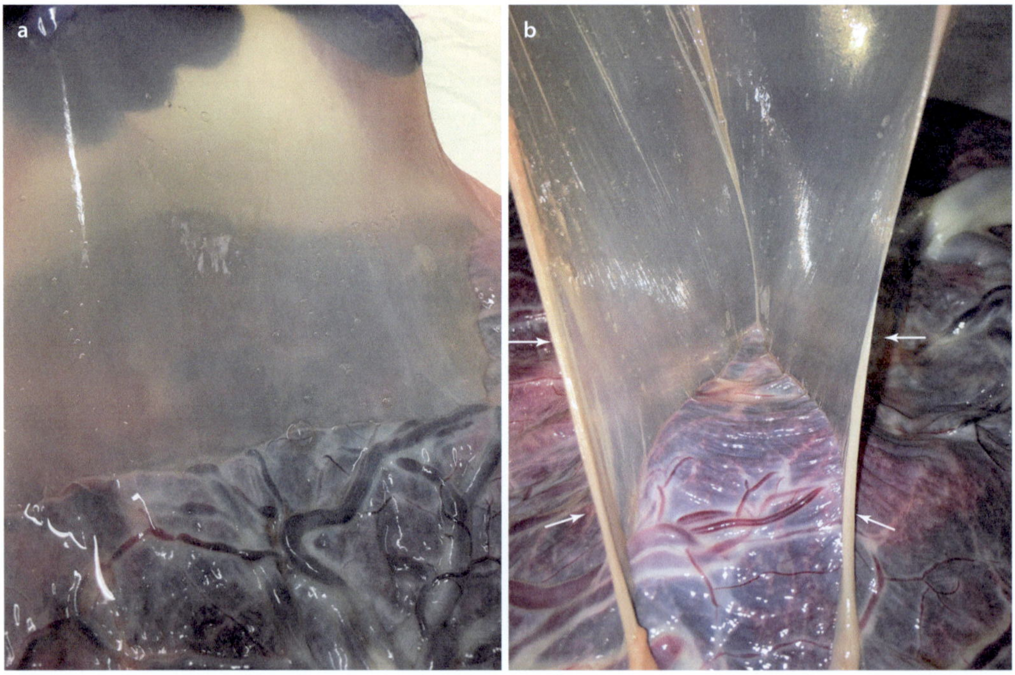

Fig. 2.2 **a** Details of the septum of a monochorionic twin placenta. The septum is thin and translucent. **b** Image of the septum of a monochorionic twin placenta after the separation of the amniotic membranes (thin arrows). There is no intervening chorion and we can easily peel off the entire septum from the chorionic septum

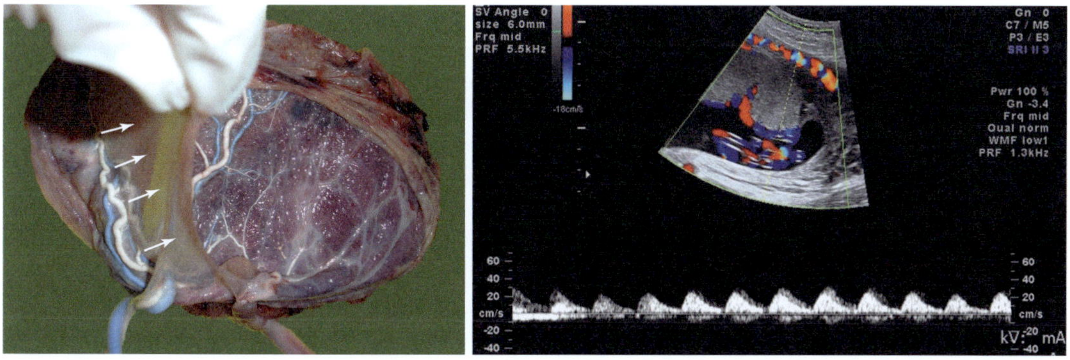

■ **Fig. 2.3** Image of a monoamniotic placenta with proximate cord insertions and a partial biamniotic septum (arrow). Insert: ultrasound image of the same pregnancy at 15 weeks demonstrating the cord entanglement that is typical in a monoamniotic pregnancy

the septum from the chorionic plate. Finally, monoamniotic twin placentas either entirely lack an intertwin septum or only an incomplete biamniotic septum is present between the two cord insertions (■ Fig. 2.3).

2.2.2 Microscopic Chorionicity Determination After Birth

The pathologist assigns the chorionicity according to the microscopic differences of the intertwin septum. In monochorionic diamniotic placentas, the intertwin septum is made up by two layers of amnion (epithelium and underlying connective tissue) (■ Fig. 2.4). In contrast, the dichorionic septum contains a chorionic layer in between the two amniotic layers. The space between the amnion and chorion is all that remains of the extraembryonic coelomic cavity after fusion of amnion and chorion (■ Fig. 2.5).

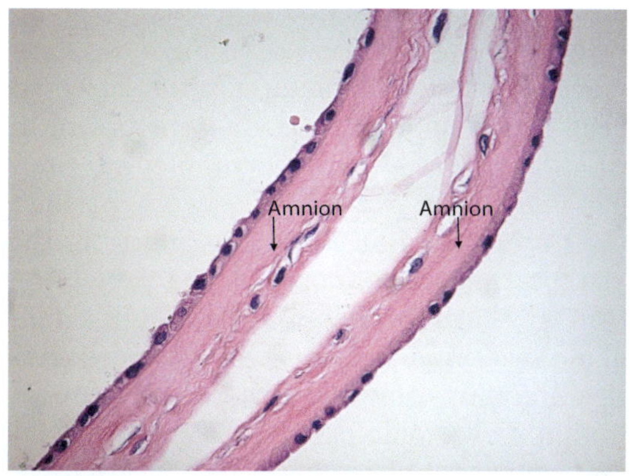

■ **Fig. 2.4** Microscopic image of the septum of a monochorionic diamniotic placenta. There are two layers of amnion without interposing chorionic connective tissue or trophoblast

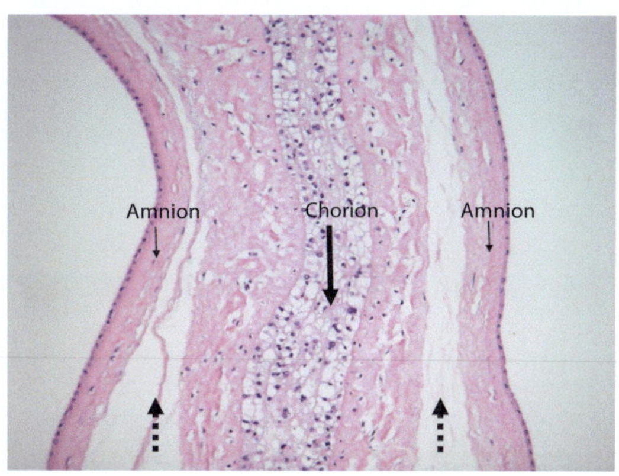

■ **Fig. 2.5** Microscopic image of the septum of a dichorionic placenta. Two layers of amnion can be seen on line the septum on the outside (thin arrows). In the middle are the intermediate trophoblastic cells of the chorion leave (thick arrow) with on either side chorionic connective tissue (interrupted arrows)

2.3 Specific Problems in Twin Placentas: Placenta Previa and Discordant Lesions

2.3.1 Placenta Previa

Placenta previa is more common in dichorionic pregnancies than in monochorionic and singleton pregnancies [3]. This increased risk is due to the implantation of two placentas, as well as to the increased use of in vitro fertilization, a known risk factor for placenta previa [4]. We diagnose placenta previa on the second trimester ultrasound scan when the edge of the placenta is within 2 cm from the internal os. However, it is essential to counsel patients that the overall majority of low-lying placentas resolve by the time of birth [3].

2.3.2 Placental Lesions

2.3.2.1 Pathologic Placental Findings

Placental pathology is crucial to document inflammatory and vascular lesions that can explain adverse neonatal outcome [5, 6]. In twin pregnancies, these lesions are more common, as the risk of preterm labor, ruptured membranes, and poor growth is increased. In chorioamnionitis, the histopathological findings may differ between the twins. Because most result from an ascending infection, the placenta and membranes of the presenting twin may be more affected in dichorionic than in monochorionic pairs [7]. In advanced chorioamnionitis, only the non-presenting twin from a dichorionic pair with a separate placenta appears to be at lower risk. In contrast, monochorionic twins are more often equally affected.

Data on the vascular lesions in twin placentas are limited. The ESPRIT study examined the occurrence of pathological lesions in twin placentas. They reported that 42% of monochorionic and 33% of dichorionic placentas had at least one of the following lesions: infarction, chorioangioma, subchorial fibrin deposition, retroplacental hematoma, or abnormal villus maturation [8]. All these lesions – except for a chorioangioma – were significantly more common in monochorionic placentas. In dichorionic placentas, however, placental lesions were observed more often in the smaller twin and in twins with growth below the fifth centile, whereas no such association was found in monochorionic twins.

Fetal vessel thrombosis is also more common in monochorionic than in dichorionic placentas (5–8% vs. 3%) [9, 10]. However, in dichorionic twins, vessel thrombosis is associated with hypertensive disorders, whereas in monochorionic twins, it is associated with growth restriction and even fetal demise. As such, a thrombosis of an anastomosis may trigger an acute transfusion imbalance and therefore cause demise in a previously uncomplicated monochorionic pair.

2.3.2.2 Complete Hydatidiform Mole and Placental Mesenchymal Dysplasia

In a dizygotic twin, a normal fetus can coexist with a complete hydatidiform mole (46 chromosomes, diploid, all paternally derived) (▪ Fig. 2.6a). These pregnancies have a high risk of developing severe complications, such

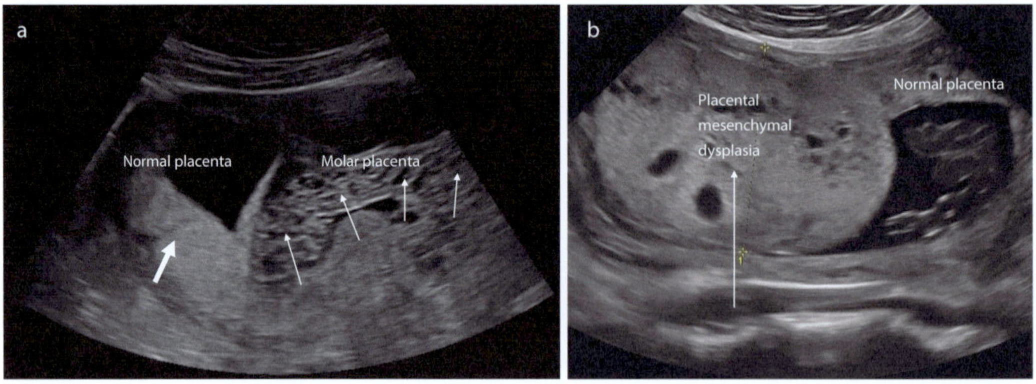

▪ **Fig. 2.6** **a** Ultrasound image of a molar (small arrow) and normal placenta (thick arrow) in a dichorionic twin pregnancy at 11 weeks. **b** Ultrasound image of placental mesenchymal dysplasia in the placental share (small arrow) of a growth restricted twin in a monochorionic diamniotic pregnancy at 20 weeks

as pre-eclampsia, growth restriction, and malignant trophoblastic disease [11, 12]. A few case studies report on a partial mole (69 chromosomes, triploid, extra set of paternal chromosomes) in monochorionic and dichorionic pairs, which is a lethal anomaly [13–15].

Placental mesenchymal dysplasia (◘ Fig. 2.6b) (placental mosaicism confined to the chorionic mesoderm, 46 chromosomes, diploid, all from paternal origin) can mimic a partial mole on prenatal ultrasound scan. It can exist in a dichorionic, but also in a monochorionic setting, affecting the entire placenta or only one placental share [16–18]. In contrast to partial moles, this condition is limited to the placenta and may result in a good outcome, albeit with increased risks of growth restriction, genetic syndromes, and fetal demise. We can differentiate placental mesenchymal dysplasia from a partial mole by amniocentesis [16, 19].

2.4 Vascular Anastomoses in Monochorionic Twin Placentas

2.4.1 The Vascular Anastomoses

The monochorionic placenta is unique in that the placenta is shared by the two fetuses whose blood circulations are almost invariably connected via placental vascular anastomoses. Sporadically, vascular anastomoses can also be found in dichorionic placentas, but this occurrence is extremely rare [20, 21]. Vascular anastomoses in monochorionic placentas can often easily be detected after birth on macroscopic examination as they lie on the surface of the fetal side of the placenta. However, sometimes the anastomoses are very small and difficult to see with the naked eye. Color dye injection of the vessels may then facilitate the detection of these minuscule anastomoses and help characterize the type, number, and size of the anastomoses [22, 23]. Placental evaluation using color dye injection has also played an essential role in elucidating the pathophysiology of the various complications and detection of new disorders in monochorionic twins. Vascular anastomoses are the basis for the development of twin-twin transfusion syndrome (TTTS) and twin anemia-polycythemia sequence (TAPS) [24]. Both TTTS and TAPS develop from a net imbalance of blood flow through the vascular anastomoses. However, there are striking differences in the placental angioarchitecture, number and size of anastomoses, and therefore in the amount and direction of blood flow, resulting in different clinical presentations and complications (see below).

There are three different types of vascular anastomoses: arterio-arterial (AA), veno-venous (VV), and arterio-venous (AV) anastomoses. AA and VV anastomoses are superficial, bidirectional, and have a low vascular resistance. They form direct connections between the two fetal circulations. After color dye injection, AA and VV anastomoses can clearly be seen as direct vascular connections running on the surface of the chorionic plate: dye flows very easily from one side of the placenta to the other due to the low vascular resistance. In contrast, AV anastomoses are deep, unidirectional, and have a high vascular resistance. AV anastomoses consist of an artery from one twin and the vein of the other twin that are connected by a capillary network below the chorionic plate. They can be visualized as a supplying artery and a draining vein that pierce the chorionic plate in close proximity to each other. As a result of the unidirectional flow in AV anastomoses, an imbalance in the net transfusion of blood can occur. After dye injection, the color in the injected artery does not mix with the color in the injected vein, because dye cannot pass through the capillary network. An example of the different types of anastomoses in an uncomplicated monochorionic placenta after dye injection is shown in ◘ Fig. 2.7. An example of a dichorionic placenta after dye injection showing the absence of anastomoses is depicted in ◘ Fig. 2.8.

Various complications may occur in monochorionic twin pregnancies, posing major diagnostic and therapeutic challenges for fetal surgeons. To continue improving our under-

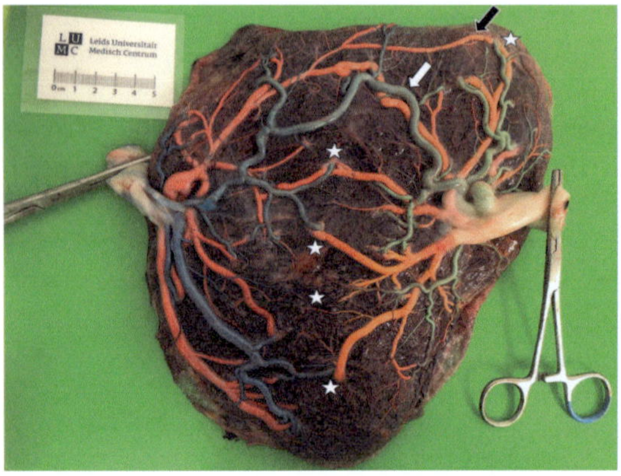

Fig. 2.7 Placenta of an uncomplicated monochorionic twins, delivered at 35 weeks. Birthweight of twin 1 was 2400 g and twin 2 2720 g. Blue and green dyes are used to inject arteries, pink and yellow for veins. Note the large AA anastomosis (white arrow), VV anastomosis (black arrow), and several AV anastomoses (white stars)

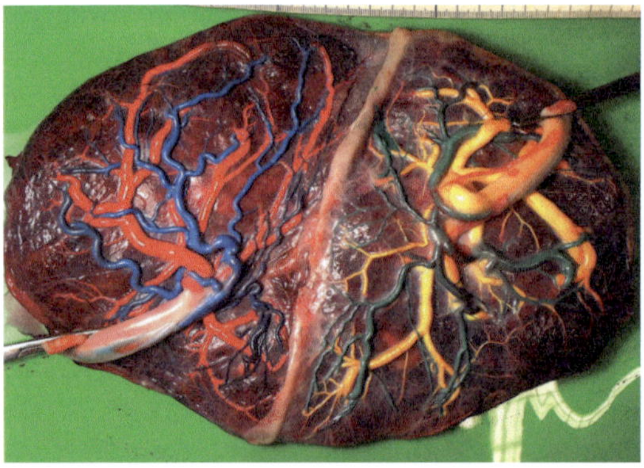

Fig. 2.8 Dichorionic placenta. Note the thick intertwin membrane, which, in the dichorionic placenta, cannot be removed manually. In contrast, the intertwin membrane in a monochorionic placenta can always easily be removed

standing of the pathogenesis of these complications, routine injection of all placentas is of paramount importance. The differences in placental angioarchitecture between the various complications in monochorionic twins, including TTTS, TAPS, and sFGR, are highlighted and illustrated in the following sections.

2.4.2 Placentas in Twin-Twin Transfusion Syndrome (TTTS)

Usually blood flow across placental anastomoses in monochrionic placentas is balanced. However, in TTTS, there is chronic and unbalanced feto-fetal transfusion from the donor-twin to the recipient-twin. Although placental anastomoses are ubiquitous in monochorionic placentas, TTTS develops only in approximately 10% of monochorionic twins. Extensive placental research during the last two decades has led to a clearer understanding of the pathogenesis of TTTS. The pathophysiology of TTTS is described as resulting from a net imbalance of blood flow between the fetuses through communicating placental anastomoses. TTTS only develops in the presence of unidirectional AV anastomoses, when blood from one twin (the donor) is pumped through the artery to the shared cotyledon and then drains through a vein to the other twin (the recipient). TTTS develops therefore in the presence of at least one AV anastomosis, unless blood is pumped back to the donor through another AV anastomosis in the opposite direction or through a bidirectional AA or VV anastomosis.

Another crucial finding in TTTS placentas is related to the presence, or rather absence, of arterio-arterial (AA) anastomoses. The prevalence of AA anastomoses is significantly lower in TTTS placenta compared to uncomplicated monochorionic placentas, 35–45% versus 95%, suggesting a protective role of AA anastomoses in preventing the development of TTTS [25, 26]. As mentioned previously, AA anastomoses are bidirectional and have a low resistance and may therefore compensate for hemodynamic imbalances by creating an equilibrating shift. However, it is still not clear why TTTS may still develop in the presence of an AA anastomosis. We previously found that the diameter of the AA anastomosis in TTTS placentas was smaller than in a control group of uncomplicated monochorionic placentas. We hypothesized that a smaller diameter of the AA anastomosis (with a higher vascular resistance) may prevent adequate equilibration of the intertwin hemodynamic imbalances, hence leading to the development of TTTS [26].

Although the role of AA and AV anastomoses in the development of TTTS has been widely investigated, the role of VV anastomoses remains unclear and has received little attention. VV anastomoses, in analogy to AA anastomoses, are superficial anastomoses and allow bidirectional flow. However, in contrast to AA anastomoses, VV anastomoses are found more frequently in TTTS placentas than in uncomplicated monochorionic placentas, 36% in TTTS placentas versus 25% in uncomplicated monochorionic placentas [27]. The presence of VV anastomoses in monochorionic twin pregnancies is therefore thought to be a potential risk factor for the development of TTTS. A possible hypothesis is that the development of TTTS can be prompted by hemodynamic changes in the shared venous system, as the venous system is more susceptible to external pressure changes. Whether other placental factors, besides the type and size of vascular anastomoses, may also play a role in the development of TTTS remains to be elucidated. Unequal placental sharing and abnormal cord insertion (velamentous or marginal) have been suggested to play a role in the development of TTTS, but the (causal) relation remains controversial and the pathophysiological mechanism still not clear [28–30]. However, when unequal placenta sharing or velamentous cord insertion is present, it is usually the donor that has the smaller placenta portion and the abnormally inserted cord. An example of a TTTS placenta is shown in ◻ Fig. 2.9.

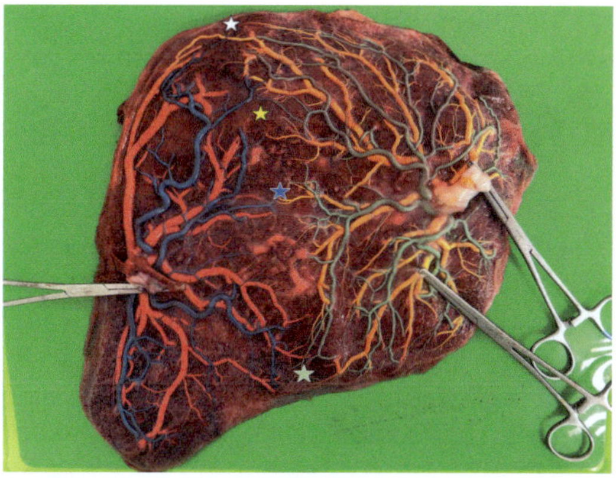

◻ **Fig. 2.9** A TTTS placenta (stage 3) not treated with laser surgery and delivered at 31 + 6 weeks gestational age. Note the VV anastomosis (white star), small AA anastomosis (yellow star), and several AV (blue star), and VA (green star) anastomoses

2.4.3 Placentas in Twin-Twin Transfusion Syndrome (TTTS) After Fetoscopic Laser Surgery

Injection studies with color dye allow accurate detection of residual anastomoses and gives invaluable feedback information to the fetal surgeons in regard to the success or completeness of the laser coagulation intervention. Placental injection studies should therefore be regarded as standard postnatal evaluation in all complicated monochorionic twin pregnancies after fetoscopic surgical intervention. This is important for a number of reasons, including, to evaluate the success of the operation and the operator performance as a type of quality control. This is not only necessary for the outcome of a single operation, but also to improve the techniques of fetal surgery in general and eventually create a benchmark or standard of practice. Residual anastomoses can result in recurrent TTTS or post-laser TAPS. The reported rate of residual anastomoses after selective fetoscopic laser surgery is between 4% and 33% [31]. The large variance is probably due to different laser surgery techniques as well as different placental injection techniques. The advent of the Solomon laser surgery method, a technique requiring laser coagulation of the whole vascular equator, has showed a reduction in residual anastomoses from 39% to 12% compared to selective laser coagulation [31, 32]. An example of a TTTS placenta successfully treated with laser surgery is shown in ◘ Fig. 2.10. An example of a TTTS placenta after incomplete laser surgery and various small residual anastomoses is shown in ◘ Fig. 2.11a, b. The patient developed post-laser TAPS and was treated with an intrauterine blood transfusion. The twins were delivered at a gestational age of 27 + 5 weeks, with hemoglobin levels in the donor and recipient of 8 g/dL and 21.5 g/dL, respectively.

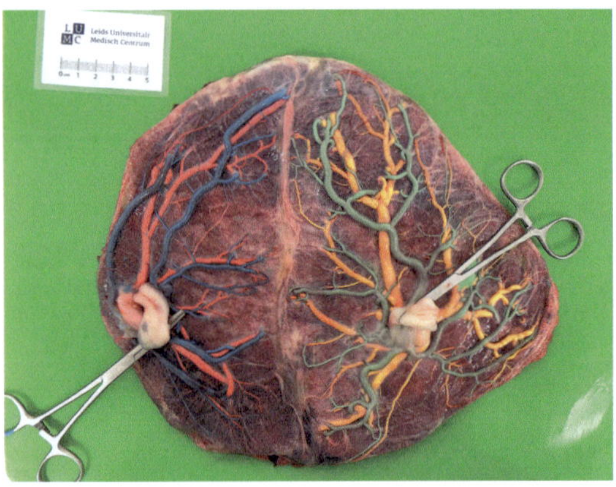

◘ **Fig. 2.10** TTTS placenta treated with laser surgery. Note the demarcation line along the vascular equator after using the Solomon laser coagulation technique, from one margin to the other

2.4.4 Placentas in Twin Anemia-Polycythemia Sequence (TAPS)

TAPS placentas are characterized by the presence of only few miniscule AV anastomoses. On average, spontaneous TAPS placentas have only 4–5 anastomoses compared to 10 in uncomplicated monochorionic placentas, whereas post-laser TAPS placentas have even fewer residual anastomoses (on average 2 per placenta) [24, 33]. The diameter of these tiny anastomoses is <1 mm and makes it difficult for unexperienced eyes to be able to detect them, especially without careful dye injection. The small size and small number of these anastomoses is the basis of the pathogenesis of TAPS as it allows only a very slow transfer of blood from the donor to the recipient and does not lead to the associated amniotic fluid imbalance as seen in TTTS. Most TAPS cases (80–90%) are also characterized

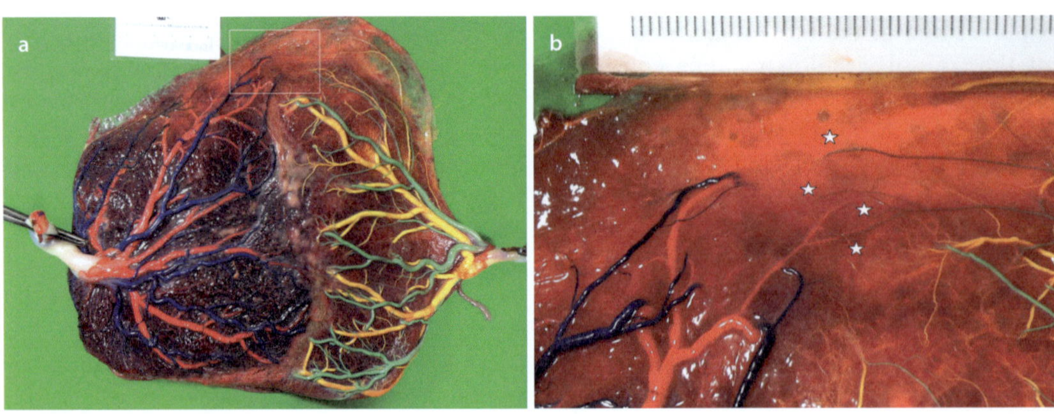

◘ **Fig. 2.11** **a** TTTS placenta treated with laser surgery, but developed post-laser TAPS due to incomplete treatment. Note the difference in color between the two placental shares: plethoric color of the placenta share of the recipient (left side) and pale color of the donor (right side). A few minuscule residual anastomoses were left patent at the top margin of the placenta (white rectangle; see enlargement in ◘ Fig. 2.11b). **b** Enlargement of the top margin of the placenta in ◘ Fig. 2.11a. Note the minuscule residual anastomoses, almost barely visible with the naked eye (white stars)

by the absence of AA anastomoses [34]. The low prevalence of AA anastomoses in TAPS supports the hypothesis that AA anastomoses have a protective effect and prevent not only the development of TTTS but also of TAPS. However, in a minority of TAPS cases (10–20%), an AA anastomosis can be detected [35]. In these cases, the size of AA anastomoses is typically small with a diameter <1 mm, just like the AV anastomoses. The small diameter of the AA anastomosis probably prevents adequate intertwin blood equilibration.

A typical aspect of TAPS is the striking difference in color between the plethoric placental share of the recipient and the pale placental share of the donor [36]. The color difference is positively correlated with the intertwin hemoglobin (Hb) difference: the larger the difference in Hb, the more striking the difference in color of the two placental shares [37]. This difference is almost pathognomonic for TAPS and may help differentiate TAPS from acute peripartum TTTS in twins with unexplained large Hb differences at birth [37].

Finally, an interesting aspect of TAPS placentas is related to the placental sharing. In monochorionic placentas in general, discrepancies in share lead to similar discrepancies in fetal growth and birth weight. The twin infant with a lower placental share often has a lower birth weight, whereas the co-twin with the larger placental share has a higher birth weight. In contrast, in twins with TAPS, birth weights seemed to be inversely related to the placental shares. In other words, the recipient twin often has a larger birth weight but a smaller placental share, whereas the donor twin, who is usually smaller, has a larger placental share [38]. This would seem to indicate that fetal growth in TAPS is determined by feto-fetal blood transfusion and not by placental share. One could speculate that this chronic loss of blood and nutrients from the donor to the recipient leads to diminished fetal growth. However, the conversely larger placental share has yet to be explained. One possible explanation is that the chronic anemia, chronic hypoxia, and loss of nutrients stimulate expansion of the placental territory and therefore a relatively larger placental share. An example of a TAPS placenta is demonstrated in ◘ Fig. 2.11a.

2.4.5 Placentas in Selective Fetal Growth Restriction (sFGR)

sFGR results primarily from unequal placental sharing. Typically, the growth-restricted fetus often has a small placental share and a velamentous cord insertion, while the larger fetus has a larger placental share and a (para-) central cord insertion. Placental characteristics in sFGR vary according to the type and severity of sFGR [39, 40]. Type I sFGR placentas are characterized by the invariable presence of an average-sized AA and mild to moderate unequal sharing. Type II is also characterized by unequally shared placenta, but AA anastomoses may be absent or small. In contrast, type III sFGR placentas have larger AA anastomoses (almost double the size compared to type I) and a higher degree of sharing discordance. More research in monochorionic twins with sFGR according to the umbilical artery Doppler measurements is urgently needed and may lead to a better understanding of how the placental architecture contributes to the pathophysiology and clinical outcomes. ◘ Figure 2.12 shows an example of sFGR placenta.

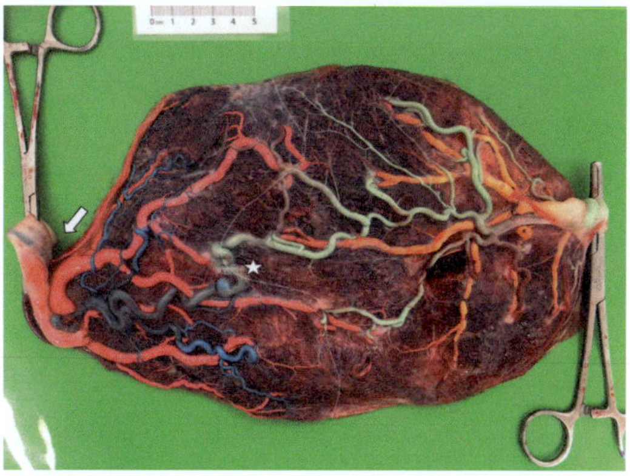

◘ **Fig. 2.12** sFGR type I placenta delivered at 36 weeks. Birth weight of twin 1 was 1870 g and twin 2 was 2450 g (birth weight discordance of 24%). Note the large AA anastomosis (white star), the velamentous cord insertion (white arrow), and the unequal placental sharing (white dotted line marks the vascular equator)

2.4.6 Placentas in Monoamniotic Twins

Monoamniotic placentas are characterized by the high prevalence of large AA anastomoses (in 98% of cases) and VV anastomoses (in 43% of cases), as well as proximate cord insertions in the majority of cases (defined as a distance between the two cords is ≤4 cm) [41]. The frequent presence of a large AA anastomosis in monoamniotic placentas may explain the low risk of TTTS or TAPS in monoamniotic twins (<5%). Most importantly, because of the single amniotic sac, umbilical cord entanglement occurs in virtually all spontaneous monoamniotic twins [42]. In twins treated with fetoscopic intervention, disruption of the intertwin dividing membrane may occur, causing iatrogenic monoamnionicity in approximately 20% of cases [43]. An example of a monoamniotic placenta is shown in ◘ Fig. 2.13.

2.4.7 Bipartite Monochorionic Placentas

It is important to know that not all monochorionic twins have a single placenta. In rare cases, monochorionic placentas can be divided in two separate placental masses and also have vascular anastomoses running through the connecting membranes [2]. These

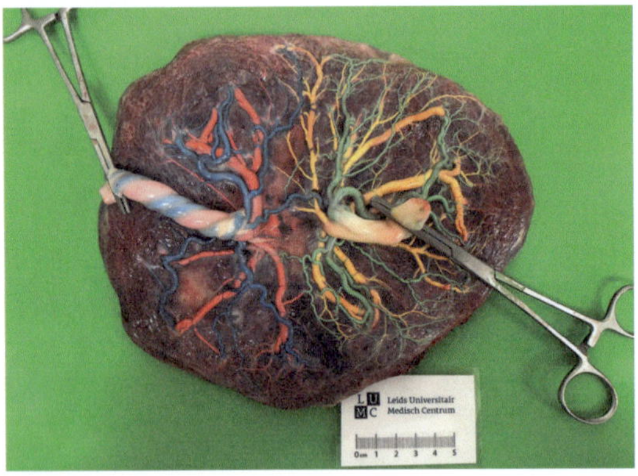

◘ **Fig. 2.13** Monoamniotic placenta delivered at 30 + 1 weeks gestational age. Note the proximate cord insertions, the blue AA anastomosis running between the two cords, and the multitude of AV and VA anastomoses

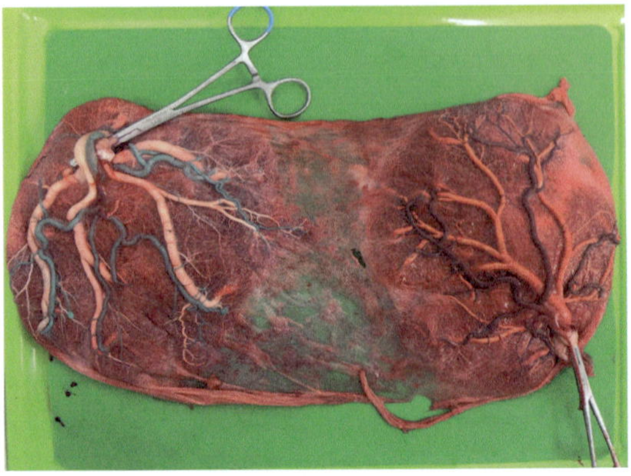

◘ **Fig. 2.14** Bipartite monochorionic placenta with two separate placental masses and without anastomoses

so-called bipartite placentas occur in 2–3% of monochorionic placentas. Monochorionic twin pregnancies with bipartite placentas may be associated with a higher rate of complications, such as TTTS, TAPS, and sFGR. In ◘ Fig. 2.14, an example of a bipartite monochorionic placenta is shown.

2.5 Umbilical Cord Abnormalities in Twin Pregnancies

2.5.1 Single Umbilical Artery

A single umbilical artery is three times as common in twins compared to singletons (3% vs. 1%), with a similar incidence in mono-and dichorionic pairs [44–46]. Usually, the smaller twin has a single umbilical artery. A single umbilical artery seems to increase the risk of very preterm birth too, even after correcting for previous preterm birth and monochorionicity [46]. Interestingly, the single umbilical artery in twins does not seem to show the same compensatory dilatation as in singletons, which may explain its association with poor growth [45].

2.5.2 Velamentous Cord Insertion

A velamentous cord insertion is also three times more common in twins than in singletons [47] and is especially prevalent in monochorionic (20%) as compared to dichorionic

(8%) twins [28, 30]. The use of artificial conception increases the chance of a velamentous insertion in dizygotic dichorionic twins [48]. A velamentous insertion increases the risks of preterm birth in both mono-and dichorionic twins [30, 47]. In dichorionic twins, a velamentous insertion inserts either directly onto the uterine wall or on the intertwin septum, whereas a velamentous insertion in a monochorionic twin pregnancy inserts only on the uterine wall, never on the intertwin septum, which typically lacks a chorionic layer. Furthermore, in a dichorionic twin pregnancy, we must always rule out a velamentous insertion on the intertwin septum, as it can cause acute exsanguination of the second twin if the intertwin septum is artificially ruptured during a vaginal birth or the velamentous vessels may be damaged during a double amniocentesis with a single entry through the intertwin septum (◘ Fig. 2.15).

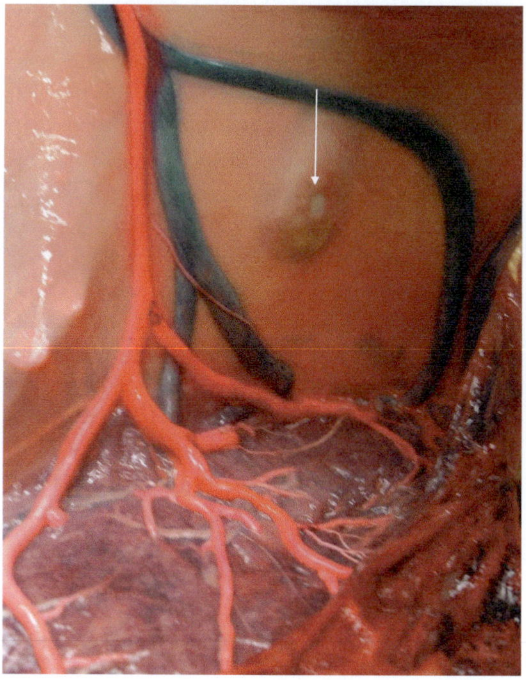

◘ **Fig. 2.15** Intertwin septum at birth of a dichorionic placenta with a velamentous cord insertion of the second twin on the intertwin septum. The patient underwent an amniocentesis at 15 weeks with single uterine puncture through the intertwin septum. The needle avoided the velamentous vessels (arrow), but as the patient ruptured the membranes of the presenting twin at 28 weeks, both twins developed an oligohydramnios

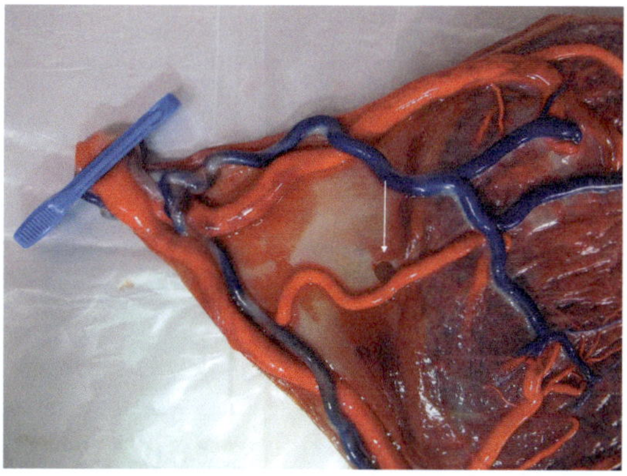

◘ **Fig. 2.16** Placenta at birth at 34 weeks after fetoscopic laser coagulation of the anastomoses for twin-twin transfusion syndrome. The placenta was anterior with a velamentous insertion of the recipient cord. The trocar insertion (arrow) was performed with the assistance of color Doppler and narrowly avoided the velamentous vessels

In monochorionic twins, a velamentous insertion also increases the risk of growth restriction and intra-uterine demise [30, 49, 50], whereas no such association could be demonstrated in dichorionic twins [30, 51]. The presence of a velamentous insertion in one or both twins increases the risk of TTTS (► Chap. 14), whereas the combination of a velamentous insertion with a more central insertion is associated with discordant growth in a monochorionic twin pair [49, 52]. In the overall majority, it is the donor and the growth-restricted twin who have the velamentous insertion. However, in the rare instances that the recipient has the velamentous cord, trocar entry, which is always in the recipient sac, can be challenging (◘ Fig. 2.16). It is thus crucial to determine the cord insertion of each twin on prenatal ultrasound scan not only to label the twins but also to assess the risk of subsequent pregnancy complications.

2.5.3 Vasa Previa

About 1 in 25 pregnancies with velamentous cord insertion have vasa previa, and 90% of pregnancies with vasa previa have a velamentous insertion [53]. Since velamentous insertions are more common in twin pregnancies, vasa previa are also more prevalent, although data on the exact incidence are lacking [54–56].

Nevertheless, given the accuracy of ultrasound scan and the potentially lethal complications, vasa previa (defined as within a 5 cm of the internal os) should be ruled out at the time of the second-trimester scan (◘ Fig. 2.17) [57]. Similar to placenta previa, these cases require follow-up, but parents must be reassured that the overall majority will resolve by the time of birth. As mentioned above, in a dichorionic twin pregnancy, we should also exclude a velamentous insertion of the second twin's cord on the intertwin septum, as this may behave as vasa previa during a vaginal twin birth (◘ Fig. 2.18).

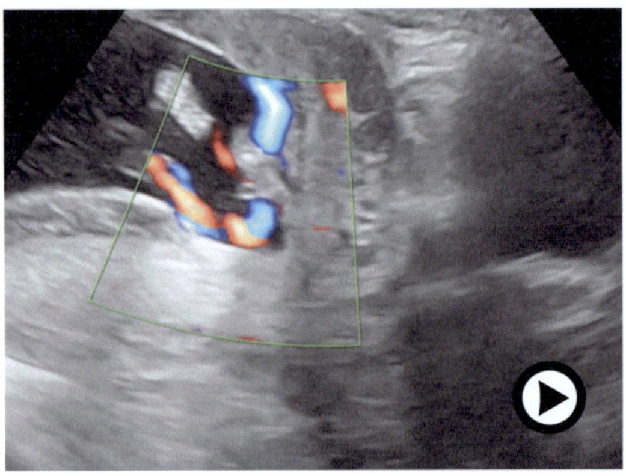

◘ **Fig. 2.17** Ultrasound image of vasa previa in a spontaneous monochorionic twin pregnancy at 19 weeks. The placenta is anterior, but the cord of one of the twins is velamentous on the posterior uterine wall with the umbilical stem vessels crossing over the internal os (https://doi.org/10.1007/000-2sx)

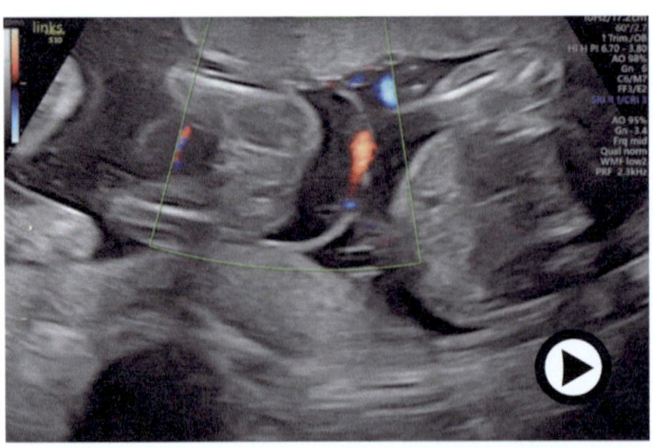

◘ **Fig. 2.18** Ultrasound image of a velamentous insertion of one of the twins on the intertwin septum at 20 weeks. The placenta is posterior but the cord inserts anteriorly on the intertwin septum with the umbilical stem vessels traversing the intertwin septum. It will be important to ascertain that there are no vasa previa if this twin is second presenting before a vaginal birth is attempted (https://doi.org/10.1007/000-2sy)

Finally, ruptured vasa previa in a monochorionic setting may lead to a rapid exsanguination of both twins as they are connected to one another through vascular anastomoses [58].

2.5.4 Cord Coiling

Both hypo- and hypercoiled cords are associated with adverse perinatal outcomes [59]. In monochorionic twin pregnancies, there is a known association between the difference in coiling index and growth difference [60]. In addition, in TTTS, the donor usually has the more hypocoiled cord and the recipient the more hypercoiled cord [61, 62]. However, it is uncertain to what degree the coiling index is useful in clinical practice.

2.5.5 Proximate Cord Insertions in Monochorionic Twin Pregnancies

As mentioned above, proximate cord insertions – a distance between the cord insertions of <4 cm – are more typically seen in monoamniotic twins and are rare in monochorionic diamniotic twins (53% vs. 3%) [41, 63]. AA anastomoses are present in virtually all cases of proximate cord insertion [41, 63, 64], and the incidence of VV anastomoses is twice as high compared to placentas without proximate cord insertions (56% vs. 26%) [41].

While the incidence of TTTS appears to be lower in monochorionic twins with proximate cord insertions [41, 63], the large intertwin anastomoses may predispose these pregnancies to more acute transfusion imbalances. Especially in cases of fetal demise or neurological damage, it is important to document whether the umbilical cords insert close together and whether there are large anastomoses, as this may explain sudden hypoperfusion. Also, in the event of fetal demise, the surviving co-twin may recruit the entire placenta through the large AA and VV anastomosis [65].

Whenever TTTS develops in a pregnancy with proximate cord insertions, laser separa-

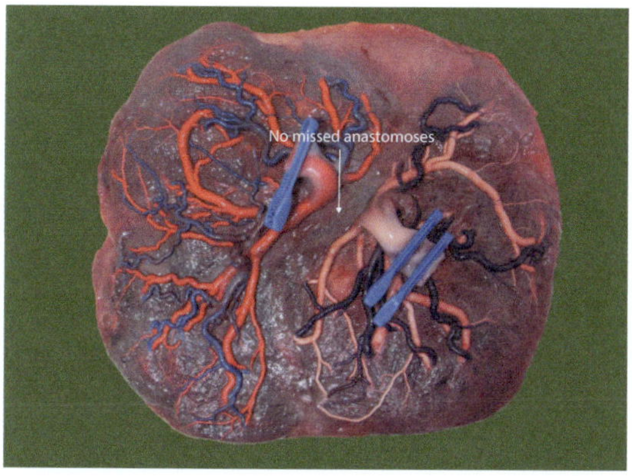

■ **Fig. 2.19** Monoamniotic placenta after birth at 34 weeks with proximate cord insertions, successfully treated with laser coagulation of the anastomoses at 19 weeks for twin-twin transfusion syndrome

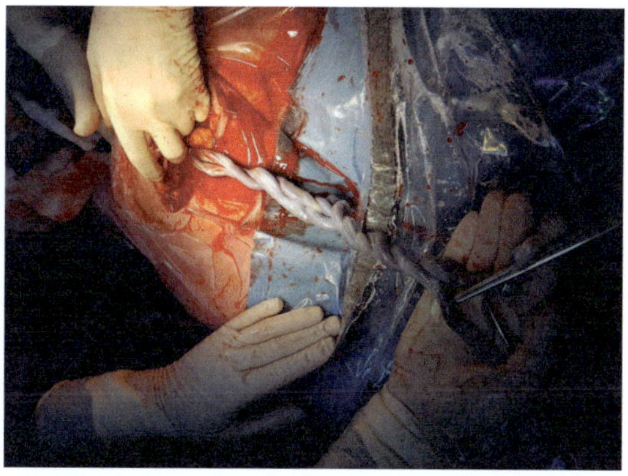

■ **Fig. 2.20** Cord entanglement at the time of elective cesarean section at 33 weeks in a monoamniotic twin pregnancy

tion may be technically not possible because of the large communications. However, in advanced disease, we usually evaluate the feasibility fetoscopically, because frequently large anastomoses are lacking and separation is possible to cure the disease (■ Fig. 2.19) [66]. In addition, whenever proximate cords are diagnosed in a diamniotic setting, it is relevant always to confirm the intertwin septum is between both babies, as rarely, the proximate insertions point to a partial monoamniotic twin pregnancy [67].

2.5.6 Cord Entanglement

Cord entanglement (■ Fig. 2.20) can only be present when the intertwin septum is incomplete. As mentioned above, it is typically seen in monoamniotic pairs but can also occur after spontaneous or iatrogenic septostomy in diamniotic twins (■ Fig. 2.21) [68–72]. The cord entanglement in itself does not appear to increase the mortality in monoamniotic twins [68]. Probably, the combination of pressure on the entangled cord, in combination with the large AA anastomoses, accounts for the sudden and often double demise in monoamniotic twin pairs [73]. Moreover, in the case of single fetal demise and cord entanglement, the demised twin's cord becomes autolytic. As a result, this fibrotic umbilical cord may tie off the healthy co-twin's cord, resulting in double fetal demise at a later point in pregnancy. In these instances, a cord transection avoids a remote, unexpected demise of the co-twin [74].

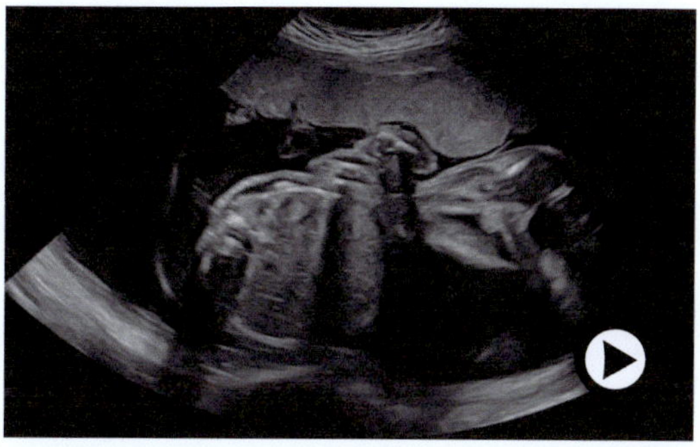

■ **Fig. 2.21** Ultrasound image at 23 weeks, 3 days after laser coagulation for twin-twin transfusion syndrome performed after septostomy. The patient presented with decreased fetal movements on the right sac. On ultrasound, the sac of the recipient on the right side was empty as the recipient moved to the left-sided donor sac (https://doi.org/10.1007/000-2sz)

2.6 Conclusion

Placental examination after birth is not only essential to confirm the chorionicity but also provides essential information to explain any adverse perinatal outcome in twin pregnancies. Especially, the placental examination and color injection studies in monochorionic twin pregnancies help us to understand the pathophysiology of TTTS and TAPS, and serve as a quality control to detect any missed anastomoses after fetoscopic laser coagulation of the anastomoses. No monochorionic placenta is the same, and differences in sharing, placental function, and vascular anastomoses may explain the myriad of monochorionic complications. Further placental studies in fetal growth restriction in monochorionic twin pregnancies may be helpful to understand better its underlying pathophysiology. A better understanding will ultimately improve our management of these high-risk pregnancies.

2.6.1 Review Questions

1. How is chorionicity determined after birth?

2. What are the specific problems in twin placentas?

3. What is the role of the vascular anastomoses in the typical complications of monochorionic twin pregnancies?

4. Which abnormalities of the umbilical cord may occur in twin pregnancies?

2.6.2 Multiple-Choice Questions

1. Which of the following statements on chorionicity determination is correct?
   - (a) Separate placental masses indicate dichorionic placentation.
   - (b) The absence of visible anastomoses excludes monochorionicity.
   - (c) In a monochorionic diamniotic placenta, the septum can be removed from the chorionic plate.
   - (d) In monoamniotic placentas, the intertwin septum is always entirely absent.

Answer: (c)

2. In placental mesenchymal dysplasia:
   - (a) Both placental shares are always affected equally in a monochorionic setting.
   - (b) The fetus has 46 chromosomes, all paternally derived.
   - (c) The fetus usually has a normal karyotype.
   - (d) There is an increased risk of malignant trophoblastic disease.

Answer: (c)

3. Vascular anastomoses play a crucial role in the typical complications in monochorionic twin pregnancies. Which of the following statements is correct?
   - (a) In twin-twin transfusion syndrome, fewer placentas have a unidirectional artery-to-artery anastomosis.
   - (b) In twin anemia-polycythemia sequence, typically only few, tiny unidirectional artery-to-vein anastomoses are present.
   - (c) In acute peripartum twin-twin transfusion, there is a striking difference in color between the placental shares of donor and recipient.
   - (d) In selective growth restriction type II in monochorionic pairs, the placenta is very unequally shared, but typically, there is a very large artery-to-artery anastomosis present.

Answer: (b)

4. Twins more commonly have abnormal cords. Which of the following statements is correct:
   - (a) In monochorionic diamniotic twins, it is crucial to exclude a cord insertion and velamentous vessels on the intertwin septum, as these may rupture during birth.
   - (b) A velamentous cord insertion increases the risk of vasa previa, which in monochorionic twins may

cause the exsanguination of both twins.
(c) In twin-twin transfusion syndrome, the donor's cord shows greater coiling than the recipient's cord.
(d) In twin-twin transfusion syndrome, we cannot perform a laser coagulation of the anastomoses if the cords insert close to one another on the placenta.

Answer: (b)

Disclosure Statement

The authors report no conflict of interest.

Financial Support

L. Lewi is the recipient of a grant of "Fonds voor Wetenschappelijk Onderzoek" (FWO grantnr: 1804718N).

References

1. Loos RJ, Derom C, Derom R, Vlietinck R. Birthweight in liveborn twins: the influence of the umbilical cord insertion and fusion of placentas. BJOG. 2001;108(9):943–8.
2. Lopriore E, Sueters M, Middeldorp JM, Klumper F, Oepkes D, Vandenbussche FP. Twin pregnancies with two separate placental masses can still be monochorionic and have vascular anastomoses. Am J Obstet Gynecol. 2006;194(3):804–8.
3. Weis MA, Harper LM, Roehl KA, Odibo AO, Cahill AG. Natural history of placenta previa in twins. Obstet Gynecol. 2012;120(4):753–8.
4. Qin JB, Wang H, Sheng X, Xie Q, Gao S. Assisted reproductive technology and risk of adverse obstetric outcomes in dichorionic twin pregnancies: a systematic review and meta-analysis. Fertil Steril. 2016;105(5):1180–92.
5. Ptacek I, Sebire NJ, Man JA, Brownbill P, Heazell AE. Systematic review of placental pathology reported in association with stillbirth. Placenta. 2014;35(8):552–62.
6. Roescher AM, Timmer A, Erwich JJ, Bos AF. Placental pathology, perinatal death, neonatal outcome, and neurological development: a systematic review. PLoS One. 2014;9(2):e89419.
7. Phung DT, Blickstein I, Goldman RD, Machin GA, LoSasso RD, Keith LG. The Northwestern Twin Chorionicity Study: I. Discordant inflammatory findings that are related to chorionicity in presenting versus nonpresenting twins. Am J Obstet Gynecol. 2002;186(5):1041–5.
8. Kent EM, Breathnach FM, Gillan JE, McAuliffe FM, Geary MP, Daly S, et al. Placental pathology, birthweight discordance, and growth restriction in twin pregnancy: results of the ESPRiT Study. Am J Obstet Gynecol. 2012;207(3):220.e1–5.
9. Sato Y, Benirschke K. Increased prevalence of fetal thrombi in monochorionic-twin placentas. Pediatrics. 2006;117(1):e113–7.
10. Chan MP, Hecht JL, Kane SE. Incidence and clinicopathologic correlation of fetal vessel thrombosis in mono- and dichorionic twin placentas. J Perinatol. 2010;30(10):660–4.
11. Lin LH, Maesta I, Braga A, Sun SY, Fushida K, Francisco RPV, et al. Multiple pregnancies with complete mole and coexisting normal fetus in North and South America: a retrospective multicenter cohort and literature review. Gynecol Oncol. 2017;145(1):88–95.
12. Wee L, Jauniaux E. Prenatal diagnosis and management of twin pregnancies complicated by a co-existing molar pregnancy. Prenat Diagn. 2005;25(9):772–6.
13. Benirschke K, Spinosa JC, McGinniss MJ, Marchevsky A, Sanchez J. Partial molar transformation of the placenta of presumably monozygotic twins. Pediatr Dev Pathol. 2000;3(1):95–100.
14. Nugent CE, Punch MR, Barr M Jr, LeBlanc L, Johnson MP, Evans MI. Persistence of partial molar placenta and severe preeclampsia after selective termination in a twin pregnancy. Obstet Gynecol. 1996;87(5 Pt 2):829–31.
15. Steller MA, Genest DR, Bernstein MR, Lage JM, Goldstein DP, Berkowitz RS. Clinical features of multiple conception with partial or complete molar pregnancy and coexisting fetuses. J Reprod Med. 1994;39(3):147–54.
16. Gheysen W, Strybol D, Moerman P, Steylemans A, Corveleyn A, De Catte L, et al. Discordance for placental mesenchymal dysplasia in a monochorionic diamniotic twin pregnancy: a case report. Clin Case Rep. 2018;6(8):1557–60.
17. Surti U, Hill LM, Dunn J, Prosen T, Hoffner L. Twin pregnancy with a chimeric androgenetic and biparental placenta in one twin displaying placental mesenchymal dysplasia phenotype. Prenat Diagn. 2005;25(11):1048–56.
18. Robertson M, Geerts LT, de Jong G, Wainwright H. Mesenchymal dysplasia in a monochorionic diamniotic twin pregnancy with review of the differential diagnosis of cystic changes in the placenta. J Ultrasound Med. 2007;26(5):689–93.
19. Fukunaga M. Immunohistochemical characterization of p57(KIP2) expression in early hydatidiform moles. Hum Pathol. 2002;33(12):1188–92.
20. Zhao D, Lipa M, Wielgos M, Cohen D, Middeldorp JM, Oepkes D, et al. Comparison between monochorionic and dichorionic placentas with special attention to vascular anastomoses and placental share. Twin Res Hum Genet. 2016;19(3):191–6.
21. Lanna M, Faiola S, Casati D, Rustico MA. Twin-twin transfusion syndrome in dichorionic twin

pregnancy: rare but not impossible. Ultrasound Obstet Gynecol. 2019;54(3):417–8.
22. Couck I, Aertsen M, Jespers A, Deneckere S, Lewi L. The assessment of placental sharing using X-ray angiogram versus digital photograph: a prospective study. Placenta. 2019;83:1–4.
23. Lopriore E, Slaghekke F, Middeldorp JM, Klumper FJ, van Lith JM, Walther FJ, et al. Accurate and simple evaluation of vascular anastomoses in monochorionic placenta using colored dye. J Vis Exp. 2011;(55):e3208.
24. Couck I, Lewi L. The placenta in twin-to-twin transfusion syndrome and twin anemia polycythemia sequence. Twin Res Hum Genet. 2016;19(3):184–90.
25. de Villiers SF, Slaghekke F, Middeldorp JM, Walther FJ, Oepkes D, Lopriore E. Arterio-arterial vascular anastomoses in monochorionic placentas with and without twin-twin transfusion syndrome. Placenta. 2012;33(8):652–4.
26. Zhao DP, de Villiers SF, Slaghekke F, Walther FJ, Middeldorp JM, Oepkes D, et al. Prevalence, size, number and localization of vascular anastomoses in monochorionic placentas. Placenta. 2013;34(7):589–93.
27. Zhao DP, Cambiaso O, Otano L, Lewi L, Deprest J, Sun LM, et al. Veno-venous anastomoses in twin-twin transfusion syndrome: a multicenter study. Placenta. 2015;36(8):911–4.
28. Couck I, Mourad Tawfic N, Deprest J, De Catte L, Devlieger R, Lewi L. Does site of cord insertion increase risk of adverse outcome, twin-to-twin transfusion syndrome and discordant growth in monochorionic twin pregnancy? Ultrasound Obstet Gynecol. 2018;52(3):385–9.
29. Cambiaso O, Zhao DP, Abasolo JI, Aiello HA, Oepkes D, Lopriore E, et al. Discordance of cord insertions as a predictor of discordant fetal growth in monochorionic twins. Placenta. 2016;47:81–5.
30. Costa-Castro T, Zhao DP, Lipa M, Haak MC, Oepkes D, Severo M, et al. Velamentous cord insertion in dichorionic and monochorionic twin pregnancies – does it make a difference? Placenta. 2016;42:87–92.
31. Knijnenburg PJC, Slaghekke F, Tollenaar LSA, van Klink JM, Zhao DP, Middeldorp JM, et al. Incidence of and risk factors for residual anastomoses in twin-twin transfusion syndrome treated with laser surgery: a 15-year single-center experience. Fetal Diagn Ther. 2019;45(1):13–20.
32. Slaghekke F, Lewi L, Middeldorp JM, Weingertner AS, Klumper FJ, Dekoninck P, et al. Residual anastomoses in twin-twin transfusion syndrome after laser: the Solomon randomized trial. Am J Obstet Gynecol. 2014;211(3):285.e1–7.
33. de Villiers SF, Slaghekke F, Middeldorp JM, Walther FJ, Oepkes D, Lopriore E. Placental characteristics in monochorionic twins with spontaneous versus post-laser twin anemia-polycythemia sequence. Placenta. 2013;34(5):456–9.
34. de Villiers S, Slaghekke F, Middeldorp JM, Klumper FJ, Walther FJ, Oepkes D, et al. Arterio-arterial vascular anastomoses in monochorionic twin placentas with and without twin anemia-polycythemia sequence. Placenta. 2012;33(3):227–9.
35. van Meir H, Slaghekke F, Lopriore E, van Wijngaarden WJ. Arterio-arterial anastomoses do not prevent the development of twin anemia-polycythemia sequence. Placenta. 2010;31(2):163–5.
36. Tollenaar LS, Zhao DP, Middeldorp JM, Slaghekke F, Oepkes D, Lopriore E. Color difference in placentas with twin anemia-polycythemia sequence: an additional diagnostic criterion? Fetal Diagn Ther. 2016;40(2):123–7.
37. Tollenaar LSA, Zhao DP, Middeldorp JM, Oepkes D, Slaghekke F, Lopriore E. Can color difference on the maternal side of the placenta distinguish between acute peripartum twin-twin transfusion syndrome and twin anemia-polycythemia sequence? Placenta. 2017;57:189–93.
38. Tollenaar LS, Slaghekke F, Middeldorp JM, Klumper FJ, Haak MC, Oepkes D, et al. Twin anemia polycythemia sequence: current views on pathogenesis, diagnostic criteria, perinatal management, and outcome. Twin Res Hum Genet. 2016;19(3):222–33.
39. Groene SG, Tollenaar LSA, Slaghekke F, Middeldorp JM, Haak M, Oepkes D, et al. Placental characteristics in monochorionic twins with selective intrauterine growth restriction in relation to the umbilical artery Doppler classification. Placenta. 2018;71:1–5.
40. Lewi L, Gucciardo L, Huber A, Jani J, Van Mieghem T, Done E, et al. Clinical outcome and placental characteristics of monochorionic diamniotic twin pairs with early- and late-onset discordant growth. Am J Obstet Gynecol. 2008;199(5):511.e1–7.
41. Zhao DP, Peeters SH, Middeldorp JM, Klumper FJ, Duan T, Oepkes D, et al. Monochorionic placentas with proximate umbilical cord insertions: definition, prevalence and angio-architecture. Placenta. 2015;36(2):221–5.
42. Dias T, Mahsud-Dornan S, Bhide A, Papageorghiou AT, Thilaganathan B. Cord entanglement and perinatal outcome in monoamniotic twin pregnancies. Ultrasound Obstet Gynecol. 2010;35(2):201–4.
43. Peeters SH, Stolk TT, Slaghekke F, Middeldorp JM, Klumper FJ, Lopriore E, et al. Iatrogenic perforation of intertwin membrane after laser surgery for twin-to-twin transfusion syndrome. Ultrasound Obstet Gynecol. 2014;44(5):550–6.
44. Heifetz SA. Single umbilical artery. A statistical analysis of 237 autopsy cases and review of the literature. Perspect Pediatr Pathol. 1984;8(4):345–78.
45. Klatt J, Kuhn A, Baumann M, Raio L. Single umbilical artery in twin pregnancies. Ultrasound Obstet Gynecol. 2012;39(5):505–9.

46. Stout MJ, Odibo AO, Longman R, Shanks AL, Cahill AG. The incidence of isolated single umbilical artery in twins and adverse pregnancy outcomes. Prenat Diagn. 2013;33(3):269–72.
47. Ebbing C, Kiserud T, Johnsen SL, Albrechtsen S, Rasmussen S. Prevalence, risk factors and outcomes of velamentous and marginal cord insertions: a population-based study of 634,741 pregnancies. PLoS One. 2013;8(7):e70380.
48. Delbaere I, Goetgeluk S, Derom C, De Bacquer D, De Sutter P, Temmerman M. Umbilical cord anomalies are more frequent in twins after assisted reproduction. Hum Reprod. 2007;22(10):2763–7.
49. Couck I, Mourad Tawfic N, Deprest J, De Catte L, Devlieger R, Lewi L. Does the site of the cord insertion increase the risk of adverse outcome, twin-to-twin transfusion syndrome and discordant growth in monochorionic twin pregnancies? Ultrasound Obstet Gynecol. 2018;52(3):385–9.
50. Kent EM, Breathnach FM, Gillan JE, McAuliffe FM, Geary MP, Daly S, et al. Placental cord insertion and birthweight discordance in twin pregnancies: results of the national prospective ESPRiT Study. Am J Obstet Gynecol. 2011;205(4):376.e1–7.
51. Kalafat E, Thilaganathan B, Papageorghiou A, Bhide A, Khalil A. Significance of placental cord insertion site in twin pregnancy. Ultrasound Obstet Gynecol. 2018;52(3):378–84.
52. Saito M, Tokunaka M, Takita H, Goto M, Koyano M, Sekiya B, et al. Impact of first trimester determination of abnormal cord insertion on twin-to-twin transfusion syndrome and other adverse outcomes in monochorionic diamniotic twins: a retrospective cohort study. Prenat Diagn. 2020;40(4):507–13.
53. Vintzileos AM, Ananth CV, Smulian JC. Using ultrasound in the clinical management of placental implantation abnormalities. Am J Obstet Gynecol. 2015;213(4 Suppl):S70–7.
54. Baulies S, Maiz N, Munoz A, Torrents M, Echevarria M, Serra B. Prenatal ultrasound diagnosis of vasa praevia and analysis of risk factors. Prenat Diagn. 2007;27(7):595–9.
55. Bronsteen R, Whitten A, Balasubramanian M, Lee W, Lorenz R, Redman M, et al. Vasa previa: clinical presentations, outcomes, and implications for management. Obstet Gynecol. 2013;122(2 Pt 1):352–7.
56. Catanzarite V, Cousins L, Daneshmand S, Schwendemann W, Casele H, Adamczak J, et al. Prenatally diagnosed vasa previa: a single-institution series of 96 cases. Obstet Gynecol. 2016;128(5):1153–61.
57. Oyelese Y. Vasa previa: time to make a difference. Am J Obstet Gynecol. 2019;221(6):539–41.
58. van Steenis A, Zhao DP, Steggerda SJ, Kist WJ, Haak MC, Oepkes D, et al. Double fatal outcome after ruptured vasa previa in monochorionic twins: case report and review of the literature. J Matern Fetal Neonatal Med. 2016;29(15):2523–6.
59. Pergialiotis V, Kotrogianni P, Koutaki D, Christopoulos-Timogiannakis E, Papantoniou N, Daskalakis G. Umbilical cord coiling index for the prediction of adverse pregnancy outcomes: a meta-analysis and sequential analysis. J Matern Fetal Neonatal Med. 2020;33(23):4022–9.
60. Degani S, Lewinsky RM, Aharoni A, Gonen R, Ohel G. Differences between twin umbilical coiling indices correlate to differences in twin weight and Doppler indices. J Matern Fetal Investig. 1998;8(3):130–3.
61. Cromi A, Ghezzi F, Durig P, Di Naro E, Raio L. Sonographic umbilical cord morphometry and coiling patterns in twin-twin transfusion syndrome. Prenat Diagn. 2005;25(9):851–5.
62. Bamberg C, Diemert A, Glosemeyer P, Tavares de Sousa M, Hecher K. Discordance of umbilical coiling index between recipients and donors in twin-twin transfusion syndrome. Placenta. 2019;76:19–22.
63. Umur A, van Gemert MJ, Nikkels PG. Monoamniotic-versus diamniotic-monochorionic twin placentas: anastomoses and twin-twin transfusion syndrome. Am J Obstet Gynecol. 2003;189(5):1325–9.
64. Bajoria R. Abundant vascular anastomoses in monoamniotic versus diamniotic monochorionic placentas. Am J Obstet Gynecol. 1998;179(3 Pt 1):788–93.
65. Deneckere S, Couck I, Devlieger R, de Catte L, Deprest J, Chantraine F, et al. Placental vascular recruitment after single intrauterine demise: a newly diagnosed phenomenon unique to monochorionic pregnancies. Prenat Diagn. 2019;39(5):409–12.
66. Zhao DP, Peeters SH, Middeldorp JM, Klumper FJ, Oepkes D, Lopriore E. Laser surgery in twin-twin transfusion syndrome with proximate cord insertions. Placenta. 2013;34(12):1159–62.
67. Galjaard S, Moerman P, Corveleyn A, Devlieger R, Lewi L. Partial monochorionic and monoamniotic twin pregnancies: a report of two cases. Ultrasound Obstet Gynecol. 2014;44(6):722–4.
68. Rossi AC, Prefumo F. Impact of cord entanglement on perinatal outcome of monoamniotic twins: a systematic review of the literature. Ultrasound Obstet Gynecol. 2013;41(2):131–5.
69. Gordon BJ, Chon AH, Korst LM, Llanes A, Miller DA, Chmait RH. Incidental septostomy after laser surgery for twin-twin transfusion syndrome: perinatal outcomes and antenatal management. Fetal Diagn Ther. 2018;44(4):285–90.
70. Bevilacqua E, Aliberti C, D'Ambrosio V, Giancotti A, Perrone G, La Torre R. Spontaneous septostomy in monochorionic diamniotic twins: difficult diagnosis, difficult management. J Obstet Gynaecol. 2014;34(4):359.
71. Fleming T, Miller T. Spontaneous septostomy in monochorionic diamniotic twins resulting in cord entanglement and fetal demise. Aust J Ultrasound Med. 2012;15(3):103–6.

72. Jeanty C, Newman E, Jeanty P, Rodts-Palenik S. Prenatal diagnosis of spontaneous septostomy in dichorionic diamniotic twins and review of the literature. J Ultrasound Med. 2010;29(3):455–63.
73. Lewi L. Cord entanglement in monoamniotic twins: does it really matter? Ultrasound Obstet Gynecol. 2010;35(2):139–41.
74. Molina FS, Gomez LF, Gonzalia DA, Fresneda MD, Padilla MC, Lewi L. Cord transection in monoamniotic twins: use of a 1000-micron fiber with conical tip. Ultrasound Obstet Gynecol. 2014;44(1):116–8.

Key Reading

Couck I, Mourad Tawfic N, Deprest J, De Catte L, Devlieger R, Lewi L. Does site of cord insertion increase risk of adverse outcome, twin-to-twin transfusion syndrome and discordant growth in monochorionic twin pregnancy? Ultrasound Obstet Gynecol. 2018;52(3):385–9.

Lewi L, Deprest J, Hecher K. The vascular anastomoses in monochorionic twin pregnancies and their clinical consequences. Am J Obstet Gynecol. 2013;208(1):19–30.

Slaghekke F, Lewi L, Middeldorp JM, Weingertner AS, Klumper FJ, Dekoninck P, et al. Residual anastomoses in twin-twin transfusion syndrome after laser: the Solomon randomized trial. Am J Obstet Gynecol. 2014;211(3):285.e1–7.

Zhao DP, de Villiers SF, Slaghekke F, Walther FJ, Middeldorp JM, Oepkes D, et al. Prevalence, size, number and localization of vascular anastomoses in monochorionic placentas. Placenta. 2013;34(7):589–93.

Zhao D, Lipa M, Wielgos M, Cohen D, Middeldorp JM, Oepkes D, et al. Comparison between monochorionic and dichorionic placentas with special attention to vascular anastomoses and placental share. Twin Res Hum Genet. 2016;19(3):191–6.

Biology and Genetics of Dizygotic and Monozygotic Twinning

Jeffrey J. Beck, Susanne Bruins, Hamdi Mbarek, Gareth E. Davies, and Dorret I. Boomsma

Contents

A. Khalil et al. (eds.), *Twin and Higher-order Pregnancies*,
https://doi.org/10.1007/978-3-030-47652-6_3

Trailer

This chapter summarizes what is known and what remains unknown about the human twinning process. The interest of this chapter is a description of the processes underlying twinning, with a specific focus on the biological and genetic aspects. While the mechanisms and contributory factors to dizygotic twinning are becoming well established, much remains unknown about the etiology of monozygotic twinning. Here we provide an overview of the incidence of twinning across the globe and present what is known about the influences of twinning based on the findings of historical, epidemiological, and more recent molecular studies.

Definitions

1. Zygosity – The number of zygotes that become fertilized leading to a multiple birth, or the genetic makeup of the pregnancy.
2. Dizygotic twins – Non-identical or fraternal twins that are the result of two independent ova that are fertilized by two separate spermatozoa.
3. Monozygotic twins – Identical twins that arise from a single fertilized ovum.

Learning Objectives

- Define and differentiate between the biological mechanisms that give rise to monozygotic and dizygotic twins.
- Compare and contrast the composition of fetal membranes of monozygotic and dizygotic twins.
- Describe the genetic and non-genetic factors that are associated with spontaneous dizygotic twinning events.
- Explain the strengths and weaknesses of zygosity assessment methods.
- Describe the differences in rates of monozygotic and dizygotic twins.
- Introduce the first genome-wide association study of dizygotic twinning.

3.1 Introduction

Twins and higher-order multiples have piqued the interest of humankind for many centuries. The remarkable similar resemblance often ascribed to twins has been observed in many literary texts and philosophical works. Twins with similar outward appearance but with noticeable personality differences have been well characterized throughout history. Observations of twins are noted as far back in time as the Biblical accounts of Jacob and Esau, by philosophers Augustine of Hippo and Aristotle, and by poets like Shakespeare (e.g., *The Comedy of Errors* and *Twelfth Night*).

From a scientific perspective, it was in the nineteenth century that the Scottish obstetrician J Matthews Duncan recognized and documented that two types of twins existed, now commonly referred to as identical and fraternal (non-identical) twins [2]. Sir Francis Galton was the first the recognize the value of studying twins to elucidate the genetic contribution to variation in human traits [3]; however, he was not aware of the distinction between monozygotic (MZ or identical) and dizygotic (DZ or fraternal) twins. Even in the early twentieth century, the existence of two types of twins was debated with the famous statistician Sir Ronald Fisher (who was the second of twins himself) proving mathematically that it was highly unlikely that there was more than one type of twin [4]. Nevertheless, the idea put forth by Galton was to compare trait concordance in twins in an attempt at disentangling the genetic (nature) and environmental (nurture) influences. Galton's proposal laid the foundation for modern era twin studies aimed at discerning the genetic contribution of complex traits and etiology of disease.

The theoretical basis of quantitative genetics proved to be fundamental to the creation and application of the classical twin design, which builds on the – by now firmly established – differential genetic relatedness of MZ and DZ twin pairs. Realizing the enormous potential of quantitative genetic theory to studies that apply the classical twin design for studying human traits, large twin registries were established in the 1950s [5], although studies of twins had already been done in Russia [6–8] and elsewhere. The first scientific studies of twins in medicine were by Poll [9] and Siemens [10] who investigated the different levels of similarity between MZ and DZ twins for mole counts. Findings from their work suggested that MZ twin pairs were nearly genetically identical, whereas DZ twin pairs shared on average 50% of their genetic variation; this was reflected in the twice as large resemblance for mole counts in MZ than in DZ twin pairs. By now, twin registries are increasingly popular, and have proven strengths in longitudinal data collection and inclusion of biological samples to evaluate the genetic variation in susceptibility to disease.

Remarkably, despite the rapid gain in knowledge about the importance of genetic variation due to advancements in genotyping technology combined with the development of powerful linkage and genetic association studies, there is not a comprehensive understanding of the twinning process. For example, there are no estimates for the heritability of twinning. A number of factors influencing the DZ twinning process are well described, and the first genetic factors for DZ twinning have been characterized [11]. However, the heritability of DZ twinning remains unknown, and the knowledge regarding the etiology of MZ twinning is even more limited.

This chapter summarizes the current body of knowledge surrounding the epidemiological, biological, and genetic aspects of human twinning. Included are explanations of the biological mechanisms of twinning, descriptions of the underlying genetic contributions to the twinning process, and details on the frequency of twinning within populations.

3.2 Zygosity, Chorionicity, Placentation of Twinning

Zygosity refers to the genetic makeup of the pregnancy, or the number of zygotes that become fertilized leading to a multiple birth. Twins, in rarer cases triplets, quadruplets (four), quintuplets (five), arising from a single fertilized ovum are termed monozygotic (MZ). The first identical quintuplets known to have survived their infancy were the Canadian Dionne quintuplets, all five of which survived to adulthood (◘ Fig. 3.1).

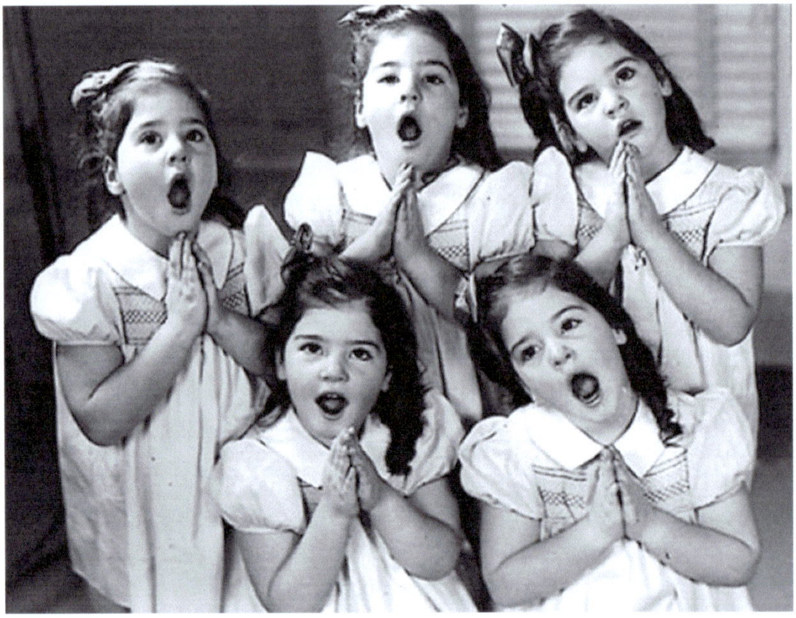

◘ **Fig. 3.1** The Dionne quintuplets. *The Dionne quintuplets, born May 28, 1934, outside of Callander, Ontario, Canada. Despite being born 2 months premature, all five quintuplets survived to adulthood.* (Source: ▸ https://commons.wikimedia.org/wiki/File:Dionne_quintuplets.jpg)

Alternatively, twins or multiples originating from two or more ova that are fertilized by separate spermatozoa are called dizygotic (DZ) [12], or trizygotic in the case of triplets. Nowadays, higher-order births of non-identical twins often are the result of assisted reproductive technologies (ART).

Multiple gestation pregnancies are inherently high risk to both the mother and the developing fetuses. Certain twin pregnancies, specifically those possessing a single chorion (monochorionic), exhibit an even higher risk for numerous pre- and peri-natal complications. Therefore, information about the status of the developing fetal membranes is helpful for monitoring and improving the outcome of a multiple gestation pregnancy.

In early stage human development, the membranes of the placenta begin to form around day 4. Examination of placental membranes by ultrasound imaging serves as a non-invasive method for determining zygosity/twin status [13–16]. According to the traditional models of twinning (◘ Fig. 3.2), DZ twins have distinct placentas and fetal membranes and are therefore dichorionic diamniotic, although fused membranes are possible. Approximately two-thirds of all MZ twins share one placenta with monochorionic diamniotic membranes, while roughly one-third have completely dis-

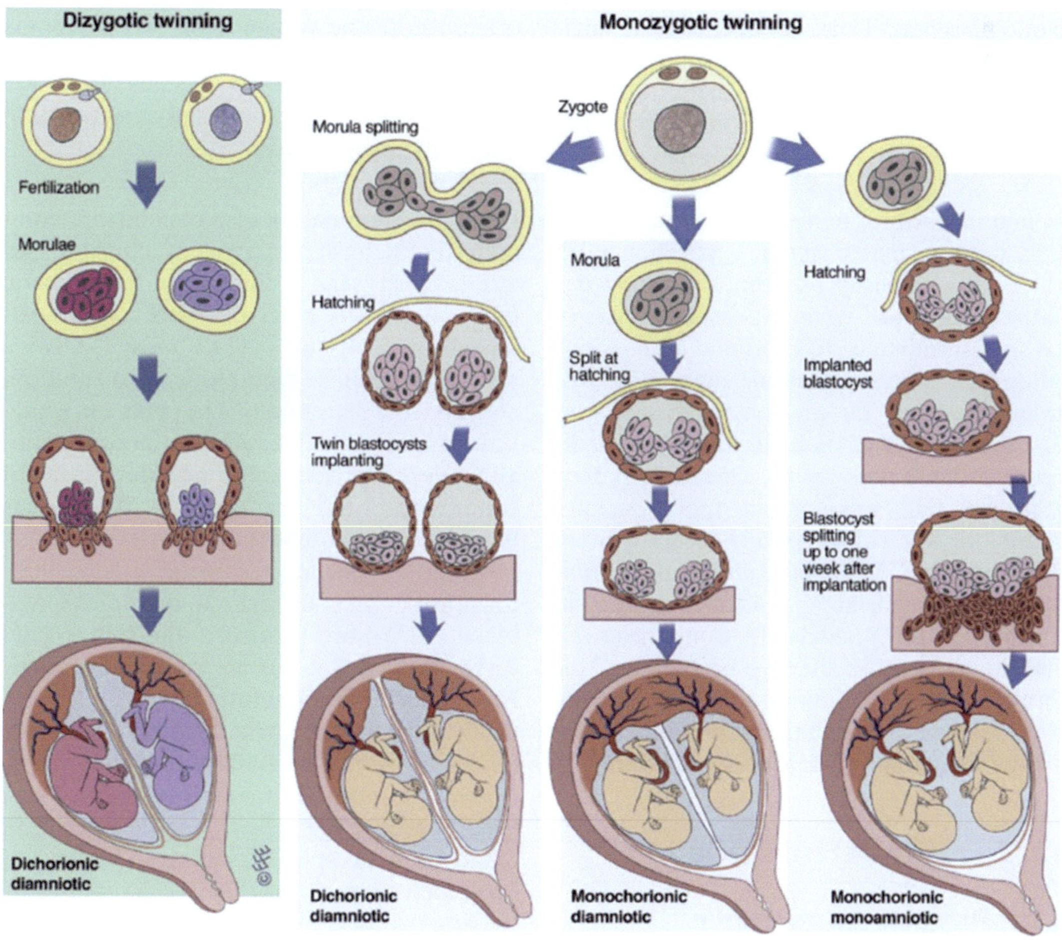

◘ **Fig. 3.2** The traditional model of twinning. *The formation of the two main types of twins according to the traditional model of twinning. DZ twins are the result of two distinct fertilization events and are dichorionic and diamniotic. MZ twins result from the postzygotic splitting of a single embryo early in gestation with varying numbers of fetal membranes depending on the timing of embryo splitting.* (This figure was obtained from McNamara et al. [21])

tinct placentas and membranes (dichorionic diamniotic). Only about 1% of MZ twins have one set of membranes and one placenta, making them monochorionic monoamniotic. The latter case poses highest risk for pre- and perinatal morbidity and mortality.

The placenta and membranes of a multiple gestation pregnancy represent a first means of identifying some MZ twins due to the presence of a single chorion. Although MZ twins will be of the same sex, not all same-sex twins are MZ. Therefore, for all same-sex twin pairs, DNA typing is the most useful and reliable method for determining zygosity [17]. Challenging the assumption that a single chorion indicates monozygosity, it is also possible for DZ twins to possess monochorionic diamniotic placentas. Thus, the dogma of a single chorion being synonymous with monozygosity is no longer proper due to chimeric DZ twins [18], a phenomenon in which one individual is composed of cells from two or more zygotes.

In normal embryogenesis, the chorionic membrane begins to form at about day 3. It is believed that if zygote separation takes place early, typically between day 1 and day 3, the result is MZ twins with separate placentas and membranes (dichorionic diamniotic). Alternatively, monochorionic diamniotic MZ twins result after the chorion has formed (day 3), but before the amnion has formed (typically between day 6 and day 8). Therefore, postzygotic splitting resulting in monochorionic diamniotic MZ twins typically occurs between day 3 and day 8. MZ twins with monochorionic monoamniotic membranes likely arise by splitting between day 8 and day 13. Conjoined twins are thought to arise after the beginning of the formation of the primitive streak, likely after day 14. However, the timing and mechanism(s) are not clear and empirical evidence is rare.

3.3 Zygosity Determination

3.3.1 Physical Appearance

For research purposes, twin zygosity is often times and most easily determined from questionnaires regarding similarity of physical characteristics. For instance, twins that are equal on most physical features and that are often times confused for one another are typically judged to be MZ. Alternatively, twins that differ on two or more physical characteristics and/or are not often mistaken for one another are often classified as DZ. As a whole, zygosity assessment from survey responses of physical traits corresponds rather well with zygosity determination through DNA typing [19, 20]. Apart from DNA testing, other basic rules that are routinely employed for zygosity determination are if the twins are opposite sex – DZ, of discordant blood groups – DZ, or possess a single, non-fused, placenta – MZ (please note the presence of two placentas does not imply DZ).

3.3.2 Placentation

Placental examination of a twin birth is common to establish the type of chorion and infer zygosity. DZ twins, except for chimeric twins, have two placentas with two chorions and two amnions. Thus, most DZ twins have dichorionic diamniotic placentation, although the placentas of DZ twins can sometimes appear as fused; yet they are functionally independent and with no inter-placental communication. Placentation in MZ twins is thought to vary depending on the timing of postzygotic splitting following a single fertilization event. Dichorionic diamniotic MZ twins (~33%) are formed if the split occurs early, on days 1–3, up to the morula stage. Monochorionic diamniotic MZ twins (~66%) result if the split happens between days 3 and 8, during which blastocyst hatching starts. Monochorionic monoamniotic MZ twins (~1%) occur if the split occurs between days 8 and 13. If no split has occurred by day 13, conjoined twins form [12, 21]. Examples of varying numbers of fetal membranes are also observed in triplets and higher-order multiples as shown in ◘ Fig. 3.3 (images adapted from Lamb et al. [22]).

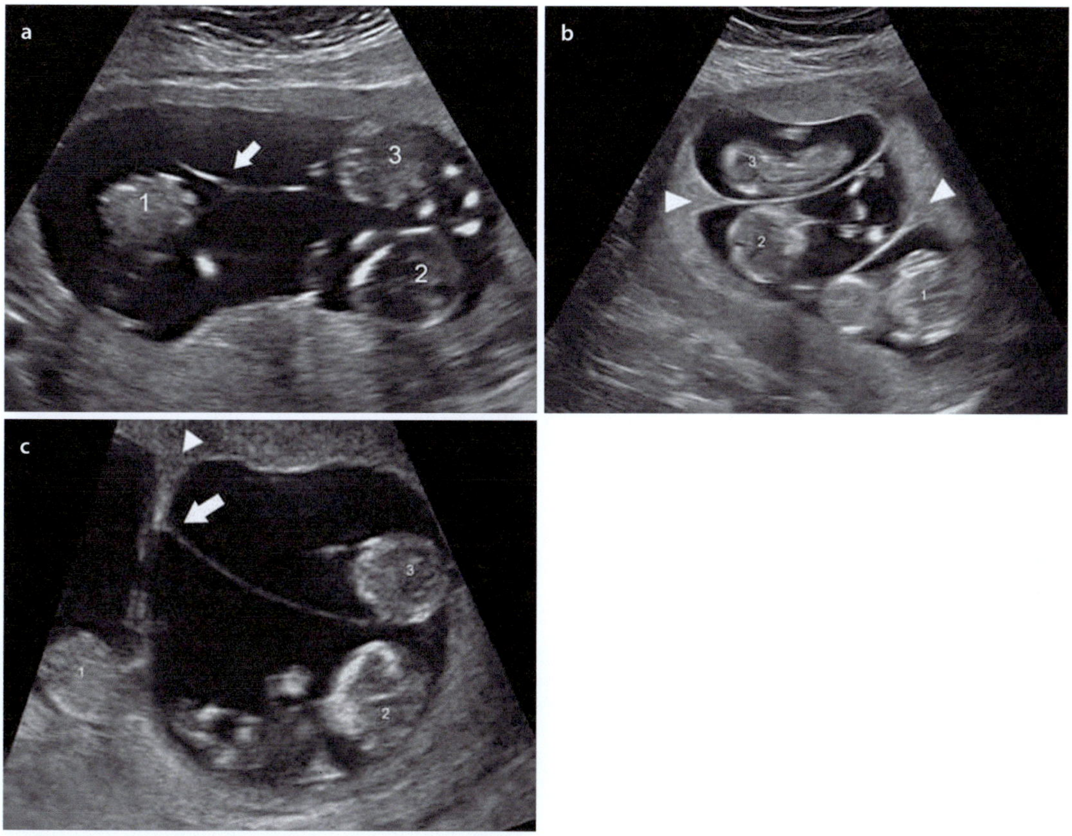

Fig. 3.3 Ultrasound images of triplets with varying numbers of fetal membranes. **a** *Monochorionic and therefore monozygotic triplets at 12 weeks of gestational age. The arrow indicates the meeting point of three amniotic membranes. Numbers indicate the three fetuses.* **b** *Trichorionic triplets at 12 weeks gestational age. The arrowheads indicate the separation between each fetus. These three fetuses do not share their placentas. This set of triplets can be trizygotic, dizygotic (one identical pair), or monozygotic. Numbers indicate the three fetuses.* **c**. *Dichorionic, triamniotic triplets at 13 weeks gestational age. The arrowhead indicates the separation of the chorionic membranes, which proves that this fetus does not share a placenta with fetuses 2 or 3. The arrow indicates the amniotic membarnes of fetuses 2 and 3, which are a monzygotic pair. At this point in time, it is unsure if fetus 1 shares zygosity with fetuses 2 and 3. Numbers indicate the three fetuses.*(This figure was adapted from Lamb et al. [22] with written permission from Cambridge University Press)

3.3.3 DNA Typing

The most robust and reliable way of determining zygosity is by DNA typing. The advent of cost-effective DNA genotyping has allowed for the opportunity to accurately determine zygosity through quantitative measures of allele sharing between twins when biological samples are available [23, 24]. Genetically, MZ twins will share (close to) 100% of their alleles and on average, DZ twins will share 50% of their alleles: similar to the allele sharing pattern of siblings. The recommended minimum number of single nucleotide polymorphisms (SNPs) needed to assess zygosity is around 50 [24]; however, utilization of around 20,000–30,000 SNPs bolsters confidence in zygosity determination. Procedurally, after genotyping and quality control, an optimal number of SNPs are selected and allele sharing in all pairs is determined. Sharing is reported as a proportion of markers for which a pair shares zero alleles (Z_0), one allele (Z_1), and two alleles (Z_2). From the proportions, total allele sharing (represented by $\hat{\neq}$) is calculated with the following formula: $\hat{\neq} = Z_2 + 0.5 * Z_1$. MZ pairs are identified by finding pairs with a $\hat{\neq}$ > 0.90, allowing for some measurement error.

DZ pairs are defined as pairs with a $\hat{\neq}$ and Z_1 between ~0.30 and ~0.70 [23].

3.4 Etiology of Twinning

3.4.1 Genetic Causes of MZ Twins

There have been several reports of families in which MZ twinning occurs more frequently than expected [25–30], although there is no compelling evidence to support an underlying genetic contribution to MZ twinning. Instances of familial MZ twinning from both maternal and paternal lineages have been documented, yet it has also been suggested that, independent of the sex of the parent transmitting the gene, a single gene is responsible for MZ twinning [29, 31]. There is additional evidence to suggest that there is no paternal effect on familial MZ twinning [32].

More recently, a gene thought to likely play a role in MZ twinning is *PITX2*. The *PITX2* gene was found as a candidate of monozygotic twinning in a molecular screening of an "experimental twinning" model in chickens [33]. *PITX2* encodes a protein that acts as a transcription factor, regulating the expression of genes involved with the formation of the embryonic axis.

3.4.2 Generation of MZ Twins

The universally accepted model of MZ twinning, often times referred to as the "fission model," rests on the hypothesis of postzygotic splitting of the conceptus within the first 2 weeks of development [21]. As exemplified by the model, the number of fetuses, chorions, and amnions are the result of the timing of embryo division. An alternative model of MZ twinning, sometimes called the "fusion model," challenges the traditional postzygotic splitting conjecture. The fusion model has been suggested due to criticisms of the traditional model lacking scientific evidence and the lack of specification of cleavage initiating factors [34]. The proposed alternate theory is based on two premises: (1) – MZ twinning occurs during the first cleavage division, resulting in twin zygotes and (2) – the structure of the fetal membranes is dependent on the various modes of fusion of the fetal membranes within the zona pellucida. Despite the two theories, the embryological processes that govern MZ twinning are still largely unknown and up for debate [35].

3.4.3 Genetic Causes of DZ Twins

DZ twinning is a complex trait that is likely under the influence of multiple genes. In the last decade, astonishing progress in characterizing the genes responsible for DZ twinning has been made. However, a comprehensive understanding of the genetic factors underlying the human tendency to conceive DZ twins is still lacking. Bearing this in mind, there are a number of genes with known roles in ovulation, female fertility, and DZ twinning in humans [36]. For example, mutations resulting in amino acid changes of the follicle-stimulating hormone receptor (FSHR) protein have been shown to influence DZ twinning [37]. Additionally, a variant within the promoter region of the *FSHR* gene was found to segregate with DZ twinning in a large family [38]; however, other studies have not replicated the involvement of this gene [39]. Several other candidate gene studies have provided evidence suggesting the involvement of other genes in the DZ twinning process, namely, serpin family A member 1 (*SERPINA1*) commonly referred to as alpha-1-antitrypsin [40, 41], peroxisome proliferator activated receptor gamma (*PPARG*) [42], and the fragile X "premutation" (*FRAXA*) [43, 44], although results were not replicated in future studies.

Linkage studies in family-based study designs have not provided evidence of enhanced genetic sharing among affected family members over chromosomal regions harboring the previously described candidate genes [38, 45]. However, linkage studies have indicated chromosomal regions that may possess novel candidate genes for DZ twinning [38, 45, 46]. For example, a study of 525 Australian and Dutch families of DZ twinning demonstrated the presence of new candidate DZ twinning genes on chromosomes 6, 12, and 20 [38]. The results reaffirmed the notion that DZ twinning is a complex phenotype influenced by numerous genes. Mutations in growth differentiation factor-9 (*GDF9*) appear to influence DZ twinning in humans, albeit such mutations appear to be rare. Screening in large numbers of families with a rich history of DZ twinning revealed a two-base deletion in *GDF9* in heterozygous form resulting in a loss-of-function mutation in three families [47, 48]. It was also discovered that overall genetic variation in *GDF9* is more prevalent in mothers of DZ twins compared to controls [48]. Findings from non-human studies (e.g., sheep) of DZ twinning have implicated bone morphogenetic protein 15 (*BMP15*) and bone morphogenetic protein receptor 1B (*BMPR1B*) in the DZ twinning process; however, similar effects have not been found when studying *BMP15* [49] or *BMPR1B* [50] in humans. Both *GDF9* and *BMP15* are expressed in the oocyte and are essential for follicular development and have been implicated in premature ovarian failure [51]. *BMPR1B* is expressed in multiple cell types of the ovary and is the cognate receptor for *BMP15*. Surprisingly, while heterozygous mutations (one copy present) in *GDF9* and *BMP15* increase twinning rates, homozygous mutations (two copies present) result in female infertility.

More recently, genome-wide association studies (GWAS) have made it possible to scan the entire human genome for SNPs that are associated with a trait of interest in humans (e.g., twinning). In 2016, the first meta-analysis of GWAS in European-ancestry populations (Netherlands, Australian, Minnesota [United States of America]) identified the first common genetic variants associated with spontaneous DZ twinning [11]. Three statistically significant SNPs were found: in the upstream region of the follicle-stimulating hormone beta subunit (*FSHB*) gene, within an intron of the mothers against decapentaplegic homolog 3 (*SMAD3*) gene, and in an intergenic region on chromosome 1. The two SNPs near *FSHB* and within *SMAD3* were replicated in an independent Icelandic cohort. The former encodes the beta subunit of FSH, while the gene product of the latter is transcription factor involved in gonadal responsiveness to FSH. Sixty-three candidate genes of DZ twinning [52] were also tested, but only *FSHB* was associated with DZ twinning in gene-based tests. Interestingly, the replicated SNPs associated with twinning were also found to be associated with higher serum FSH levels, and with multiple aspects of female fertility, including earlier age at menarche, earlier age at first child, higher lifetime parity, earlier age at menopause, and later age at last child. Polygenic risk scores for DZ twinning were found to be significantly associated with DZ twinning in the independent Icelandic cohort, with a higher likelihood of having children, higher lifetime number of children, and an earlier age at first child. Together these findings corroborate the link between fertility and DZ twinning.

3.4.4 Generation of DZ Twins

Mechanisms leading to dizygotic twins operate on the selection of developing follicles within the ovary when instead of one ovum being released mid-cycle, two follicles mature, and both oocytes are released for fertilization. The subsequent fertilization of two eggs by two sperm during a pregnancy result in DZ twins. The processes of ovarian folliculogenesis and dominant follicle selection are governed by both circulating and intra-ovarian concentrations of FSH. Spontaneous DZ twinning tends to run in families and is associated with elevated concentrations of FSH in the mother [53]. FSH amounts seem to vary with geography, season, ethnic origin, and increasing parity, and are increased in tall, heavy, and older mothers with a peak at around 37 years of age [54]. Following this logic, it has been proposed that age-dependent twinning may also be due to natural selection favoring double ovulation events in response to declining fertility with increasing age [55]. It has also been documented that mothers of DZ twins have an increased number of FSH pulses during the early follicular phase, without a concurrent luteinizing hormone (LH) pulse [56].

It is well known that improved nutrition is a contributing factor for increases in multiple ovulation (i.e., twinning frequency) in other species [57, 58], yet this has not been demonstrated in humans. In fact, human twinning rates do not appear to reflect average nutritional status as established from longitudinal studies of countries experiencing extended periods of starvation, such as the Dutch hunger winter [1]. In general, above a specific, yet undetermined, threshold, nutrition seems to be of minimal importance for twinning and reproduction in general.

3.5 Incidence of Twins

In the early twentieth century Wilhelm Weinberg postulated a method, referred to as the "Weinberg differential rule," for approximating population estimates of the number of MZ versus DZ twins [59]. Weinberg's proposal assumed that all MZ twins and half of DZ twins would be of the same sex, with the other half of DZ twins being of opposite sex. Therefore, he suggested multiplying the number of opposite-sex twins by two, which served as an estimate for the total number of DZ twins. The excess of same-sex twins would then be the number of MZ twins. Thought of in a different way, subtracting the total number of opposite-sex twins from the number of same-sex twins would yield an estimate of the number of MZ twins. Weinberg's calculation has been widely adopted because it serves as a simple method for estimating twinning frequency in populations; however, it rests on the assumption that the frequency of same-sex twins is the same as that of opposite-sex twin pairs, which may not always be the case [60, 61].

The rate of twinning includes stillbirths (≥28 weeks) and live births and is defined as the number of twin maternities per 1000 maternities. Differences in twinning rates between geographical regions have been studied extensively. In the 1970s, Bulmer studied twinning frequencies in three distinct geographical regions: Europe/North Africa, Sub-Saharan Africa, and Asia [62]. Bulmer found that the highest rate of twinning occurred in Sub-Saharan Africa (~23 per 1000 maternities), while the lowest rate occurred in Asia (~5–6 per 1000 maternities). Twinning rates exhibit considerable temporal and spatial variation (see ◘ Fig. 3.4). Provided that

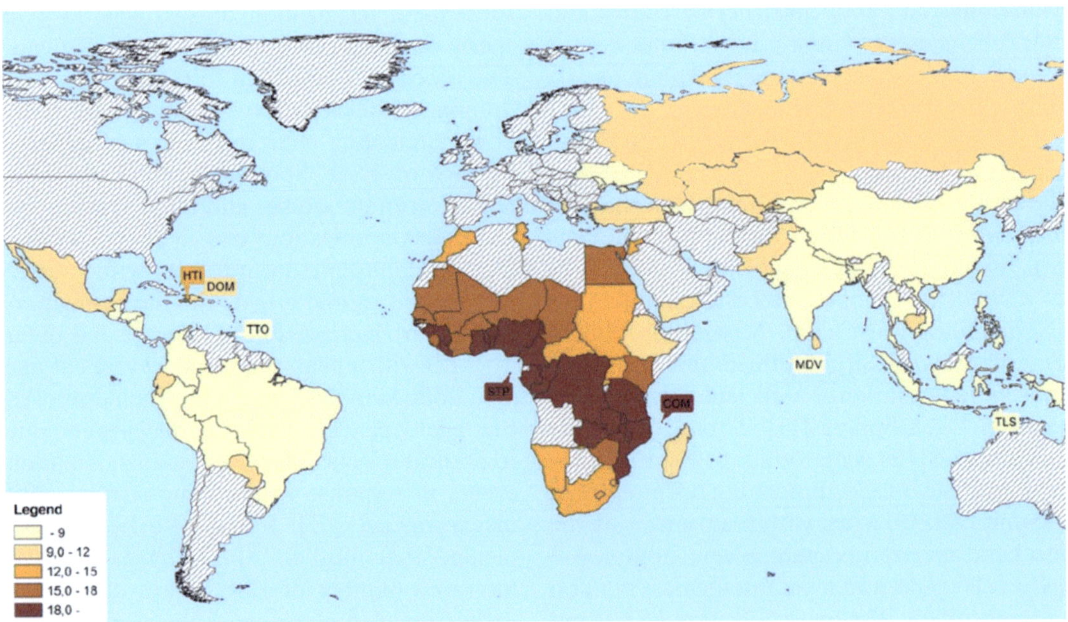

◘ **Fig. 3.4** Rates of twinning worldwide. *Heatmap showing the number of twins per 1000 births in 77 countries. Huge variation in twinning rates can be observed across the different regions of the developing world.* (The figure was adapted from Smits and Monden [76] by Veronika Odintsova to include 2011 Russian twinning rates.)

Table 3.1 Multiple births in Russian Federation in 2017

		Total number			Proportion in all deliveries			Birth rate per 1000		
	All deliveries, including born outside clinic	Multiple (all)	Twins	Triplets and higher order	Multiple (all)	Twins	Triplets and higher order	Multiple (all)	Twins	Triplets and higher order
Russian Federation	1,649,782	20,239	19,938	301	1.23	1.21	0.02	12.27	12.09	0.18

Table 3.1 was created and provided by Veronika Odintsova based on Russian national statistics [63]

the MZ twinning rate is known to be fairly constant around the world, the variation in overall twinning rate is generally attributed to the variation in DZ twinning rates.

Global twinning rates have predominantly been reported from Western countries with less being known about twinning rates in Eastern countries. In 2017, data received from open resources of national statistics of the Ministry of Health of the Russian Federation report a multiple birth rate of 12.27 births per 1000 deliveries (alive or stillbirth) as seen in Table 3.1 [63]. The overall twinning rate during this time was reported to be 12.09 per 1000 and the rate of higher-order multiples occurred at a rate of 0.18 per 1000.

3.5.1 Incidence of MZ Twins

Worldwide, and across all races, MZ twin birth rates occur at a constant rate of approximately 4 in every 1000 pregnancies [64]. The remarkable consistency in MZ twinning rates among all populations suggests that identical twinning is an occurrence that is not influenced by genetics. Unlike DZ twinning, the incidence of MZ twins is independent of maternal age, height, weight, or parity [65]. Although MZ twinning appears to be a sporadic event, instances of familial MZ twinning of varying modes of inheritance have been reported, with one report of autosomal dominant inheritance with variable penetrance [66]. The introduction of assisted reproductive technologies (ART) greatly enhances rates of DZ twinning and to some extent MZ twinning [67]. The increase in MZ twinning rates due to ART has been attributed to mechanical forces affecting the zona pellucida, or to the effects of incubation media and late implantation in in vitro fertilization procedures [68–70].

3.5.2 Incidence of DZ Twins

DZ twinning is common, yet large regional differences in DZ twinning rates exist around the world. The rate of DZ twins range from approximately 6 per 1000 maternities in Asia, to 10–20 per 1000 in Europe and the United States, to as high as 40 per 1000 in certain regions of Africa [12]. DZ twinning rates also vary substantially over time. In the United States, the observed incidence of twin births increased by a factor of 1.9 between 1971 and 2009 [71]. A considerable portion of the increase is attributable to fertility treatments, with an estimated 36% of all twins born in the United States in 2011 resulting from ART [71, 72]. DZ twinning rates peaked in the mid-2000s, following the number of ART pregnancies. In developed countries, with technological advancements and careful monitoring, DZ twinning rates due to ART have dropped substantially. In contrast to MZ twinning, spontaneous (i.e., no ART) DZ twinning is also very dependent on many maternal factors including age, nationality, parity, height, weight, and family history [36, 54].

3.5.3 Triplets and Higher-Order Multiples

The pattern of variation in triplet rates across the world is remarkably similar to that observed for twin births. That is, rates of triplet births are highest in African countries, intermediate in European populations, and lowest in Asian countries. More generally, the rate of triplets is in accordance with Hellin's law [73], which states that there is on average one twin maternity per N singleton maternities and that there is one X-tuplet maternity per $N^{(X-1)}$ [74, 75]. Thus, if the number of twin maternities is one in N singleton maternities, then the number of triplets is one in $N^{(3-1)}$. It follows that quadruplets (see Fig. 3.5) would occur at a rate of $N^{(4-1)}$. According to this logic, if there is one twin in every 80.05 births, this predicts that triplets occur at a rate of about 1 in ever 6408 births, which is only 4% higher than the incidence actually observed [76].

3.6 Factors Affecting Twinning

Many of the risk factors for DZ twinning are rather well established and include assisted reproductive technologies (ART), higher maternal age, parity, body composition, and smoking [12, 36, 77]. For MZ twinning, there is little to no agreement regarding the involved risk factors and/or causes [78]. Given that the two types of twinning are biologically distinct phenomena, it is not surprising that many of the factors involved in DZ twinning are not,

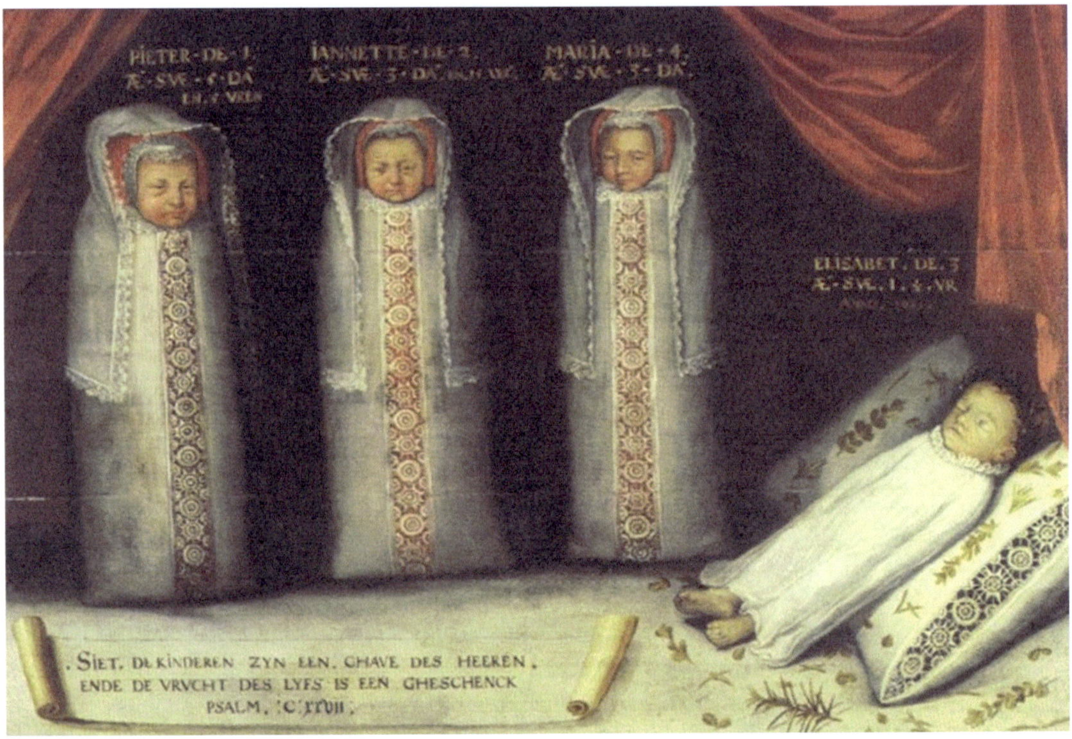

Fig. 3.5 Painting of Dutch quadruplets. *"Vierling Costerus" – Painting of quadruplets born on June 9, 1621, in Dordrecht, the Netherlands. Remarkably, the birth of the first (Pieter) and the last (Maria) was separated by 53 hours indicating an extremely difficult birthing process. Prior to the quad birth of one boy and three girls as pictured here, the parents mention the birth of twins 7 years before. Sadly, due to the high infant mortality rate in the seventeenth century, about 40–50% of children did not reach the age of 18, and the chance of survival was even smaller for multiple births. In the case of the quadruplets pictured here, one died an hour and a half after birth (Elisabet), and two others deceased within the first year.* (This figure was obtained by written permission from the Dordrecht Museum. The Noordbrabants Museum in 's-Hertogenbosch received this painting as a gift in 1925 and presented it on loan to the Dordrechts Museum in 1986. Painter and client are unknown.)

or to a lesser extent, found in MZ twinning. Below we describe established risk factors involved in multiple pregnancy and multiple birth.

3.6.1 Assisted Reproductive Technologies (ART)

Assisted reproductive technologies, especially in vitro fertilization (IVF) and ovulation induction (OI), are well-established risk factors for DZ and to some extent MZ twinning [78]. Ovulation inducing agents such as clomiphene citrate, human pituitary gonadotropins, and human menopausal gonadotropins are known to increase ovulation rate and hence the probability of multiple pregnancy [79]. In case of IVF, increased multiple pregnancy and multiple birth are due to the transfer of multiple embryos [12, 80]. Although less well understood, there is also a slight increase in MZ twinning after IVF and other ART, with estimates ranging from a two- to 12-fold increase in MZ twinning rate after ART procedures [78] and a two- to fivefold increase in MZ twinning following IVF [81, 82]. Notably, OI agents are often used in concert with IVF; thus, the increased chance of multiple pregnancy following IVF cannot be merely attributed to multiple embryo transfer [36].

3.6.2 Other Risk Factors

Higher maternal age is another well-established risk factor for DZ twinning [36, 62]; however, conflicting reports have been made for MZ twinning [62, 83, 84]. Paradoxically, while fertility decreases with age, the spontaneous twinning rate increases. Both polyovulation and embryonic survival rate increase with maternal age, suggesting that increased ovulation rate and decreased spontaneous abortion of potentially unhealthy offspring could act together as an insurance system to produce one last round of reproduction, with twinning being merely a by-product [55, 85]. Additionally, increased parity (the number or maternities prior to twin pregnancy) is associated with a higher risk of DZ, but not MZ twinning [12, 86], independent of maternal age [36, 87]. Moreover, maternal body composition has been reported rather consistently in relation to DZ twinning, with both obesity and tall stature increasing the risk of DZ twinning [53, 84, 88]. Furthermore, an unexpected relation between maternal smoking and higher probability of DZ twinning is sometimes observed although the mechanism behind this observation remains unclear [77, 89, 90].

3.7 Endocrinology of DZ Twinning

Mothers of spontaneous DZ twins have a predisposition to multiple ovulation events due to interference with selection of a single dominant follicle. Multiple follicle growth and subsequent multiple ovulation events have been observed in mothers of hereditary dizygotic twins [91, 92]. Follicular recruitment, selection, and dominance is controlled by a complex regulatory network within the hypothalamic-pituitary-ovarian axis (◘ Fig. 3.6). The two main pituitary-derived hormones essential for reproductive function are FSH and LH and are secreted in response to the pulsatile secretion of gonadotropin-releasing hormone. FSH is the main hormone controlling follicular growth and its secretion is controlled by the main secretory products of the large dominant follicle(s), namely, estradiol and inhibin. Circulating concentrations of FSH, other intra-ovarian factors (e.g., GDF9 and BMP15), and their cognate receptors physiologically regulate ovarian folliculogenesis and ovulation quota. Transcriptional regulators of *FSH*, such as SMAD3, also regulate gonadal responsiveness to FSH. Ongoing development of a single follicle takes place when a certain threshold level of plasma FSH is marginally exceeded [93, 94]. When FSH levels are much higher than the threshold level, or exceed the threshold for an extended duration, multiple follicle growth can result [95]. In accordance with the endocrine model of dizygotic twinning [96], high levels of pituitary gonadotropins (i.e., FSH) are responsible for increased multiple ovulation in mothers of DZ twins.

3

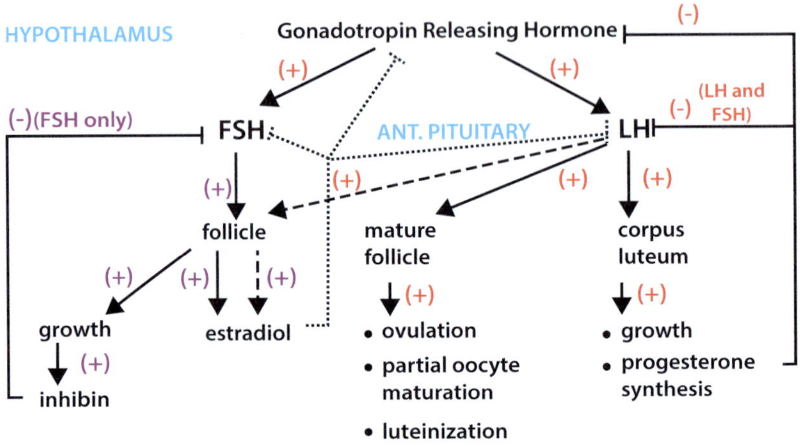

Fig. 3.6 Hormonal feedback and endocrine regulation of female reproductive physiology. + *signs denote positive feedback, whereas blunted arrows indicate negative feedback*. (This figure was obtained by written permission from the lecture materials of Dr. Kathleen Eyster (University of South Dakota, United States))

A number of studies, but not all [91], have shown increased levels of plasma gonadotropins in mothers of DZ twins [56, 97–99].

3.8 Non-human Twinning

Studies of non-human species have revealed several genes that contribute to DZ twinning. For example, in sheep, which are typically uniparous, certain breeds have higher incidences of multiple births [100]. Several genes, namely, *GDF9*, *BMP15*, and *BMPR1B*, have been confirmed to influence twinning rates in sheep by increasing follicle development and oocyte maturation [50, 101–103]. Major genes that increase ovulation rate and litter size in sheep and humans have been shown to have implications in other species. Evidence exists for genetic effects on twinning in cattle [104], the marmoset monkey [105], and on hormone-induced ovulation rate in mice [106].

Genes specific to MZ twinning remain elusive. Animal studies (originally in rabbit and roe deer) have suggested that MZ twinning results from disturbances to developmental thresholds and that delayed fertilization/implantation play a role [62]. These hypotheses have been further tested in nine-banded armadillos (*Dasypus novemcinctus*), which bear obligate MZ quadruplets each and every time they breed [107–110].

3.9 Sex Ratio

Sex ratio is defined as the ratio of males to total births. For DZ twins and singletons the ratio is 0.514, meaning a slight excess of males [62, 111]. For spontaneous MZ twins, triplets, and quadruplets, the sex ratio is lower (0.496) due to a slight excess of females [61, 111]. The value is even lower for monoamniotic twins, including conjoined twins, with a sex ratio of 0.2 [111]. There does not seem to be an excess of males in aborted twins. Dichorionic MZ twins exhibit the smallest increase in females, whereas monochorionic diamniotic MZ twins show the largest increase; thus, the rise may be due to later twinning events. Monochorionic monoamniotic twins and conjoined twins show an even greater increase in the number of females.

3.10 Discussion and Conclusion

Twinning is a common and multifactorial phenomenon, and elements of the twinning process remain poorly uncharacterized. Improved understanding of the underlying biological and genetic aspects of MZ and DZ twins and of the twinning process as a whole has been enhanced by the development of molecular and cytogenetic techniques. The influences on

DZ twinning are well studied, including contributions of numerous maternal (age, height, weight, parity, family history), environmental (ART), and associated genetic factors (most notably common variants near *FSHB* and within *SMAD3*). However, despite the robust associations with DZ twinning, the ability to predict DZ twinning events remains imprecise due to the myriad of genetic and non-genetic contributions. Likewise, comprehensive models of MZ twinning lack compelling evidence and are challenged by instances of atypical twinning. MZ twinning is likely influenced by some equivocal combination of non-genetic and genetic factors that likely result in delayed fertilization, embryo development, implantation, or some form of mechanical disruption of the early embryo. Further elucidation of the mechanisms by which twinning processes occur will have significant merit for predicting, managing, and improving the outcomes of multiple gestation pregnancies.

3.10.1 Review Questions

1. What are the etiological similarities and differences of monozygotic and dizygotic twins?

2. What is the role played by assisted reproductive technologies in the incidence of twinning over time?

3.10.2 Multiple-Choice Questions

1. What is the most conclusive method for determining zygosity status of twins?
   (a) Examination of placentation
   (b) Sex status (same or opposite sex)
   (c) Evaluation of survey responses
   (d) DNA testing
   (e) Assessment of outward physical appearance

Answer: (d). Although the other methods are convenient and relatively robust approaches for determining zygosity status of twins, only DNA testing provides a quantitative and accurate assessment of allele sharing for all twins, including same-sex twin pairs.

2. What is another term for dizygotic twins?
   (a) Identical twins
   (b) Fraternal twins
   (c) Typical twins
   (d) Atypical twins

Answer: (b). Dizygotic, or non-identical twins, develop from separate ova and are therefore genetically distinct. Thus, because their genetic relatedness is the same as for other sibling pairs, dizygotic twins are commonly referred to as fraternal twins.

3. The rarest form of monozygotic twins (with the exception of conjoined twins) exhibit which of the following fetal membrane states?
   (a) Dichorionic diamniotic
   (b) Dichorionic monoamniotic
   (c) Monochorionic diamniotic
   (d) Monochorionic monoamniotic

Answer: (d). Monochorionic monoamniotic monozygotic twins represent about 1% of all twin pregnancies. Approximately 66% of monozygotic twins are monochorionic diamniotic, whereas 33% are dichorionic diamniotic.

4. Genome-wide association studies have identified common genetic variants associated with spontaneous dizygotic twinning and female fertility in which genes?
   (a) *FSHB* and *SMAD3*
   (b) *GDF9* and *BMP15*
   (c) *BMP4* and *WFIKKN1*
   (d) *FSHR* and *BMPR1B*

Answer: (a). Single nucleotide polymorphisms near *FSHB* and within *SMAD3* are significantly associated with a higher rate of spontaneous dizygotic twinning and several other aspects of female fertility (e.g., earlier age at menarche, earlier age at first child, and higher lifetime parity).

3

5. In order of highest to lowest incidence, which of the following captures the large regional differences that are observed for dizygotic twinning?
   (a) Asia, Africa, Europe
   (b) Africa, Europe, Asia
   (c) Europe, Asia, Africa
   (d) Europe, Africa, Asia

Answer: (b). Whereas monozygotic twinning rates are relatively constant worldwide (~3 per 1000 births), large regional differences exist in dizygotic twinning rates with the highest incidence in African populations (~40 per 1000 births), followed by European populations (~10–20 per 1000 births), and the lowest incidence in Asian populations (~6 per 1000 births).

6. Which of the following is *not* a known non-genetic risk factor for spontaneous dizygotic twinning?
   (a) Parity
   (b) Maternal age
   (c) Nutritional status
   (d) Smoking status
   (e) Body mass index
   (f) Height

Answer: (c). Spontaneous dizygotic twinning is associated with parity, as well as increased maternal age, increased body mass index, increased height, and smoking status prior to pregnancy. Nutritional status is not known to be a direct contributor to dizygotic twinning as longitudinal studies in countries that experienced periods of starvation demonstrated consistent rates of twinning (e.g., Dutch hunger winter [1]).

Acknowledgments We are grateful to Veronika Odintsova for the generous contribution of the multiple birth data from the Russian Federation, which was obtained from the Federal Research Institute for Health Organization and Informatics, Ministry of Health of Russian Federation, Moscow, Russia.

References

1. Eriksson AW, Bressers WM, Kostense PJ, Pitkanen KJ, Mielke JH, Jorde LB, et al. Twinning rate in Scandinavia, Germany and The Netherlands during years of privation. Acta Genet Med Gemellol. 1988;37(3–4):277–97.
2. Duncan JM. Fertility, sterility and allied topics. 2nd ed. New York: William Wood and Co.; 1871. 498 p.
3. Galton F. The history of twins, as a criterion of the relative powers of nature and nurture. Fraser's Magazine. 1875:566–76.
4. Fisher RA. The genesis of twins. Genetics. 1919;4(5):489–99.
5. Skytthe A, Kyvik KO, Holm NV, Christensen K. The Danish twin registry. Scand J Public Health. 2011;39(7 Suppl):75–8.
6. Levit SG. Twin investigations in the U.S.S.R. Character and Personality. 1935;3:188–93.
7. Sukhanov S. Opsihozah u bliznetsov [On psychosis in twins]. Klinicheskij jurnal. 1900;4:341–52.
8. Yudin TI. O shodstve psihoza u bratjev i sester. [On similarity of psychosis in brothers and sisters]. Sovremennaya psihiatria. 1907;10:337–42.
9. Poll H. Über Zwillingsforschung als Hilfsmittel menschlicher Erbkunde. Z Ethnol. 1914;46:87–105.
10. Siemens HW. Die Zwillingspathologie. Mol Gen Genet. 1924;35:311–2.
11. Mbarek H, Steinberg S, Nyholt DR, Gordon SD, Miller MB, McRae AF, et al. Identification of common genetic variants influencing spontaneous dizygotic twinning and female fertility. Am J Hum Genet. 2016;98(5):898–908.
12. Hall JG. Twinning. Lancet. 2003;362(9385):735–43.
13. Benirschke K, Masliah E. The placenta in multiple pregnancy: outstanding issues. Reprod Fertil Dev. 2001;13(7–8):615–22.
14. Benirschke K, Kim CK. Multiple pregnancy. 1. N Engl J Med. 1973;288(24):1276–84.
15. Benirschke K, Kim CK. Multiple pregnancy. 2. N Engl J Med. 1973;288(25):1329–36.
16. Benirschke K. The placenta in twin gestation. Clin Obstet Gynecol. 1990;33(1):18–31.
17. Cutler TL, Murphy K, Hopper JL, Keogh LA, Dai Y, Craig JM. Why accurate knowledge of Zygosity is important to twins. Twin Res Hum Genet. 2015;18(3):298–305.
18. Umstad MP, Short RV, Wilson M, Craig JM. Chimaeric twins: why monochorionicity does not guarantee monozygosity. Aust N Z J Obstet Gynaecol. 2012;52(3):305–7.
19. Wray NR, Ripke S, Mattheisen M, Trzaskowski M, Byrne EM, Abdellaoui A, et al. Genome-wide

association analyses identify 44 risk variants and refine the genetic architecture of major depression. Nat Genet. 2018;50(5):668–81.
20. Forget-Dubois N, Perusse D, Turecki G, Girard A, Billette JM, Rouleau G, et al. Diagnosing zygosity in infant twins: physical similarity, genotyping, and chorionicity. Twin Res. 2003;6(6):479–85.
21. McNamara HC, Kane SC, Craig JM, Short RV, Umstad MP. A review of the mechanisms and evidence for typical and atypical twinning. Am J Obstet Gynecol. 2016;214(2):172–91. https://doi.org/10.1016/j.ajog.2015.10.930.
22. Lamb DJ, Vink JM, Middeldorp CM, van Beijsterveldt CE, Haak MC, Overbeek LI, et al. Effects of chorionicity and zygosity on triplet birth weight. Twin Res Hum Genet. 2012;15(2):149–57. https://doi.org/10.1375/twin.15.2.149.
23. Odintsova VV, Willemsen G, Dolan CV, Hottenga JJ, Martin NG, Slagboom PE, et al. Establishing a twin register: an invaluable resource for (behavior) genetic, epidemiological, biomarker, and 'Omics' studies. Twin Res Hum Genet. 2018;21(3):239–52.
24. Hannelius U, Gherman L, Makela VV, Lindstedt A, Zucchelli M, Lagerberg C, et al. Large-scale zygosity testing using single nucleotide polymorphisms. Twin Res Hum Genet. 2007;10(4):604–25.
25. Cyranoski D. Developmental biology: two by two. Nature. 2009;458(7240):826–9.
26. Barban N, Jansen R, de Vlaming R, Vaez A, Mandemakers JJ, Tropf FC, et al. Genome-wide analysis identifies 12 loci influencing human reproductive behavior. Nat Genet. 2016;48(12):1462–72.
27. Machin G. Familial monozygotic twinning: a report of seven pedigrees. Am J Med Genet C Semin Med Genet. 2009;151C(2):152–4.
28. Shapiro LR, Zemek L, Shulman MJ. Familial monozygotic twinning: an autosomal dominant form of monozygotic twinning with variable penetrance. Prog Clin Biol Res. 1978;24(Pt B):61–3.
29. Shapiro LR, Zemek L, Shulman MJ. Genetic etiology for monozygotic twinning. Birth Defects Orig Artic Ser. 1978;14(6A):219–22.
30. St Clair JB, Golubovsky MD. Paternally derived twinning: a two century examination of records of one Scottish name. Twin Res. 2002;5(4):294–307.
31. Michels VV, Riccardi VM. Twin recurrence and amniocentesis: male and MZ heritability factors. Birth Defects Orig Artic Ser. 1978;14(6A):201–11.
32. Lichtenstein P, Kallen B, Koster M. No paternal effect on monozygotic twinning in the Swedish twin registry. Twin Res. 1998;1(4):212–5.
33. Torlopp A, Khan MA, Oliveira NM, Lekk I, Soto-Jimenez LM, Sosinsky A, et al. The transcription factor Pitx2 positions the embryonic axis and regulates twinning. elife. 2014;3:e03743.
34. Herranz G. The timing of monozygotic twinning: a criticism of the common model. Zygote. 2013;23(1):27–40.
35. Denker HW. Comment on G. Herranz: the timing of monozygotic twinning: a criticism of the common model. Zygote (2013). Zygote. 2013;23(2):312–4.
36. Hoekstra C, Zhao ZZ, Lambalk CB, Willemsen G, Martin NG, Boomsma DI, et al. Dizygotic twinning. Hum Reprod Update. 2008;14(1):37–47.
37. Al-Hendy A, Moshynska O, Saxena A, Feyles V. Association between mutations of the follicle-stimulating-hormone receptor and repeated twinning. Lancet. 2000;356(9233):914.
38. Painter JN, Willemsen G, Nyholt D, Hoekstra C, Duffy DL, Henders AK, et al. A genome wide linkage scan for dizygotic twinning in 525 families of mothers of dizygotic twins. Hum Reprod. 2010;25(6):1569–80.
39. Montgomery GW, Duffy DL, Hall J, Kudo M, Martin NG, Hsueh AJ. Mutations in the follicle-stimulating hormone receptor and familial dizygotic twinning. Lancet. 2001;357(9258):773–4.
40. Boomsma DI, Frants RR, Bank RA, Martin NG. Protease inhibitor (Pi) locus, fertility and twinning. Hum Genet. 1992;89(3):329–32.
41. Lieberman J, Borhani NO, Feinleib M. Twinning as a heterozygous advantage for alpha1-antitrypsin deficiency. Prog Clin Biol Res. 1978;24(Pt B):45–54.
42. Duffy D, Montgomery G, Treloar S, Birley A, Kirk K, Boomsma D, et al. IBD sharing around the PPARG locus is not increased in dizygotic twins or their mothers. Nat Genet. 2001;28(4):315.
43. Fryns JP. The female and the fragile X. A study of 144 obligate female carriers. Am J Med Genet. 1986;23(1–2):157–69.
44. Kenneson A, Warren ST. The female and the fragile X reviewed. Semin Reprod Med. 2001;19(2):159–65.
45. Derom C, Jawaheer D, Chen WV, McBride KL, Xiao X, Amos C, et al. Genome-wide linkage scan for spontaneous DZ twinning. Eur J Hum Genet. 2006;14(1):117–22.
46. Busjahn A, Knoblauch H, Faulhaber HD, Aydin A, Uhlmann R, Tuomilehto J, et al. A region on chromosome 3 is linked to dizygotic twinning. Nat Genet. 2000;26(4):398–9.
47. Montgomery GW, Zhao ZZ, Marsh AJ, Mayne R, Treloar SA, James M, et al. A deletion mutation in GDF9 in sisters with spontaneous DZ twins. Twin Res. 2004;7(6):548–55.
48. Palmer JS, Zhao ZZ, Hoekstra C, Hayward NK, Webb PM, Whiteman DC, et al. Novel variants in growth differentiation factor 9 in mothers of dizygotic twins. J Clin Endocrinol Metab. 2006;91(11):4713–6.

3

49. Zhao ZZ, Painter JN, Palmer JS, Webb PM, Hayward NK, Whiteman DC, et al. Variation in bone morphogenetic protein 15 is not associated with spontaneous human dizygotic twinning. Hum Reprod. 2008;23(10):2372–9.
50. Luong HT, Chaplin J, McRae AF, Medland SE, Willemsen G, Nyholt DR, et al. Variation in BMPR1B, TGFRB1 and BMPR2 and control of dizygotic twinning. Twin Res Hum Genet. 2011;14(5):408–16.
51. Dixit H, Rao L, Padmalatha V, Raseswari T, Kapu AK, Panda B, et al. Genes governing premature ovarian failure. Reprod Biomed Online. 2010;20(6):724–40.
52. Harris RA, Tardif SD, Vinar T, Wildman DE, Rutherford JN, Rogers J, et al. Evolutionary genetics and implications of small size and twinning in callitrichine primates. Proc Natl Acad Sci U S A. 2014;111(4):1467–72.
53. Nylander PP. The factors that influence twinning rates. Acta Genet Med Gemellol. 1981;30(3): 189–202.
54. Campbell DM, Campbell AJ, MacGillivray I. Maternal characteristics of women having twin pregnancies. J Biosoc Sci. 1974;6(4):463–70.
55. Hazel WN, Black R, Smock RC, Sear R, Tomkins JL. An age-dependent ovulatory strategy explains the evolution of dizygotic twinning in humans. Nat Ecol Evol. 2020;4:987–92.
56. Lambalk CB, Boomsma DI, De Boer L, De Koning CH, Schoute E, Popp-Snijders C, et al. Increased levels and pulsatility of follicle-stimulating hormone in mothers of hereditary dizygotic twins. J Clin Endocrinol Metab. 1998;83(2):481–6.
57. Montgomery GW, Hawker H. Seasonal reproduction in ewes selected on seasonal changes in wool growth. J Reprod Fertil. 1987;79(1):207–13.
58. Hunter MG, Robinson RS, Mann GE, Webb R. Endocrine and paracrine control of follicular development and ovulation rate in farm species. Anim Reprod Sci. 2004;82–83:461–77.
59. Weinberg W. Beiträge zur physiologie und der pathologie der mehrlingsgeburten beim menschen. Arch Physiol. 1902;88:346–30.
60. Cameron AH. The Birmingham twin survey. Proc R Soc Med. 1968;61(3):229–34.
61. James WH. Excess of like sexed pairs of dizygotic twins. Nature. 1971;232(5308):277–8.
62. Bulmer MG. The biology of twinning in man. Clarendon Press, Oxford; 1970.
63. Polikarpov AVAGA, Golubev NA, Turina EM, Ogryzko EV, Shelepova EA. Key indicators of the health of the mother and child, the activities of the service for childhood and obstetrics in the Russian Federation. Moscow: The Ministry of Health of the Russian Federation; 2018. p. 164.
64. Tong S, Caddy D, Short RV. Use of dizygotic to monozygotic twinning ratio as a measure of fertility. Lancet. 1997;349(9055):843–5.
65. Bressers WM, Eriksson AW, Kostense PJ, Parisi P. Increasing trend in the monozygotic twinning rate. Acta Genet Med Gemellol. 1987;36(3): 397–408.
66. Harvey MA, Huntley RM, Smith DW. Familial monozygotic twinning. J Pediatr. 1977;90(2): 246–7.
67. Alikani M, Cekleniak NA, Walters E, Cohen J. Monozygotic twinning following assisted conception: an analysis of 81 consecutive cases. Hum Reprod. 2003;18(9):1937–43.
68. Abusheikha N, Salha O, Sharma V, Brinsden P. Monozygotic twinning and IVF/ICSI treatment: a report of 11 cases and review of literature. Hum Reprod Update. 2000;6(4): 396–403.
69. Milki AA, Jun SH, Hinckley MD, Behr B, Giudice LC, Westphal LM. Incidence of monozygotic twinning with blastocyst transfer compared to cleavage-stage transfer. Fertil Steril. 2003;79(3):503–6.
70. Steinman G. Mechanisms of twinning. VI. Genetics and the etiology of monozygotic twinning in in vitro fertilization. J Reprod Med. 2003;48(8):583–90.
71. Kulkarni AD, Jamieson DJ, Jones HW Jr, Kissin DM, Gallo MF, Macaluso M, et al. Fertility treatments and multiple births in the United States. N Engl J Med. 2013;369(23):2218–25.
72. Fauser BC, Devroey P, Macklon NS. Multiple birth resulting from ovarian stimulation for subfertility treatment. Lancet. 2005;365(9473): 1807–16.
73. Hellin D. Die Ursache der Multiparitat der uniparen Tiere uberhaupt und der Zwillingsschwangerschaft beim Menschen insbesondere (The causes ofmultiple maternities among uniparous animals and in man). Seitz & Schauer. 1895;
74. Fellman J, Eriksson AW. On the history of Hellin's law. Twin Res Hum Genet. 2009;12(2):183–90.
75. Fellman J, Eriksson AW. Statistical analyses of Hellin's law. Twin Res Hum Genet. 2009;12(2): 191–200.
76. Smits J, Monden C. Twinning across the developing world. PLoS One. 2011;6(9):e25239.
77. Hoekstra C, Willemsen G, van Beijsterveldt CE, Lambalk CB, Montgomery GW, Boomsma DI. Body composition, smoking, and spontaneous dizygotic twinning. Fertil Steril. 2010;93(3): 885–93.
78. Aston KI, Peterson CM, Carrell DT. Monozygotic twinning associated with assisted reproductive technologies: a review. Reproduction. 2008;136(4): 377–86.
79. Lamont JA. Twin pregnancies following induction of ovulation: a literature review. Acta Genet Med Gemellol. 1982;31(3–4):247–53.
80. Ananth CV, Chauhan SP. Epidemiology of twinning in developed countries. Semin Perinatol. 2012;36(3):156–61.

81. Sills ES, Tucker MJ, Palermo GD. Assisted reproductive technologies and monozygous twins: implications for future study and clinical practice. Twin Res. 2000;3(4):217–23.
82. Edwards RG, Mettler L, Walters DE. Identical twins and in vitro fertilization. J In Vitro Fert Embryo Transf. 1986;3(2):114–7.
83. Steinman G. Mechanisms of twinning. II. Laterality and intercellular bonding in monozygotic twinning. J Reprod Med. 2001;46(5):473–9.
84. Bortolus R, Parazzini F, Chatenoud L, Benzi G, Bianchi MM, Marini A. The epidemiology of multiple births. Hum Reprod Update. 1999;5(2):179–87.
85. Varella M, Fernandes E, Arantes J, Acquaviva T, Lucci T, Hsu R, David V, Bussah V, Valentova J, Segal N, Otta E. Twinning as an evolved age-dependent physiological mechanism: evidence from large Brazilian Samples. Multiple pregnancy (new challenges). United Kingdom: IntechOpen; 2018.
86. Hankins GV, Saade GR. Factors influencing twins and zygosity. Paediatr Perinat Epidemiol. 2005;19(Suppl 1):8–9.
87. Tong S, Short RV. Dizygotic twinning as a measure of human fertility. Hum Reprod. 1998;13(1):95–8.
88. Basso O, Nohr EA, Christensen K, Olsen J. Risk of twinning as a function of maternal height and body mass index. JAMA. 2004;291(13):1564–6.
89. Olsen J, Bonnelykke B, Nielsen J. Tobacco smoking and twinning. Acta Med Scand. 1988;224(5):491–4.
90. Parazzini F, Chatenoud L, Benzi G, Di Cintio E, Dal Pino D, Tozzi L, et al. Coffee and alcohol intake, smoking and risk of multiple pregnancy. Hum Reprod. 1996;11(10):2306–9.
91. Gilfillan CP, Robertson DM, Burger HG, Leoni MA, Hurley VA, Martin NG. The control of ovulation in mothers of dizygotic twins. J Clin Endocrinol Metab. 1996;81(4):1557–62.
92. Martin NG, Shanley S, Butt K, Osborne J, O'Brien G. Excessive follicular recruitment and growth in mothers of spontaneous dizygotic twins. Acta Genet Med Gemellol. 1991;40(3–4):291–301.
93. Schoemaker J, van Weissenbruch MM, Scheele F, van der Meer M. The FSH threshold concept in clinical ovulation induction. Baillieres Clin Obstet Gynaecol. 1993;7(2):297–308.
94. Brown JB. Pituitary control of ovarian function--concepts derived from gonadotrophin therapy. Aust N Z J Obstet Gynaecol. 1978;18(1):46–54.
95. Baird DT. A model for follicular selection and ovulation: lessons from superovulation. J Steroid Biochem. 1987;27(1–3):15–23.
96. Milham S Jr. Pituitary gonadotrophin and dizygotic twinning. Lancet. 1964;2(7359):566.
97. Martin NG, Olsen ME, Theile H, El Beaini JL, Handelsman D, Bhatnagar AS. Pituitary-ovarian function in mothers who have had two sets of dizygotic twins. Fertil Steril. 1984;41(6):878–80.
98. Martin NG, Robertson DM, Chenevix-Trench G, de Kretser DM, Osborne J, Burger HG. Elevation of follicular phase inhibin and luteinizing hormone levels in mothers of dizygotic twins suggests nonovarian control of human multiple ovulation. Fertil Steril. 1991;56(3):469–74.
99. Nylander PP. Serum levels of gonadotrophins in relation to multiple pregnancy in Nigeria. J Obstet Gynaecol Br Commonw. 1973;80(7):651–3.
100. Montgomery GW, McNatty KP, Davis GH. Physiology and molecular genetics of mutations that increase ovulation rate in sheep. Endocr Rev. 1992;13(2):309–28.
101. Demars J, Fabre S, Sarry J, Rossetti R, Gilbert H, Persani L, et al. Genome-wide association studies identify two novel BMP15 mutations responsible for an atypical hyperprolificacy phenotype in sheep. PLoS Genet. 2013;9(4):e1003482.
102. Reader KL, Haydon LJ, Littlejohn RP, Juengel JL, McNatty KP. Booroola BMPR1B mutation alters early follicular development and oocyte ultrastructure in sheep. Reprod Fertil Dev. 2012;24(2):353–61.
103. Vage DI, Husdal M, Kent MP, Klemetsdal G, Boman IA. A missense mutation in growth differentiation factor 9 (GDF9) is strongly associated with litter size in sheep. BMC Genet. 2013;14:1.
104. Komisarek J, Dorynek Z. Genetic aspects of twinning in cattle. J Appl Genet. 2002;43(1):55–68.
105. Marmoset Genome S, Analysis C. The common marmoset genome provides insight into primate biology and evolution. Nat Genet. 2014;46(8):850–7.
106. Spearow JL. Major genes control hormone-induced ovulation rate in mice. J Reprod Fertil. 1988;82(2):787–97.
107. Enders AC. Implantation in the nine-banded armadillo: how does a single blastocyst form four embryos? Placenta. 2002;23(1):71–85.
108. Prodohl PA, Loughry WJ, McDonough CM, Nelson WS, Avise JC. Molecular documentation of polyembryony and the micro-spatial dispersion of clonal sibships in the nine-banded armadillo, Dasypus novemcinctus. Proc Biol Sci. 1996;263(1377):1643–9.
109. Storrs EE, Williams RJ. A study of monozygous quadruplet armadillos in relation to mammalian inheritance. Proc Natl Acad Sci U S A. 1968;60(3):910–4.
110. Blickstein I, Keith LG. On the possible cause of monozygotic twinning: lessons from the 9-banded

armadillo and from assisted reproduction. Twin Res Hum Genet. 2007;10(2):394–9.

111. James WH. Sex ratio and placentation in twins. Ann Hum Biol. 1980;7(3):273–6.

Key Reading

Bulmer MG. The biology of twinning in man. Clarendon Press, Oxford; 1970. An overview of multiple births in humans

Hall JG. Twinning. Lancet. 2003;362(9385):735–43. https://doi.org/10.1016/S0140-6736(03)14237-7. A report focused on the biological and genetic aspects of twinning

Hoekstra C, Zhao ZZ, Lambalk CB, Willemsen G, Martin NG, Boomsma DI, Montgomery GW. Dizygotic twinning. Hum Reprod Update. 2008;14(1):37–47. https://doi.org/10.1093/humupd/dmm036. A summary of the genetic and non-genetic risk factors associated with conception of spontaneous dizygotic twins

Mbarek H, Steinberg S, Nyholt DR, Gordon SD, Miller MB, McRae AF, Boomsma DI. Identification of common genetic variants influencing spontaneous dizygotic twinning and female fertility. Am J Hum Genet. 2016;98(5):898–908. https://doi.org/10.1016/j.ajhg.2016.03.008. This paper describes the identification of common genetic variants that are strongly associated with being a mother of dizygotic twins and female fertility

McNamara HC, Kane SC, Craig JM, Short RV, Umstad MP. A review of the mechanisms and evidence for typical and atypical twinning. Am J Obstet Gynecol. 2016;214(2):172–91. https://doi.org/10.1016/j.ajog.2015.10.930. A comprehensive review and in-depth description of the biological mechanisms of typical and atypical twinning

Twin-Singleton Comparisons Across Multiple Domains of Life

Gonneke Willemsen, Veronika Odintsova, Eco de Geus, and Dorret I. Boomsma

Contents

A. Khalil et al. (eds.), *Twin and Higher-order Pregnancies*,
https://doi.org/10.1007/978-3-030-47652-6_4

4

Trailer

In this chapter, we address the question whether individuals born from a multiple pregnancy differ from singletons. The answer to this question is important for health-care professionals and researchers, as well as multiples themselves and their family members.

First, we review findings from the literature with respect to twin – non-twin differences in early life and conclude that a multiple pregnancy increases the risk of congenital problems and mortality for the unborn and newborn children.

Next, we provide an overview of the outcomes of comparing adult twins to their singleton siblings across a wide range of traits assessed in the Netherlands Twin Register (NTR). In a within-family design, comparing twins to siblings from the same family, we correct for familial confounding. Overall, hardly any evidence was found for the presence of twin-sibling differences for the five domains explored, which included body composition and physical development, personality and psychopathology, behavioral and sociodemographic traits, physiological parameters and physical disease, and cognitive function. With the exception of minor differences in body composition, twins do not seem to differ from singletons, when taking family factors into account.

In conclusion, while being a twin can be seen as special, adult twins are similar to ordinary siblings across most domains of life.

Definitions

1. Twin – An individual born after the same pregnancy of multiple zygotes leading to a multiple birth.
2. Singleton – An individual who was the single (surviving) zygote during a pregnancy and therefore not part of a multiple birth.
3. Barker hypothesis – The theory of fetal origins of adult disease.
4. Congenital disorder – A condition present at birth that results from genetic or chromosomal disorders, exposure to certain medications or chemicals, or certain infections during pregnancy.
5. Within-family design – A comparison of outcome (dependent) variables between members of the same family who may differ on the predictor (independent) variables.

Learning Objectives

- To gain insight into the risk of congenital problems and mortality in multiple pregnancy
- To understand the challenges in studying twin-singleton differences and how the study of multiples and their singleton siblings from the same family can resolve some of these problems
- To increase knowledge regarding potential differences between multiples and singletons in their development, behavior, and health

4.1 Introduction

Over the past decades, twin and higher-order multiple pregnancy rates have increased in many countries worldwide [14, 82, 112]. While the increased number of infertility treatments is often stated as the reason for this increase, the increase in maternal age is also a significant contributor [57]. Compared to singletons, that is children born from a single pregnancy originating with a single zygote, children born from a multiple pregnancy are born on average 3 weeks earlier [33], and are about 4 cm shorter and 1 kilo lighter at birth [70]. Multiples, that is, twins, triplets, and higher-order multiples, may be at increased risk of complications during pregnancy, delivery, and in the postnatal period. The fetal origins hypothesis and the developmental origins of health and disease hypothesis, often referred to as the Barker hypothesis, poses that low birth weight reflects intra-uterine growth retardation that may affect later development and increases the risk of disease development and earlier mortality [4]. Numerous studies in the general population have indeed found evidence for an association of low birth weight with diseases including hypertension, cardiovascular disease, and diabetes [55], and with all-cause mortality [48]. An important question is whether this hypothesis extends to twins, with twins compared to singletons having a higher risk of disease development and early mortality due to their on average lower birth weight, which would have consequences for the health care of multiples.

Twins do not only differ from singletons in birth weight. They also shared a womb, and grew up with a sibling who is exactly of the same age and often the same sex and even, depending on the zygosity, alike in physical appearance. Growing up with such a close companion may lead to differences in behavior as it may encourage or discourage certain behaviors and lifestyles through mechanisms of social interaction [18]. Twins also tend to have older parents than non-twin children, and for a range of behavioral and cognitive outcomes the children of older parents do somewhat better than children of younger fathers and mothers [102, 113].

The above inference raises the important question of whether twins are similar to singletons, both with regard to health and non-health-related traits. The answer to this question is relevant to health-care professionals but also to researchers making use of the twin design in studies to unravel the influence of genetic and environmental factors on traits of interest. The generalization of findings based on twin research rests on the assumption that twins do not differ from non-twin individuals. For example, in studies of gene-by-environment interaction, twins should not differ from singletons regarding their exposure to the environment under study. While this seems a reasonable assumption, for example in case of the death of parents, this may be different for some other life events such as divorce or having an intimate relationship with others, because twin relations may discourage such relationships [66, 67, 69]. Importantly, in addition to health-care professionals and scientists, twins themselves and their family members are interested in the question whether and how twins are different from singletons.

In this chapter, we first discuss findings from the literature with respect to twin – non-twin differences in early life, e.g., birth weight, pre- and perinatal mortality differences, and congenital problems. In the second part, we provide the results for adult twin – non-twin comparisons across a wide range of traits assessed in the Netherlands Twin Register (NTR), including a large series of biomarkers.

4.2 Congenital Disorders and Infant Mortality

When the proportion of multiple births in Europe increased from 1.9% (1984–1988) to 3.1% (2004–2008), the prevalence of congenital anomaly from multiple births also increased [15]. A multiple pregnancy carries extra risk for fetuses and neonates. Twins grow slower during the third trimester than singletons [23], experience more intrauterine growth restriction [19], and are more likely to have a low birth weight [72]. This may influence both twins but may also be limited to one of the members in a twin pair, in the case of selective fetal growth restriction [35]. Compared to singletons, multiple birth children show a substantially higher rate of overall perinatal mortality [91, 99] and stillbirth [24, 42], though some studies report lower perinatal mortality rates in preterm twin pregnancies, possibly due to increased medical surveillance in the case of a multiple pregnancy [3, 47].

In about 60% of twin pregnancies, malpresentation occurs, with one or both of the twins not optimally positioned for birth [40]. Surgical delivery and assisted interventions during vaginal delivery are common in multiple pregnancies [45, 88, 99] and multiple birth is a risk factor for low Apgar scores [97, 98]. While preterm delivery and low birth weight explain part of the higher perinatal mortality and morbidity rates in twins, the risk of adverse outcomes is still higher when comparing twins with normal birthweight to singletons of the same birthweight [112].

The second-born twin generally faces the greatest risks as obstetric complications, such as placental separation, cord prolapse, uterine atony, prolonged intertwin delivery time, and cervical spasm, may occur after delivery of the first-born twin [88] and can cause fetal distress, low Apgar scores, and neonatal morbidity [41, 75].

Prematurity and low birthweight are also associated with neurodevelopmental disorders and cerebral injury. Cerebral palsy (CP) is reported five to ten times more often in twins compared with singletons [80, 81, 89]. The risk of CP is affected by birth asphyxia that causes cerebral impairment [81] and by neonatal death or stillbirth in the co-twin [13].

There is considerable evidence that babies from multiple pregnancies have a higher risk of total congenital anomalies than singleton babies [30, 34, 73, 81], with reports of a relative risk of 1.29 for congenital anomaly in multiple births relative to singletons [14]. Hall [39] estimated that probably 10% of monozygotic twins are born with a congenital anomaly. The most common anomalies in twins and singletons for which twins have a higher risk than singletons are cardiovascular anomalies [34, 49, 60, 62, 87, 108]. Higher rates in twins are also reported for anomalies of the central nervous system, the digestive system, in particular gut atresias, the genitourinary track, and musculoskeletal systems [34, 60]. In addition, neural tube defects have been reported more often in twins [109], and the prevalence of clubfoot is twice that of the general population [110]. Twins, however, do not seem to have an excess risk of oral cleft compared to singletons [37, 110]. With respect to chromosomal abnormalities, study results differ. Some have shown lower rates of chromosomal abnormalities in twins compared to singletons [16, 25, 49, 73, 108], while others showed no differences [34, 60]. Some chromosomal anomalies and imprinting disorders are more prevalent in MZ twins with discordant presentation. For example, in Beckwith-Wiedemann syndrome the majority of affected twins have an unaffected MZ co-twin who may have only some features of the disease, and it has been suggested that a methylation failure in the twinning process is involved [11].

Several explanations have been proposed for the higher rates of congenital anomalies and malformations in twins, including disturbances in early embryonic development, especially in MZ twinning [34, 49, 63], hemodynamic instability in monozygotic placentation [79], contribution of artificial reproductive technologies and other treatments of infertility [10, 14, 34], as well as maternal age at pregnancy [76]. In the majority of the cases, congenital anomalies occur in discordant pairs where only one twin is affected [17]. The etiology is poorly understood but may involve epigenetic factors [92] as was found in a study of monozygotic twin girls who were discordant for a caudal duplication anomaly [74]. The coding region of the *AXIN1* was sequenced in both twins and while no mutation was detected, this region was significantly more methylated in the affected twin than in the unaffected twin.

Several conditions are unique to multiple pregnancies such as monochorionic-monoamniotic condition, twin-twin transfusion syndrome (TTTS), and some rare malformations such as conjoined twins, *fetus in fetu,* and acardiac malformation [56, 65]. Many congenital anomalies in twins are more common in MZ twins than in DZ twins [73] and within the MZ twins, more common in monochorionic than dichorionic twins [34]. Together with TTTS, congenital anomalies are an additional risk for mortality and adverse neurodevelopmental outcome in monochorionic twins [38, 61, 77].

A very rare condition, which may occur in MZ twins, involves the reversal of the internal organs known as *situs inversus partialis* or *totalis* [58]. Several case reports of MZ twins with *situs inversus* are reported in the literature [2, 12, 31, 50, 90]. This may be related to the phenomenon of "mirror twins," when the features appear asymmetrical in co-twins. For example, left-handedness in one twin and right-handedness in the other twin may be the expression of an anatomical mirror image at the level of the nervous system [31]. Other explanations include conjoined twinning, a late division of the embryo leading to MZ twinning, and a malrotation of the viscera during early embryonic life [31, 58].

In conclusion, a multiple pregnancy increases the risk of congenital problems and mortality of the unborn and newborn. Still, the majority of twins are born healthy in countries with good health-care systems and develop normally. This however, does not exclude the possibility that twins differ from singletons in more subtle ways. In the next part, we therefore explore possible differences between twins and their singleton siblings.

4.3 Adult Twin-Sibling Comparisons Across a Wide Variety of Traits

4.3.1 Background and Procedure

While a twin pregnancy carries, as described above, a number of risks, the majority of twins are born healthy. One important question is whether such twins differ from singletons in their development and health at later age. To provide insight into the potential differences between multiples and singletons, it is essential to choose the correct reference group to which to compare the multiples. By selecting a group of singletons from the general population, this may introduce a bias as this population would also include individuals from one-child families, confounding the effects of being born after a singleton pregnancy with those of having no siblings. Even when choosing singletons from families with more than one child, this does not correct for potential differences across twin and non-twin families, such as parental behaviors or parental genotypes. Hence, differences observed at the population level between twins and non-twins in so-called between-family comparisons should be interpreted carefully. Differences may reflect true effects, but they may also be confounded by between-family differences in, e.g., family structure, urban-rural residency, and multiple other factors, including the maternal genotype, which is known to be associated with DZ twinning [64].

One way of eliminating these problems is by comparing twins to their own singleton siblings. This design optimally matches controls (siblings) and cases (twins), as twins and siblings come from the same family, and largely share their genetic background and family environment [20]. Within-family designs are becoming common in molecular genetics, where it is recognized that gene-outcome associations found among unrelated individuals may reflect between-family variation in genetic and environmental factors. A within-family comparison reduces confounding by these factors but does require statistical approaches that take into account the dependencies in the data such as paired-sample tests. Alternatively, differences due to genetic and environmental factors can be assessed in genetic structural equation models that simultaneously model the mean and the covariance structure in the data [83]. This approach is often taken in behavioral genetic studies, when the aim of the study is to estimate genetic and non-genetic contribution to the observed variance in a trait of interest. These studies, however, do not always report the outcomes of twin-sibling comparisons and sometimes assume that twins are similar to non-twin siblings.

In the following, we employed the within-family design in an adult sample from the Netherlands Twin Register. The Netherlands Twin Register (NTR) is one of the larger twin registers and also includes family members of twins, collecting data on twins as well as siblings, parents, spouses, and offspring. The NTR conducts longitudinal survey and experimental studies with the help of registered twins and their family members. Information on young twins is obtained from parents and teacher reports, while adolescent and adult twins and their registered family members provide the data themselves [123]. Here, we compare adult twin individuals to their singleton siblings for a wide range of variables collected in survey and biobanking studies. To this aim, we selected at random one twin and a sibling from the same family, with the sibling of the same sex as the twin. We also selected only those siblings of twins who did not differ more than 6 years in age from the twin.

For more detailed information on the methodology, please see the Appendix. The focus of most previous NTR studies has been on the quantification of genetic and non-genetic influences for a wide domain of traits, and while siblings were often included in the study design, relatively few studies reported the outcomes of twin-sibling comparisons. We identified the NTR studies that explicitly tested and reported the outcomes of twin-sibling comparisons and added these results to our discussion of twin-sibling differences in traits from various domains.

4.3.2 The Outcomes of Twin-Sibling Comparisons Across Multiple Domains in the NTR

◘ Tables 4.1 and ◘ 4.2 summarize the findings for the twin-sibling comparisons for survey and biobank data, respectively.

▪ Body Composition and Physical Development

Our findings for body composition as presented in ◘ Tables 4.1 and ◘ 4.2 show that adult twins differed significantly from their singleton siblings in height and body mass index, with twins being somewhat smaller and lighter than their non-twin brothers and sisters. This was seen when data were obtained in the survey and a trend was also present for the data collected during the home visit, when weight was measured. In line with the trend for lower body mass index, twins also tended to have a smaller waist circumference at the time of the home visit.

Our results are in line with another large study in childhood and adolescence in the NTR, where twins were shown to be shorter and have a lower BMI than their siblings [28]. In a subset of this sample, they found the expected the twin-sibling difference in birth length and birth weight, with the effect still present at the age of 1 year but found no evidence for twin-sibling difference for height, weight, and BMI at age 4. For this sample, no significant twin-sibling differences in body composition were seen at the young adult age, though there was a trend for twins to have a somewhat lower weight and shorter leg length. Additional components of physical development have also been examined. While differences in growth hormone levels were seen, with average lower levels of DHEAS and IGF-I levels in twins compared to their siblings [26], male twins did not differ from their siblings in testis size [29] and female twins did not differ for age at menarche [8].

These results and those of previous studies indicate that twins, who are more often born after a shorter gestation period and weigh less at birth than their singleton siblings, remain somewhat shorter and lighter well into adulthood, but in other aspects develop in the same way as their siblings.

▪ Personality and Psychopathology

◘ Table 4.1 presents the data for our matched twin-sibling comparison for five personality traits. Few differences are apparent, with only a trend for a personality trait called "openness to experience," where twin seems to score somewhat lower than the siblings. For sensation-seeking traits, twins and siblings are similar, and twins also did not differ from siblings in their perception of support, life satisfaction, or loneliness. Several NTR studies previously tested and reported on adult twin-sibling differences in personality, in large samples that did not employ within-family designs, and reported no twin-singleton differences for the traits studied, which included sensation seeking [95], neuroticism [106] life satisfaction [96] or trait anger (Distel et al. [21].

With respect to psychopathology, ◘ Table 4.1 shows twins did not differ from their siblings in ADHD symptoms in adults. They also did not differ in borderline personality total scores, confirming previous findings in an overlapping sample [21], nor for anxious depression. Depression, anxiety, and a combined anxious depression score were the subject of several previous studies in large samples of adult twins and singleton siblings, but no matter the definition, the two groups did not differ [66, 68, 93]. Adult twins and singleton siblings were also similar in the prevalence of burnout

Table 4.1 Outcomes of within-family twin-sibling comparisons for body size, personality, mental health, demographics, and lifestyle data collected in adult participants (survey 8) from the Netherlands Twin Register. Twins and siblings from the same family were selected to be of the same sex and of similar ages (not more than 6 years apart in age)

	Pairs	Twin		Sibling		Twin-sibling comparison results	
	N	Mean	SD	Mean	SD	T-test value	P-value
Continuous traits							
Age (years)	685	30.41	12.86	32.14	12.20	−15.347	0.000
Height (cm)	655	173.73	8.93	174.40	8.50	−2.480	0.013
Body mass index (BMI, kg/m^2)	634	22.73	3.12	23.89	3.82	−7.365	0.000
NEO neuroticism	613	29.38	7.60	29.90	7.29	−1.400	0.162
NEO extraversion	613	42.97	5.94	42.50	6.00	1.510	0.132
NEO openness to experience	613	36.59	5.78	37.37	5.82	−2.734	0.006
NEO agreeableness	613	45.54	4.97	45.01	4.84	2.206	0.028
NEO conscientiousness	613	44.76	5.78	45.04	5.54	−0.948	0.344
SSS total sensation seeking	411	11.22	2.41	11.13	2.45	0.711	0.478
SSS thrill adventure seeking	605	9.16	3.65	8.83	3.69	1.942	0.053
SSS experience seeking	418	16.00	4.46	16.33	4.58	−1.205	0.229
SSS boredom susceptibility	593	18.22	4.79	18.30	4.82	−0.303	0.762
SSS disinhibition	593	13.45	3.70	13.18	3.52	1.566	0.118
UNC-FSSQ confidant support	561	23.28	2.81	22.98	3.06	1.782	0.075
UNC-FSSQ affective support	559	13.81	1.97	13.72	1.99	0.745	0.457
SWLS general satisfaction with life	649	27.67	4.91	27.34	5.17	1.299	0.194
TILS loneliness	633	3.90	1.20	3.96	1.26	−0.920	0.358
CAARS ADHD index	599	8.11	4.12	8.44	3.93	−1.554	0.121
PAI-BOR total borderline personality	603	15.16	8.37	15.92	8.22	−1.775	0.076
PAI-BOR affect instability	603	4.40	3.00	4.59	3.00	−1.225	0.221
PAI-BOR identity problems	603	3.82	2.72	4.05	2.90	−1.562	0.119
PAI-BOR negative relationships	602	4.14	2.85	4.62	2.75	−3.244	0.001
PAI-BOR self-harm	602	2.81	2.40	2.65	2.31	1.242	0.215
ASR anxious-depressed scale	526	4.93	5.15	5.29	5.46	−1.183	0.237

(continued)

Table 4.1 (continued)

		Twin		Sibling		Test statistics	
Dichotomous traits	*N*	**N yes**	**% yes**	**N yes**	**% yes**	**Chi-square**	**p-value**
Being in good subjective health	657	590	89.8	575	87.5	1.675	0.196
Ever been in contact with mental health services	532	128	24.1	160	30.1	5.339	0.021
Regular sport participation	634	415	65.5	399	62.9	0.945	0.331
Regular alcohol use (2 or more times per week)	618	233	37.7	248	40.1	0.912	0.340
Current smoker	613	217	35.4	203	33.1	0.929	0.335
Ever tried hash	591	167	28.3	178	30.1	0.578	0.447
Being in a steady relationship, when 30 years or older	312	275	88.1	280	89.7	0.271	0.603
Living together with partner, when 30 years or older	312	258	82.7	268	85.9	1.095	0.295

Abbreviations: *NEO* NEO Five-Factor Inventory, *SSS* Sensation Seeking Scale, *UNC-FSSQ* Duke-UNC Functional Social Support Questionnaire, *SWLS* Satisfaction With Life Scale, *TILS* Three-Item *Loneliness Scale*, *CAARS* Conners' Adult ADHD Rating Scales, *PAI-BOR* Personality Assessment Inventory-Borderline Features scale, *ASR* Adult Self-Report

[68, 69]. Earlier NTR studies did not show evidence for differences between twins and siblings for obsessive-compulsive symptoms in adults [36] nor, in sample of young adults, for autistic traits [43]. A comparison of younger twins and siblings with respect to psychopathology showed no differences in ADHD symptoms between adolescent twins and singleton siblings [84]. Table 4.1 also shows twins and singleton siblings were similar in their reports of being in good health and in ever having been in contact with mental health services.

Considering the overall picture of these findings, twins do not seem to differ from their siblings in personality and psychopathology. Any differences found were very small.

Behavioral and Sociodemographic Traits

Table 4.1 also presents the results of the twin-sibling comparison for various health behaviors, which show twins to be similar to their singleton siblings in their reports of regularly sport participation, regular alcohol drinking, current smoking behavior, and ever having tried hash. This is in line with NTR studies, in which the prevalence of problem drinking [71] and cannabis use initiation [22] was similar in twins and their siblings. Likewise, previous NTR studies which examined aspects of childhood behavior have not found differences between twins and siblings for bullying and victimization in 9-year-old twins and siblings [101] and for truancy during secondary education [1].

With respect to sociodemographic traits, Table 4.1 indicates there are no differences between twins and siblings for being in a relationship, and for living together with a partner. As age may play a role, we limited our comparison for relationship status to those aged 30 or older. A previous study by [67] showed that at the age of 27 years MZ female twins were less often in a relationship than siblings. NTR studies on other sociodemographic traits did not find any twin-sibling differences for employment status [68] and

Table 4.2 Within-family twin-sibling comparison for biomarkers as assessed in the Netherlands Twin register. Twins and siblings from the same family were selected to be of the same sex and of similar ages (not more than 6 years apart in age)

	Pairs	Twin		Sibling		Correlation of trait difference with		Twin-sibling comparison results using standardized scores[a]	
	N	Mean	SD	Mean	SD	Difference in age	Difference in BMI	T-test value	P-value
Age (years)	382	36.30	12.28	37.37	11.98	1.00	0.084	−6.586	0.000
Height (cm)	378	174.37	9.02	175.58	9.13	−0.041	−0.089	−3.855	0.000
Body mass index (BMI)	374	24.37	4.05	25.29	4.37	0.084	1.00	−3.399	0.001
Waist circumference (cm)	373	83.30	11.26	85.72	12.23	0.062	0.809***	−3.153	0.002
Fasting total cholesterol (mmol/l)	323	4.85	1.02	4.94	0.94	0.103	0.074	−0.911	0.363
Fasting HDL (mmol/l)	323	1.40	0.35	1.41	0.37	0.053	−0.258***	−2.118	0.035
Fasting LDL (mmol/l)	323	2.93	0.92	2.95	0.84	0.089	0.096	−0.223	0.824
Triglycerides (mmol/l)	323	1.16	0.57	1.27	0.63	0.033	0.277***	−1.450	0.148
Fasting glucose (mmol/l)	321	5.30	0.73	5.41	0.88	−0.000	0.266***	−1.140	0.255
Fasting insulin (μIU/ml	315	8.41	4.83	9.82	7.94	0.055	0.392***	−1.539	0.125
Hba1c (%)	318	5.26	0.51	5.33	0.64	0.116	0.051	−1.388	0.166
White blood cell count (10^{12}/L)	346	6.33	1.72	6.58	1.94	0.020	0.165**	−1.690	0.092
Red blood cell count (10^{12}/L)	347	4.68	0.48	4.66	0.46	0.022	0.164**	1.470	0.143
C-reactive protein (mg/L)	353	2.69	4.18	3.47	5.00	0.030	0.299***	−1.726	0.085
Interleukin 6 (pg/mL)	347	1.42	1.27	1.97	5.24	0.093	0.043	−1.758	0.080
AST (U/L)	293	20.83	6.92	20.68	7.22	0.075	0.113	0.701	0.484
ALT (U/L)	275	10.93	7.39	11.02	9.19	0.085	0.072	0.314	0.754
GGT (U/L)	293	28.03	24.47	29.87	24.00	0.081	0.184***	−0.399	0.690
Creatinine (U/L)	293	85.52	13.95	85.28	14.26	−0.058	0.046	0.420	0.674
Telomere length	289	2.78	0.69	2.66	0.49	−0.209***	−0.045	3.491	0.001

Abbreviations: *ALT* alanine aminotransferase, *AST* aspartate aminotransferase, *GGT* gamma-glutamyltransferase
*<0.05, **<0.01, ***<0.001
[a]Age and sex standardized scores were used in the paired sample t-tests for height, BMI, and waist circumference. For all other variables, age, sex, and BMI standardized scores were used

the prevalence of being in a creative profession [100]. However, compared to their singleton siblings, twins more often lived in highly urbanized areas in two younger age cohorts, though no difference was seen for the oldest age cohort [107]. It is possible that in the younger cohorts the age difference between twins and siblings was of importance, as the on average older sibling may already have had the financial means or the motive of an own increasing family to move to less populated areas.

Overall, twin status does not affect choices related to health behavior and most other behaviors, though particular aspects of social behavior such as being in a relationship and residential choices deserve more attention to provide definite answers.

▪ Biomarkers and Disease

The results for our twin-sibling comparisons for biomarkers can be seen in ◘ Table 4.2. For total cholesterol, HDL cholesterol, LDL cholesterol, and triglyceride levels, there were no significant differences between twins and siblings. With respect to glucose metabolism, looking at the data the pattern seems to suggest a trend for siblings to have higher values, in particular for insulin. However, differences in BMI between twins and siblings are strongly related to differences in glucose metabolism parameters and when comparing scores after the effects of BMI are taken into account, twins and siblings were similar in glucose metabolism. We further compared twins and siblings on C-reactive protein (CRP), white and red blood cell count, and IL6 level and found no significant differences for any of these variables. This is in line with a previous small-scale study including 222 twins and 85 siblings in which no differences between twins and siblings were observed for the cytokine response to ex vivo amyloid-beta stimulation [86]. ◘ Table 4.2 also summarizes the twin-sibling data for liver enzymes and creatinine, which were similar for the two groups. This extends the findings by van Beek et al. [5], who in a larger sample that included this subset, also reported no differences in the liver enzymes aspartate aminotransferase (AST) and alanine aminotransferase (ALT) but did not comment on gamma-glutamyl transferase (GGT).

While the majority of our comparisons did not reveal any twin-sibling differences, there was a trend for twin and siblings to differ in telomere length, with shorter telomere length in the siblings compared to the twins, even when correcting for age effects using standardized scores. Further studies would be needed to determine whether this represents a meaningful twin-sibling difference.

A series of previous NTR studies focused on cardiovascular functioning in adult twins and their siblings. No differences were seen for blood pressure, whether measured in a laboratory setting [46], ambulatory during everyday life [53], or defined as hypertensive state [32]. For cardiac functioning, operationalized as heart rate or heart rate variability, again no significant differences between twins and their siblings were found [52, 54]. Twin-sibling differences were also not present for respiration rate [52] or cortisol [51].

With respect to other physical diseases, NTR studies in adult women showed twins did not differ from their singleton siblings in the occurrence of polycystic ovary syndrome based on survey information [104], nor in the presence of cervix smear abnormalities as determined by cervical screening [103]. Twin-sibling differences were also not reported for asthma in a study including more than 11,000 adult male and female twins and siblings, but surprisingly siblings reported somewhat higher rates of allergy than twins (23.3% vs. 18.2%, [105]).

In summary, these studies show that, while there may be a few exceptions pointing to a disadvantage in singletons, twins and their singleton siblings are generally very similar in biomarkers and disease.

▪ Cognitive Function

We did not apply a within-family test for cognitive function in this study, but here we summarize the results from previous NTR studies. A number of studies in young twins have shown differences in cognitive abilities. In samples of twins and siblings with average age between 9 and 13, twins scored lower on full scale, verbal and performance IQ [94] and on IQ, reading performance, and verbal working memory [59]. De Zeeuw et al. [111] tested cognitive function in the largest sample yet, including 1375 twins and 1375 siblings and again showed lower scores for specific aspects of cognitive function (IQ, reading performance, and verbal working memory) at age 9 in twins compared to their siblings. However, twins are often not the first-born children in a family. After taking birth order into account, the cognitive disadvantage of twins dissipated. Lower scores for cognitive function were only seen when comparing the twins to older siblings. When comparing the scores of twins at age 9 with the scores of their younger siblings at age 9, twins no longer differed from their singleton siblings. Twins did not differ from older or younger siblings with respect to for visuospatial working memory, verbal, and spatial short-term memory. Interestingly, twins scored higher on physical education than their older and younger singleton siblings [111]. Note that not all studies on cognition in young twins showed lower scores in twins compared to their singleton siblings. A recent study including more than 11,000 twins and 262 of their siblings at age 7.5 showed that reading ability in twins was comparable to that in siblings and to national norms [7]. Two smaller NTR studies provided information on the twin-sibling comparison for adult cognitive function: Van den Berg et al. [9] found no twin-sibling differences for reading vocabulary, and Posthuma et al. [85] showed no difference in intelligence between twins and siblings.

Overall, while lower scores for cognitive ability in twins have been reported, these effects seem related to the position (birth order) in the nuclear family. Those first born in the family more often score higher on cognitive tests than those later born, an effect which is independent of whether they are born from a singleton or multiple pregnancy. As not all studies in children showed lower scores across the cognitive domains and studies in adults did not show any twin-singleton differences, a twin-singleton difference for cognitive function seems modest and likely limited to specific domains.

4.4 Concluding Remarks

A twin or multiple pregnancy carries an increased risk of prenatal mortality and congenital abnormalities. However, the majority of children born from a multiple pregnancy are healthy at birth and develop into healthy individuals. Still, multiples could differ from singletons in other ways, due to their lower gestational age and birthweight or due to growing up with a sibling of the same age and often same sex and looks, i.e., the close companionship hypothesis. Our studies indicate that twins do not differ from their singleton siblings across a wide range of behavioral and lifestyle parameters, biomarkers, or diseases.

The one aspect on which twins differed from non-twins was body composition. Twins remained smaller and lighter compared to their singleton siblings, even as adults, attaining about 1 point lower BMI lower than singletons. As very few physiological differences were seen, the difference in body composition seems to be a lasting and likely beneficial aspect of being a twin.

Very little evidence was found for the close companionship hypothesis: twins did not differ from their singleton siblings across a wide range of behavioral and psychological traits. Twins did do better than singletons in physical education classes at school, which could indicate the effect of always having a playmate during childhood. In adults, no differences in regular sport participation are seen, suggesting that the effect, if confirmed, may only be present at younger ages. We did not test for effects of zygosity and we cannot exclude the possibility that specific twin effects may still occur for specific groups, especially monozygotic twins, as implied by the finding of [70] that MZ female twins were less often in a relationship than others. However, as our study included a large number of monozygotic twins the effects are likely to be small and limited to specific situations and groups.

We did not investigate effects of fertility treatment. Many of the studies presented here were conducted in twins who were born before ART and IVF became frequently used in the Netherlands, but it may have occurred in the younger twins participating in the studies. Still, many of these twins will not have had a sibling, as fertility problems occurred in these families, and the number of IVF twin-sibling pairs will thus be very limited. A previous study by the NTR matching IVF with DZ naturally conceived twins showed no differences in growth, attainment of motor milestones, or in behavioral development, leading to the conclusion that for nearly all aspects, development in these groups of children is similar [6].

While twins and siblings born in the same family do not differ, it is still possible that individuals born in twin families differ from singletons born within non-twin families due to the genetic background of their parents. This may be especially so in DZ twin families, as we know that mothers of DZ twins are somewhat taller and heavier than mothers of monozygotic twins [44], and genes found to be related to twinning are also related to increased body mass [64]. In a study of 5-year-old Dutch twin children, female twins were as tall as singleton children, while male twins were still somewhat shorter than children from the general population and twins overall had a lower BMI than the general population [27]. In a separate study, Estougie et al. [28] reported no differences in height between young adult twins and their siblings and their height was comparable to the general population. For BMI, no differences were observed between 18-year-old twins and 18-year-olds from the general population, whereas the siblings of twins had increased BMI values. A Finnish study among 17-year-old twins reported that twins were as tall as singletons, but that boy twins were still leaner, though an American twin study showed no twin effects on weight and height at age 8 [78]. It is possible that, when it comes to body weight and body height, twins on average reach their full potential at a later age than singletons. Alternatively, twins may never reach their full potential for height and weight. As a large number of the genetic variants involved in body composition are now known, this hypothesis could be tested in the near future. Other factors may also differ within families for twins and non-twins. Maternal age at birth and parity are higher on average for DZ twins, and twins differ from singletons in gestational age. Also, the rearing environment is different for two children than for a single child, though this is not specifically limited to multiples but is the case for any family including multiple children.

Another aspect that may deserve additional attention is the position of multiples in the family. For a number of cognitive traits, the differences between twins and siblings could be explained by position within the family. This has not been systematically studied for other traits, which may reveal similar position-in-family effects. In addition to the position in the family, whether twins were born first or second, also requires more attention. In this study, there was an equal distribution of twins born first and second by design. As birth complications more often occur for the second born twin, this may be another factor leading to small differences between twins and singletons.

Our results regarding a large number of traits and common disorders are fairly optimistic, indicating that twins do not differ from singletons. By comparing the twins to their non-twin siblings, we avoid confounding by between-family factors. We note, however, that our work did not look at rare disorders and that despite the large number of participants in the Netherlands Twin Register some forms of bias may be present. Parents of twins who presented with serious complications at birth may decide against participation. Adolescent and adult twins with health problems, whether mental or physical, may be less inclined to enroll in the longitudinal study or may drop out during the study. In addition, the decision to enroll and continue participation is also influenced by other factors such as educational attainment. Still, twins are born in all strata of society and tend to be motivated to take part in medical and scientific studies and, though we have seen that NTR participation is related to educational attainment, participants with lower educational levels are also present in the sample.

In conclusion, with the exception of congenital disorders and body composition, twins do not seem to differ from singletons, when taking family factors into account. While being a twin can be seen as special, for most traits twins are just like ordinary siblings.

4.5 Quotes by Twins

In the ninth NTR survey to adult participants [123], twins were asked whether they liked being a twins. The following quotes are a selection from answers provided by more than 5000 multiples. Their comments are in line with the findings in our chapter.

They highlight that a multiple pregnancy carries risk:

- "I did not grow up as twins. Twin sister died at birth."

Many of the multiples view their multiple status as something special, though not everyone responds positively.

- "I like it as long as people see us as separate individuals. It is in any case not ordinary and I do like that."
- "Sad for all those singletons…honestly."
- "Quite nice. I have different (closer) contact with my twin brother than with my other brothers."
- "Quite nice; as twin you are never alone."
- "Being a twin has two sides. A very nice side because we got along very well as sisters and because being a twin is also somewhat special. The disadvantage of being a twin is that I have the feeling I am constantly compared to my twin sister and that I do this also."
- "Still somewhat special. We do have another connection with each other than with my other brothers (4)."
- "Super great! I feel that there is someone who always has my back and who understand me. I think this is because we are also friends."
- "In general it is nice, because we understand each other very well and are strongly connected. But sometimes it is also a bit suffocating since you were and are always compared to each other and we also compare ourselves and never want to do under for the other."
- "Nice. You have a special connection with each other which you do not have with brother or sister. A bit difficult to learn to make friends and keep them, because I always had my sister and never had to do this."

However, comments also indicate that the multiples do not see much difference with ordinary brothers and sisters, especially not as adults.

- "We are a dizygotic twin pair, so I do not see it as very special. I do not connect more with him than with my other brothers."
- "We have a very different life. I view him just like my other brother."
- "It's OK. Not very special. The connection with my younger sister is no less, my younger sister and my twin sister are just as important for me. The one is not more important than the other. Sometimes it is nice to be a twin, sometimes less nice. It has (in the past) advantages and disadvantages."
- "Quite nice, not very special."
- "Quite nice but not as special as people often expect."
- "It is nice that you can race to see who finishes his study first, but noting more."
- "It is somewhat more special than other brothers/sisters, but for the rest not much difference."
- "In the past special to do everything together, now I do not notice much. It is just like an ordinary brother."
- "In the past very nice, now it just seems as if we are normal sisters."
- "OK. In the past I did a lot together with my twin brothers Now it is just like with my other brother or sister."
- "Normal. No differences with people who are not a twin."
- "Not different than having my other 2 brothers."

4

4.6 Review Questions

Open Questions:

1. Question: How would two major hypotheses explain differences between twins and singletons?

Answer: A somatic and a social hypothesis. First, twins are born earlier and have smaller body size at birth. This may be associated with a range of later outcomes. Second, growing up with a close companion since birth and mechanisms of social interaction may lead to differences in behavioral outcomes between twins and non-twins.

2. Question: What type of design optimizes testing for differences between twins and non-twins?

Answer: A so-called within-family design in which outcomes in twins are compared to outcomes in their non-twin siblings.

3. Question: What is the empirical evidence for twin non-twin differences (as a function of developmental stage)?

Answer: Multiples have an increased risk of congenital problems but with exception of being lighter and having a lower body mass index; there are few differences between adult twins and singletons.

4.6.1 Multiple-Choice Questions

1. For which class of diseases/disorders do we observe prominent differences between twins and non-twins?
   (a) Psychiatric diseases
   (b) Congenital anomalies
   (c) Cardiovascular disease
   (d) Neoplasia

Answer: (b)

2. What is the average pregnancy duration for twins?
   (a) 32 weeks
   (b) 35 weeks
   (c) 37 weeks
   (d) 40 weeks

Answer: (c)

3. Which of the following is true about multiple pregnancy in comparison to singleton pregnancy?
   (a) Shorter gestational age
   (b) More intrauterine growth restriction and lower weight at birth
   (c) Higher risk of complications during pregnancy and malpresentation at birth
   (d) All the above

Answer: (d)

4. Which disorders are more prevalent in MZ twins in comparison to singletons and DZ twins?
   (a) Down syndrome
   (b) Beckwith-Wiedemann syndrome
   (c) Cri du chat syndrome
   (d) Huntington's disease

Answer: (b)

5. In adulthood, what is the domain in which some twin-singleton differences are found?
   (a) Body composition and physical development
   (b) Personality and psychopathology
   (c) Cognitive function
   (d) Behavioral and sociodemographic traits
   (e) Physiological parameters and physical disease

Answer: (a)

4.7 Appendix: Within-Family Twin – Non-Twin Comparisons Across a Wide Range of Traits Assessed in the Netherlands Twin Register

4.7.1 Participants and Selection Procedure

To compare twins to their siblings, we made use of the data from two separate projects: (1) the eighth NTR survey on health, lifestyle and personality, which was sent out to adult participants between 2004 and 2009 [120, 123]; (2) a large-scale blood collection project carried out between 2004 and 2009 in which participants were visited at home to obtain blood samples and health information [125].

For each of the two datasets, we followed the same procedure. We first selected all twins and their singleton siblings with known age, sex, birth year, and, in the case of twins, zygosity. Known half-siblings and non-biological siblings were excluded. Next, we randomly selected one of the twins in case a twin pair both participated and assessed whether there was a same-sex singleton sibling in the family who was born within 6 years from the twin. This sibling was then selected, if at the time of participating he or she was within 6 years of the age of the twin. In the case multiple singleton siblings of a twin met the criteria, we selected the same-sex sibling closest in birth year. We made two exceptions to this procedure. In the case of an opposite-sex twin pair, when a male twin-sibling pair could be formed in the dataset, we selected the male pair. This was done to maximize the presence of male pairs in the analyses as fewer males participated than females. When both older and younger siblings within the 6-year time frame were present, preference was given to the sibling younger than the twin, as twins more often have older siblings than younger siblings. Even applying these criteria, our sample selections included more female pairs than male pairs and more older than younger singleton siblings.

4.7.2 NTR Survey 8

As part of a longitudinal survey study, this survey was sent out to adult twins registered with the NTR. It was completed by 10,176 multiples and 2,142 siblings and collected information on a wide range of traits [120]. After applying the selection criteria, the sample for the present analyses consisted of 685 twin-sibling pairs, 177 (26%) being male. Average age (sd) of the twins at the time of survey completion was 30.4 (12.9) and of the siblings 32.1 (12.2) years. In 142 (21%) of the pairs, the twin was older than the sibling. We compared the twins and their singleton siblings on the following continuous traits: self-reported height and body mass index (BMI, calculated as $\text{weight}_{(kg)}/\text{height}^2_{(m)}$); the big five personality dimensions (openness, conscientiousness, extraversion, agreeableness, neuroticism) as measured with the NEO Five-Factor Inventory [117, 121]; borderline personality components measured with the Personality Assessment Inventory-Borderline Features scale (PAI-BOR; [124]); sensation seeking score and its subscales thrill and adventure seeking, boredom susceptibility, disinhibition and experience seeking as measured with the Sensation Seeking Scale [119, 126]; attention deficit hyperactivity disorder (ADHD) as measured with the Conners' Adult ADHD Rating Scales (CAARS; [116]); the anxious depression scale of the Adult Self-Report which combines elements of depression and anxiety [114]; dimensions of social support (confidant and affective) as measured with the Duke-UNC Functional Social Support Questionnaire; and life satisfaction as measured with the Satisfaction With Life Scale [118]; loneliness as measured with the Three-Item Loneliness Scale [122]. In addition, we compared twins and siblings on categorical traits with outcomes operationalized as yes versus no, including the following traits: being in good health (reports of good or excellent health were coded as yes), ever been in contact with mental health services, being a current smoker, drinking alcohol regularly (reports of drinking alcohol 2 or more times per week were classified as yes), ever tried hash, being in a relationship (data only included for those age 30 years and older), and living together with a partner (data only included for those aged 30 years and older).

4.7.3 NTR Biobank

Between 2004 and 2010, 9530 individuals provided a blood sample and health-related information as part of a large-scale biobank project [125]. When conducting the selection procedure as described above, this resulted in 382 twin-sibling pairs, of which 144 (38%) were male-male pairs. The average age of the twins was 36.3 (12.3) and of the siblings 37.4 (12.0). In 265 pairs, the singleton sibling was older than the twin. We compared twins and their singleton siblings on the following variables: lipid profile (total cholesterol, HDL, LDL, and triglyceride levels), glucose metabolism (glucose, insulin, and HbA1c levels), white and red blood cell counts, C-reactive protein as indicator of general inflammation, liver enzymes alanine transaminase (ALT), aspartate transaminase (AST), and gamma-glutamyltransferase (GGT), creatinine as measure of kidney function and telomere length. For lipid profile and glucose metabolism, data were only included if the participant had kept to the instruction to be fasting at the time of blood collection (see [125]).

4.7.4 Analyses

All analyses were conducted in IBM SPSS Statistics version 25. To compare the twins with their singleton sibling, we conducted a paired-sample t-test for continuous traits and a McNemar chi-squared test for categorical traits. As age and BMI may be important factors in the physiological parameters, we here correlated the differences in age and BMI for the twins and siblings with their differences in physiological parameters and present the test outcomes for age, sex, and BMI standardized residuals. Considering the large number of comparisons conducted, we consider a trend when p-values are between 0.010 and 0.001 and p-values <0.001 as significant.

References

1. van der Aa N, Rebollo-Mesa I, Willemsen G, Boomsma DI, Bartels M. Frequency of truancy at high school: evidence for genetic and twin specific shared environmental influences. J Adolesc Health. 2009;45(6):579–86.
2. Agirbasli M, Hamid R, Jennings HS 3rd, Tiller GE. Situs inversus with hypertrophic cardiomyopathy in identical twins. Am J Med Genet. 2000;91(5):327–30.
3. Alexander GR, Slay Wingate M, Salihu H, Kirby RS. Fetal and neonatal mortality risks of multiple births. Obstet Gynecol Clin N Am. 2005;32(1):1–16. vii
4. Barker DJ, Barker DJ. In utero programming of chronic disease. Clin Sci. 1998;2:115–28.
5. van Beek JH, de Moor MH, de Geus EJ, Lubke GH, Vink JM, Willemsen G, Boomsma DI. The genetic architecture of liver enzyme levels: GGT, ALT and AST. Behav Genet. 2013;43(4):329–39.
6. van Beijsterveldt CE, Bartels M, Boomsma DI. Comparison of naturally conceived and IVF-DZ twins in the Netherlands twin registry: a developmental study. J Pregnancy. 2011;2011:517614.
7. van Bergen E, Snowling MJ, de Zeeuw EL, van Beijsterveldt CEM, Dolan CV, Boomsma DI. Why do children read more? The influence of reading ability on voluntary reading practices. J Child Psychol Psychiatry. 2018;59(11):1205–14.
8. van den Berg SM, Boomsma DI. The familial clustering of age at menarche in extended twin families. Behav Genet. 2007;37(5):661–7.
9. van den Berg SM, Posthuma D, Boomsma DI. A longitudinal genetic study of vocabulary knowledge in adults. Twin Res. 2004;7(3):284–91.
10. Bergh T, Ericson A, Hillensjö T, Nygren KG, Wennerholm UB. Deliveries and children born after in-vitro fertilisation in Sweden 1982-95: a retrospective cohort study. Lancet. 1999;354(9190):1579–85.
11. Bliek J, Alders M, Maas SM, Oostra RJ, Mackay DM, van der Lip K, Callaway JL, Brooks A, van't Padje S, Westerveld A, Leschot NJ, Mannens MM. Lessons from BWS twins: complex maternal and paternal hypomethylation and a common source of haematopoietic stem cells. Eur J Hum Genet. 2009;17(12):1625–34.
12. Bondavalli W, Bondavalli G, La Bella G, Nizzoli A. Un caso di destrocardia con Situs Viscerum Inversus Totalis concordante in coppie di gemelle DZ. Acta Genet Med Gemellol. 1959;8:201–14.

13. Bonellie SR, Currie D, Chalmers J. Comparison of risk factors for cerebral palsy in twins and singletons. Dev Med Child Neurol. 2005;47(9):587–91.
14. Boyle BB, Helen D, McConkey R. The epidemiology of congenital anomalies in multiple births: a European registry based study. Pediatr Res. 2011;70(5):408.
15. Boyle B, McConkey R, Garne E, Loane M, Addor MC, Bakker MK, Boyd PA, Gatt M, Greenlees R, Haeusler M, Klungsøyr K, Latos-Bielenska A, Lelong N, McDonnell R, Métneki J, Mullaney C, Nelen V, O'Mahony M, Pierini A, Rankin J, Rissmann A, Tucker D, Wellesley D, Dolk H. Trends in the prevalence, risk and pregnancy outcome of multiple births with congenital anomaly: a registry-based study in 14 European countries 1984–2007. BJOG. 2013;120(6):707–16.
16. Boyle B, Morris JK, McConkey R, Garne E, Loane M, Addor MC, Gatt M, Haeusler M, Latos-Bielenska A, Lelong N, McDonnell R, Mullaney C, O'Mahony M, Dolk H. Prevalence and risk of Down syndrome in monozygotic and dizygotic multiple pregnancies in Europe: implications for prenatal screening. BJOG. 2014;121(7):809–20.
17. Bryan E, Little J, Burn J. Congenital anomalies in twins. Baillieres Clin Obstet Gynaecol. 1987;1(3):697–721.
18. Carey G. Twin imitation for antisocial behavior: implications for genetic and family environment research. J Abnorm Psychol. 1992;101:18–25.
19. Cunningham FG. Fetal-growth disorders. In: Williams obstetrics. 22nd ed. New York: McGraw Hill; 2001. p. 893–910. Available at: https://accessmedicine.mhmedical.com/content.aspx?bookid=1918&sectionid=171807435 (Accessed: 28 November 2019).
20. Dick DM, Johnson JK, Viken RJ, Rose RJ. Testing between-family associations in within-family comparisons. Psychol Sci. 2000;11(5):409–13.
21. Distel MA, Roeling MP, Tielbeek JJ, van Toor D, Derom CA, Trull TJ, Boomsma DI. The covariation of trait anger and borderline personality: a bivariate twin-siblings study. J Abnorm Psychol. 2012;121(2):458–66.
22. Distel MA, Vink JM, Bartels M, van Beijsterveldt CE, Neale MC, Boomsma DI. Age moderates non-genetic influences on the initiation of cannabis use: a twin-sibling study in Dutch adolescents and young adults. Addiction. 2011;106(9):1658–66.
23. Doom EC, Delbaere I, Martens G, Temmerman M. Birth weight for gestational age among Flemish twin population. Facts Views Vis Obgyn. 2012;4(1):42–9.
24. Doyle P. The outcome of multiple pregnancy. Hum Reprod. 1996;11(Suppl 4):110–20.
25. Doyle PE, et al. Congenital malformations in twins in England and Wales. J Epidemiol Community Health. BMJ Publishing Group Ltd. 1990;45(1):43–8. https://doi.org/10.1136/jech.45.1.43.
26. Estourgie-van Burk GF, Bartels M, Boomsma DI. A twin-sibling study on early growth and hormone levels in adolescents. Behav Genet. 2015;45(3):283–93.
27. Estourgie-van Burk GF, Bartels M, van Beijsterveldt TC, Delemarre-van de Waal HA, Boomsma DI. Body size in five-year-old twins: heritability and comparison to singleton standards. Twin Res Hum Genet. 2006;9(5):646–55.
28. Estourgie-van Burk GF, Bartels M, Boomsma DI, Delemarre-van de Waal HA. Body size of twins compared with siblings and the general population: from birth to late adolescence. J Pediatr. 2010;156(4):586–91.
29. Estourgie-van Burk GF, Bartels M, Delemarre-van de Waal HA, Boomsma DI. Heritability of testis size. Twin Res Hum Genet. 2009;12(4):351–5.
30. Euro-Peristat P. European perinatal health report. Core indicators of the health and care of pregnant women and babies in Europe in 2015. 2018. Available at: www.europeristat.com. Accessed: 17 November 2019.
31. Gedda L, Sciacca A, Brenci G, Villatico S, Bonanni G, Gueli N, Talone C. Situs viscerum specularis in monozygotic twins. Acta Genet Med Gemellol. 1984;33(1):81–5.
32. de Geus EJ, Posthuma D, Ijzerman RG, Boomsma DI. Comparing blood pressure of twins and their singleton siblings: being a twin does not affect adult blood pressure. Twin Res. 2001;4(5):385–91.
33. Gielen M, van Beijsterveldt CE, Derom C, Vlietinck R, Nijhuis JG, Zeegers MP, Boomsma DI. Secular trends in gestational age and birthweight in twins. Hum Reprod. 2010;25(9):2346–53.
34. Glinianaia SV, Rankin J, Wright C. Congenital anomalies in twins: a register-based study. Hum Reprod. 2008;23(6):1306–11.
35. Groene SG, Tollenaar LSA, Oepkes D, Lopriore E, van Klink JMM. The impact of selective fetal growth restriction or birth weight discordance on long-term neurodevelopment in Monochorionic twins: a systematic literature review. J Clin Med. 2019;8(7):944.
36. van Grootheest DS, Cath DC, Beekman AT, Boomsma DI. Genetic and environmental influences on obsessive-compulsive symptoms in adults: a population-based twin-family study. Psychol Med. 2007;37(11):1635–44.
37. Grosen D, Bille C, Petersen I, Skytthe A, JV H, Pedersen JK, Murray JC, Christensen K. Risk of oral clefts in twins. Epidemiology. 2011;22(3):313–9.
38. Hack KE, Derks JB, Elias SG, Franx A, Roos EJ, Voerman SK, Bode CL, Koopman-Esseboom C, Visser GH. Increased perinatal mortality and morbidity in monochorionic versus dichorionic twin pregnancies: clinical implications of a large Dutch cohort study. BJOG. 2008;115(1):58–67.
39. Hall JG. Twinning. Lancet. 2003;362(9385):735–43.

4

40. Hansen M, Colvin L, Petterson B, Kurinczuk JJ, de Klerk N, Bower C. Twins born following assisted reproductive technology: perinatal outcome and admission to hospital. Hum Reprod. 2009;24(9):2321–31.
41. Hartley RS, Hitti J. Birth order and delivery interval: analysis of twin pair perinatal outcomes. J Matern Fetal Neonatal Med. 2005;17(6):375–80.
42. Heino A, Gissler M, Hindori-Mohangoo AD, Blondel B, Klungsøyr K, Verdenik I, Mierzejewska E, Velebil P, Sól Ólafsdóttir H, Macfarlane A, Zeitlin J, Euro-Peristat Scientific Committee. Variations in multiple birth rates and impact on perinatal outcomes in Europe. PLoS One. 2016;11(3):e0149252.
43. Hoekstra RA, Bartels M, Verweij CJ, Boomsma DI. Heritability of autistic traits in the general population. Arch Pediatr Adolesc Med. 2007;161(4):372–7.
44. Hoekstra C, Willemsen G, van Beijsterveldt CE, Lambalk CB, Montgomery GW, Boomsma DI. Body composition, smoking, and spontaneous dizygotic twinning. Fertil Steril. 2010;93(3):885–93.
45. Hofmeyr GJ, Barrett JF, Crowther CA. Planned caesarean section for women with a twin pregnancy. Cochrane Database Syst Rev. 2011;7(12):CD006553.
46. Hottenga JJ, Boomsma DI, Kupper N, Posthuma D, Snieder H, Willemsen G, de Geus EJ. Heritability and stability of resting blood pressure. Twin Res Hum Genet. 2005;8(5):499–508.
47. Kahn B, Lumey LH, Zybert PA, Lorenz JM, Cleary-Goldman J, D'Alton ME, Robinson JN. Prospective risk of fetal death in singleton, twin, and triplet gestations: implications for practice. Obstet Gynecol. 2003;102(4):685–92.
48. Kajantie E, Osmond C, Barker DJ, Forsén T, Phillips DI, Eriksson JG. Size at birth as a predictor of mortality in adulthood: a follow-up of 350 000 person-years. Int J Epidemiol. 2005;34(3):655–63.
49. Källén B. Congenital malformations in twins: a population study. Acta Genet Med Gemellol (Roma). 1986;35(3–4):167–78.
50. Kean BH. Complete transposition of the viscera in both of one-egg twins. J Hered. 1942;33(6):217–21.
51. Kupper N, de Geus EJ, van den Berg M, Kirschbaum C, Boomsma DI, Willemsen G. Familial influences on basal salivary cortisol in an adult population. Psychoneuroendocrinology. 2005a;30(9):857–68.
52. Kupper N, Willemsen G, Posthuma D, de Boer D, Boomsma DI, de Geus EJ. A genetic analysis of ambulatory cardiorespiratory coupling. Psychophysiology. 2005b;42(2):202–12.
53. Kupper N, Willemsen G, Riese H, Posthuma D, Boomsma DI, de Geus EJ. Heritability of daytime ambulatory blood pressure in an extended twin design. Hypertension. 2005c;45(1):80–5.
54. Kupper NH, Willemsen G, van den Berg M, de Boer D, Posthuma D, Boomsma DI, de Geus EJ. Heritability of ambulatory heart rate variability. Circulation. 2004;110(18):2792–6.
55. Kwon EJ, Kim YJ. What is fetal programming?: a lifetime health is under the control of in utero health. Obstet Gynecol Sci. 2017;60(6):506–19.
56. Lancaster P, Kucera J, Knudsen L, Botting B, Robert-Gnansia E, Goujard J, Elek C, Mastroiacovo P, Cocchi G, Borman B, Irgens L, Castilla E, Martinez-Frias M-L, et al. Conjoined twins–an epidemiological study based on 312 cases. The International Clearinghouse for Birth Defects Monitoring Systems. Acta Genet Med Gemellol (Roma). 1991;40(3–4):325–35.
57. Lambalk CB, De Koning CH, Braat DD. The endocrinology of dizygotic twinning in the human. Mol Cell Endocrinol. 1998;145(1–2):97–102.
58. Layton WM. Situs inversus in conjoined twins. Am J Med Genet. 1989;34(2):297.
59. van Leeuwen M, van den Berg SM, Peper JS, Hulshoff Pol HE, Boomsma DI. Genetic covariance structure of reading, intelligence and memory in children. Behav Genet. 2009;39(3):245–54.
60. Li SJ, Ford N, Meister K, Bodurtha J. Increased risk of birth defects among children from multiple births. Birth Defects Res A Clin Mol Teratol. 2003;67(10):879–85.
61. Lopriore E, Nagel HT, Vandenbussche FP, Walther FJ. Long-term neurodevelopmental outcome in twin-to-twin transfusion syndrome. Am J Obstet Gynecol. 2003;189(5):1314–9.
62. Mastroiacovo P, Castilla EE, Arpino C, Botting B, Cocchi G, Goujard J, Marinacci C, Merlob P, Métneki J, Mutchinick O, Ritvanen R, Rosano A. Congenital malformations in twins: an international study. Am J Med Genet. 1999;83(2):117–24.
63. Melnick M, Myrianthopoulos NC. The effects of chorion type on normal and abnormal developmental variation in monozygous twins. Am J Med Genet. 1979;4(2):147–56.
64. Mbarek H, Steinberg S, Nyholt DR, Gordon SD, Miller MB, McRae AF, Hottenga JJ, Day FR, Willemsen G, de Geus EJ, Davies GE, Martin HC, Penninx BW, Jansen R, McAloney K, Vink JM, Kaprio J, Plomin R, Spector TD, Magnusson PK, Reversade B, Harris RA, Aagaard K, Kristjansson RP, Olafsson I, Eyjolfsson GI, Sigurdardottir O, Iacono WG, Lambalk CB, Montgomery GW, McGue M, Ong KK, Perry JRB, Martin NG, Stefánsson H, Stefánsson K, Boomsma DI. Identification of common genetic variants influencing spontaneous dizygotic twinning and female fertility. Am J Hum Genet. 2016;98(5):898–908.
65. Meyers C, Elias S, Arrabal P. Congenital anomalies and pregnancy loss. In: Keith LG, Papiernik E, editors. Multiple pregnancy: epidemiology, gestation, and perinatal outcome. London: Parthenon Publishing Group; 1995. p. 73–8.
66. Middeldorp CM, Birley AJ, Cath DC, Gillespie NA, Willemsen G, Statham DJ, de Geus EJ, Andrews JG, van Dyck R, Beem AL, Sullivan PF, Martin NG, Boomsma DI. Familial clustering of

major depression and anxiety disorders in Australian and Dutch twins and siblings. Twin Res Hum Genet. 2005a;8(6):609–15.
67. Middeldorp CM, Cath DC, Vink JM, Boomsma DI. Twin and genetic effects on life events. Twin Res Hum Genet. 2005b;8(3):224–31.
68. Middeldorp CM, Cath DC, Boomsma DI. A twin-family study of the association between employment, burnout and anxious depression. J Affect Disord. 2006;90(2–3):163–9.
69. Middeldorp CM, Stubbe JH, Cath DC, Boomsma DI. Familial clustering in burnout: a twin-family study. Psychol Med. 2005c;35(1):113–20.
70. Mook-Kanamori DO, van Beijsterveldt CE, Steegers EA, Aulchenko YS, Raat H, Hofman A, Eilers PH, Boomsma DI, Jaddoe VW. Heritability estimates of body size in fetal life and early childhood. PLoS One. 2012;7(7):e39901.
71. de Moor MH, Vink JM, van Beek JH, Geels LM, Bartels M, de Geus EJ, Willemsen G, Boomsma DI. Heritability of problem drinking and the genetic overlap with personality in a general population sample. Front Genet. 2011;2:76.
72. Muhlhausler BS, Hancock SN, Bloomfield FH, Harding R. Are twins growth restricted? Pediatr Res. 2011;70(2):117–22.
73. Myrianthopoulos NC. Congenital malformations in twins. Acta Genet Med Gemellol (Roma). 1976;25:331–5.
74. Oates NA, van Vliet J, Duffy DL, Kroes HY, Martin NG, Boomsma DI, Campbell M, Coulthard MG, Whitelaw E, Chong S. Increased DNA methylation at the AXIN1 gene in a monozygotic twin from a pair discordant for a caudal duplication anomaly. Am J Hum Genet. 2006;79(1):155–62.
75. Odintsova VV, Dolan CV, van Beijsterveldt CEM, de Zeeuw EL, van Dongen J, Boomsma DI. Pre- and perinatal characteristics associated with Apgar scores in a review and in a new study of Dutch twins. Twin Res Hum Genet. 2019;22(3):164–76.
76. Ooki S. Maternal age and birth defects after the use of assisted reproductive technology in Japan, 2004–2010. Int J Womens Health. 2013;5:65–77.
77. Ortibus E, Lopriore E, Deprest J, Vandenbussche FP, Walther FJ, Diemert A, Hecher K, Lagae L, De Cock P, Lewi PJ, Lewi L. The pregnancy and long-term neurodevelopmental outcome of monochorionic diamniotic twin gestations: a multicenter prospective cohort study from the first trimester onward. Am J Obstet Gynecol. 2009;200(5):494.e1–8.
78. Pietiläinen KH, Kaprio J, Rissanen A, Winter T, Rimpelä A, Viken RJ, Rose RJ. Distribution and heritability of BMI in Finnish adolescents aged 16y and 17y: a study of 4884 twins and 2509 singletons. Int J Obes Relat Metab Disord. 1999;23(2):107–15.
79. Pharoah PO. Causal hypothesis for some congenital anomalies. Twin Res Hum Genet. 2005;8(6):543–50.
80. Pharoah PO. Risk of cerebral palsy in multiple pregnancies. Clin Perinatol. 2006;33(2):301–13.
81. Pharoah PO, Dundar Y. Monozygotic twinning, cerebral palsy and congenital anomalies. Hum Reprod Update. 2009;15(6):639–48.
82. Pison P, Monden C, Smits J. Twinning rates in developed countries: trends and explanations. Popul Dev Rev. 2015;41(4):629–49.
83. Posthuma D, Beem AL, de Geus EJ, van Baal GC, von Hjelmborg JB, Iachine I, Boomsma DI. Theory and practice in quantitative genetics. Twin Res. 2003;6(5):361–76.
84. Polderman TJ, van Dongen J, Boomsma DI. The relation between ADHD symptoms and fine motor control: a genetic study. Child Neuropsychol. 2011;17(2):138–50.
85. Posthuma D, De Geus EJ, Bleichrodt N, Boomsma DI. Twin-singleton differences in intelligence? Twin Res. 2000;3(2):83–7.
86. Posthuma D, Meulenbelt I, de Craen AJ, de Geus EJ, Slagboom PE, Boomsma DI, Westendorp RG. Human cytokine response to ex vivo amyloid-beta stimulation is mediated by genetic factors. Twin Res Hum Genet. 2005;8(2):132–7.
87. Pradat P. Epidemiology of major congenital heart defects in Sweden, 1981–1986. J Epidemiol Community Health. BMJ Publishing Group. 1992;46(3):211–5.
88. Rossi AC, Mullin PM, Chmait RH. Neonatal outcomes of twins according to birth order, presentation and mode of delivery: a systematic review and meta-analysis. BJOG. 2011;118(5):523–32.
89. Scher AI, Petterson B, Blair E, Ellenberg JH, Grether JK, Haan E, Reddihough DS, Yeargin-Allsopp M, Nelson KB. The risk of mortality or cerebral palsy in twins: a collaborative population-based study. Pediatr Res. 2002;52(5):671–81.
90. Segal NL. Situs Inversus Totalis in twins: a brief review and a life history / twin research: twin studies of trisomy 21; monozygotic twin concordance for bilateral coronoid hyperplasia; prenatal hormonal effects in mixed-sex non-human primate litters; insurance mandates and twinning after in vitro fertilization / news reports: first report of identical twin puppies; twins sisters turn 100; remembering an identical twin production designer; New York City Marathon quadruplets. Twin Res Hum Genet. 2017;20(1):90–5.
91. Sheay W, Ananth CV, Kinzler WL. Perinatal mortality in first- and second-born twins in the United States. Obstet Gynecol. 2004;103(1):63–70.
92. Singh SM, Murphy B, O'Reilly R. Epigenetic contributors to the discordance of monozygotic twins. Clin Genet. 2002;62(2):97–103.
93. Smit DJ, Posthuma D, Boomsma DI, De Geus EJ. The relation between frontal EEG asymmetry and the risk for anxiety and depression. Biol Psychol. 2007;74(1):26–33.
94. van Soelen IL, Brouwer RM, van Leeuwen M, Kahn RS, Hulshoff Pol HE, Boomsma DI. Heritability of verbal and performance intelligence in a pediatric longitudinal sample. Twin Res Hum Genet. 2011;14(2):119–28.

95. Stoel RD, De Geus EJ, Boomsma DI. Genetic analysis of sensation seeking with an extended twin design. Behav Genet. 2006;36(2):229–37.
96. Stubbe JH, Posthuma D, Boomsma DI, De Geus EJ. Heritability of life satisfaction in adults: a twin-family study. Psychol Med. 2005;35(11):1581–8.
97. Svenvik M, Brudin L, Blomberg M. Preterm birth: a prominent risk factor for low Apgar scores. Biomed Res Int. 2015;2015:978079.
98. Thorngren-Jerneck K, Herbst A. Low 5-minute Apgar score: a population-based register study of 1 million term births. Obstet Gynecol. 2001;98(1):65–70.
99. Vasak B, Verhagen JJ, Koenen SV, Koster MP, de Reu PA, Franx A, Nijhuis JG, Bonsel GJ, Visser GH. Lower perinatal mortality in preterm born twins than in singletons: a nationwide study from The Netherlands. Am J Obstet Gynecol. 2017;216(2):161.e1–9.
100. Roeling MP, Willemsen G, Boomsma DI. Heritability of working in a creative profession. Behav Genet. 2017;47:298–304.
101. Veldkamp SA, van Bergen E, de Zeeuw EL, van Beijsterveldt CE, Boomsma DI, Bartels M. Bullying and victimization: the effect of close companionship. Twin Res Hum Genet. 2017;20(1):19–27.
102. Veldkamp SAM, Zondervan-Zwijnenburg MAJ, van Bergen E, Barzeva SA, Tamayo-Martinez N, Becht AI, van Beijsterveldt CEM, Meeus W, Branje S, Hillegers MHJ, Oldehinkel AJ, Hoijtink HJA, Boomsma DI, Hartman C. Parental age in relation to offspring's neurodevelopment. J Clin Child Adolesc Psychol. 2020:1–13. https://doi.org/10.1080/15374416.2020.1756298. (online ahead of print)
103. Vink JM, van Kemenade FJ, Meijer CJ, Casparie MK, Meijer GA, Boomsma DI. Cervix smear abnormalities: linking pathology data in female twins, their mothers and sisters. Eur J Hum Genet. 2011;19(1):108–11.
104. Vink JM, Sadrzadeh S, Lambalk CB, Boomsma DI. Heritability of polycystic ovary syndrome in a Dutch twin-family study. J Clin Endocrinol Metab. 2006;91(6):2100–4.
105. Willemsen G, van Beijsterveldt TC, van Baal CG, Postma D, Boomsma DI. Heritability of self-reported asthma and allergy: a study in adult Dutch twins, siblings and parents. Twin Res Hum Genet. 2008;11(2):132–42.
106. Willemsen G, Boomsma DI. Religious upbringing and neuroticism in Dutch twin families. Twin Res Hum Genet. 2007;10(2):327–33.
107. Willemsen G, Posthuma D, Boomsma DI. Environmental factors determine where the Dutch live: results from the Netherlands twin register. Twin Res Hum Genet. 2005;8(4):312–7.
108. Windham GC, Bjerkedal T. Malformations in twins and their siblings, Norway, 1967–79. Acta Genet Med Gemellol. 1984;33(1):87–95.
109. Windham GC, Sever LE. Neural tube defects among twin births. Am J Hum Genet. 1982;34(6):988–98.
110. Yu Y, Cozen W, Hwang AE, Cockburn MG, Zadnick J, Hamilton AS, Mack T, Figueiredo JC. Birth anomalies in monozygotic and dizygotic twins: results from the California twin registry. J Epidemiol. 2019;29(1):18–25.
111. de Zeeuw EL, van Beijsterveldt CE, de Geus EJ, Boomsma DI. Twin specific risk factors in primary school achievements. Twin Res Hum Genet. 2012;15(1):107–15.
112. Zeitlin J, Mohangoo A, Cuttini M, EUROPERISTAT Report Writing Committee, Alexander S, Barros H, Blondel B, Bouvier-Colle MH, Buitendijk S, Cans C, Correia S, Gissler M, Macfarlane A, Novak-Antolic Z, Zeitlin J, Zhang WH, Zimbeck M. The European perinatal health report: comparing the health and care of pregnant women and newborn babies in Europe. J Epidemiol Community Health. 2009;63(9):681–2.
113. Zondervan-Zwijnenburg MAJ, Veldkamp SAM, Neumann A, Barzeva SA, Nelemans SA, van Beijsterveldt CEM, Branje SJT, Hillegers MHJ, Meeus WHJ, Tiemeier H, Hoijtink HJA, Oldehinkel AJ, Boomsma DI. Parental age and offspring childhood mental health: a multi-cohort, population-based investigation. Child Dev. 2020;91(3):964–82.

Appendix: Within-Family Twin – Non-Twin Comparisons Across a Wide Range of Traits Assessed in the Netherlands Twin Register

114. Achenbach TM, Rescorla LA. Manual for the ASEBA adult forms & profiles. Burlington: Research Center for Children, Youth, & Families, University of Vermont; 2003.
115. Broadhead WE, Gehlbach SH, de Gruy FV, Kaplan BH. The Duke-UNC Functional Social Support Questionnaire. Measurement of social support in family medicine patients. Med Care. 1988;26(7):709–23.
116. Conners CK, Erhardt D, Sparrow EP. Conners' Adult ADHD Rating Scales (CAARS). Technical Manual. Toronto: Multi-Health Systems Inc.; 1999.
117. Costa PT, MacCrae RR. Revised NEO Personality Inventory (NEO-PI-R) and NEO Five-Factor Inventory (NEO-FFI): professional manual. Odessa: Psychological Assessment Resources; 1992.
118. Diener E, Emmons RA, Larsen RJ, Griffin S. The satisfaction with life scale. J Pers Assesss. 1985;49:71–5.

119. Feij JA, van Zuilen RW. Handleiding bij de spanningsbehoeftelijst (SBL). Lisse: Swets & Zeitlinger; 1984.
120. Geels LM, Vink JM, van Beek JH, Bartels M, Willemsen G, Boomsma DI. Increases in alcohol consumption in women and elderly groups: evidence from an epidemiological study. BMC Public Health. 2013;13:207.
121. Hoekstra H, Ormel J, De Fruyt F. NEO persoonlijkheidsvragenlijsten NEO-PI-R en NEO-FFI, Handleiding. Lisse: Swets & Zeitlinger; 1996.
122. Hughes ME, Waite LJ, Hawkley LC, Cacioppo JT. A short scale for measuring loneliness in large surveys results from two population-based studies. Res Aging. 2004;26:655–72.
123. Ligthart L, van Beijsterveldt CEM, Kevenaar ST, de Zeeuw E, van Bergen E, Bruins S, Pool R, Helmer Q, van Dongen J, Hottenga JJ, Van't Ent D, Dolan CV, Davies GE, Ehli EA, Bartels M, Willemsen G, de Geus EJC, Boomsma DI. The Netherlands twin register: longitudinal research based on twin and twin-family designs. Twin Res Hum Genet. 2019;31:1–14.
124. Morey LC. The personality assessment inventory: professional manual. Odessa: Psychological Assessment Resources; 1991.
125. Willemsen G, de Geus EJ, Bartels M, van Beijsterveldt CE, Brooks AI, Estourgie-van Burk GF, Fugman DA, Hoekstra C, Hottenga JJ, Kluft K, Meijer P, Montgomery GW, Rizzu P, Sondervan D, Smit AB, Spijker S, Suchiman HE, Tischfield JA, Lehner T, Slagboom PE, Boomsma DI. The Netherlands Twin Register biobank: a resource for genetic epidemiological studies. Twin Res Hum Genet. 2010;13(3):231–45.
126. Zuckerman M. Dimensions of sensation seeking. J Consult Clin Psychol. 1971;36:45–52.

Key Reading

Alexander GR, Slay Wingate M, Salihu H, Kirby RS. Fetal and neonatal mortality risks of multiple births. Obstet Gynecol Clin North Am. 2005;32(1):1–16. vii

Dick DM, Johnson JK, Viken RJ, Rose RJ. Testing between-family associations in within-family comparisons. Psychol Sci. 2000;11(5):409–13.

Estourgie-van Burk GF, Bartels M, Boomsma DI. Delemarre-van de Waal HA. Body size of twins compared with siblings and the general population: from birth to late adolescence. J Pediatr. 2010;156(4):586–91.

Kahn B, Lumey LH, Zybert PA, Lorenz JM, Cleary-Goldman J, D'Alton ME, Robinson JN. Prospective risk of fetal death in singleton, twin, and triplet gestations: implications for practice. Obstet Gynecol. 2003;102(4):685–92.

Middeldorp CM, Cath DC, Vink JM, Boomsma DI. Twin and genetic effects on life events. Twin Res Hum Genet. 2005;8(3):224–31.

Antenatal Care in Twins and Multiple Pregnancy

Contents

Dating of Twin Pregnancies

Pierre Macé, Houman Mahallati, and Laurent J. Salomon

Contents

A. Khalil et al. (eds.), *Twin and Higher-order Pregnancies*,
https://doi.org/10.1007/978-3-030-47652-6_5

5

Trailer

Dating of the pregnancy is one of the main aims of first trimester ultrasound in twin pregnancies. The main objective of dating in multiple pregnancies is to make ultrasound examinations later in pregnancy more effective in the screening and management of complications either specific or more frequent in these pregnancies. The dating of twin pregnancies should ideally be based on that of singletons and should be performed when the crown-rump length (CRL) measurement is between 45 and 84 mm (i.e., 11 + 0 to 13 + 6 weeks of gestation) using the same reference charts, at the time of the routine first trimester ultrasound scan. If the woman presents after 14 weeks of GA and with a CRL measurement above 84 mm, the dating of pregnancy should be based on the head circumference measurement. One of the recurrent questions is the choice of the fetus upon which to base dating, especially when there is a significant difference between the sizes of the two twins. The recent ISUOG guidelines on the role of ultrasound in twin pregnancies have outlined the most common practice: the larger CRL should be used for pregnancy dating as it may protect against overlooking the diagnosis of a subsequent selective IUGR of the smaller twin. As is the case for singleton pregnancies, twin pregnancies conceived via ART should be dated using the oocyte retrieval date or the embryonic age from fertilization.

Definitions

ART: Assisted reproductive technologies

CRL: Crown-rump length

GA: Gestational age

sIUGR: Selective intra-uterine growth restriction

TTTS: Twin-to-twin transfusion syndrome

Learning Objectives

After reading this chapter, the reader should know the following:

- How to date a twin pregnancy
- How to date a twin pregnancy conceived via ART
- What is considered the significant threshold for CRL measurement discrepancy
- How to deal with a significant discrepancy in CRL measurements

5.1 Introduction

In addition to determining chorionicity and amnionicity, and screening for aneuploidies and structural defects, dating of the pregnancy is one of the important goals of ultrasound in twin pregnancies, especially when exams are done in the first trimester.

The primary purpose of dating in twin pregnancies is not entirely the same as with that of singletons, in which the estimation of a due date is not as relevant in the context of multiple pregnancies as most deliveries take place before 40 weeks of gestation, either spontaneously or due to a medical indication.

The main objective of dating in multiple pregnancies is therefore rather to make subsequent ultrasound examinations at later term more effective in the screening and management of complications either specific to twin pregnancies (TTTS or selective intra-uterine growth restriction (IUGR)) or more frequent in these pregnancies (IUGR, structural defects, and aneuploidies).

One of the recurrent questions is therefore the choice of the fetus upon which to base dating, especially when there is a significant difference between the size of the two twins. This must be done in a manner as to not ignore these potential complications and at the same time not generate unnecessary parental anxiety or result in further unnecessary investigations.

5.2 When and How to Date Twin Pregnancies?

Routine dating of pregnancy from a measurement of the crown-rump length (CRL) at the time of first trimester ultrasound has been shown to be superior to the use of menstrual dates or dating after 14 weeks of GA [1] and should therefore be used in singleton pregnancies [2]. It is likely that the same should apply in twins, although there have been no specific studies demonstrating that it performs better than last menstrual period. The question is therefore whether the CRL reference charts used in singletons can also be used in twin pregnancies.

The dating of twin pregnancies should ideally be based on that of singletons and should be performed when the crown-rump length (CRL) measurement is between 45 and 84 mm (i.e., 11 + 0 to 13 + 6 weeks of gestation) [3, 4] using the same reference charts, at the time of the routine first trimester examination (◘ Fig. 5.1).

Indeed, a study by Dias et al. [4] compared the dating of twin and singleton pregnancies (controls) conceived following assisted reproductive technologies (ART) by measuring the CRL (*Robinson charts*) [5] and compared with the known date of conception. They showed that the variation in CRL between singleton and twins was unlikely to be clinically relevant, with a maximum variation of about 2 mm, or 1 day of gestational age (GA), well within the first trimester ultrasound accuracy range for dating pregnancy, and probably consistent with normal physiological variation .

If the woman presents after 14 weeks of GA and with a CRL measurement above 84 mm, the dating of pregnancy should be based on the head circumference measurement [2, 3], which appeared to produce the most reliable prediction, even based on most recent predictive reference charts [6].

As for singleton pregnancies, twin pregnancies conceived via ART should be dated using the oocyte retrieval date or the embryonic age from fertilization [3].

5.3 The Choice of the Fetus Upon Which to Base Dating

While it is likely that dating in the first trimester is desirable, there is less consensus on whether pregnancy should be dated on measurements taken on the smallest twin, the largest twin, or on the mean measurements of the two twins [3, 4, 7, 8].

Theoretically, the choice of the smallest twin has the advantage of not creating unnecessary parental anxiety about possible growth restriction as early as the first trimester. The exception to this would be cases with significant and obviously pathological CRL discordances (see below). There are three potential disadvantages to this strategy: (1) ignoring a potential growth restriction in the small fetus that appears to be growing appropriately and is "appropriate" for gestational age due to the "a priori" designation of dates based on that smaller fetus, (2) the potential to incorrectly assume there is fetal macrosomia of the larger twin at a later term, and (3) the risk of neglecting a post-term twin pregnancy.

These risks and the relative infrequency of large-for gestational age fetus in twin pregnancies explain the common practice of dating the pregnancy based on the larger twin.

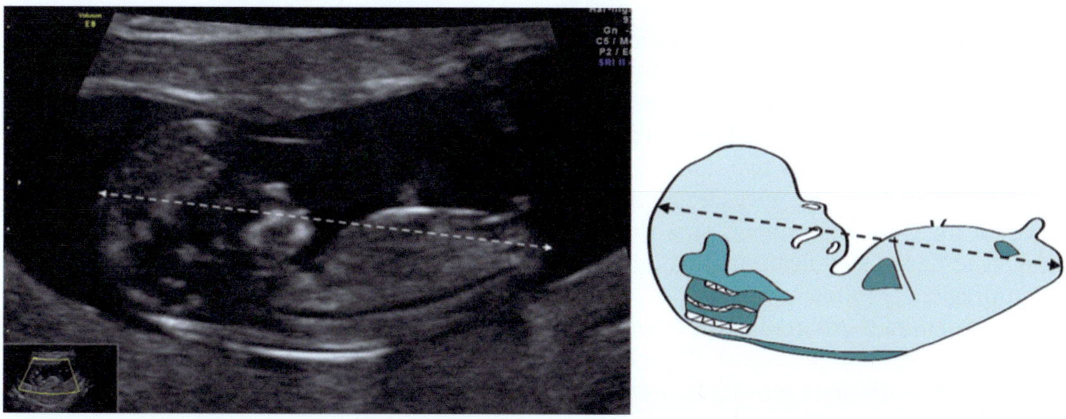

◘ **Fig. 5.1** Crown-rump length measurement, left: ultrasound view, right: schematic view

In this situation, the choice is effectively that of increasing the sensitivity of screening for selective growth restriction, while recognizing the increased risk of a higher number of false positives and potentially unnecessary testing and parental anxiety.

The choice could therefore be based on the most accurate measurement in this context, but unfortunately the literature is inconsistent as to what constitutes the most accurate measurement, with several authors finding a higher performance of either the smallest CRL [7, 9], or the mean of the two measurement [4], while the largest CRL often leads to the greatest difference with the assumed (assisted reproductive technologies) date of pregnancy.

However, all this must be put into perspective.

Given that CRL discordance in twin pregnancies is rare (less than 10% of twins have a discordance of more than 10% [7, 10], the mean discrepancy between twins at the time of first trimester ultrasound would therefore be expected to be very low.

In a prospective study including 182 twin pregnancies, Salomon et al. [7] showed that the mean difference in the CRL measurement between the two twins was 3.4 mm, or 1.2 days of GA. This was supported in a large retrospective study on 6225 twin pregnancies [10], which stated that the mean difference in the CRL measurement was 3.2 mm in dichorionic pregnancies and 3.6 mm in monochorionic diamniotic pregnancies (statistically significant difference). In this sense, using the formula reported by Robinson et al. [5], a 3 mm difference in CRL measurements is at most equivalent to a difference of 2 days of GA. As mentioned later, this difference may simply reflect different growth patterns and/or measurement errors of two normal fetuses and is well below the measurement error reported for CRL assessment. It is therefore unlikely to have a significant impact on subsequent pregnancy follow-up.

The situation is different in the presence of a major discrepancy between CRL measurements. Several different cut-offs of significant CRL discrepancy have been proposed, which is itself a concern as the association between CRL discordance and adverse outcomes is highly dependent on the threshold adopted. It is therefore important to set a threshold to define a significant discrepancy that could impact the pregnancy outcome. The ≥10 mm or 15% CRL discordance is the most commonly used to represent the higher centiles of discordance and the 95th percentile for CRL discrepancy seems to be around 10 mm, which is a 14% difference in CRL measurement or 3.6 days of GA [7].

Again, according to Robinson et al. [5], a 10 mm difference is equivalent to a difference of between 4 and 6 days of GA depending on the GA at the time of measurement.

Above these limits, the dating of the pregnancy should definitely be based on the larger twin's CRL, as this major discrepancy probably indicates a very early-onset growth restriction of the smallest twin which may have the same significance as in a singleton pregnancy and reveal a chromosomal defect [7] or structural abnormalities. However, it is to be noted that the role of CRL discordance in screening for aneuploidy is probably limited with the introduction of non-invasive prenatal testing.

A significant CRL discordance has also been reported as an early predictor of adverse pregnancy outcomes such as significant birth weight discrepancy [11], selective IUGR, fetal loss before 20 or 24 weeks of gestation, preterm birth [10, 12], fetal loss after 24 weeks of gestation [12] or with a moderate strength of association, TTTS in monochorionic twins [10, 13–15] despite a too poor prediction accuracy to form a clinically relevant screening test for these adverse outcomes [10, 12].

In cases of pregnancy conceived either spontaneously or via ART, every significant discrepancy between the two twins (>10 mm, >15%) should lead to additional investigations of the smallest twin, which is the twin at higher risk of aneuploidy or IUGR, and closer follow-up of the pregnancy should be instituted. This is despite the poor screening performance for adverse pregnancy outcomes as stated above. An additional earlier scan, at 14 weeks of GA for monochorionic pregnancies and 16 weeks of GA for dichorionic pregnancies, should still be offered. With regard to the risk of aneuploidy, future research should investigate the relevance of major CRL discrepancy in the era of cfDNA testing.

In the vast majority of twin pregnancies for which the discordance is less than 15% (i.e., in practice less than 7–12 mm), the question of which twin to date remains thus debatable.

While the smaller twin, which appears closer to the actual age in ART-conceived pregnancies [7, 9], could be used for dating, this will decrease the IUGR detection rate later in pregnancy. The use of the average CRL will reduce the random error of the measurements. Finally, the use of the larger twin allows for a simple and consistent practice, since it applies even in the case of a major discrepancy related to aneuploidy or structural defects of the smaller one, and increases the sensitivity of subsequent selective-IUGR screening. This recommendation has also recently been stated in the ISUOG guidelines on the role of ultrasound in twin pregnancies [3] and is likely to ensure, through its simplicity, a much-needed standardization of practices. To add emphasis, such a recommendation can be applied in all cases, regardless of the discrepancy in CRL between the twins.

If the woman presents after 14 weeks of GA, the larger head circumference should be used for dating pregnancy.

The flow chart summarizes the management options for the dating of twin pregnancies (◘ Fig. 5.2).

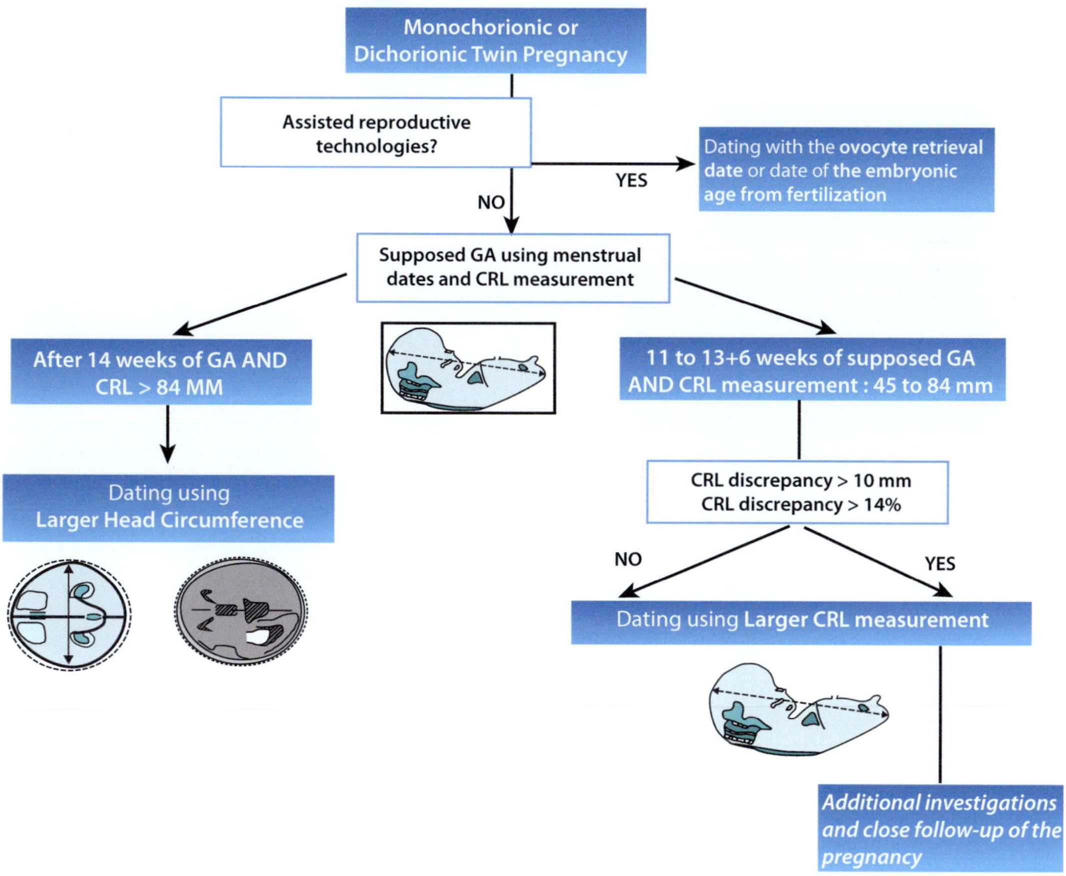

◘ **Fig. 5.2** Management flow chart for dating of twin pregnancies

5

Key Points

1. Dating of the pregnancy is one of the main objective of first trimester ultrasound in twin pregnancies.
2. Due to a usually earlier delivery date, the main objective of dating pregnancy is to increase the screening of twin pregnancy complications, especially selective intra-uterine growth restriction.
3. The dating of twin pregnancies should be based on that of singletons and be performed when the crown-rump length (CRL) measurement is between 45 and 84 mm (i.e., 11 + 0 to 13 + 6 weeks of gestation) using the same reference charts.
4. The mean discrepancy between twins at the time of first trimester ultrasound appears to be clinically irrelevant, and unlikely to have a significant impact on subsequent pregnancy follow-up.
5. Dating of pregnancy using the largest CRL measurement, as advised by ISUOG guidelines, is the most common practice and allows high sensitivity for the screening of selective intra-uterine growth restriction.
6. If the CRL measurement discrepancy is >10 mm or >15%, additional investigation should be conducted on the smallest twin which is at high risk of aneuploidy or IUGR.
7. Twin pregnancies conceived via ART should be dated using the oocyte retrieval date or the embryonic age from fertilization.
8. After 14 weeks of GA or if the CRL measurement is above 84 mm, the larger head circumference should be used for dating pregnancy.

5.3.1 Review Questions

1. What do twin and singleton pregnancies have in common in terms of pregnancy dating?

2. What are the rationales for using the CRL measurement of the largest twin for dating twin pregnancies?

3. What are the possible causes of CRL measurement discrepancy between twins during the first trimester?

4. What follow-up and monitoring should be planned if there is a significant CRL discordance between the twins during the first trimester ultrasound?

5.3.2 Multiple-Choice Questions

1. About dating in twin pregnancies, the most common practice is:
   (a) To date using the smallest CRL measurement
   (b) To date using the mean CRL measurement
   (c) To date using the largest CRL measurement except for pregnancy conceived via ART
   (d) To use "specific twin-pregnancy" reference charts for CRL measurement
   (e) To date using the larger head circumference if the woman presents after 14 weeks of GA

Answer: (c, e)

2. In cases of discrepancy between CRL measurements of twins during the first trimester examination
   (a) The threshold of significance is likely to be 10 mm or 14%.
   (b) In cases of significant discrepancy, dating should be based upon the smallest twin.
   (c) A significant discrepancy should lead to a closer follow up of the pregnancy.
   (d) Most of CRL measurement discrepancies are unlikely to have significant clinical impact.
   (e) Whatever the discrepancy, twin pregnancies conceived via ART should be dated using the oocyte retrieval date or the embryonic age from fertilization.

Answer: (a, c, d, e)

References

1. Whitworth M, Bricker L, Mullan C. Ultrasound for fetal assessment in early pregnancy. Cochrane Pregnancy and Childbirth Group, editor. Cochrane Database of Systematic Reviews [Internet]. 2015 Jul 14 [cited 2019 Apr 11]; Available from: http://doi.wiley.com/10.1002/14651858.CD007058.pub3.
2. ISUOG. Practice guidelines: performance of first-trimester fetal ultrasound scan: ISUOG guidelines. Ultrasound Obstet Gynecol. 2013;41(1):102–13.
3. Khalil A, Rodgers M, Baschat A, Bhide A, Gratacos E, Hecher K, et al. ISUOG practice guidelines: role of ultrasound in twin pregnancy. Ultrasound Obstet Gynecol. 2016;47(2):247–63.
4. Dias T, Mahsud-Dornan S, Thilaganathan B, Papageorghiou A, Bhide A. First-trimester ultrasound dating of twin pregnancy: are singleton charts reliable? BJOG Int J Obstet Gynaecol. 2010;117(8):979–84.
5. Robinson HP, Fleming JEE. A critical evaluation of sonar "crown-rump length" measurements. Br J Obstet Gynaecol. 1975;82(9):702–10.
6. Papageorghiou AT, Kemp B, Stones W, Ohuma EO, Kennedy SH, Purwar M, et al. Ultrasound-based gestational-age estimation in late pregnancy. Ultrasound Obstet Gynecol. 2016;48(6):719–26.
7. Salomon LJ, Cavicchioni O, Bernard JP, Duyme M, Ville Y. Growth discrepancy in twins in the first trimester of pregnancy. Ultrasound Obstet Gynecol. 2005;26(5):512–6.
8. Sebire NJ, D'Ercole C, Soares W, Nayar R, Nicolaides KH. Intertwin disparity in fetal size in monochorionic and dichorionic pregnancies. Obstet Gynecol. 1998;91(1):82–5.
9. Chaudhuri K, Su L-L, Wong P-C, Chan Y-H, Choolani MA, Chia D, et al. Determination of gestational age in twin pregnancy: which fetal crown-rump length should be used?: gestational dating in twins. J Obstet Gynaecol Res. 2013;39(4):761–5.
10. Litwinska E, Syngelaki A, Cimpoca B, Sapantzoglou I, Nicolaides KH. Intertwin discordance in fetal size at 11–13 weeks' gestation and pregnancy outcome. Ultrasound in Obstetrics & Gynecology [Internet]. 2019 Nov 11 [cited 2019 Nov 28]; Available from: https://obgyn-onlinelibrary-wiley-com.lama.univ-amu.fr/doi/10.1002/uog.21923.
11. Kalish RB, Chasen ST, Gupta M, Sharma G, Perni SC, Chervenak FA. First trimester prediction of growth discordance in twin gestations. Am J Obstet Gynecol. 2003;189(3):706–9.
12. D'Antonio F, Khalil A, Pagani G, Papageorghiou AT, Bhide A, Thilaganathan B. Crown–rump length discordance and adverse perinatal outcome in twin pregnancies: systematic review and meta-analysis. Ultrasound Obstet Gynecol. 2014;44(2):138–46.
13. Mackie FL, Hall MJ, Morris RK, Kilby MD. Early prognostic factors of outcomes in monochorionic twin pregnancy: systematic review and meta-analysis. Am J Obstet Gynecol. 2018;219(5):436–46.
14. Stagnati V, Zanardini C, Fichera A, Pagani G, Quintero RA, Bellocco R, et al. Early prediction of twin-to-twin transfusion syndrome: systematic review and meta-analysis: early prediction of TTTS. Ultrasound Obstet Gynecol. 2017;49(5):573–82.
15. Memmo A, Dias T, Mahsud-Dornan S, Papageorghiou AT, Bhide A, Thilaganathan B. Prediction of selective fetal growth restriction and twin-to-twin transfusion syndrome in monochorionic twins. BJOG Int J Obstet Gynaecol. 2012;119(4):417–21.

Key Reading

Khalil A, Rodgers M, Baschat A, Bhide A, Gratacos E, Hecher K, et al. ISUOG practice guidelines: role of ultrasound in twin pregnancy. Ultrasound Obstet Gynecol. 2016;47(2):247–63.

Determining Chorionicity and Amnionicity

Mieke Vanoppen and Liesbeth Lewi

Contents

Electronic Supplementary Material The online version of this chapter (https://doi.org/10.1007/978-3-030-47652-6_6) contains supplementary material, which is available to authorized users. The videos can be accessed by scanning the related images with the SN More Media App.

A. Khalil et al. (eds.), *Twin and Higher-order Pregnancies*,
https://doi.org/10.1007/978-3-030-47652-6_6

Trailer

Knowledge of the correct chorionicity is essential to distinguish the high-risk monochorionic from the lower-risk dichorionic twin pregnancies. As monochorionic twins are connected by vascular anastomoses during their intrauterine life, transfusion imbalances may occur. Also, if one twin dies, the other twin may bleed into its demised co-twin across the anastomoses, leading to double demise or brain damage in the surviving twin. All twins should have their chorionicity determined in the first trimester and for monochorionic twins the amnionicity, as it will determine the follow-up frequency, the risk assessment for chromosomal anomalies, and the management of discordant anomalies and fetal growth restriction. In this chapter, we describe the sonographic markers for chorio-amnionicity determination in the first trimester as well as the pitfalls that may lead to a wrong chorio-amnionicty assignment.

Definitions

Lambda or twin peak sign: refers to the triangular extension of placental tissue into the base of the intertwin membrane

T or empty lambda sign: refers to the apposition of the two amniotic membranes at the insertion of the intertwin membrane to the placental surface

Learning Objectives

- To understand the importance of determining chorio-amnionicity to plan adequate clinical surveillance
- To know the adequate timing to determine chorio-amnionicity
- To provide an overview of the ultrasound markers for chorio-amnionicity in early and advanced pregnancy
- To acknowledge possible pitfalls in determining chorio-amnionicity

6.1 Introduction

Antenatal determination of chorio-amnionicity in twin pregnancies is essential, as antenatal and perinatal complications are more common in monochorionic compared with dichorionic twin pregnancies. Because of the vascular anastomoses connecting the two fetal circulations, monochorionic gestations have a higher risk due to some unique complications such as twin-to-twin transfusion syndrome, twin anemia-polycythemia sequence, and demise or neurological damage of the surviving twin if the co-twin dies during pregnancy [1]. Monoamniotic twins are at an even higher risk because of their almost universal cord entanglement and extensive intertwin anastomoses, with a risk of an acute transfusion imbalance between the twins [2]. The fetal loss rate before 24 gestational weeks is four times higher in monochorionic than in dichorionic pregnancies, and the perinatal mortality rate is twice as high [3, 4]. Consequently, chorio-amnionicity is the earliest and most accurate predictor of risk when multiple gestations are involved, and early first-trimester distinction between high-risk monochorionic and lower-risk dichorionic pregnancies is the key to appropriate clinical management and planning of care [5, 6]. This chapter provides an overview of ultrasound markers for chorionicity determination and their pitfalls.

6.2 Chorio-amnionicity Determination

6.2.1 Timing of Chorio-amnionicity Determination

The distinction between high-risk monochorionic and lower-risk dichorionic twin pregnancies can be accurately achieved at the time of the first-trimester scan because amnion and chorion are still separated from one another [7, 8]. The earliest gestation to determine the chorionicity is 5 weeks, the fetal number 6 weeks, and the amnionicity 8 weeks [9]. Chorionicity early in gestation can be determined by counting the gestational or chorionic sacs. If there are two completely separated gestational sacs, one can assume it is a dichorionic pregnancy. At 6 weeks, the fetal poles are visible and fetal number can be counted. From a gestational age of 8 weeks and with the availability of high-resolution ultrasound, the thin amniotic membranes are visible [10, 11]. Therefore, the ideal timing in the first trimester to determine chorio-amnionicity would be at a gestational age between 8 and 13 + 6 weeks, because amnion and chorion are still separated from one another and the amniotic membranes and layers of the intertwin membrane can be clearly visualized with high-resolution ultrasound.

6.2.2 Ultrasound Markers of Chorionicity

Chorio-amnionicity can be determined by counting the layers that separate the twins and by the appearance of the junction between the intertwin membrane and the placenta [12]. With this, one can recognize the twin peak and empty lambda sign. These are the most reliable ultrasound markers and best-examined markers to determine chorio-amnionicity. The accuracy of high-resolution abdominal or transvaginal sonography in first or early second trimester using these markers ranges from 95% to 100% [7, 8, 13, 14].

- *Twin peak or "full" lambda sign*
  In dichorionic diamniotic (DCDA) twin pregnancies, there is a triangular extension of placental tissue into the base of the intertwin membrane, hence separating them by three layers: two thin amniotic membranes, and one thick layer of chorion (amnion – chorion – amnion). This gives the sonographic appearance of a "full" lambda sign [5, 12] (◘ Fig. 6.1, Video 6.1). The lambda sign was first described in 1981 (Bessis and Papernik). The echogenic chorionic villi between the two layers of amnion are also referred to as the "twin peak" sign [9, 15].
- *"Empty" lambda or T sign*
  In monochorionic diamniotic (MCDA) twin pregnancies, the twins are separated by only two thin layers of amniotic membrane, giving the sonographic image referred to as the T sign. However, in the first trimester, the term T sign might be confusing because with the current high-resolution ultrasound imaging, the two amniotic sacs and their insertion at the placental surface form a lambda, rather than a T. As there is no chorion frondosum extending into the intertwin membrane at the placental insertion site, it is looks more like lambda than a T sign and it seems preferable to speak of an "empty" lambda sign to distinguish it from the "full" lambda in dichorionic pregnancies [5, 12] (◘ Fig. 6.2, Video 6.2).

One should be aware that some conditions can mimic a "false" full lambda sign or twin peak sign in a monochorionic pregnancy,

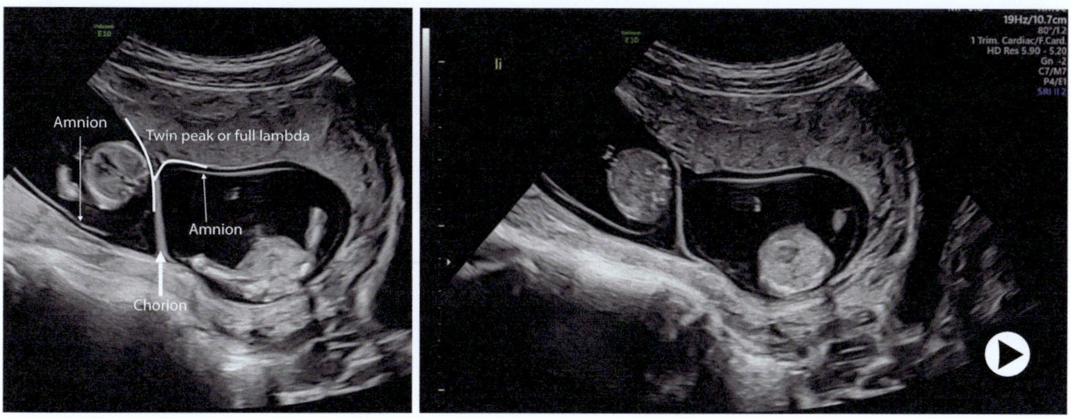

◘ **Fig. 6.1** Sonographic image of a dichorionic twin pregnancy at 13 weeks. The fetuses are separated by three layers: one thick chorionic layer (thick arrow) with on each side a thin amniotic layer (thin arrows) (amnion-chorion-amnion). The twin peak or "full" lambda sign is visible at the insertion of the intertwin septum on the placenta (https://doi.org/10.1007/000-2t0)

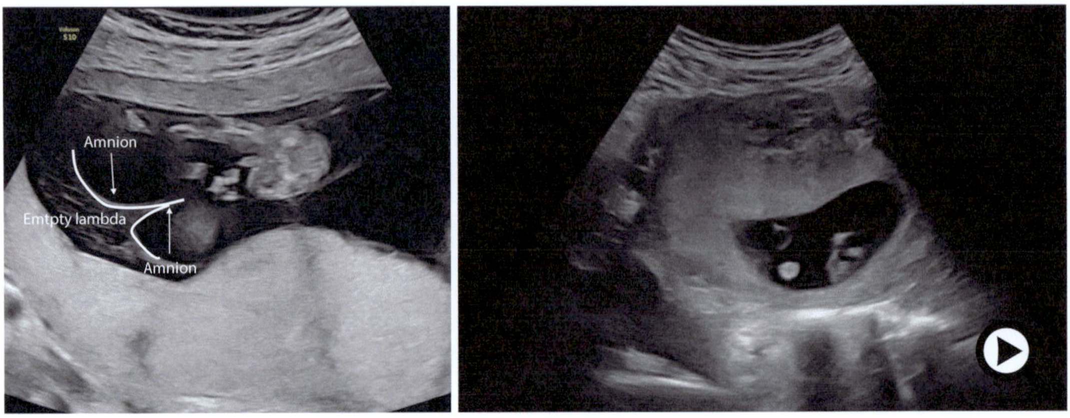

Fig. 6.2 Sonographic image of a monochorionic diamniotic twin pregnancy at 11 weeks. The fetuses are separated by only two thin layers of amnion (thin arrows) (amnion-amnion). An "empty lamda" sign can be seen at the insertion of the intertwin septum on the placenta (https://doi.org/10.1007/000-2t1)

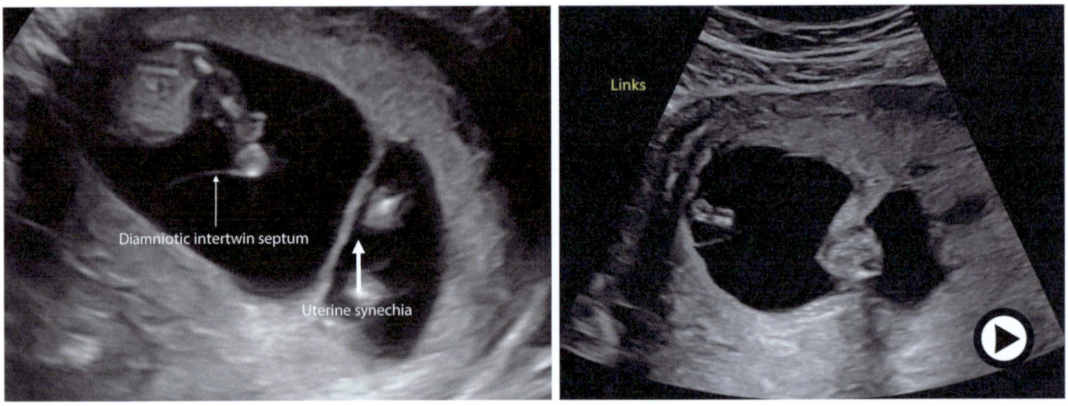

Fig. 6.3 Image of a monochorionic diamniotic twin pregnancy at 13 weeks. The patient had a uterine synechia (thick arrow) due to a curettage for placental retention in her previous pregnancy. The synechia creates a false twin peak sign, but the diamniotic septum (thin arrow) in not connected to the synechia. This patient developed a stage I twin-twin transfusion syndrome in combination with twin anemia polycythemia sequence treated with fetoscopic laser surgery and intrauterine transfusion (https://doi.org/10.1007/000-2t2)

such as an intrauterine synechia (Fig. 6.3, Video 6.3), a hematoma along with the insertion of the intertwin septum, or a regressing yolk sac at the junction between the intertwin membrane and the placenta. In this case, higher-risk monochorionic pregnancies may be mislabeled as dichorionic. Hence, it is essential to do a continuous sweep of the entire membrane insertion site during the first-trimester ultrasound examination to distinguish a full from an empty lambda sign. A true full lambda sign should always be seen along the entire insertion area, whereas a false full lambda sign would appear as a more focal or segmental projection [13].

With advancing gestational age, the determination of chorionicity becomes increasingly tricky. After 14 weeks, amnion and chorion fuse, making it more difficult to count the layers. The chorion frondosum also regresses within the intertwin septum in dichorionic pregnancies [13]. On the other hand, folding of the chorionic plate at later gestational age can mimic a "false-positive" lambda sign in a monochorionic pregnancy [12], which makes it more challenging to differentiate between a MC and DC gestation.

Other sonographic markers that have been described to determine chorionicity are the fetal gender, the number of placental masses, and the intertwin membrane thickness. Especially in advanced gestational age, where the lambda and T sign have disappeared, these markers can still be helpful to assess chorionicity as reliable as possible. Discordant fetal gender or the presence of two separate placentas suggests dichorionic twinning. However, there are exceptions to this rule that we will address later in this chapter. Further, fetal sex cannot be reliably determined by early ultrasound scans, and more than 50% of dichorionic twins are also of the same sex [13]. The third marker that has been described is measuring the thickness of the intertwin membranes. When both fetuses have the same sex, and there is only a single placenta, the appearance of the junction between the intertwin membrane and the placenta remains the most critical sign for determining chorionicity. The intertwin membrane is thicker in DC compared with MC twin pregnancies because there are more layers, including the thick chorionic layer in a DC intertwin septum. However, there is no consensus on the cutoff value of the measurement (ranging from 1.5 mm in the first trimester to 2 mm in the second trimester). Together with poor reproducibility and a higher inter- and intra-observer variation, this is undoubtedly a less reliable indicator [5, 7, 8, 13].

6.2.3 Ultrasound Markers of Amnionicity in Monochorionic Twin Pregnancies

Dichorionic twins are always diamniotic, whereas 95% of the monochorionic twins are diamniotic, and 5% are monoamniotic. The determination of amnionicity in monochorionic gestations is challenging because of the late appearance and the thin nature of the amniotic membranes. As previously mentioned, with high-resolution transabdominal and transvaginal ultrasound and appropriate experience of the clinician, amniotic membranes can be visualized from a gestational age of 8 weeks [10]. From this time, it is essential to establish whether MC pregnancies are mono- or diamniotic.

In a MCDA twin pregnancy, there is the empty lambda sign and two thin amniotic membranes separating the two fetuses, whereas, in a monochorionic mono-amniotic (MOMA) twin pregnancy, there is a single amniotic cavity and no dividing intertwin septum (◘ Fig. 6.4, Video 6.4). More specific sonographic findings to confirm the diagnosis of a MOMA pregnancy in the first trimester are the two umbilical cords that insert close to each other into the placenta and the almost universal cord entanglement [16, 17]. Further diagnostic clues include the proximity of the

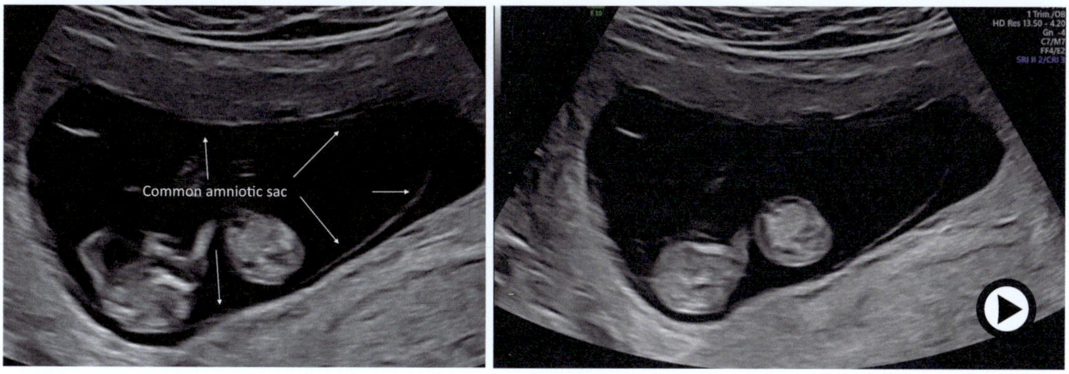

◘ **Fig. 6.4** Image of a monochorionic monoamniotic twin pregnancy. The fetuses are encircled by a single amniotic membrane (thin arrow) and move freely within the same monochorionic cavity (https://doi.org/10.1007/000-2t3)

two fetuses and the possibility of embracing fetal parts [2, 18, 19]. If there is any uncertainty regarding the presence or absence of the intertwin membrane in early pregnancy, a repeat scan in later gestation is recommended. Further, the thin intertwin amniotic membrane is easily missed if the ultrasound beam is parallel to the membrane or if the ultrasound gain is too low. Changing the angle of insonation and increasing the gain might facilitate the visualization of the thin amniotic membranes [13].

If there is difficulty in determining chorio-amnionicity in the first trimester, the patient needs to be referred for a second opinion in a tertiary center. In the absence of a definite assignment, the pregnancy should be considered monochorionic and monitored as such [6]. It is strongly recommended to store the images of the intertwin septum as proof of chorionicity, should there be any doubt later on [12].

6.2.4 Pitfalls in Determining Chorio-amnionicity Determination

1. *The number of yolk sacs does not predict amnionicity*

   In the majority of cases, the number of yolk sacs in early first-trimester monochorionic gestation reflects the number of amniotic sacs later in pregnancy. However, there are exceptions. In diamniotic pregnancies, 85% have two yolk sacs in early pregnancy, and 15% have only one yolk sac [11]. In monoamniotic pregnancies, there is almost always one yolk sac, but there have been case reports about the early presence of two yolk sacs in MOMA pregnancies as well [20, 21]. Hence, the yolk sac number in early pregnancy should not be regarded as a reliable marker to predict amnionicity [21, 22].
2. *Separate placental masses do not always indicate a dichorionic twin pregnancy*

   Two separate placental masses in twin pregnancies are reported to indicate dichorionic twinning. Counting the number of masses may be especially useful if chorionicity is determined later in pregnancy when amnion and chorion are already fused. However, about 3% of monochorionic placentas are bipartite. Suspicion is warranted when two separate placental masses are detected on the first-trimester ultrasound scan in combination with a T or empty lambda sign at the intertwin membrane-placental junction. Macroscopic examination and color dye studies of these monochorionic placentas reveal that vascular anastomoses may connect the two lobes, which explains the possibility of transfusion imbalances in these monochorionic bipartite placentas. Therefore, the number of placental masses is not always reliable to assess chorionicity. In the case of two separate placental masses, careful ultrasound examination of the number and aspect of the layers separating the twins is necessary to identify the monochorionic twin pregnancies at risk of hemodynamic intertwin complications [23, 24] (◘ Fig. 6.5).
3. *Partial monochorionic and mono-amniotic twinning*

   Intermediate forms of chorionicity and amnionicity may arise due to zygotic cleavage within the time interval just between di- and monochorionic and di- and mono-amniotic twinning. In order to detect these forms, it is crucial to scan the entire intertwin septum during the first-trimester ultrasound examination [25].

   (a) *Partial monochorionic pregnancy*

   In a partial MC pregnancy, a monochorionic part and a dichorionic part co-exist in the same intertwin membrane. During the ultrasound scan, one can identify two parts over the length of the intertwin membrane: one with an amnion-amnion constitution and the other with an amnion-chorion-amnion constitution. Hence, one sees an empty lambda (or T sign) and full lambda sign occurring together at different sites of the intertwin insertion zone at the placental surface (◘ Fig. 6.6, Video 6.5). Follow-up of partial MC pregnancies should be identical to that

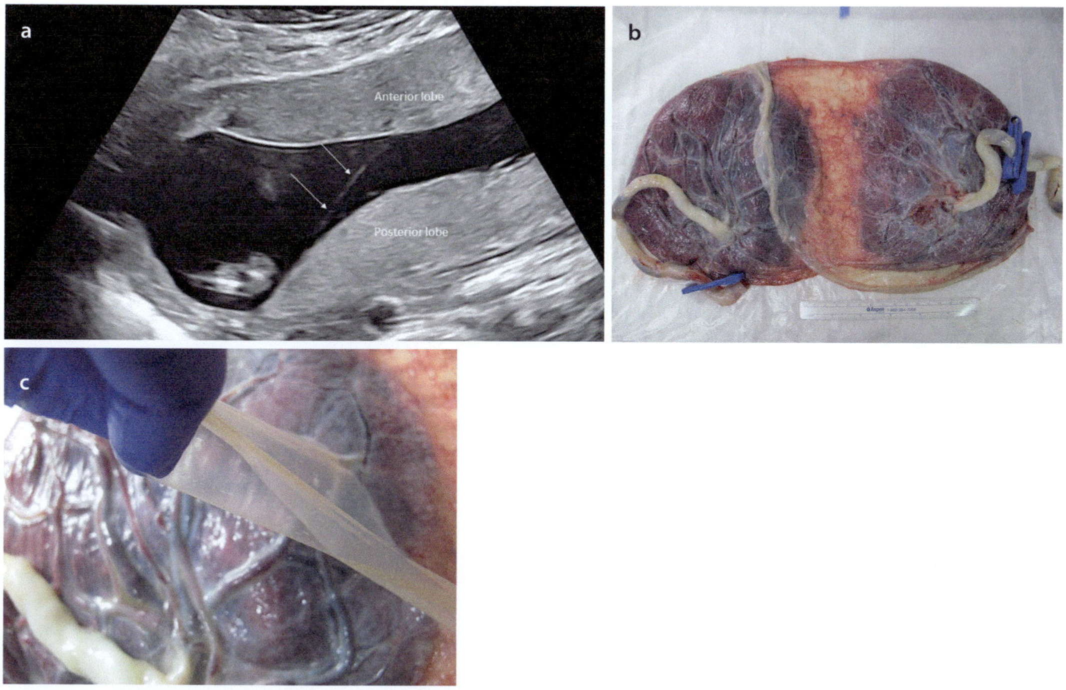

Fig. 6.5 **a** Ultrasound image of a bilobar monochorionic diamniotic placenta. The patient was referred with a dichorionic twin pregnancy based on the presence of two separate placental masses. However, because of the thin intertwin septum and concordant sex, a monochorionic twin pregnancy was suspected and the pregnancy was followed as such. She ruptured the membranes at 34 weeks and went into spontaneous labor. **b** At birth, the placenta was confirmed to be a bilobar monochorionic placenta. **c** The intertwin septum consisted of only two thin amniotic membranes. There were no vascular communications present

of a MC twin pregnancy, as vascular anastomoses can run across the MC part of the septum [25].

(b) *Partial monoamniotic pregnancy*

In a partial MA pregnancy, the dividing intertwin septum is incomplete. This type of partial twinning has not been reported as a diagnosis in early pregnancy, because a disruption in the septum may be difficult to recognize on the first-trimester scan. However, with advancing gestational age, both twins will appear on the same side of the dividing septum with their cords entangled, while on the first-trimester scan, two thin amniotic membranes were visualized (as is typical in a MCDA pregnancy). If the intertwin septum no longer separates the twins, this suggests a partial MA twin and also implies that initial diagnosis of a MCDA pregnancy changes to a partial MA pregnancy. Hence, it is essential to verify on each ultrasound exam that the intertwin septum still separates the twins in order to detect these rare partial forms [25]. Discontinuity of the intertwin membrane or septostomy can also be caused by invasive procedures such as fetoscopic laser therapy, leading to "iatrogenic" MOMA twins [26] (Fig. 6.7). Several case reports describe a spontaneous rupture of the intertwin membrane, with "pseudo-MOMA" twins as a result [27–29]. However, the septum may well be incomplete from the start, and these may well be partial MOMA twins from the start. Once a partial MA pregnancy is diagnosed, it seems prudent to manage these cases as real MA pairs because of the vascular anastomoses in combination with cord entanglement, as seen in MA pregnancies [25].

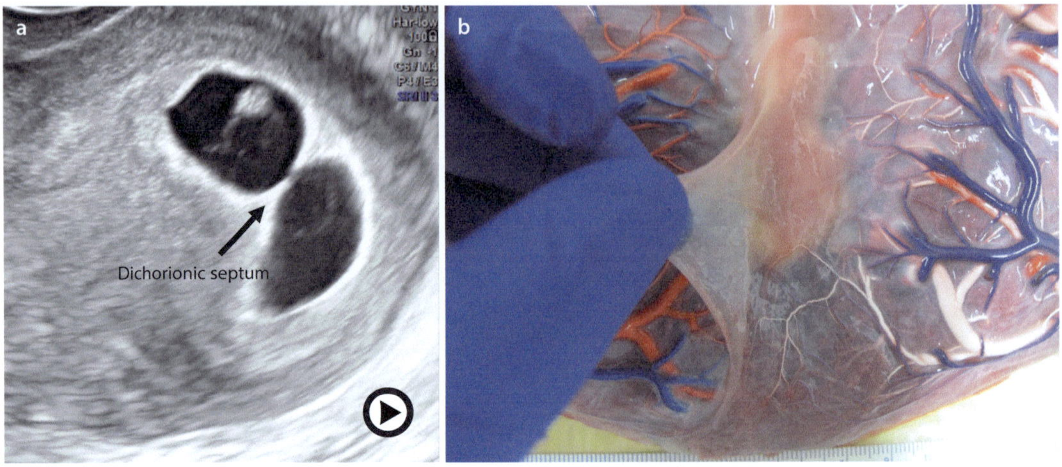

Fig. 6.6 **a** At 7 weeks, the pregnancy was labelled as dichorionic. However, at 13 weeks, part of the intertwin septum consisted of three layers (amnion-chorion-amnion) with twin peak sign, whereas the other part had only two layers with an "empty lambda sign" (Video 6.5). The pregnancy was considered to be a partial monochorionic placenta and followed as monochorionic twin pregnancy. She was delivered by an elective repeat cesarean section at 36 weeks. Most of the intertwin septum was diamniotic as confirmed on pathology. **b** A small part of the septum was dichorionic and could not be removed from the placenta (https://doi.org/10.1007/000-2t4)

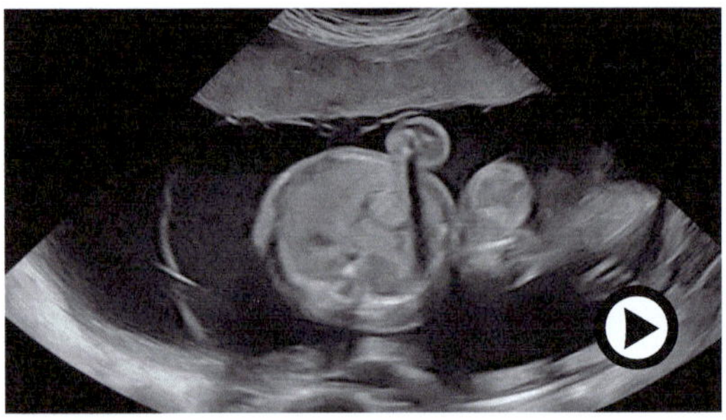

Fig. 6.7 Image of an iatrogenic monoamniotic twin pregnancy after laser surgery with septostomy at 23 weeks. Day 4 after the surgery, the patient consulted because of no fetal movements of the right twin. On ultrasound scan, both babies were in the same, left-sided amniotic sac, whereas the right sac was empty (https://doi.org/10.1007/000-2t5)

The incidence of these intermediate forms of twinning, partial MC, and partial MA, is not known but is probably rare. However, in order to detect these partial forms, it is vital to inspect the entire intertwin septum during the first-trimester ultrasound and also to verify that the septum still separates the twins with every follow-up scan [25].

4. *Discordant fetal sex is not always indicative for dichorionic twins*

   Traditionally, discordant fetal sex is thought to indicate dizygosity, and therefore dichorionicity. However, several case reports have mentioned a discordant fetal sex phenotype in monozygotic or monochorionic twins, especially after assisted reproductive technology. Although rare, sex discordance in twin pregnancies is not necessarily proof of dichorionicity [13, 23].

   (a) *Discordant fetal sex in monozygotic monochorionic twins due to mosaicism*

   Mosaicism may arise due to a postzygotic nondisjunction error during the early embryonic cell divisions or meiosis, followed by a correction of aneuploidy. Sex chromosome mosaicisms are often in combination with a Turner syndrome (45,X0) [30]. In the case of discordant fetal sex in monochorionic twin pregnancies, the phenotype depends on the proportion of sex chromosomes that dominate in the mosaicism of each twin.

   - *45, X0/46, XY in monochorionic twins*

     Postzygotic nondisjunction leading to the loss of a Y-chromosome in one twin will result in Turner syndrome with female external genitalia, while the co-twin is male. Alternatively, postzygotic nondisjunction can also lead to 45, X0/46, XY mosaicism in a monozygotic embryo, with various proportions of 45, X0, and 46, XY cells in the monochorionic twins [13].

- *46, XX/46, XY mosaicism in monochorionic twins*

  Trisomy rescue of a trisomic 47, XXY zygote can develop into a pair of diploid XX/XY mosaicism in monochorionic twins if one loses the extra X and other loses its Y chromosome [31].

- *45, X0/47 XYY monochorionic twins*

  Postzygotic nondisjunction of a 46, XY zygote involving the Y chromosome during anaphase can result in a 45, X0, and 47, XYY embryo [32].

(b) *Discordant fetal sex in monozygotic monochorionic twins due to a monogenic disorder*

Single gene defects in the sex-determining region of the Y gene can result in a discordant external sex phenotype in monozygotic twins with normal 46, XY karyotype. Theoretically, prezygotic defects in sex-determining autosomal dominant genes (e.g., SOX9) can cause discordant phenotype in monozygotic twin pairs due to variable penetrance. Another mechanism is the postzygotic mutation of an autosomal dominant gene affecting only one twin [13].

(c) *Ambiguous genitals*

Malformed external genitalia that are unrelated to chromosomal or genetic disorders can cause confusion in determining fetal sex in monochorionic twins. For example, hypospadias in a male fetus can mimic female genitalia, while a cloacal malformation with a phallus-like structure in a female fetus can mimic male genitalia [13].

(d) *Discordant fetal sex in dizygotic monochorionic twins due to chimerism*

Rarely, a pair of dizygotic twins form a monochorionic placenta. The fusion of separately fertilized embryos at the late-morula stage can result in a dizygotic MCDA twin pregnancy. As these twins originate from two different embryos, they are chimeric and can have discordant fetal sex. Due to vascular communications in their monochorionic placenta, the hematopoietic cells can intermix, causing blood chimerism. High levels of blood chimerism in dizygotic twins can lead to an erroneous assignment of monozygosity [33]. In these exceptional cases, a blood test for zygosity is unreliable, and testing should be performed on somatic tissues, such as on amniotic fluid cells, skin biopsy samples, or buccal cells [34]. Although monochorionic dizygotic twins are extremely rare, they seem to be more common after in vitro fertilization due to the associated risk of embryonic fusion before implantation [33, 35]. Monochorionic dizygotic twins are genetically and structurally healthy and must be carefully differentiated from the other causes [13].

In conclusion, not all sex-discordant twins are dichorionic, and not all monochorionic twins are monozygotic. If the first-trimester scan confirms monochorionicity, but the twins appear to be discordant in sex, an amniocentesis should be offered because of the possibility of underlying chromosomal and genetic anomalies. These pitfalls stress the importance of first-trimester determination of chorio-amnionicity, as the sonographic markers used at advanced gestational ages are not always reliable.

6.3 Conclusion

The prenatal distinction between high-risk monochorionic and lower-risk dichorionic pregnancies is essential in the follow-up and management of a twin pregnancy. Chorio-amnionicity determination is highly accurate in the first trimester and is based on the number and aspect of the layers that constitute the intertwin septum separating the twins. The diagnosis of a twin pregnancy should always specify the chorionicity and for monochorionic pairs, also the amnionicity. A photograph should be taken of the intertwin septum and kept in the case notes should doubt arise later on. In case of doubt, it is best to refer the patient to a tertiary care center in the first trimester. Other sonographic markers to determine the chorionicity after the first trimester include fetal sex, number of placental masses, and the thickness of the intertwin membranes. However, one should be aware of the associated pitfalls that make these markers less reliable.

6.3.1 Review Questions

1. What is the best time to determine the chorionicity and amnionicity on prenatal ultrasound scan?

6

2. What are the best ultrasound markers?

3. What are potential pitfalls?

6.3.2 Multiple-Choice Questions

1. A 30-year-old para 3 presents at 28 weeks for the first ultrasound scan and is diagnosed with twins. Which of the following statements is correct?
   (a) Since there are two placental masses, the pregnancy must be dichorionic.
   (b) As the babies have the same sex, chorionicity cannot be accurately determined and the pregnancy is best managed as monochorionic.
   (c) The thickness of the intertwin membrane is a reliable method to determine the chorionicity.
   (d) If no vascular anastomoses are visualized, the pregnancy is likely to be dichorionic.

Answer: (b)

2. A patient is referred at 6 weeks 4 days with suspected monoamniotic twins. You tell the patient that:
   (a) As there is only one yolk sac, monoamnionicity is confirmed.
   (b) There is no cord entanglement, the pregnancy is likely to diamniotic.
   (c) The pregnancy is likely diamniotic, but this needs confirmation after 8 weeks.
   (d) As there are two yolk sacs present, the pregnancy is diamniotic.

Answer: (c)

Disclosure Statement

The authors report no conflict of interest.

Financial Support

LL is the recipient of a grant of "Fonds voor Wetenschappelijk Onderzoek" (FWO grantnr: 1804718N).

References

1. Lewi L, Van Schoubroeck D, Gratacos E, Witters I, Timmerman D, Deprest J. Monochorionic diamniotic twins: complications and management options. Curr Opin Obstet Gynecol. 2003;15: 177–94.
2. Sebire NJ, Souka A, Skentou H, Geerts L, Nicolaides KH. First trimester diagnosis of monoamniotic twin pregnancies. Ultrasound Obstet Gynecol. 2000;16:223–5.
3. Hack KE, Derks JB, Elias SG, et al. Increased perinatal mortality and morbidity in monochorionic versus dichorionic twin pregnancies: clinical implications of a large Dutch cohort study. BJOG. 2008;115:58–67.
4. Litwinska E, Syngelaki A, Cimpoca B, Frei L, Nicolaides KH. Outcome of twin pregnancy with two live fetuses at 11–13 weeks' gestation. Ultrasound Obstet Gynecol. 2020;55:32–8. https://doi.org/10.1002/uog.21892. [Epub ahead of print].
5. D'Antonio F, Bhide A. Early pregnancy assessment in multiple pregnancies. Best Pract Res Clin Obstet Gynaecol. 2014;28(2):201–14.
6. Khalil A, Rodgers M, Baschat A, et al. ISUOG practice guidelines: role of ultrasound in twin pregnancy. Ultrasound Obstet Gynecol. 2016;47: 247–63.
7. Stenhouse E, Hardwick C, Maharaj S, Webb J, Kelly T, Mackenzie FM. Chorionicity determination in twin pregnancies: how accurate are we? Ultrasound Obstet Gynecol. 2002;19(4):350–2.
8. Carroll SGM, Soothill PW, Abdel-Fattah SA, Porter H, Montague I, Kyle PM. Prediction of chorionicity in twin pregnancies at 10–14 weeks of gestation. BJOG. 2002;109(2):182–6.
9. Shetty A, Smith PM. The sonographic diagnosis of chorionicity. Prenat Diagn. 2005;25:735–9.
10. Bora SA, Papageorghiou AT, Bottomley C, Kirk E, Bourne T. Reliability of transvaginal ultrasonography at 7–9 weeks' gestation in the determination of chorionicity and amnionicity in twin pregnancies. Ultrasound Obstet Gynecol. 2008;32(5):618–21.

11. Shen O, Samueloff A, Beller U, Rabinowitz R. Number of yolk sacs does not predict amnionicity in early first-trimester monochorionic multiple gestations. Ultrasound Obstet Gynecol. 2006;27(1):53–5.
12. Lewi L, Gucciardo L, Van Mieghem T, et al. Monochorionic diamniotic twin pregnancies: natural history and risk stratification. Fetal Diagn Ther. 2010;27(3):121–33.
13. Lu J, Cheng YKY, Ting YH, Law KM, Leung TY. Pitfalls in assessing chorioamnionicity: novel observations and literature review. Am J Obstet Gynecol. 2018;219(3):242–54.
14. Maruotti GM, Saccone G, Morlando M, Martinelli P. First-trimester ultrasound determination of chorionicity in twin gestations using the lambda sign: a systematic review and meta-analysis. Eur J Obstet Gynecol Reprod Biol. 2016;202: 66–70.
15. Finberg HJ. The "twin peak" sign: reliable evidence of dichorionic twinning. J Ultrasound Med. 1992;11:571–7.
16. Arabin B, Laurini RN, Van Eyck J. Early prenatal diagnosis of cord entanglement in monoamniotic multiple pregnancies. Ultrasound Obstet Gynecol. 1999;13:191–86.
17. Hack KE, Van Gemert MJ, Lopriore E, et al. Placental characteristics of monoamniotic twin pregnancies in relation to perinatal outcome. Placenta. 2009;30:62–5.
18. Lewi L. Cord entanglement in monoamniotic twins: does it really matter? Ultrasound Obstet Gynecol. 2010;35:139–41.
19. Rossi AC, Prefumo F. Impact of cord entanglement on perinatal outcome of monoamniotic twins: a systematic review of the literature. Ultrasound Obstet Gynecol. 2013;41:131–5.
20. Murakoshi T, Ishii K, Matsushita M, Shinno T, Naruse H, Torii Y. Monochorionic monoamniotic twin pregnancies with two yolk sacs may not be a rare finding: a report of two cases. Ultrasound Obstet Gynecol. 2010;36(3):384–6.
21. Corbett SL, Shmorgun D. Yolk sac number does not predict reliably amnionicity in monochorionic twin pregnancies: a case of a monochorionic monoamniotic twin pregnancy with two distinct yolk sacs on early first-trimester ultrasound. Ultrasound Obstet Gynecol. 2012;39(5):607–8.
22. Bishop DK. Yolk-sac number in monoamniotic twins. Obstet Gynecol. 2010;116(2):504–7.
23. Lopriore E, Sueters M, Middeldorp JM, Klumper F, Oepkes D, Vandenbussche F. Twin pregnancies with two separate placental masses can still be monochorionic and have vascular anastomoses. Am J Obstet Gynecol. 2006;194:804–8.
24. Machin GA. Why is it important to diagnose chorionicity and how do we do it? Best Pract Res Clin Obstet Gynaecol. 2004;18(4):515–30.
25. Galjaard S, Moerman P, Corveleyn A, Devlieger R, Lewi L. Partial monochorionic and monoamniotic twin pregnancies: a report of two cases. Ultrasound Obstet Gynecol. 2014;44(6):722–4.
26. Ting YH, Lao TT, Law KM, Cheng YKY, Lau TK, Leung TY. Pseudoamniotic band syndrome after in utero intervention for twin-to-twin transfusion syndrome: case reports and literature review. Fetal Diagn Ther. 2016;40:67–72.
27. Lee KJ, Kim MK, Lee SY, Lee WS, Lee YH. Spontaneous rupture of the dividing membrane in a monochorionic pregnancy resulting in a pseudo-monoamniotic pregnancy with cord entanglement. J Obstet Gynaecol Res. 2012;38:863–6.
28. Fleming T, Miller T. Spontaneous septostomy in monochorionic diamniotic twins resulting in cord entanglement and fetal demise. Australas J Ultrasound Med. 2012;15:103–6.
29. Nasrallah FK, Faden YA. Antepartum rupture of the intertwin-dividing membrane in monochorionic diamniotic twins: a case report and review of the literature. Prenat Diagn. 2005;25:856–60.
30. Grati F. Chromosomal mosaicism in human feto-placental development: implications in prenatal diagnosis. J Clin Med. 2014;3(3):809–37.
31. Zech NH, Wisser J, Natalucci G, Riegel M, Baumer A, Schinzel A. Monochorionic-diamniotic twins discordant in gender from a naturally conceived pregnancy through post-zygotic sex chromosome loss in a 47, XXY zygote. Prenat Diagn. 2008;28:759–63.
32. Bohec C, Douet-Guilbert N, Basinko A, et al. Difficult diagnosis and management of a hetero-karyotypic monochorionic twin pregnancy with discordant fetal sex and 45,X/47,XYY karyotypes. Fetal Pediatr Pathol. 2010;29:424–30.
33. Souter VL, Kapur RP, Nyholt DR, et al. A report of dizygous monochorionic twins. N Engl J Med. 2003;349:154–8.
34. Redline RW. Nonidentical twins with a single placenta – disproving dogma in perinatal pathology. N Engl J Med. 2003;349(2):111–4.
35. Miura K, Niikawa N. Do monochorionic dizygotic twins increase after pregnancy by assisted reproductive technology? J Hum Genet. 2005;50:1–6.

Key Reading

D'Antonio F, Bhide A. Early pregnancy assessment in multiple pregnancies. Best Pract Res Clin Obstet Gynaecol. 2014;28(2):201–14.

Galjaard S, Moerman P, Corveleyn A, Devlieger R, Lewi L. Partial monochorionic and monoamniotic twin pregnancies: a report of two cases. Ultrasound Obstet Gynecol. 2014;44(6):722–4.

Lu J, Cheng YKY, Ting YH, Law KM, Leung TY. Pitfalls in assessing chorioamnionicity: novel observations and literature review. Am J Obstet Gynecol. 2018;219(3):242–54.

Twin Labelling, Timing, Frequency and Content of Ultrasound Assessment

Laoreti Arianna, Faiola Stefano, and Lanna Mariano

Contents

A. Khalil et al. (eds.), *Twin and Higher-order Pregnancies*,
https://doi.org/10.1007/978-3-030-47652-6_7

Trailer

A reproducible method for antenatal labelling of twins is important in the management of all twin pregnancies. When dichorionic, 70% of twins are heterozygotes, and that makes easier to name them properly. The question is more complicated for monozygotic twins. The first fundamental moment for labelling is when screening for aneuploidy is undertaken: there must be a reliable and accurate system in place to ensure that invasive prenatal diagnosis or selective fetal reduction is carried out on the at-risk or affected twin, respectively. The identification of each fetus by the position of its placenta is of limited value. The proposed strategy of labelling twins by their proximity to the cervix also carries limitations, since fetuses are free to move independently of each other, resulting in varying presentation throughout pregnancy. Clear labelling around the time of birth is also important when communicating with the neonatal team. Antenatal labelling according to twins' site, either left or right, or upper/top and lower/bottom ensures continuity of assessment during follow-up scans and precludes any misconception regarding which twin will be born first. The frequency of monitoring with ultrasound scanning differs according to chorionicity and amnionicity. Monochorionic (MC) twins must be monitored more frequently than dichorionic (DC) twins to detect complications of shared placenta in a timely manner. Uncomplicated monochorionic twins should have a first-trimester scan and, thereafter, scans should be performed every 2 weeks starting from 16 weeks, in order to detect promptly twin-to-twin transfusion syndrome (TTTS) and twin anaemia-polycythemia sequence (TAPS). In addition to the above-mentioned parameters of fetal biometry and indices of TTTS/TAPS, ultrasound evaluation in twin pregnancies must include also the identification of patients at higher risk of preterm birth.

Definition

Labelling: identification of characteristics and position of each twin in a multiple pregnancy.

Monozygotic twins: fetuses derived from a single oocyte fertilized by a single sperm, resulting in a single zygote.

Heterozygotic twins: fetuses derived from two zygotes (see above).

Dichorionic twins: fetuses with two separate placental masses, which could be both heterozygotic and monozygotic.

Monochorionic twins: fetuses that share the same placenta, the majority of them are monozygotic.

Twin-to-twin transfusion syndrome: a typical complication of monochorionic twins where placental blood flows from one fetus, called donor, to the other, called recipient, giving a high percentage of perinatal mortality if untreated. The diagnosis is based on the evidence of oligohydramnios in donor sac and polyhydramnios in the recipient one.

Twin anemia-polycythemia sequence: the coexistence of sign of anemia in one fetus and of polycythemia in the other in a monochorionic twin pregnancies, without sign of twin-to-twin transfusion syndrome; it could arise as a spontaneous complication or after in utero treatment for TTTS.

Learning Objectives

- To learn how to identify correctly fetuses in a multiple pregnancy
- To know how to perform a prenatal management of monochorionic pregnancy
- To identify complication of a monochorionic twin pregnancy

7.1 Twin Labelling

The most challenging problems of multiple pregnancies derive from a conflict between twins (or triplets): they share the same mother, the same uterus, sometimes the same placenta, in case of monochorionicity, or even the same sac, if monoamniotic, but they are different individuals. In this context, twins deserve to be recognized and correctly identified both during prenatal and postnatal life, since for each of them there might be a different management option.

A reproducible method for antenatal labelling of twins is important in the management of all twin pregnancies to ensure that biometric measurements from longitudinal growth scans are consistently allocated to the same twin at each visit. Failure to do so may result in fluctuation of fetal growth data as smaller and larger twin sizes are swapped repeatedly during the course of the pregnancy.

When dichorionic, 70% of twins are heterozygotes, and that makes easier to name them properly, because of sex discordance or different placenta position. In the remaining 30% of dichorionic homozygotic ones, the identification could be more challenging, unless there are complications for just one twin, such as growth restriction or premature rupture of membrane and subsequent oligohydramnios.

The issue is more complicated for monozygotic twins, moreover if monochorionic: they have interdependent circulations deriving from placental vascular anastomoses [1, 2] which may give rise to specific complications such as twin-to-twin transfusion syndrome (TTTS), twin anaemia-polycythemia sequence (TAPS) and twin reversed arterial perfusion (TRAP) sequence, related to a high risk of perinatal mortality and morbidity.

In these cases, each twin has its own characteristic features (recipient, donor, etc.), and longitudinal ultrasound assessment is of a paramount importance, in order to reach an early diagnosis of complications, and carry out timely interventions for the improvement of outcomes.

The first fundamental moment for labelling is when screening for aneuploidy is undertaken: there must be a reliable and accurate system in place to ensure that invasive prenatal diagnosis or selective fetal reduction is carried out on the at-risk or affected twin, respectively [3]. In this occasion, description of site of placenta insertion (anterior/posterior), fetuses' characteristics (crown-rump length; nuchal translucency width; sex, if discordant) and their relative position in the uterus (upper/lower, left/right) is mandatory.

Nevertheless, identifying each fetus by the position of its placenta is of limited value as not only does placental position change with advancing gestation, but this technique cannot be used with twin pregnancies where the placenta is either monochorionic or fused dichorionic [4].

Furthermore, ultrasound determination of fetal sex as a discriminator is limited by unreliable fetal sexing in early pregnancy and is of no value in same-sex twin pregnancies [5].

Another proposed strategy is the labelling by twin's proximity to the cervix.

Nevertheless, it has to be considered that this nomenclature approach carries limitations and is error-prone.

In fact, while the gestational sac's position relative to the cervix remains constant throughout the pregnancy because the base of the intertwin membrane is immobile, fetuses are free to move independently of each other, resulting in varying presentation and their position relative to the cervix can change considerably, especially in early pregnancy (Fig. 7.1).

Dias et al. retrospectively demonstrated that at 11–14 weeks' gestation approximately 90% of twins have a left/right orientation, and

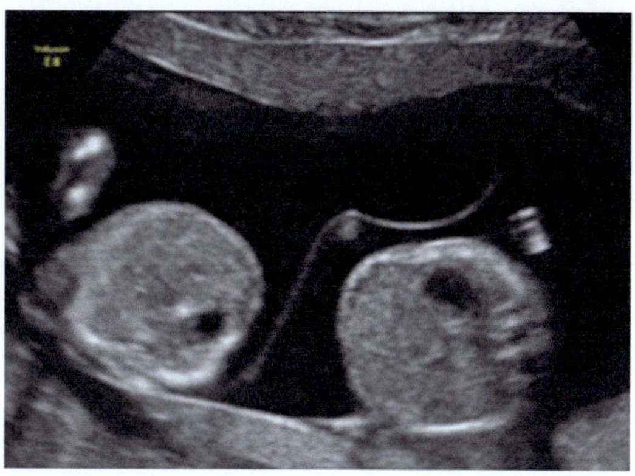

Fig. 7.1 The intertwine membrane is positioned in such a way as to divide the uterine cavity in a left/right or top/bottom orientation

the remainder are positioned in a top/bottom manner [3]. By the time of the last ultrasound scan at 34 weeks, approximately 8.5% of the left/right oriented twins have changed their presenting order, such that the fetus in the sac, further away from the cervix, is deemed to be the presenting twin. None of the top/bottom twins changed their order of presentation during the course of the pregnancy.

Clear labelling around the time of birth is also important when communicating with the neonatal team.

Ideally, the antenatal and the postnatal labelling of twins should not be conflicting and should have a standardized approach that minimizes the chances for confusion. This is particularly important in cases of twins with discordant anomalies that may not be obvious externally or when trying to correlate antenatal growth rates with postnatal growth patterns.

Paediatricians conventionally label as 'Twin 1' the first-born twin and as 'Twin 2' the second baby, irrespective of mode of delivery.

Dias et al., analysing twins of discordant sex, demonstrated that a significant number of twins switch label or nomenclature at the time of birth, and that this was influenced by the mode of delivery [3].

Fetuses designated as 'Twin 2' at the 34-week ultrasound scan were born first in approximately 25% of cases delivered by Caesarean section. This may be due to the fact that a lower-segment uterine incision may offer preferential access to the fetus designated as 'Twin 2' rather than to 'Twin 1'. In addition, the same finding occurred in about 5% of twin pregnancies delivered vaginally.

This phenomenon may be explained by a switch of the presenting twin in the 2-week interval between ultrasound assessment and delivery, resulting in the delivery of Twin 2 'through', as it were, a fold in the intertwin membrane (◘ Fig. 7.2).

In a series where a large regional database of twin ultrasound scans was considered, there was a discrepancy between antenatal labelling and the anticipated birth order in 37.6% of cases when judged by sex discordance and in 36% of cases when judged by weight discordance [6].

Multiple logistic regression analyses demonstrated that weight discordance, but not chorionicity, scan-to-delivery interval, gestation at scan or gestation at delivery, significantly influenced the change in birth order.

In the majority of normal twin pregnancies, this 'perinatal switch phenomenon' will be of no significant medical consequence.

However, it is important to alert parents and healthcare professionals attending the delivery to this fact, in order to avoid the parents' perception of apparent 'error' and in order to guide paediatricians in cases of twins discordant for structural abnormalities that are not obvious by external examination (e.g. cardiac defect, congenital diaphragmatic hernia or other internal abnormality).

When dealing with such high-risk pregnancies, standard clinical operating procedures must include an ultrasound scan performed just prior to delivery and immediate postnatal verification of the affected twin requiring further management.

In summary, accurate antenatal labelling of the twins following a reliable, consistent strategy is mandatory, and this information should be clearly documented in the woman's notes. Antenatal labelling according to twins' site, either left or right, or upper/top and lower/bottom, ensures continuity of assessment during follow-up scans and precludes any misconception regarding which twin will be born first.

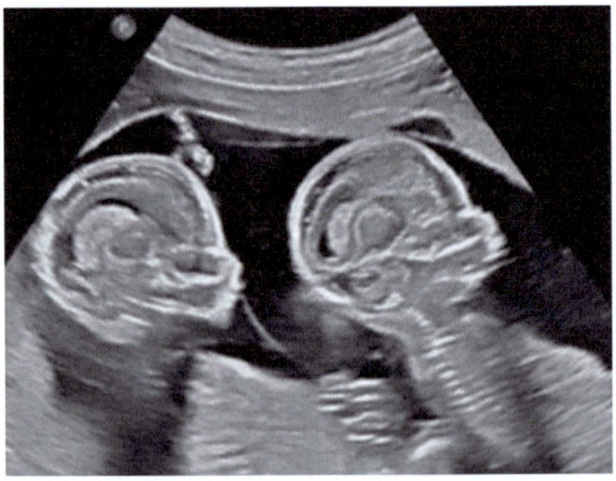

◘ **Fig. 7.2** Monochorionic twins with the same presentation, divided from a membrane, the right one is nearest to cervix the second is nearest to the uterine wall: which one will be delivered first?

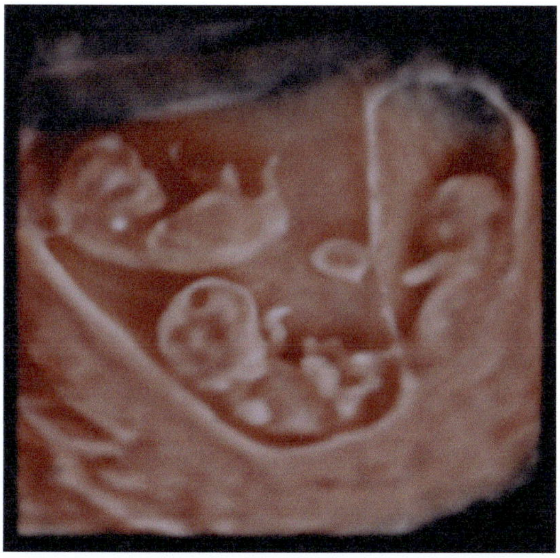

Fig. 7.3 A triplet pregnancy, dichorionic triamniotic, at 11 weeks gestation: labelling is mandatory to properly identify twins during the course of the pregnancy

The only limitation of this technique is in monoamniotic twin pregnancies, where the lack of an intertwin membrane results in both universal cord entanglement and continuously variable fetal position.

Mapping in the first trimester according to the insertion of twins' cord relative to the placental edges and membrane insertion is another option of added value.

Guidelines strongly suggest to describe each twin using as many features as possible, so as to enable others to identify them accurately (e.g. 'Twin A (female) is on the maternal right with a posterior placenta and marginal cord insertion') (Fig. 7.3).

For pregnancies with discordance, the labelling should be accompanied by a description such as 'Twin A, recipient' [7].

7.2 Timing, Frequency and Content of Ultrasound Assessment in Twin Pregnancy

The frequency of monitoring with ultrasound scanning differs according to chorionicity and amnionicity. Monochorionic (MC) twins must be monitored more frequently than dichorionic (DC) twins to detect complications of shared placenta in a timely manner. It is recommended to provide individualized rather than conventional care from a fetal medicine specialist for twins with a shared amnion, ideally in a tertiary care centre (Fig. 7.2).

7.2.1 Uncomplicated DC Twin Pregnancy

In uncomplicated dichorionic twin pregnancy, ultrasound imaging should be performed in the first trimester, again at around 20 weeks' gestation (second-trimester anomaly scan), and every 4 weeks thereafter (unless a complication is detected which might require more frequent scans).

At each ultrasound assessment, the following should be assessed: fetal biometry, amniotic fluid volume and umbilical artery Doppler (from 20 weeks' gestation) for both twins [7].

Discordance in estimated fetal weight (EFW) should be calculated and documented at each scan from 20 weeks (Fig. 7.3).

In DC pregnancies, sIUGR should be followed as in growth-restricted singletons. The timing of delivery should be determined based on a risk-benefit assessment and according to the wishes of the parents, guided by obstetric and neonatal counselling. As these twins have separate circulations, the pregnancy can be followed as in growth-restricted singleton pregnancy, monitoring for progressive deterioration of umbilical artery, MCA and DV Doppler, and of biophysical profile scores. These pregnancies should be managed in specialist centres with the relevant expertise.

Cervical length assessment should also be performed ideally at the same visit as the anomaly scan in the second trimester using a cut-off of 25 mm, in order to identify women at risk of extreme preterm birth.

7.2.2 Monochorionic (MC) Twin Pregnancy

In uncomplicated MC twin pregnancy, ultrasound fetal surveillance is intended to detect complications of shared placenta in a timely manner.

International Guidelines recommend that uncomplicated monochorionic twins have a first-trimester scan and, thereafter, scans should be performed every 2 weeks starting from 16 weeks, in order to detect promptly TTTS and TAPS [7].

Indeed, intensive monitoring is required since TTTS and TAPS may complicate abruptly and unpredictably these pregnancies, and also the progression of stage in TTTS is not predicted accurately [8].

The optimal interval between ultrasound scans has been object of studies [9–11].

Thorson et al. retrospectively examined the association between interval from previous ultrasound to diagnosis of TTTS and stage at diagnosis according to Quintero.

The interval was categorized as 14 days or less or greater than 14 days.

The authors found that twin-twin transfusion syndrome was more likely to be diagnosed at advanced stage with an ultrasound interval greater than 14 days (p = .004). In the group scanned with an interval ≤14 days, there were only two cases (13.3%) of late twin-twin transfusion syndrome (Quintero Stage ≥ III) compared to 16 cases (59%) in the group scanned with an interval >14 days. These data suggested that a maximum surveillance interval of 14 days for monochorionic twins might lead to earlier stage at diagnosis, earlier intervention, and better outcomes [11].

These findings were recently supported by a retrospective study by McDonald et al. [9].

Authors found a trend towards a longer interval for cases with advanced TTTS compared to early TTTS. The interval between ultrasound scans was longer in cases with unexplained fetal demise in utero and advanced TTTS than early TTTS (3.4 weeks vs. 0.9 weeks, $p < 0.05$), supporting current recommendations for fortnightly ultrasound surveillance.

Two sets of parameters must be evaluated at each ultrasound assessment: fetal biometry, in order to identify growth disorders, and indices of TTTS and TAPS.

With regard to these latter complications, at every scan the operator should note and record evidence of membrane folding, measure the deepest vertical pocket (DVP) of amniotic fluid for each fetus, evaluate bladder sizes and fetal Doppler indices starting from 16 weeks for the umbilical artery (UA) and from 20 weeks for the middle-cerebral artery (MCA).

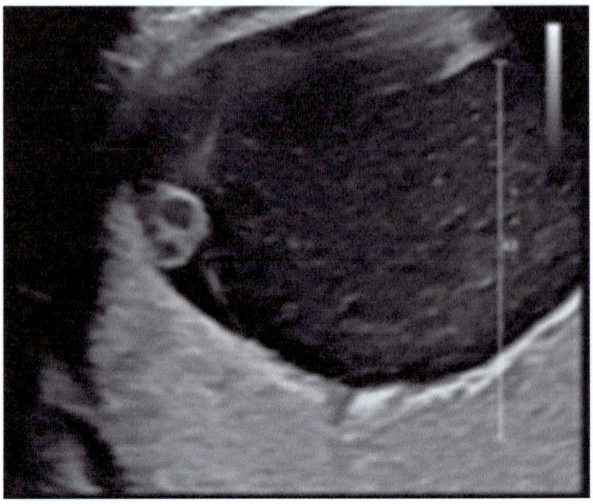

Fig. 7.4 A polyhydramnios-oligohydramnios sequence that define a twin-to-twin transfusion syndrome (TTTS)

If significant inequality in DVP exists or there is membrane infolding, then more frequent ultrasound surveillance may be warranted (Figs. 7.4 and 7.5a, b).

Complicated monochorionic twins should be scanned more frequently, depending on the condition and its severity [7, 12].

According to the National Institute for Health and Care Excellence guidance, EFW discordance should be calculated and documented at every scan from 20 weeks onwards.

If this discordance reaches 25% or more, a referral should be made to a tertiary-level Fetal Medicine Unit for assessment, increased fetal surveillance, including fetal Doppler, and planning of delivery when appropriate.

EFW charts that include a combination of head, abdomen and femur measurements perform best in both singleton and twin pregnancy [7].

Currently, the charts used to monitor fetal growth in twin pregnancy are the same as those used for singletons.

However, studies have shown a reduction in fetal growth in twin compared with singleton pregnancy, particularly in the third trimester.

Stirrup et al. [13] provided ultrasound biometry charts in a large group of normal

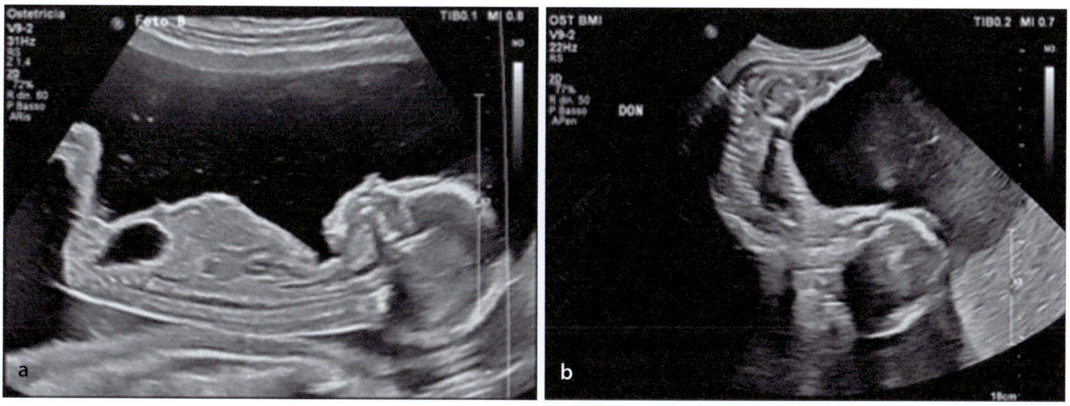

Fig. 7.5 **a** A recipient twin with a large bladder, compared to **b** a 'stuck' donor twin

twin gestations showing a reduced growth rate in monochorionic compared to dichorionic sets. Notably in this study, parental factors have not been considered in constructing the nomograms.

More recently, a retrospective multicentre study including 1781 uncomplicated twin pregnancies (1289 DC and 492 MCDA) was performed with the aim to construct reference charts for gestation of fetal biometric parameters, stratified by chorionicity and customized for obstetrical and parental characteristics [14].

Authors confirmed the previously reported finding of a different growth pattern in comparison with singleton fetuses, with a flattening of the biometric curve starting at 26–28 weeks of gestation for all biometric parameters.

Differences with singleton charts were larger in monochorionic twins, progressively increasing during the third trimester for some parameters such as abdominal circumference.

Moreover, as previously shown in singletons, a relationship between fetal biometric data and parental characteristic and fetal gender was documented in both dichorionic and monochorionic twins, supporting the use of customized nomograms.

In clinical practice, the use of specific twin growth charts is controversial due to the concern that the reduced growth in the third trimester observed in most twin pregnancies might be caused by some degree of placental insufficiency, warranting close observation [7].

A prospective validation study is needed to prove that customized twin growth chart curves are superior to singleton or non-customized twin curves.

Doppler ultrasound investigation of umbilical and fetal circulation is widely used for fetal surveillance in high-risk pregnancies, with proven efficacy for identifying fetal compromise and improving pregnancy outcome.

Doppler assessment in MC twins has been proved useful in diagnosing and managing fetal anaemia, sIUGR and TTTS [15–17].

International Guidelines recommend the assessment of fetal Doppler indices starting from 16 weeks for the umbilical artery (UA) and from 20 weeks for the middle-cerebral artery (MCA). In MC twin pregnancy complicated by sIUGR, fetal Doppler (UA and MCA) should be assessed at least weekly. If the UA Doppler is abnormal, assessment of the ductus venosus (DV) blood flow should be undertaken [7].

Fetal Doppler velocimetry can be evaluated in both a qualitative and a quantitative manner. In clinical practice, qualitative waveform assessment is mostly used, e.g. absent or reverse umbilical artery (ARED-UA) or ductus venosus (DV) a-wave end-diastolic flow (Fig. 7.6a–c).

Quantitative reference values for UA, MCA and DV Doppler velocimetry in MC twins are lacking, leading to increased difficulty in the interpretation of ominous quantitative findings such as an increased UA-Pulsatility Index (UA-PI) value referred to singleton nomograms.

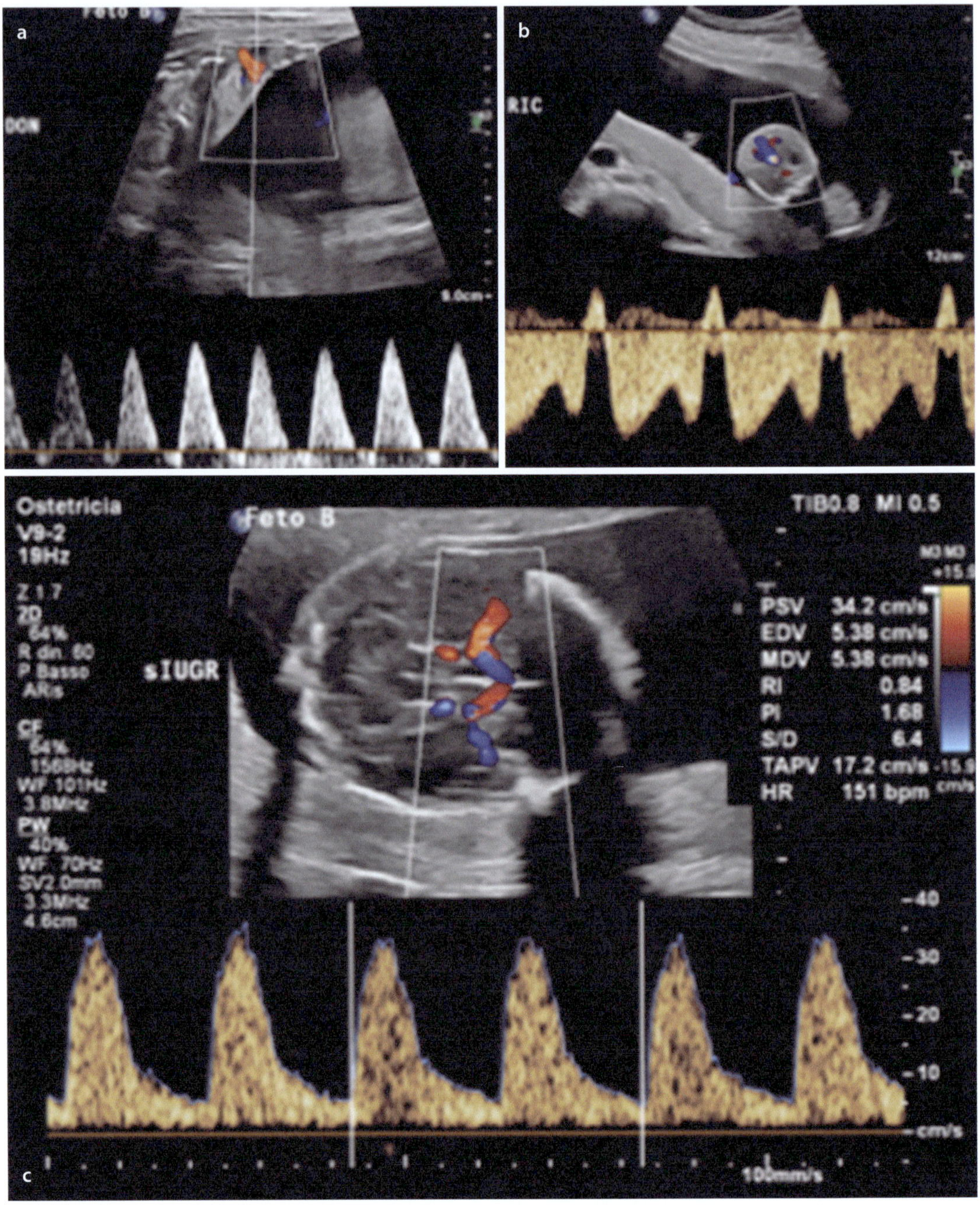

Fig. 7.6 **a** Doppler velocimetry on umbilical artery in a donor twin, with absent-reversed end-diastolic flow. **b** Doppler velocimetry on ductus venosus in a recipient twin, with reversed '**a**' wave. **c** Doppler velocimetry on middle cerebral artery

As for intrauterine growth charts, some authors have suggested that singleton Doppler nomograms are not appropriate for interpreting findings in twins [18, 19].

Mulcahy et al. performed a prospective multicentre cohort study in Ireland and reported the longitudinal references for UA-PI and UA-Resistance Index (UA-RI), MCA-PI and MCA-peak systolic velocity (PSV) and cerebroplacental ratios (CPR) derived from 508 DC and 110 MC twin pregnancies from 24 to 38 weeks of gestation.

They found that both in DC and MC twins, UA-PI and UA-RI appeared to be higher than in singletons, while MCA-PI, MCA-PSV and CPR appeared lower [18].

Klaritsch et al. prospectively examined 50 uncomplicated MC pregnancies, aiming at establishing gestational age-specific reference ranges for MCA-PSV in MC twin. Authors found that MCA-PSV increased with advancing gestational age, showing measurements comparable to singletons between 18 and 37 weeks. However, before 18 weeks MCA-PSV values were higher in MC twin pregnancies compared to singleton pregnancies, possibly leading to increased number of false-positive diagnoses of presumed fetal anaemia if singletons references are used [19].

Our unit has recently conducted a retrospective study on 150 uncomplicated MC twin pairs to construct specific longitudinal Doppler references for UA-PI, MCA-PI and MCA-PSV and DV-PI. Estimated centiles (3rd, 5th, 10th, 50th, 90th, 95th, 97th) of UA-PI, MCA-PI, MCA-PSV and DV-PI according to the gestational age were presented. The comparison with singletons showed substantial differences, with higher UA-PI and lower MCA-PI and PSV median values in MC twins. Median DV-PI values were similar to the values for singletons, while the upper centiles were higher in MC twins. The comparison with singleton reference values underscores the deviation from physiology that is intrinsic to these unique pregnancies and supports the need for MC twin-specific charts [20].

In addition to the above-mentioned parameters of fetal biometry and indices of TTTS/TAPS, ultrasound evaluation in MC twin pregnancy must include also the identification of patients at higher risk of preterm birth.

Cervical length measurement is the preferred method of screening for preterm birth in twins and is performed ideally at the same visit as the anomaly scan in the second trimester.

A cervical length <25 mm at 18–24 weeks' gestation in twin pregnancy is a moderate predictor of preterm birth before 34 weeks, but not before 37 weeks [21].

Conde-Agudelo et al. [21] showed that in asymptomatic women a cervical length ≤20 mm at 20–24 weeks is the most accurate predictor of preterm birth before 32 and before 34 weeks (pooled sensitivities, specificities and positive and negative likelihood ratios were 39% and 29%; 96% and 97%; 10.1 and 9.0; and 0.64 and 0.74, respectively).

A cervical length ≤25 mm at 20–24 weeks has a pooled positive likelihood ratio of 9.6 for the prediction of preterm birth before 28 weeks.

7.3 Triplets and Higher-Order Multifetal Pregnancy

Triplet and higher-order multiple pregnancies are associated with significantly increased risks of maternal and neonatal morbidity compared with both twin and singleton gestations, and close surveillance is required in this setting [22].

Determination of chorionicity and amnionicity, ideally performed in the first trimester, is the first critical step for risk assessment, counselling (including options of fetal reduction) and pregnancy management.

As for twin pregnancies, it is important to use a consistent strategy for identifying and labelling each fetus over serial ultrasound examinations [23].

In trichorionic triplet pregnancies, recognition of distinctive placental masses, different placental position and sex discordance may be helpful in naming the fetuses properly.

In dichorionic triplet pregnancies, a monochorionic pair is identified (possibly sharing the same amniotic sac) and mapping in the first trimester according to the insertion of fetuses' cord relative to the placental edges, and membrane insertion is an option of additional value.

Antenatal labelling according to fetuses' site, either left or right, or upper/lower, is based on the fact that the gestational sac's position relative to the cervix remains constant throughout the pregnancy and ensures continuity of assessment during follow-up scans.

Guidelines strongly recommend to describe each fetus using as many features as possible (e.g. dichorionic triamniotic triplet pregnancy. Twin A, independent fetus, female, is on the maternal left with a posterior placenta and marginal cord insertion'; monochorionic pair: Twin B, male, is on maternal top right, with an anterior placenta and a central cord insertion; Twin C, male, is on maternal bottom right, with an anterior placenta and a marginal cord insertion).

Documentation of chorionicity, amnionicity and labelling must be included clearly in the woman's notes.

Ultrasound surveillance differs according to chorionicity and amnionicity [23].

In uncomplicated trichorionic triamniotic triplet pregnancies, ultrasound imaging should be performed in the first trimester, again at around 20 weeks' gestation, 24, 26, 28, 30, 32 and 34 weeks (unless a complication is detected which might require more frequent scans). At each ultrasound assessment, the following should be assessed: fetal biometry, amniotic fluid volume and umbilical artery Doppler for each fetus.

Dichorionic triamniotic and monochorionic triamniotic triplets must be monitored more frequently in order to promptly detect complications of shared placenta. Ultrasound assessment should be performed in the first trimester, at 16 weeks and every 2 weeks thereafter (18, 20, 22, 24, 26, 28, 30, 32, and 34 weeks). Fetal biometry and indices of TTTS and TAPS must be assessed at each scan.

Triplets with a shared amnion should require individualized care from a fetal medicine specialist in a tertiary care centre.

Despite the high incidence of preterm birth in triplet pregnancies (with a mean gestational age of approximately 32 weeks), cervical length measurement is not a sensitive screening test in higher-order gestations, and there is no strong evidence that any intervention (e.g. progesterone supplementation, cerclage) is beneficial for preventing preterm birth in women with multifetal gestations and short cervical length [24].

7.3.1 Review Questions

1. What is the benefit of antenatal ultrasound labelling in multiple pregnancies?
2. What is the most reproducible and reliable method of antenatal labelling in multiple pregnancies?
3. Describe the 'perinatal switch phenomenon' and the potential clinical consequences related to this.
4. What is the recommended timing and frequency of ultrasound scans in uncomplicated monochorionic twin pregnancies?
5. Describe the parameters that must be evaluated at each ultrasound scan in monochorionic twin pregnancies.
6. What are the main differences reported by studies in UA-PI and MCA-PSV in monochorionic twin compared to singleton pregnancies?

7. Describe the recommended pathway of ultrasound surveillance in trichorionic triamniotic triplet pregnancy.

7.3.2 Multiple-Choice Questions

1. What is the most reliable method for antenatal labeling in twin pregnancies?
   A. Determination of placenta position
   B. Determination of fetal sex
   C. Determination of twin's proximity to the cervix
   D. Determination of twins' site, either left or right, or upper/top and lower/bottom

Answer is D. Identifying each fetus by the position of its placenta is of limited value because this technique cannot be used with twin pregnancies where the placenta is either monochorionic or fused dichorionic. Ultrasound determination of fetal sex as a discriminator is limited by unreliable fetal sexing in early pregnancy and is of no value in same-sex twin pregnancies. Assessment of twin's proximity to the cervix also carries limitations and is error-prone. In fact, while the gestational sac's position relative to the cervix remains constant throughout the pregnancy because the base of the intertwin membrane is immobile, fetuses are free to move independently of each other, resulting in varying presentation, and their position relative to the cervix can change considerably, especially in early pregnancy.

2. Which is the optimal interval between scans (after first trimester scan) in uncomplicated monochorionic twin pregnancies?
   A. Every 2 weeks starting from 18 weeks
   B. Every 4 weeks starting from 16 weeks
   C. Every 2 weeks starting from 16 weeks
   D. Weekly starting from 16 weeks

Answer is C. Studies on uncomplicated monochorionic twins have shown that a maximum surveillance interval of 14 days, starting from 16 weeks, might lead to earlier stage of TTTS at diagnosis, earlier intervention, and better outcomes.

Complicated monochorionic twins should be scanned more frequently, depending on the condition and its severity

3. Which parameters should NOT be evaluated routinely at each ultrasound assessment in monochorionic twin pregnancies?
   A. Fetal biometry
   B. Deepest vertical pocket (DVP) of amniotic fluid for each fetus
   C. Bladder sizes for each fetus
   D. Fetal Doppler indices starting from 16 weeks
   E. Tricuspid valve regurgitation

Answer is E. Fetal biometry must be assessed at each visit and estimated fetal weight (EFW) discordance should be calculated and documented at every scan. If this discordance reaches 25% or more, a referral should be made to a tertiary-level Fetal Medicine Unit for assessment and increased fetal surveillance. In addition to this, indices of TTTS and TAPS must be evaluated at each scan, and the operator should note and record evidence of membrane folding, measure the DVP of amniotic fluid for each fetus, evaluate bladder sizes and fetal Doppler indices starting from 16 weeks for the umbilical artery (UA) and from 20 weeks for the middlec-Cerebral artery (MCA).

4. Which is the preferred method of screening of preterm birth in twin pregnancies?
   A. Fetal fibronectin testing alone
   B. Cervical length measurements
   C. Home uterine activity monitoring
   D. sFLT1/PLGF

Answer is B. Cervical length measurement is the preferred method of screening for preterm birth in twins; 25 mm is the cutoff most commonly used in the second trimester. A cervical length $\leq$25 mm at

20–24 weeks has a pooled positive likelihood ratio of 9.6 for the prediction of preterm birth before 28 weeks.

5. Which is the recommended timing and frequency of ultrasound in uncomplicated dichorionic twin pregnancies?
   - A. In the first trimester and every 2 weeks starting from 18 weeks
   - B. In the first trimester and every 4 weeks starting from 18 weeks
   - C. In the first trimester and every 4 weeks starting from 20 weeks
   - D. In the first trimester and every 3 weeks starting from 20 weeks

Answer is C. In uncomplicated dichorionic twin pregnancy, ultrasound imaging should be performed in the first trimester, again at around 20 weeks' gestation (second-trimester anomaly scan), and every 4 weeks thereafter (unless a complication is detected which might require more frequent scans). At each ultrasound assessment, the following should be assessed: fetal biometry, amniotic fluid volume and umbilical artery Doppler (from 20 weeks' gestation) for both twins.

Acknowledgments We thank Dr. Mariangela Rustico for her leading role in managing monochorionic twins at our centre.

References

1. Zhao DP, de Villiers SF, Slaghekke F, Walther FJ, Middeldorp JM, Oepkes D, Lopriore E. Prevalence, size, number and localization of vascular anastomoses in monochorionic placentas. Placenta. 2013;34(7):589–93.
2. Lanna MM, Consonni D, Faiola S, Schena V, Ratti M, Ferrazzi E, Rustico MA. Color-dye injection of monochorionic placentas and correlation with pregnancy complications. Placenta. 2015;36: 1095e1099e.
3. Dias T, Ladd S, Mahsud-Dornan S, Bhide A, Papageorghiou A, Thilaganathan B. Systematic labelling of twin pregnancies on ultrasound. Ultrasound Obstet Gynecol. 2011;38:130–3.
4. Oppenheimer L, Holmes P, Simpson N, Dabrowski A. Diagnosis of low-lying placenta: can migration in the third trimester predict outcome? Ultrasound Obstet Gynecol. 2001;18:100–2.
5. Harrington K, Armstrong V, Freeman J, Aquilina J, Campbell S. Fetal sexing by ultrasound in the second trimester: maternal preference and professional ability. Ultrasound Obstet Gynecol. 1996;8:318–21.
6. D'Antonio F, Dias T. B. Thilaganathan on behalf of the Southwest Thames Obstetric Research Collaborative (STORK). Does antenatal ultrasound labeling predict birth order in twin pregnancies? Ultrasound Obstet Gynecol. 2013;41(3):274–7.
7. Khalil A, Rodgers M, Baschat A, Bhide A, Gratacos E, Hecher K, Kilby MD, Lewi L, Nicolaides KH, Oepkes D, Raine-Fenning N, Reed K, Salomon LJ, Sotiriadis A, Thilaganathan B, Ville Y. ISUOG practice guidelines: role of ultrasound in twin pregnancy. Ultrasound Obstet Gynecol. 2016;47:247–63.
8. Dickinson JE, Evans SF. The progression of disease stage in twin-twin transfusion syndrome. J Matern Fetal Neonatal Med. 2004;16(2):95–101.
9. McDonald R, Hodges R, Knight M, Teoh M, Edwards A, Neil P, Wallace EM, DeKoninck P. Optimal interval between ultrasound scans for the detection of complications in MonochorionicTwins. Fetal Diagn Ther. 2017;41(3):197–201.
10. Sueters M, Middeldorp JM, Lopriore E, Oepkes D, Kanhai HH, Vandenbussche FP. Timely diagnosis of twin-to-twin transfusion syndrome in monochorionic twin pregnancies by biweekly sonography combined with patient instruction to report onset of symptoms. Ultrasound Obstet Gynecol. 2006;28(5):659–64.
11. Thorson HL, Ramaeker DM, Emery SP. Optimal interval for ultrasound surveillance in monochorionic twin gestations. Obstet Gynecol. 2011; 117(5):1227.
12. Kilby MD. Bricker L on behalf of the Royal College of Obstetricians and Gynaecologists. Management of monochorionic twin pregnancy. BJOG. 2016;124:e1–e45.
13. Stirrup OT, Khalil A, D'Antonio F, Thilaganathan B. Southwest Thames Obstetric Research C. Fetal growth reference ranges in twin pregnancy: analysis of the Southwest Thames Obstetric Research Collaborative (STORK) multiple pregnancy cohort. Ultrasound Obstet Gynecol. 2015;45: 301–7.
14. Ghi T, Prefumo F, Fichera A, Lanna M, Periti E, Persico N, Viora E, Rizzo G. Società Italiana di Ecografia Ostetrica e Ginecologica Working Group on fetal biometric charts. Development of customized fetal growth charts in twins. Am J Obstet Gynecol. 2017;216(5):514.e1–514.e17.
15. Gratacós E, Lewi L, Carreras E, Lewi L, Carreras E, Becker J, Higueras T, Deprest J, Cabero L. Incidence and characteristics of umbilical artery intermittent absent and/or reversed end-diastolic flow in complicated and uncomplicated monochorionic twin pregnancies. Ultrasound Obstet Gynecol. 2004;23:456–60.

16. Quintero RA, Morales WJ, Allen MH, Bornick PW, Johnson PK, Kruger M. Staging of twin-twin transfusion syndrome. J Perinatol. 1999 Dec;19(8):550–5.
17. Tollenaar LSA, Lopriore E, Middeldorp JM, Haak MC, Klumper FJ, Oepkes D, Slaghekke F. Improved prediction of twin anemia-polycythemia sequence by delta middle cerebral artery peak systolic velocity: new antenatal classification system. Ultrasound Obstet Gynecol. 2019;53(6):788–93.
18. Mulcahy C, McAuliffe FM, Breathnach F, Geary M, Daly S, Higgins J, Hunter A, Morrison J, Burke G, Higgins S, Dicker P, Mahony R, Tully E, Malone F. Umbilical and fetal middle cerebral artery Doppler reference ranges in a twin population followed longitudinally from 24 to 38 weeks' gestation. Ultrasound Obstet Gynecol. 2014;44(4):461–7.
19. Klaritsch P, Deprest J, Van Mieghem T, Gucciardo L, Done E, Jani J, Lewi P, Rasmussen S, Lewi L. Reference ranges for middle cerebral artery peak systolic velocity in monochorionic diamniotic twins: a longitudinal study. Ultrasound Obstet Gynecol. 2009;34:149–54.
20. Casati D, Pellegrino M, Cortinovis I, Spada E, Lanna M, Faiola S, Cetin I, Rustico MA. Longitudinal Doppler references for monochorionic twins and comparison with singletons. PLoS One. 2019;14(12):e0226090.
21. Conde-Agudelo A, Romero R. Prediction of preterm birth in twin gestations using biophysical and biochemical tests. Am J Obstet Gynecol. 2014;211:583–95.
22. Luke B, Brown MB. Maternal morbidity and infant death in twin vs triplet and quadruplet pregnancies. Am J Obstet Gynecol. 2008;198:401.e1.
23. National Institute for Health and Care Excellence (NICE) guideline [NG137]. Twin and triplet pregnancy. September: Published date; 2019.
24. Fichera A, Pagani G, Stagnati V, Cascella S, Faiola S, Gaini C, Lanna M, Pasquini L, Raffaelli R, Stampalija T, Tommasini A, Prefumo F. Cervical-length measurement in mid-gestation to predict spontaneous preterm birth in asymptomatic triplet pregnancy. Ultrasound Obstet Gynecol. 2018;51(5):614.

Key Reading

Casati D, Pellegrino M, Cortinovis I, Spada E, Lanna M, Faiola S, Cetin I, Rustico MA. Longitudinal Doppler references for monochorionic twins and comparison with singletons. PloS One. 2019;14(12): e0226090.

D'Antonio F, Dias T, Thilaganathan B. on behalf of the Southwest Thames Obstetric Research Collaborative (STORK). Does antenatal ultrasound labeling predict birth order in twin pregnancies? Ultrasound Obstet Gynecol. 2013;41(3):274–7.

Dias T, Ladd S, Mahsud-Dornan S, Bhide A, Papageorghiou A, Thilaganathan B. Systematic labelling of twin pregnancies on ultrasound. Ultrasound Obstet Gynecol. 2011;38:130–133.

Khalil A, Rodgers M, Baschat A, Bhide A, Gratacos E, Hecher K, Kilby MD, Lewi L, Nicolaides KH, Oepkes D, Raine-Fenning N, Reed K, Salomon LJ, Sotiriadis A, Thilaganathan B, Ville Y. ISUOG practice guidelines: role of ultrasound in twin pregnancy. Ultrasound Obstet Gynecol. 2016;47: 247–263.

Thorson HL, Ramaeker DM, Emery SP. Optimal interval for ultrasound surveillance in monochorionic twin gestations. Obstet Gynecol. 2011;117(5):1227.

Prenatal Screening for and Diagnosis of Aneuploidy in Twin Pregnancies

Alexandra Matias, Beatriz Teixeira, and Miguel Macedo

Contents

A. Khalil et al. (eds.), *Twin and Higher-order Pregnancies*,
https://doi.org/10.1007/978-3-030-47652-6_8

Trailer

Prenatal screening poses specific challenges in multiple pregnancies but is in high demand due to the increased prevalence of multiple pregnancies. Both ultrasound and biochemical screening methods are available, although they are less accurate than in singleton pregnancies. The introduction of non-invasive prenatal testing has been a big step forward with higher sensitivities and lower false-positive rates. In this chapter, we present an overview of the methods and implications of screening for aneuploidy in multiple pregnancies, which will aid in the counseling of prospective parents.

Definitions

Combined screening: a combination of nuchal translucency and biochemical markers (serum-free β-human chorionic gonadotropin (β-hCG) and pregnancy-associated plasma protein-A (PAPP-A)) at 11–14 weeks of gestation

Contingent screening: the individual risk for trisomy 21 is classified as high, low, or intermediate, with only those in the intermediate group requiring additional screening with a non-invasive prenatal test

NIPT: non-invasive prenatal test

cff DNA: cell-free fetal DNA

Learning Objectives

- To understand the difference between screening and diagnosis
- To understand the different ultrasound and biochemical modalities available for prenatal screening in twins and multiple pregnancies
- To understand the superiority of non-invasive prenatal testing in the screening for major aneuploidies in twins
- To understand the importance of counseling of prospective parents when faced with the complexities of twin or higher-order multiple pregnancies

Prenatal screening and diagnosis pose specific challenges in multiple pregnancies [5, 26, 36] but are in high demand due to the increased prevalence of multiple pregnancies. Both ultrasound and biochemical screening methods are available, although they are less accurate than in singleton pregnancies. The introduction of non-invasive prenatal testing has meant a big step forward with higher sensitivities at lower false-positive rates. Most of these tests will define a risk for the pregnancy and not a fetus-specific risk. Moreover, faced with a "screen-positive" result, there is no feature to suggest which fetus may be affected. Furthermore, invasive diagnostic tests are more complex in twins, and it may be difficult to ensure that both twins are sampled. In this chapter, we present an overview of the methods and implications of screening for aneuploidy in multiple pregnancies, which will aid in the counseling of prospective parents.

8.1 Screening Versus Diagnosis

A screening test is not equivalent to a diagnostic test. Screening is applied to a low-risk asymptomatic population in order to identify and treat individuals at higher than baseline risk for suffering from a specific disease. A diagnostic test and a preventive or curative measure must always be available or the purpose of screening will not be accomplished.

The effectiveness of screening requires a series of prerequisites to make it clinically useful. A diagnostic test, on the other hand, does not quantify the risk for a disease but rather confirms with certainty the presence or absence of the disease.

Hence, a screening test should stick to the following requirements:

- The *natural history of the disease* should be *well understood*.
- The disease should be *prevalent*.
- The test should have a low false-positive rate (*high specificity*).
- The test should have a low false-negative rate (*high sensitivity*).
- The test should be *simple*, *safe*, *reproducible*, and *reliable*.
- *Benefits* should outweigh the *risks*.
- The test should be *cost-effective*.

- The whole population should have *equal access* to the test.
- The test should be *acceptable* clinically, socially and ethically.

8.2 Screening for Aneuploidies: What Can We Offer?

In the early 1970s, *maternal age* was the only available method. Screening based on maternal age is cheap, universally available, has no intra- or inter-observer variation, is noninvasive, and is understandable by the women screened. The only drawback is its low sensitivity and high false-positive rate.

In the late 1980s, screening based on the quantification of fetoplacental markers in the maternal blood (*biochemical screening*) was introduced in the second trimester [42, 62].

The last 30 years have focused on screening for aneuploidies in the first trimester, achieving progressively higher sensitivity and lower false-positive rates (◘ Fig. 8.1). In the 1990s, screening also shifted from biochemical to fetal markers. A significant improvement was the combination of maternal age and several sonographic markers, such as fetal *nuchal translucency thickness* (NT) at 11–14 weeks. The combination of maternal age with NT measurement identified about 75% of trisomy 21 fetuses for a screen-positive rate of about 5% [55].

In 1998, ductus venosus (DV) blood flow assessment was introduced in clinical practice [35] along with nasal bone [12]. More recently, Abele and co-workers [1] published a more inclusive study on first-trimester screening for aneuploidies confirming the results from previous studies based on maternal age, fetal nuchal translucency, and different combinations of the additional markers nasal bone, tricuspid, and ductus venosus flow [1].

Twenty years later, screening for trisomy 21 in singleton pregnancies has seen a tremendous improvement with the introduction of *non-invasive prenatal test (NIPT)* using cell-free fetal DNA drawn from maternal blood [6, 28–30, 34, 60]. On the verge of 2020, the efficacy of screening for trisomy 21 reached a sensitivity of 99.9% at a false-positive rate of 0.01% (◘ Fig. 8.1).

8.3 Screening for Aneuploidies: What if There Are Two or More?

In developed countries, the incidence of multiple pregnancies has increased dramatically since the 1980s. Delayed childbearing and the more frequent use of subfertility treatment account for this clinically relevant increase. Therefore, there is an increased need for accurate screening methods in twin pregnancies. Overall, about 66% of twin pregnancies are dizygotic, and 33% are monozygotic. Monochorionic twins are always monozy-

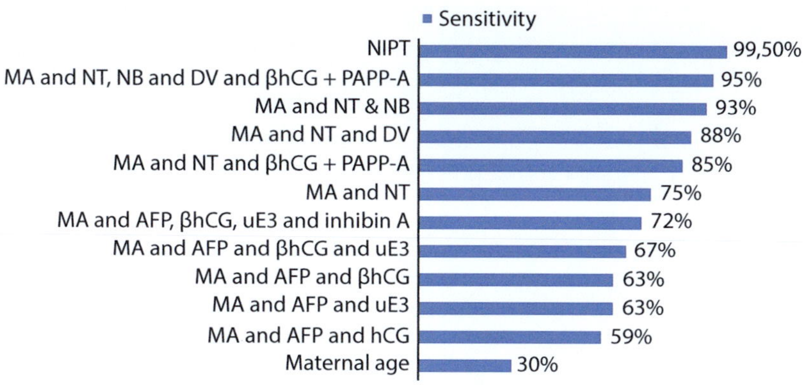

◘ **Fig. 8.1** Evolution of screening for trisomy 21 throughout the last 30 years in terms of sensitivity, for a false-positive rate of 5% (except NIPT, which has a false-positive rate of 0.1%). MA – maternal age; AFP – alfa fetoprotein; hCG – gonadotrophin hormone; uE3 – non-conjugated estriol; NT – nuchal translucency; DV – ductus venosus; NB – nasal bones; NIPT – non-invasive prenatal test

gotic, whereas about 90% of dichorionic twins are dizygotic. On prenatal ultrasound scan, we cannot determine the zygosity in same-sex dichorionic twin pregnancies.

Before parents can decide on whether to embark on screening or not in the setting of their twin pregnancy, different aspects should be discussed. As such, the issue of chorionicity, the lower sensitivity of prenatal screening for aneuploidies, the higher risk of an invasive test, and the options of selective reduction in mono-and dichorionic pregnancies and its associated risks should all be thoroughly explained to the parents-to-be.

These multiple pregnancies pose diverse challenges to what concerns the application of screening techniques. Overall, twin pregnancies are at higher risk than singleton pregnancies for aneuploidy, because of the presence of two twins. However, the risk in twin pregnancies depends on zygosity, rather than chorionicity [16]. In monozygotic pregnancies, both fetuses are usually concordant for chromosomal abnormalities, as such twins are considered to be identical. In contrast, dizygotic twins are genetically different and, therefore, may be discordant for aneuploidies.

Monochorionic pregnancies are monozygotic, and both twins are considered to have a similar risk of aneuploidy [5]. Monozygotic twins seem to have a considerably lower risk of aneuploidy than dizygotic twins and singletons. As such, a monochorionic twin has a risk that is approximately one-third of the risk in singleton pregnancies for a mother of similar age, although both fetuses are usually affected [8, 56]. Importantly, infertility treatments are associated with a 2- to 12-fold increased risk of monozygotic and mostly monochorionic twinning [7].

Dichorionic twins may be monozygotic or dizygotic. Dichorionic twins with discordant sex are always dizygotic. In the case of same-sex dichorionic twins, zygosity cannot be determined before birth unless genetic testing is performed. Dizygotic twin pregnancies were considered to have twice the risk of that of a singleton pregnancy, as both twins have an independent risk of a chromosomal abnormality [15]. However, recent studies have shown a lower incidence of fetal aneuploidy than previously expected. As such, the risk of a dizygotic pregnancy being affected by trisomy 21 is only about a third higher than a singleton pregnancy at all maternal ages up to 44 [8, 56]. One explanation for this discrepancy may be the higher rates of fetal loss in twin pregnancies. Unfortunately, there are no large studies available to give a precise estimate of the exact incidence of trisomy 21 in dizygotic twins.

8.3.1 Ultrasound Markers

8.3.1.1 Nuchal Translucency (NT)

In twin pregnancies, NT measurement combined with maternal age (Fig. 8.2a, b),

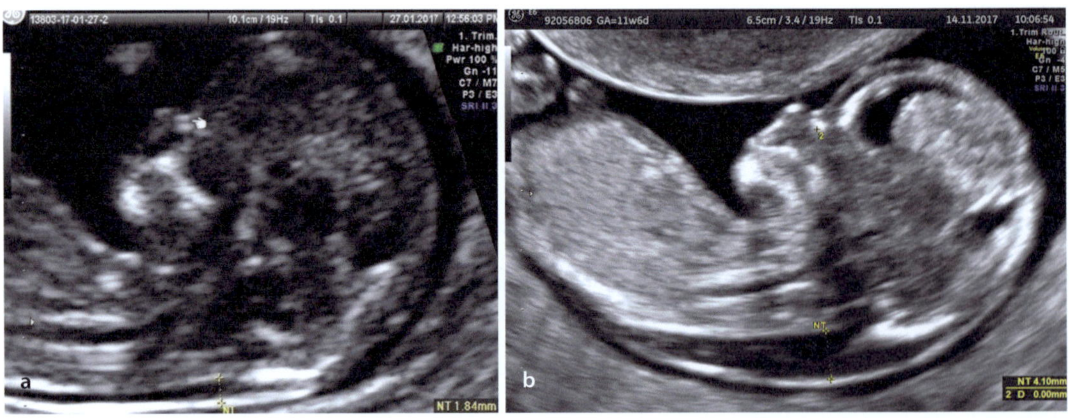

Fig. 8.2 **a** Ultrasound image of a normal nuchal translucency and nasal bones measured in a fetus at 12 weeks of gestation. **b** Ultrasound image of an increased nuchal translucency measured in a fetus at 12 weeks of gestation with trisomy 21

allows for the calculation of a separate risk for each fetus [3, 52]. Considering that the NT distribution does not differ significantly between twins and singletons, trisomy 21 detection rate in multiples should be similar to that in singletons.

In dichorionic pregnancies, each fetus is considered separately, and e fetus-specific risk is calculated by using median NT values (*summing method*). Although about 10% of dichorionic twins are actually monozygotic, this small percentage does not seem to affect the overall screening accuracy. Similarly, in higher-order multiple pregnancies, NT measurements should be assessed for each fetus separately [41].

In monochorionic pregnancies, a pregnancy-specific risk is calculated with the average of both NT measurements (*averaging method*). However, increased NT may represent the first sign of a twin-twin transfusion syndrome, and therefore, the prevalence of increased NT is considerably higher in monochorionic than in dichorionic pregnancies [53, 54]. As such, Vandecruys et al. found that the best screening performance was achieved using the average NT rather than the highest or lowest NT measured within a twin pair [61].

Overall, the combination of NT measurement and maternal age is an acceptable first-trimester screening test, with detection rates of 88% and false-positive rates of 7.3%, similar to singleton pregnancies [52]. However, the majority of the published papers suggest a more realistic estimate of 75% detection rate.

8.3.1.2 Ductus Venosus Flow (DV)

The association between reversed or absent DV flow and aneuploidy between 11 and 14 weeks was first shown in singleton pregnancies in 1998 [35]. Subsequent studies showed that the association is equally valid for cases of T18 and T13, which was confirmed in a recent meta-analysis after 20 years of application [18]. The combination of DV and NT is better than either test alone for the screening of aneuploidy [40] and should be incorporated into the first-trimester scan guidelines [39].

In dizygotic twin pairs, an abnormal DV flow assessed between 11 and 14 weeks was more frequently recorded in twins with aneuploidy, with or without cardiac defects (◘ Fig. 8.3a, b), probably related to heart dysfunction [31–33, 35, 43].

In about 1 in 6 monochorionic, and thus monozygotic pairs, the DV flow is abnormal one or both twins. Our group extensively investigated the benefit of DV flow in monochorionic twin pregnancies [38]. Similar to an increased NT, an abnormal DV flow is more common in monochorionic twins and probably indicates an early transfusion imbalance rather than the presence of aneuploidy [37, 38] (◘ Fig. 8.4). As such, Maiz et al. showed a three times higher risk of twin-twin transfusion syndrome: 30% if DV was abnormal versus 10% if DV was normal, albeit with a sensitivity of only 39% [31, 32]. Since we perform fetoscopic laser surgery only from 16 weeks onward, the need to detect TTTS in the first trimester is probably limited. However, closer surveillance of this high-risk group may allow for earlier detection and a thereby better outcome.

8.3.1.3 Nasal Bone (NB)

The addition of NB assessment to NT measurement, in combination with pregnancy-associated plasma protein-A (PAPP-A) and free beta-hCG, increased the detection rate of trisomy 21 from 79% to 89% at a 5% screen-positive rate. As in singletons, including the NB is also useful for the screening for trisomy 21 in twins [14].

8.3.2 Biochemical Markers

8.3.2.1 First-Trimester Combined Screening (Serum Markers and NT)

Currently, the first-line screening test for aneuploidy in singleton pregnancies is the first-trimester combined screening, in which the NT measurement and maternal age are combined with PAPP-A and β-hCG [3, 57]. The same screening test can also be applied in twin pregnancies, with some adjustments, as the serum biomarkers are different from those of singleton pregnancies [13, 23]. We

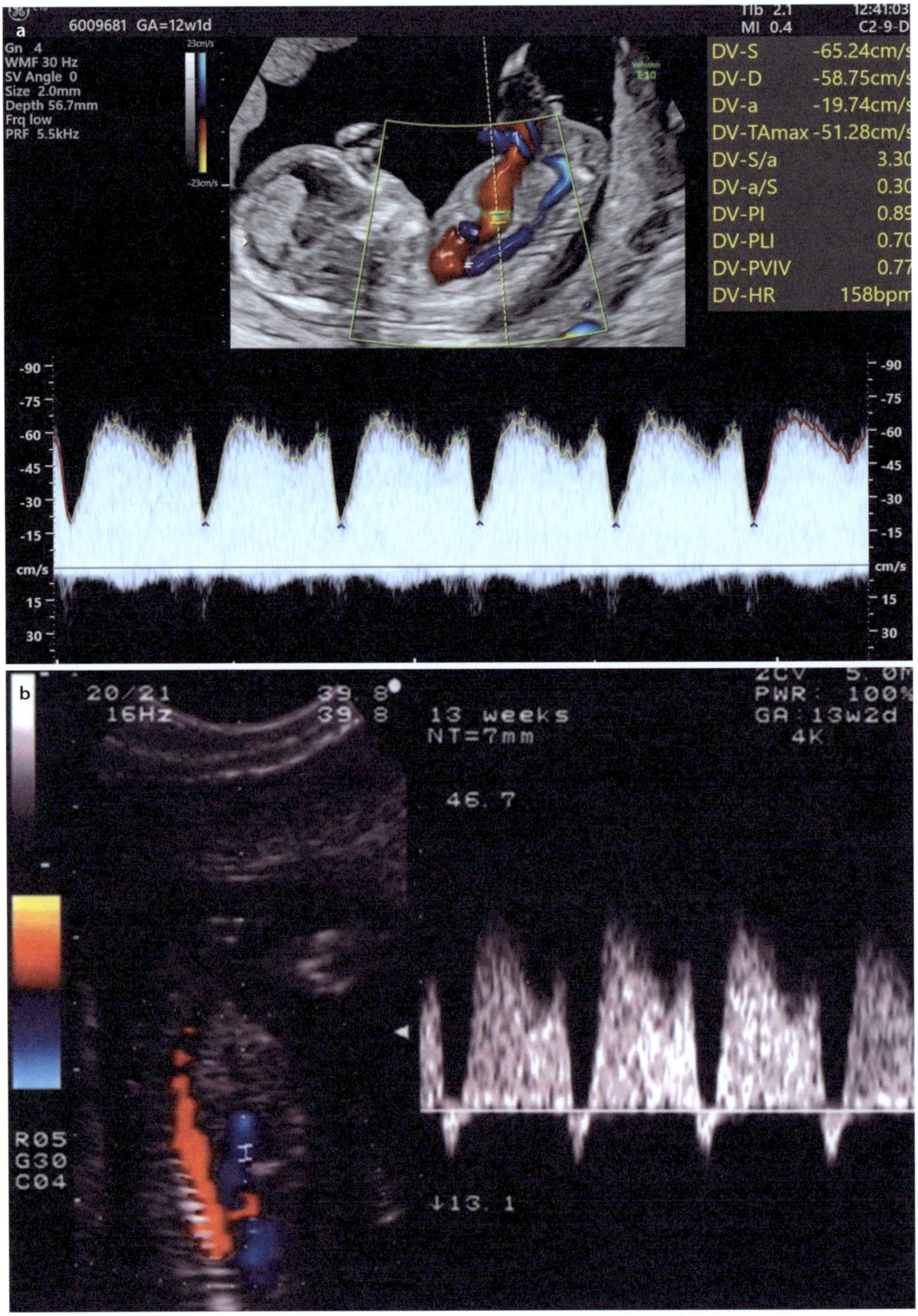

Fig. 8.3 **a** Ultrasound image of a normal ductus venosus blood flow waveform in a fetus at 12 weeks of gestation (pulsatility index of 0.87). **b** Ultrasound image of a ductus venosus with reverse blood flow waveform in a fetus with trisomy 21

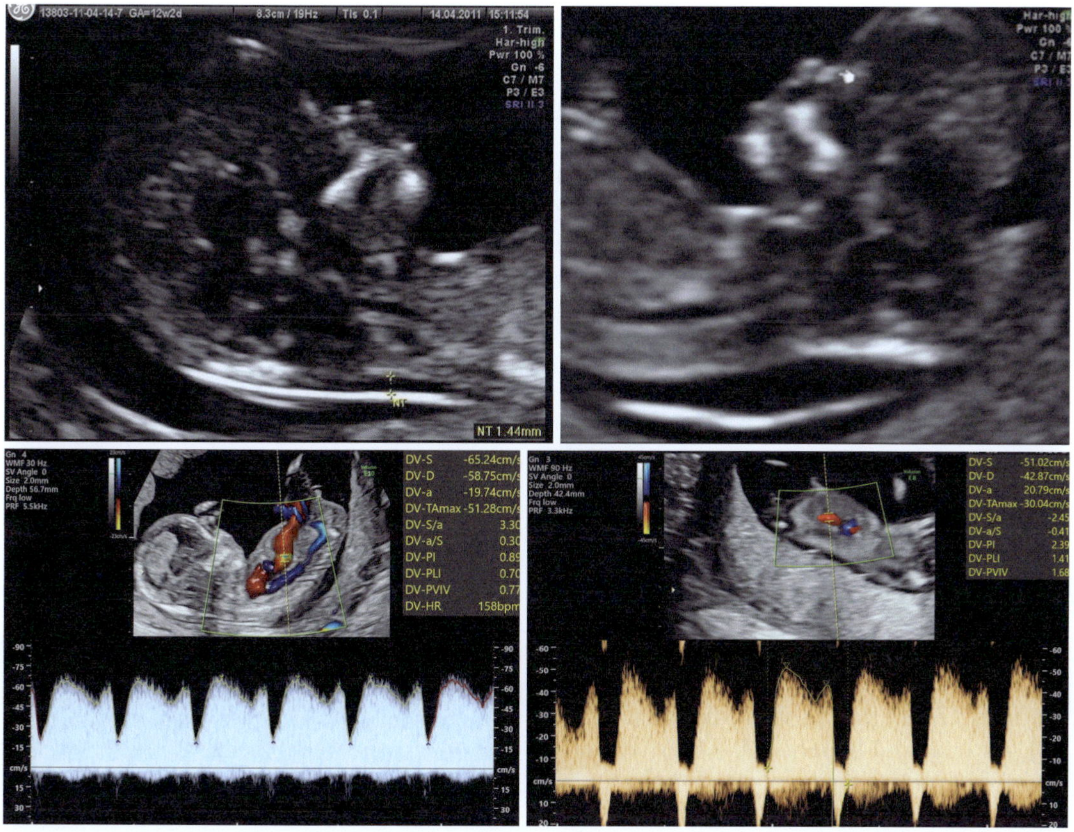

Fig. 8.4 Ultrasound images of a monochorionic twin pregnancy showing discrepant nuchal translucencies between both fetuses at 12 weeks gestation (NT of 1.44 mm and 5.1 mm, respectively). The first fetus showed a normal waveform in the ductus venosus, in contrast with fetus 2 that displayed a reverse A-wave in the ductus venosus. At 17 weeks gestation, twin-to twin transfusion eventually developed and laser ablation of arteriovenous anastomoses was performed

must also consider the effect of assisted reproductive techniques, as PAPP-A levels are uniformly decreased in such pregnancies, which may result in a higher false-positive rate in this subset of pregnancies [22].

In dichorionic twins, an unaffected fetus may mask the presence of an affected twin when calculating the risk using only serum biomarkers. However, the combination with NT and NB bone measurements, which are different for each twin, provides detection rates that approximate those of singleton pregnancies [3].

Compared with NT measurement and maternal age, the combined screening improves the accuracy by decreasing the false-positive rate (detection 87% for false-positive rate of 5%) [3, 23, 48, 63]. A recent systematic review on the combined screening test in twin pregnancies [48] demonstrated a good diagnostic performance (area under the curve: 0.817).

More and more, the combined screening test is replaced by non-invasive testing (NIPT), also in twins, and currently, in countries with universal reimbursement of NIPT, PAPP-A and beta-hCG measurements are no longer performed.

8.3.2.2 Second-Trimester Maternal Serum Screening

If NT measurement is not available or is missed because of the late diagnosis of pregnancy (after 14 weeks), the second-trimester maternal serum screening may be considered in twin pregnancies, with the measurement of alpha-fetoprotein (AFP), β-hCG, unconjugated estriol, and inhibin-A levels [3].

Although the biomarker levels are estimated to be approximately double those of singleton pregnancies, the exact distribution of serum biomarkers in twin pregnancies with trisomy 21 is not known. Furthermore, the risk estimation is pregnancy-specific, and not fetus-specific, and thus prone to errors in dichorionic pregnancies with a chromosomal abnormality in one twin. Therefore, second-trimester serum screening may be unreliable, with an estimated detection rate of 43% for dizygotic pregnancies and 73% for monozygotic pregnancies [44].

8.3.3 Non-Invasive Prenatal Testing (NIPT) or Cell-Free Fetal DNA Screening

Cell-free fetal (cff) DNA was first described in maternal plasma in 1997 [28], representing about 10% of total cff DNA in maternal blood [30]. As fetal and maternal DNA exhibit different fragmentation patterns, a ratio-based approach can be used to distinguish fetal from maternal DNA. Small increases in the DNA content of a fetal chromosome are interpreted as a high-risk result suggesting aneuploidy.

Although its effectiveness was clearly demonstrated with regard to aneuploidy screening in singleton pregnancies, with a detection rate for trisomy 21 of 99.7% and a false-positive rate of 0.04%, it was initially not clear if it could be extended to multiple pregnancies, which present certain unique procedural and interpretation challenges [9].

The main limitation of twin pregnancies is a reduced fetal fraction. Although total fetal fraction increases to 1.4 and 1.7 times for twins and triplets, respectively, the fetal fraction per fetus is reduced [10]. As a result, the 4% fetal fraction minimum requirement for singleton pregnancies would have to increase from 6% to 8% in twin pregnancies, which is difficult to achieve at 12 to 13 weeks [10]. NIPT in twins is also affected by the same limitations that apply to singleton pregnancies regarding fetal fraction: early gestational age, maternal obesity, presence of a vanishing twin, maternal cancer, and transplantation [4, 24].

Another factor to consider is the origin of the fetal DNA, which does not come from the fetus itself. In fact, it originates from the cytotrophoblast of the chorionic villi. It is, therefore, possible that the chromosomal constitution of the cytotrophoblast differs from that of the fetus. This confined placental mosaicism occurs in up to 2% of cases [47] and may result in a false-positive result.

Rarely, two other types of mosaicism may lead to false-negative results. Generalized mosaicism confined direct normality (GMDD) is characterized by abnormal chromosomes in the fetus and mesenchymal core of the placenta while the cytotrophoblast is normal. Confined fetal mosaicism, a rarer event, will have chromosomal aberrations limited to fetal cells with a chromosomally normal placenta [46].

In twin and higher-order pregnancies, the contribution from each fetus to the amount of cff DNA is not always equally distributed [20]. For example, for a fetal fraction of 10%, 8% may be derived from one twin and 2% from the other. So, in twin pregnancies, the test algorithm must be adapted to identify the lowest fetal fraction taking advantage of single nucleotide polymorphism (SNP) differences between mother and fetus [45, 59]. This technique amplifies areas where the probability of differences between mother and fetus is greatest. Other current methods used in clinical practice include shotgun massively parallel sequencing (s-MPS) and targeted (t-MPS). The same principle may be used to differentiate between fetuses in dizygotic pregnancies allowing for the calculation of the relative contribution and fraction of each fetus [50]. As such, NIPT can also be used to determine the zygosity. By doing so, it informs about the pre-test risk of aneuploidy and allows for a more complete evaluation of results and counseling. In contrast, no method currently allows for the fetal fraction calculation of monozygotic pairs, and the combined fetal fraction must be used.

Although not yet incorporated in current guidelines, several studies suggest that NIPT can be used reliably in twin pregnancies with a detection rate between 92 to 100% at a false-positive rate of 0% to 1% for the screening of trisomy 21 [27]. These values are similar to that of singleton pregnancies [17]. However, detection for trisomy 18 was 85%, and the performance in trisomy 13 could not be determined [27], limiting its use for these aneuploidies.

In a recent update from the Fetal Medicine Foundation, Gil and co-workers [21] showed that a detection rate of 98% at a false-positive rate of 0.03% for trisomy 21. For trisomy 18, the detection and false-positive rate were 89% and 0.03%, respectively. For trisomy 13, there were only three affected cases, and two were detected by the cff DNA test at a false-positive rate of 0.19%. Nevertheless, the scarce number of cases of trisomies 18 and 13 still hinders the accurate assessment of the predictive performance of the cff DNA test. Another recent study from the same group, including 959 twin pregnancies in a routine setting, demonstrated the feasibility of introducing cff DNA testing, contingent on the results of the first-trimester combined test for major trisomies [19].

If the cost of NIPT drops and reimbursement becomes available for all patients, it is foreseeable that NIPT will replace the combined first-trimester screening for aneuploidies in twins due to its higher accuracy [49, 64]. However, for higher-order multiple pregnancies, NIPT is not yet recommended. Furthermore, NIPT does not replace an invasive test as, in its present form, 100% sensitivity and specificity have not yet been reached [10]. An invasive test is always necessary to confirm a high-risk NIPT result.

8.4 Diagnostic Testing in Twin and Higher-Order Multiple Pregnancies

Twin and higher-order multiple pregnancies share common elements with singleton invasive procedures. A detailed sonographic assessment is mandatory before any invasive procedure. Fetal presentation, location, chorionicity, and cord insertions must be clearly defined and recorded. Like in singletons, amniocentesis and chorionic villus sampling (CVS) are the main diagnostic tests in twin pregnancies, but the performance is considerably more complicated. In order to perform these techniques safely with minimum fetal loss rates, only experienced operators should be involved. Ideally, if a fetal reduction is indicated and requested by the parents, this should be performed by the same operator who performed the diagnostic test.

Amniocentesis is typically performed from 16 weeks onward. The two-puncture technique is the most frequently used in twin pregnancies. It involves two consecutive punctures on each side of the intertwin membrane using two different needles. An inadvertent sampling of the same sac may occur in up to 2% of cases. Fetal loss before 24 weeks is calculated at 1.6%, which is similar to the background risk of fetal loss in screen positive twin pregnancies who refuse amniocentesis [58]. In monochorionic twin pregnancies, amniocentesis with puncture of both sacs is also recommended, especially if only one twin is affected by an increased NT or an anomaly, because the presence of heterokaryotypic monozygotic twins cannot be excluded with certainty [11, 25, 51].

CVS can be performed by a transcervical or transabdominal approach. Sampling errors were previously as high as 6%, but more recent reports place it between 2 and 4%. Sampling near the placental cord insertion, avoiding the dividing membrane, and using a combined transabdominal and transcervical approach reduce sampling errors. Fetal loss is reported at around 1% before 22 weeks above the background risk [2]. In a monochorionic setting, CVS is only performed to diagnose a monogenic disease or when both twins have a concordant anomaly. If one twin has an increased NT or has an anomaly, only a dual amniocentesis will diagnose heterokaryotypic monochorionic twins as a CVS from the shared placenta may miss the presence of the aneuploidy in one twin.

The advantages of a first-trimester diagnosis by CVS become more relevant in the context of dichorionic twin and multichorionic higher-order pregnancies as a first-trimester selective termination is associated with lower unintended rates of pregnancy loss. However, the technical challenges and higher sampling errors associated with CVS may favor amniocentesis if the risk of aneuploidy is only moderately elevated. Overall rates of pregnancy loss between the two techniques are, however, not statistically different [2].

The procedure-related risk of invasive testing in twins is higher than in singletons, and the traditional thresholds used in singletons should be weighed against the fetal loss rate of invasive procedures.

8.5 Conclusion

Prenatal screening poses specific challenges in multiple pregnancies and is presently in high demand due to the increased prevalence of multiple pregnancies. Both ultrasound and biochemical screening methods are available, though less performant than in singleton pregnancies. Recently, cff DNA testing has revolutionized the prenatal screening for fetal aneuploidy as its accuracy far exceeds that of conventional screening, also in twin pregnancies. Therefore, first-trimester NT measurement and conventional biochemical testing are likely to disappear. Parents should be counseled extensively concerning the complexities of prenatal screening in twin pregnancies, including the risks of an invasive test and fetal reduction.

8.5.1 Review Questions

1. Name five key attributes of an effective screening method.

2. Which limitations are common to NIPT in both singletons and twin pregnancies?

3. Which ultrasonographic parameters perform better in the screening of TTTS in the first trimester of pregnancy?

8.5.2 Mutiple-Choice Questions

1. What are the characteristics of a good screening test for trisomy 21?
   (a) The test should have a high specificity
   (b) The test should have a high false-negative rate
   (c) The test should have high sensitivity with a low false-positive rate
   (d) The test should have an area under the curve of 0.50 or less

Answer: (c)

2. What is currently the most accurate screening test for trisomy 21 in twin pregnancies?
   (a) The combined screening test based on maternal characteristics, nuchal translucency, PAPP-a, and β-HCG
   (b) An amniocentesis using a two-puncture technique
   (c) A chorionic villous sampling in the first trimester
   (d) Non-invasive prenatal test based on cell-free fetal DNA

Answer: (d)

3. Which statement is correct on the risk of trisomy 21 in a monochorionic twin pregnancy?
   (a) Using the combined screening test, a fetus-specific risk is calculated
   (b) Ductus venosus abnormalities are a specific marker for trisomy 21
   (c) Monochorionic twins are at a lower risk for trisomy 21 than singletons
   (d) If one twin has an increased nuchal translucency above the 99th centile, then chorionic villous sampling is the preferred diagnostic test

Answer: (d)

4. What should we tell prospective parents on the screening for trisomy 21 in a dichorionic twin pregnancy?
   (a) Non-invasive prenatal testing has the highest accuracy and is the best screening test for trisomy 21
   (b) The risk of trisomy 21 is twice as high in dichorionic twins than in

singletons, because of the presence of two babies
(c) Combined first-trimester screening has a poor accuracy to detect trisomy 21 in a twin setting
(d) In a twin setting, non-invasive prenatal testing should be considered as a diagnostic test, and an invasive test is best avoided because of the increased miscarriage risk

Answer: (a)

References

1. Abele H, Wagner P, Sonek J, Hoopmann M, Brucker S, Artunc-Ulkumen B, Kagan KO. First trimester ultrasound screening for Down syndrome based on maternal age, fetal nuchal translucency and different combinations of the additional markers nasal bone, tricuspid and ductus venosus flow. Prenat Diagn. 2015;35(12):1182–6. https://doi.org/10.1002/pd.4664. Epub 2015 Sep 7
2. Agarwal K, Alfirevic Z. Pregnancy loss after chorionic villus sampling and genetic amniocentesis in twin pregnancies: a systematic review. Ultrasound Obstet Gynecol. 2012;40(2):128–34.
3. Audibert F, Gagnon A. No. 262-prenatal screening for and diagnosis of aneuploidy in twin pregnancies. J Obstet Gynaecol Can. 2017;39(9):e347–61. https://doi.org/10.1016/j.jogc.2017.06.015.
4. Bevilacqua E, Guizani M, Cos Sanchez T, Jani JC. Concerns with performance of screening for aneuploidy by cell-free DNA analysis of maternal blood in twin pregnancy. Ultrasound Obstet Gynecol. 2016;47(1):124–5. https://doi.org/10.1002/uog.14938.
5. Bender W, Dugoff L. Screening for aneuploidy in multiple gestations: the challenges and options. Obstet Gynecol Clin N Am. 2018;45(1):41–53. https://doi.org/10.1016/j.ogc.2017.10.004.
6. Bianchi DW, Prosen T, Platt LD, Goldberg JD, Abuhamad AZ, Rava RP, Sehnert AJ, et al. Massively parallel sequencing of maternal plasma DNA in 113 cases of fetal nuchal cystic hygroma. Obstet Gynecol. 2013;121(5):1057–62. https://doi.org/10.1097/AOG.0b013e31828ba3d8.
7. Blickstein I, Verhoeven HC, Keith LG. Zygotic splitting after assisted reproduction. N Engl J Med. 1999;340:738–9.
8. Boyle B, Morris JK, McConkey R, et al. Prevalence and risk of Down syndrome in monozygotic and dizygotic multiple pregnancies in Europe: implcations for prenatal screening. British J Obstet Gynecol. 2014;121:809–19.
9. Canick JA, Kloza EM, Lambert-Messerlian GM, Haddow JE, Ehrich M, van den Boom D, Bombard AT, Deciu C, Palomaki GE. DNA sequencing of maternal plasma to identify Down syndrome and other trisomies in multiple gestations. Prenat Diagn. 2012;32:730–4.
10. Chen M, Jiang F, Guo Y, Yan H, Wang J, Zhang L, Zeng X, Li S, Li Y, Li N, Zhang C, Zhu W, Du B, Wang Y, Lan Z, Luo X, Luo F, Chen D. Validation of fetal DNA fraction estimation and its application in noninvasive prenatal testing for aneuploidy detection in multiple pregnancies. Prenat Diagn. 2019;39:1273–82.
11. Cheng PJ, Shaw SW, Shih JC, Soong YK. Monozygotic twins discordant for monosomy 21 detected by first trimester nuchal translucency screening. Obstet Gynecol. 2006;107:538–41.
12. Cicero S, Curcio P, Papageorghiou A, Sonek J, Nicolaides KH. Absence of nasal bone in fetuses with trisomy 21 at 11-14 weeks of gestation: an observational study. Lancet. 2001;358:1665–7.
13. Cleary-Goldman J, Berkowitz RL. First trimester screening for Down syndrome in multiple pregnancy. Semin Perinatol. 2005;29:395–400.
14. Cleary-Goldman J, Rebarber A, Krantz D, Hallahan T, Saltzman D. First-trimester screening with nasalbone in twins. Am J Obstet Gynecol. 2008;199(3):283.e1–3. https://doi.org/10.1016/j.ajog.2008.07.010.
15. Cuckle H. Down's syndrome screening in twins. J Med Screen. 1998;5:3–4.
16. Dube J, Dodds L, Armson BA. Does chorionicity or zygosity predict adverse perinatal outcomes in twins? Am J Obstet Gynecol. 2002;186:579–83.
17. Fosler L, Winters P, Jones KW, Curnow KJ, Sehnert AJ, Bhatt S, Platt LD. Aneuploidy screening by non-invasive prenatal testing in twin pregnancy. Ultrasound Obstet Gynecol. 2017;49(4):470–7.
18. Ge Y, Xia L, Wu Y, Cao H. Employ ductus venosus blood flow in the early detection of trisomy 21, trisomy 18 and trisomy 13. A meta-analysis. Medicine. 2019;98(12):1–6.
19. Galeva S, Konstantinidou L, Gil MM, Akolekar R, Nicolaides KH. Routine first-trimester screening for fetal trisomies in twin pregnancy: cell-free DNA test contingent on results from combined test. Ultrasound Obstet Gynecol. 2019;53(2):208–13. https://doi.org/10.1002/uog.20160. Epub 2018 Dec 7
20. Gil M, Quezada MS, Bregant B, et al. Cell-free DNA analysis for trisomy risk assessment in first-trimester twin pregnancies. Fetal Diagn Ther. 2014;35:204–11.
21. Gil MM, Galeva S, Jani J, Konstantinidou L, Akolekar R, Plana MN, Nicolaides KH. Screening for trisomies by cffDNA testing of maternal blood in twin pregnancy: update of the Fetal Medicine Foundation results and meta-analysis. Ultrasound Obstet Gynecol. 2019;53:734–42.

22. Gjerris AC, Loft A, Pinborg A, et al. First trimester screening markers are altered in pregnancies conceived after IVF/ICSI. Ultrasound Obstet Gynecol. 2009;33:8–17.
23. Goncé A, Borrell A, Fortuny A, Casals E, Martínez MA, Mercadé I, Cararach V, Vanrell JA. First-trimester screening for trisomy 21 in twin pregnancy: does the addition of biochemistry make an improvement? Prenat Diagn. 2005;25(12):1156–61.
24. Gray KJ, Wilkins-Haug LE. Have we done our last amniocentesis? Updates on cell-free DNA for Down syndrome screening. Pediatr Radiol. 2018;48(4):461–70. https://doi.org/10.1007/s00247-017-3958-y.
25. He M, Pepperell J, Gundogan F, De Paepe M, Maggio L, Lu S, Kostadinov S, O'Brien B, DeLaMonte S, Pinar H, Tantravahi U. Monochorionic twins discordant for mosaic trisomy 14. Am J Med Genetics. 2014;164A:1227–33.
26. Jenkins TM, Wapner RJ. The challenge of prenatal diagnosis in twin pregnancies. Curr Opin Obstet Gynecol. 2000;12:87–92.
27. Liao H, Liu S, Wang H. Performance of non-invasive prenatal screening for fetal aneuploidy in twin pregnancies: a meta-analysis. Prenat Diagn. 2017;37(9):874–82. https://doi.org/10.1002/pd.5118.
28. Lo YM, Corbetta N, Chamberlain PF, Rai V, Sargent IL, Redman CW, Wainscoat JS. Presence of fetal DNA in maternal plasma and serum. Lancet. 1997;350(9076):485–7.
29. Lo YM, Chiu RW. Prenatal diagnosis: progress through plasma nucleic acids. Nat Rev Genet. 2007;8(1):71–7.
30. Lo YM, Chan KC, Sun H, et al. Maternal plasma DNA sequencing reveals the genome wide genetic and mutational profile of the fetus. Sci Trans Med. 2010;2:61ra91.
31. Maiz N, Staboulidou I, Leal AM, Minekawa R, Nicolaides KH. Ductus venosus Doppler at 11 to 13 weeks of gestation in the prediction of outcome in twin pregnancies. Obstet Gynecol. 2009a;113(4):860–5.
32. Maiz N, Valencia C, Kagan KO, Wright D. NicolaidesKH. Ductus venosus Doppler in screening for trisomies 21, 18 and 13 and Turner syndrome at 11–13 weeks of gestation. Ultrasound Obstet Gynecol. 2009b;33(5):512–7.
33. Maiz N, Nicolaides KH. Ductus venosus in the first trimester: contribution to screening of chromosomal, cardiac defects and monochorionic twin complications. Fetal Diagn Ther. 2010;28(2):65–71.
34. Maron JL, Johnson KL, Bianchi DW. Cell-free fetal DNA plasma extraction and real-time polymerase chain reaction quantification. Methods Mol Med. 2007;132:51–63.
35. Matias A, Gomes C, Flack N, Montenegro N, Nicolaides KH. Screening for chromosomal defects at 11–14 weeks: the role of ductus venosus blood flow. Ultrasound Obstet Gynecol. 1998;12:380–4.
36. Matias A, Montenegro N, Blickstein I. Down syndrome screening in multiple pregnancies. Obstet Gynecol Clin N Am. 2005a;32(1):81–96.
37. Matias A, Ramalho C, Montenegro N. Search for hemodynamic compromise at 11-14 weeks in monochorionic twin pregnancy: is abnormal flow in the ductus venosus predictive of twin-twin transfusion syndrome? J Matern Fetal Neonatal Med. 2005b;18(2):79–86.
38. Matias A, Montenegro N, Loureiro T, Cunha M, Duarte S, Freitas D, Severo M. Screening for twin-twin transfusion syndrome at 11–14 weeks of pregnancy: the key role of ductus venosus blood flow assessment. Ultrasound Obstet Gynecol. 2010;35(2):142–8.
39. Matias A, Montenegro N. Ductus venosus in twins: science matters. Ultrasound Obstet Gynecol. 2016;47(6):787. https://doi.org/10.1002/uog.15927.
40. Mavrides E, Sairam S, Hollis B, Thilanagathan B. Screening for aneuplody in the first trimester by assessment of blood flow in the ductus venosus. BJOG. 2012;109:1015–9.
41. Maymon R, Dreazen E, Rozinsky S, et al. The feasibility of nuchal translucency measurement in higher order multiple gestation achieved by assisted reproduction. Hum Reprod. 1999;14:2102–5.
42. Merkatz IR, Nitowsky HM, Macri JN, Johnson WE. An association between low maternal serum alfa- fetoprotein and fetal chromosomal abnormalities. Am J Obstet Gynecol. 1984;148:886–94.
43. Montenegro N, Matias A, Areias JC, Castedo S, Barros H. Increased nuchal translucency: possible involvement of early cardiac failure. Ultrasound Obstet Gynecol. 1997;10:265–8.
44. Neveux LM, Palomaki GE, Knight GJ, et al. Multiple marker screening for down syndrome in twin pregnancies. Prenat Diagn. 1996;16:29–34.
45. Norwitz ER, McNeill G, Kalyan A, Rivers E, Ahmed E, Meng L, Vu P, Egbert M, Shapira M, Kobara K, Parmar S, Goel S, Prins SA, Aruh I, Persico N, Robins JC, Kirshon B, Demko ZP, Ryan A, Billings PR, Rabinowitz M, Benn P, Martin KA, Hedriana HL. Validation of a single-nucleotide polymorphism-based non-invasive prenatal test in twin gestations: determination of Zygosity, individual fetal sex, and fetal aneuploidy. J Clin Med. 2019;8(7):pii: E937.
46. Opstal DV, Srebniak M, Polak J, et al. False negative NIPT results: figures for chromosomes 13,18 and 21 based on chorionic villi results in 5967 cases and literature review. Plos One. 2016;11(1):e0146794. https://doi.org/10.1371/journal.pone.0146794.
47. Pittalis MC, Dalprà L, Torricelli F, Rizzo N, Nocera G, Cariati E, Santarini L, Tibiletti MG, Agosti S, Bovicelli L, et al. The predictive value of cytogenetic diagnosis after CVS based on 4860 cases with both direct and culture methods. Prenat Diagn. 1994;14(4):267–78.
48. Prats P, Rodríguez I, Comas C, Puerto B. Systematic review of screening for trisomy

21 in twin pregnancies in first trimester combining nuchal translucency and biochemical markers: a meta-analysis. Prenat Diagn. 2014;34(11):1077–83.
49. Quarello E, Jacquemard F, Ville Y. Screening of aneuploidies in twin pregnancies in 2016: we may miss the boat if we fail to take action. Gynecol Obstet Fertil. 2016;44(9):457–60. https://doi.org/10.1016/j.gyobfe.2016.05.010.
50. Qu JZZ, Leung TY, Jiang P, Liao GJW, Cheng YKY, Sun H, et al. Noninvasive prenatal determination of twin Zygosity by maternal plasma DNA analysis. Clin Chem. 2013;59:2427–35.
51. Rock KR, Millard S, Seravalli V, McShane C, Kearney J, Seitz E, Baschat AA, Miller JL. Discordant anomalies and karyotype in a monochorionic twin pregnancy: a call for comprehensive genetic evaluation. Ultrasound Obstet Gynecol. 2017;49:540–5.
52. Sebire NJ, Snijders RJM, Hughes K, Sepulveda W, Nicolaides KH. Screening for trisomy 21 in twin pregnancies by maternal age and fetal nuchal translucency thickness at 10–14 weeks of gestation. Br J Obstet Gynecol. 1996;103:999–1003.
53. Sebire NJ, D'Ercole C, Hughes K, Carvalho M, Nicolaides KH. Increased nuchal translucency thickness at 10–14 weeks of gestation as a predictor of severe twin-to-twin transfusion syndrome. Ultrasound Obstet Gynecol. 1997;10:86–9.
54. Sebire NJ, Souka A, Skentou H, Geerts L, Nicolaides KH. Early prediction of severe twin-twin trasfusion syndrome. Hum Reprod. 2000;15:2008–10.
55. Snijders RJM, Noble P, Sebire JN, Souka A, Nicolaides KH. UK multicentre project on assessment of risk of trisomy 21 by maternal age and fetal nuchal translucency thickness at 10–14 weeks of gestation. Lancet. 1998;351:343–6.
56. Sparks NT, Norton ME, Flessel M, Goldman S, Currier RJ. Observed rate of Down syndrome in twin pregnancies. Obstet Gynecol. 2016;128: 1127–33.
57. Spencer K, Nicolaides KH. Screening for trisomy 21 in twins using first trimester ultrasound and maternal serum biochemistry in a one stop clinic: a review of three years experience. Br J Obstet Gynecol. 2003;110:276–80.
58. Sperling JD, Zlatnik MG, Norton ME, Currier RJ. Pregnancy loss after amniocentesis in monochorionic and dichorionic twin pregnancies: results from a large population-based dataset. Prenat Diagn. 2019;39(10):896–900.
59. Struble CA, Syngelaki A, Oliphant A, Song K, Nicolaides KH. Fetal fraction estimate in twin pregnancies using directed cell-free DNA analysis. Fetal Diagn Ther. 2014;35:199–203.
60. Tsang JC, Lo YM. Circulating nucleic acids in plasma/serum. Pathology. 2007;39(2):197–207.
61. Vandecruys H, Faiola S, Auer M, Sebire N, Nicolaides KH. Screening for trisomy 21 in monochorionic twins by measurement of fetal nuchal translucency thickness. Ultrasound Obstet Gynecol. 2005;25:551–3.
62. Wald NJ, Cuckle HS, Densem JW, Nanchahal K, Royston P, Chard T, Haddow JE, Knight GJ, Palomaki GE, Canick JA. Maternal serum screening for Down's syndrome in early pregnancy. Br Med J. 1988;297:883–7.
63. Wald NJ, Rish S, Hackshaw AK. Combining nuchal translucency and serum markers in prenatal screening for Down syndrome in twin pregnancies. Prenat Diagn. 2003;23:588–92.
64. Yu W, Lv Y, Yin S, Liu H, Li X, Liang B, Kong L, Liu C. Screening of fetal chromosomal aneuploidy diseases using non-invasive prenatal testing in twin pregnancies. Expert Rev Mol Diagn. 2019;19(2):189–96. https://doi.org/10.1080/14737159.2019.1562906.

Key Reading

Bender W, Dugoff L. Screening for aneuploidy in multiple gestations: the challenges and options. Obstet Gynecol Clin North Am. 2018;45(1):41–53. https://doi.org/10.1016/j.ogc.2017.10.004.

Galeva S, Konstantinidou L, Gil MM, Akolekar R, Nicolaides KH. Routine first-trimester screening for fetal trisomies in twin pregnancy: cell-free DNA test contingent on results from combined test. Ultrasound Obstet Gynecol. 2019;53(2):208–13. https://doi.org/10.1002/uog.20160. Epub 2018 Dec 7

Gray KJ, Wilkins-Haug LE. Have we done our last amniocentesis? Updates on cell-free DNA for Down syndrome screening. Pediatr Radiol. 2018;48(4):461–70. https://doi.org/10.1007/s00247-017-3958-y.

Matias A, Montenegro N, Loureiro T, Cunha M, Duarte S, Freitas D, Severo M. Screening for twin-twin transfusion syndrome at 11-14 weeks of pregnancy: the key role of ductus venosus blood flow assessment. Ultrasound Obstet Gynecol. 2010;35(2): 142–8.

Norwitz ER, McNeill G, Kalyan A, Rivers E, Ahmed E, Meng L, Vu P, Egbert M, Shapira M, Kobara K, Parmar S, Goel S, Prins SA, Aruh I, Persico N, Robins JC, Kirshon B, Demko ZP, Ryan A, Billings PR, Rabinowitz M, Benn P, Martin KA, Hedriana HL. Validation of a single-nucleotide polymorphism-based non-invasive prenatal test in twin gestations: determination of zygosity, individual fetal sex, and fetal aneuploidy. J Clin Med. 2019;8(7):937.

Assessment of Fetal Growth in Twins and Multiple Pregnancy

Becky Liu and Asma Khalil

Contents

A. Khalil et al. (eds.), *Twin and Higher-order Pregnancies*,
https://doi.org/10.1007/978-3-030-47652-6_9

Trailer

Twins and higher-order multiple pregnancies are at higher risk of perinatal complications. Due to the nature of multiple pregnancies, abdominal palpation and symphysial-fundal height measurements cannot be reliably used to monitor their growth. Ultrasound is currently the best tool for growth surveillance, and due to the high complication rates, this must be performed on a regular basis. The traditional practice is to use singleton growth charts to track the growth velocity of multiples; however, these pregnancies do not follow the same trend in growth. Therefore, it is recommended to use twin-specific growth charts to ensure accurate growth assessments.

Definitions

Fetal growth: the growth of fetuses in utero.

Fetal growth restriction (FGR): a pathological restriction of the fetus in reaching its full genetic growth potential.

Selective fetal growth restriction (sFGR): in twin pregnancies, when FGR affects at least one twin.

Twin-specific growth charts: a growth chart derived specifically from twin pregnancies, which can be used to assess for growth abnormalities in twin pregnancies.

Estimated fetal weight (EFW): the approximated fetal weight calculated through the measurement of head circumference (HC), abdominal circumference (AC), and femur length (FL) using ultrasound.

Discordance: the percentage difference of the EFW between fetuses in one pregnancy.

Fetal Dopplers: pattern of blood flow through the umbilical artery (UA), middle cerebral artery (MCA), or ductus venosus (DV), that reflects placental function and fetal well-being.

9

Learning Objectives

- To understand the normal growth trajectory in twin and multiple pregnancies, and how this differs from singleton pregnancies
- To establish the best method for assessment of fetal growth in twin and multiple pregnancies
- To understand the ultrasound monitoring pathway for twin and multiple pregnancies
- To be able to identify abnormal growth and growth discordance in twin and multiple pregnancies

9.1 Introduction

Twin and higher-order multiple pregnancies are known to be associated with lower than average birth weights [1, 2]. Due to their increased risk of perinatal morbidity and mortality compared to singleton pregnancies, they require more intensive ultrasound surveillance [3–5]. Fetal growth restriction (FGR) is a well-recognized complication of multiple pregnancies. Selective fetal growth restriction (sFGR) refers to a pathological growth restriction of one (or more) fetus(es), but with normal growth of the other(s). This condition is associated with increased perinatal mortality and morbidity, and can be difficult to manage due to risks to the appropriate for gestational age (AGA) twin [6–9]. Abdominal palpation and symphysial-fundal height measurements are unreliable in detecting FGR in multiple pregnancies, and is therefore not recommended by NICE guidelines [4]. In this chapter, we aim to describe the normal growth patterns in multiples, the recommended surveillance pathways, and the identification of abnormal growth.

9.2 Normal Growth Trajectory of Multiple Pregnancies

Multiple pregnancies do not follow the same growth pattern as singleton pregnancies. Despite this, common practice continues to use singleton growth charts to monitor the growth of these pregnancies. The rationale for this practice may be due to the fact that those MC twins classified as FGR based on the classification derived from singleton growth charts, still had an increased perinatal mortality rate compared to singletons. DC pregnancies however, did not have such risks [10]. Overdiagnosis of FGR can lead to unnecessary intervention and early delivery of those pregnancies that are in fact displaying a healthy growth pattern, exposing these babies to risks of prematurity. It is therefore important to take into consideration the normal growth patterns of multiples when assessing fetal growth velocity.

9.2.1 Twin Pregnancies

Stirrup et al. performed an analysis on the growth of a large cohort of unselected twin pregnancies at different gestational ages and compared these measurements to those of singleton pregnancies [11, 12]. They found that in DC twins, the growth was similar to that of singletons until 30 weeks, and slowed down thereafter. In MC twins, the estimated fetal weight (EFW) was generally lower than that of DC twins and singletons throughout the gestations, but the biparietal diameter (BPD) and head circumference (HC) measurements recover to similar values as DC twins in the third trimester. Using these values, a twin-specific growth chart was derived [11], and is now widely available for use. When comparing the outcomes of pregnancies diagnosed as SGA according to these charts and those diagnosed using customized singleton charts, it was found that there was no difference in the stillbirth rates, but a significantly smaller number of pregnancies labelled as SGA (7.1% vs. 12.8%, respectively) [13].

The same team also studied the normal intertwin discordance between DC and MC twins in the second and third trimesters. It was found that in DC twins, the 95th percentile intertwin discordance at 20 weeks was 18.3%, and increased steadily to 21.9% by 30 weeks. In MC twins, the 95th percentile intertwin discordance was greater at 20 weeks (22.2%), and also increased by 30 weeks to 25.4% [12]. Therefore, an intertwin discordance within these ranges is considered to be part of a normal growth trajectory. ◘ Figure 9.1 demonstrates the normal growth patterns of DC compared with MC twins.

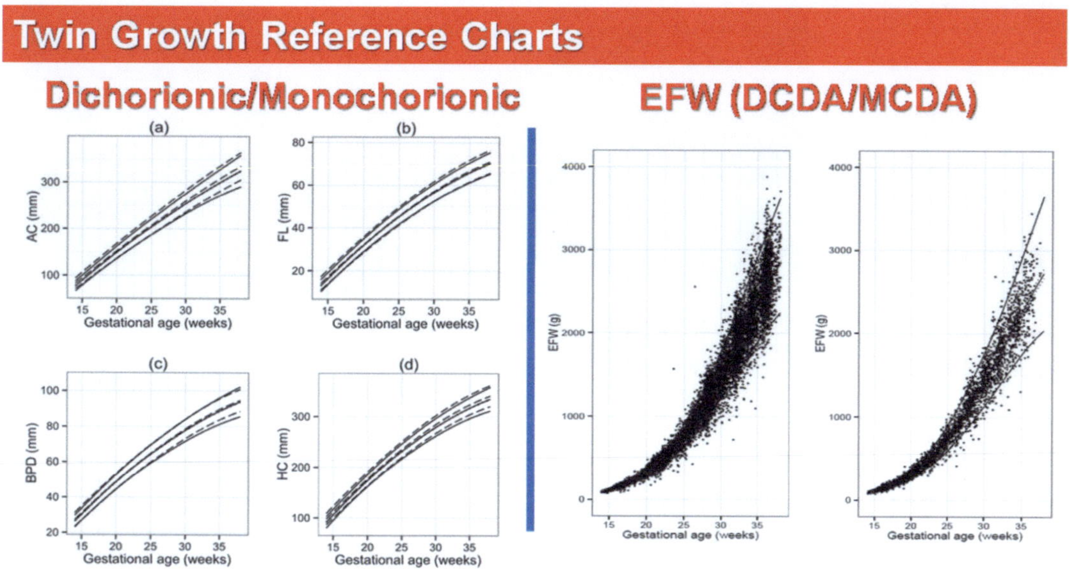

◘ **Fig. 9.1** Growth charts demonstrating the normal trend of growth of DC and MC twins. Charts on the left demonstrate the normal measurements of AC (abdominal circumference), FL (femur length), BPD (biparietal diameter), and HC (head circumference), in dichorionic (----) and monochorionic (___) twins, across increasing gestational weeks. Charts on the right demonstrate the distribution of EFW (estimated fetal weight) in DCDA (dichorionic diamniotic) and MCDA (monochorionic diamniotic) twins across increasing gestational weeks

9.2.2 Triplet Pregnancies

Few studies have looked into the normal growth patterns of triplet pregnancies. Min et al. concluded that from 30 weeks gestation, the growth of healthy triplets fell substantially below the singletons, and after 34 weeks, below the twins [2]. Other studies have also agreed that the growth of triplets was significantly less than singletons from 31 weeks [14], and after 33 weeks, the birth weights of triplets were less than those of singletons at each gestational age [15]. Efforts have been made to derive triplet-specific growth reference ranges [2, 16], but currently the use of triplet-specific growth charts remain controversial.

9.3 Timing of Ultrasound Surveillance of Fetal Growth

9

Although ultrasound assessment of fetal growth is less accurate in twins and higher-order multiple pregnancies than it is in singletons [17, 18], it remains the most reliable tool to screen for growth anomalies in multiple pregnancies. The overall predictions within ±10% and ±15% of the actual birthweight are 50% and 69% in twin pregnancies, compared to 62% and 82% in singletons, respectively. EFW calculated based on combination of head, abdomen, and femur measurements has the lowest mean absolute percentage error, in both singleton and twin pregnancies. The predictive accuracy for 25% birth-weight discordance is very good (using the Hadlock 2 formula AUC was 0.87) [17]. The formula derived by Warsof et al. is routinely used before 20 weeks [19], and Hadlock et al. after 20 weeks [20]. The ultrasound monitoring pathways in all types of multiple pregnancies are outlined in ◘ Figs. 9.2 and 9.3.

9.3.1 Dichorionic Twins

First trimester pregnancy dating in spontaneously conceived pairs should be performed

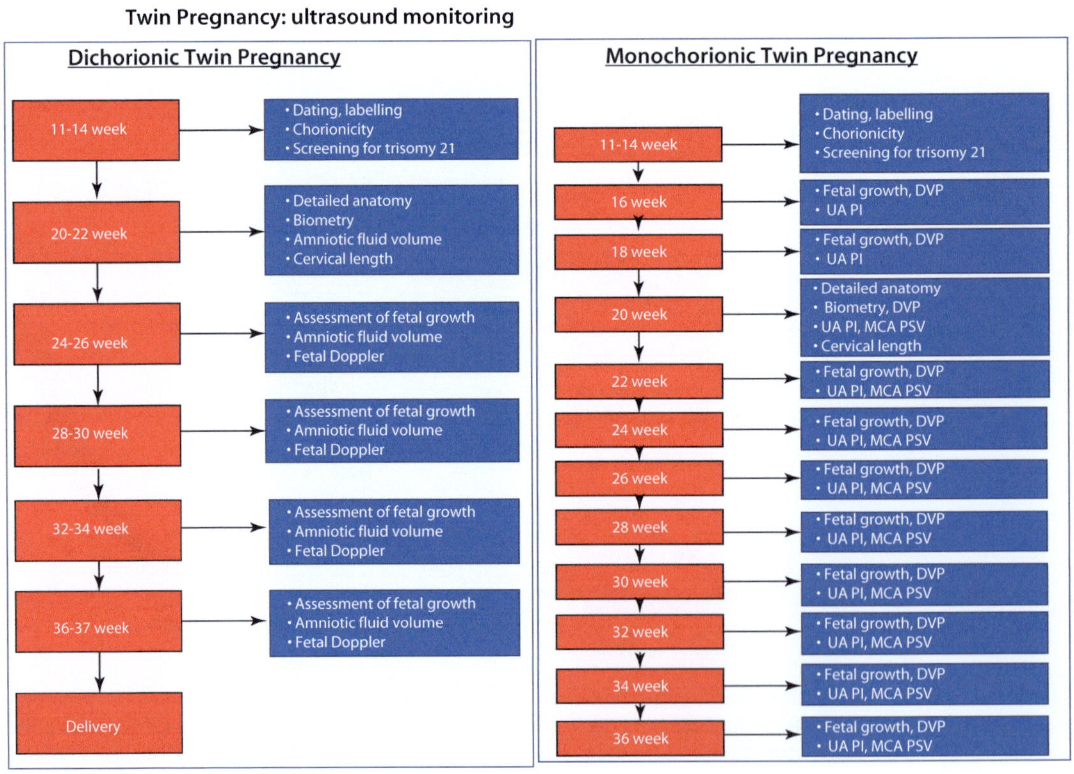

◘ **Fig. 9.2** Flowcharts demonstrating the ultrasound surveillance pathways in dichorionic twins and monochorionic twins in each gestation [21]

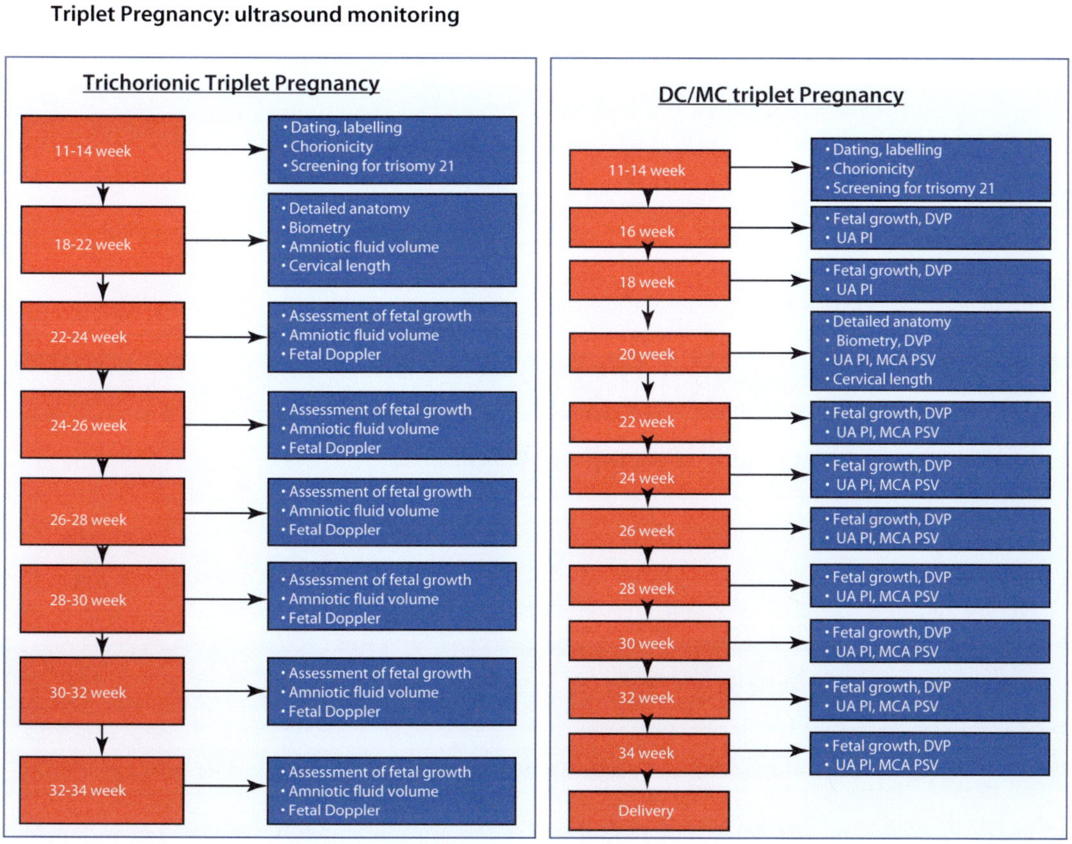

Fig. 9.3 Flowcharts demonstrating the ultrasound surveillance pathways in trichorionic triplets and dichorionic/monochorionic triplets in each gestation [4]

using the crown-rump length (CRL) of the larger twin at 11–14 weeks' gestation. A routine anomaly scan should be performed around 20 weeks (18–22 weeks) [4, 21] to assess for structural anomalies. Growth scans assessing the HC, AC, and FL should be performed 4 weekly following the anomaly scan, and the EFW using these biometries for each twin as well as the EFW discordance should be calculated at each growth scan (Fig. 9.4) [4, 21]. Cervical length measurements can be performed at the time of the anomaly scan at the clinician's discretion as the current evidence for intervention to prevent preterm delivery in those with short and open cervixes are not yet established. Figure 9.4 demonstrates the equation in which EFW discordance can be calculated.

Amniotic fluid index for each twin (measured using the deepest vertical pool (DVP)), as well as umbilical artery (UA) Doppler pulsatility index (PI) should also be assessed at each scan, to ensure adequate growth [21]. This surveillance should be increased to two weekly [21] or even weekly [4] if there is an EFW discordance >20%, or the EFW of one baby is <10th centile. Referral to a tertiary fetal medicine centre should be considered if there is an EFW discordance >25% and one baby has an EFW <10th centile [4], as this is an important indicator for sFGR.

9.3.2 Monochorionic Twins

As these twins are at higher risk of complications specific to monochorionicity (e.g. twin-to-twin transfusion syndrome (TTTS), twin-anaemia-polycythaemia sequence (TAPS)), more intensive ultrasound surveillance is required. Following the first trimester scan, ultrasound assessment should be performed 2 weekly from

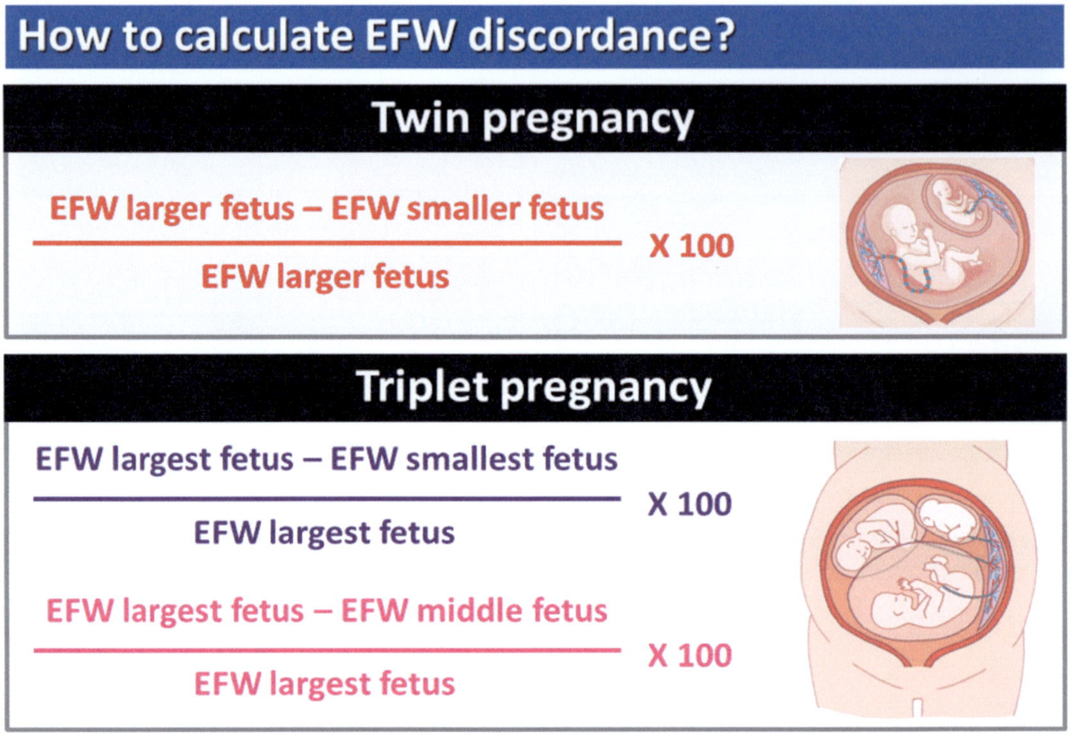

Fig. 9.4 Equations of how estimated fetal weight (EFW) discordance can be calculated for twins and triplets

16 weeks, to assess growth, DVP, UA Doppler, together with a full assessment of fetal anatomy and cardiac structure at 20 weeks [4, 21]. EFW and EFW discordance should be calculated at each scan. MCA peak systolic velocity (PSV) should be assessed from 20 weeks, to assess for signs of TAPS (▶ Chap. 17). TTTS can be diagnosed if the DVP around one twin is <2 cm, and is >8 cm around the other twin before 20 weeks, or >10 cm after 20 weeks [21] (▶ Chap. 16). Surveillance should be increased to weekly, or more frequently if clinically indicated, in a similar fashion to DC twins, and referral to a tertiary fetal medicine centre should be made when sFGR is suspected (EFW discordance >25% and EFW of one baby <10th centile) [4].

9.3.3 Triplets

Trichorionic (TC) triplets are monitored 2 weekly following the anomaly scan, in a similar manner to DC twins. Dichorionic (DC) or monochorionic (MC) triplets are monitored 2 weekly from 16 weeks, taking care to screen for monochorionic-specific conditions [4]. EFW for each triplet and EFW discordance should still be calculated at each scan, and closer surveillance carried out if sFGR is suspected. The equation above demonstrates how growth discordance can be calculated in triplet pregnancies.

9.3.4 Fetal Dopplers

Fetal blood flow can help us to assess the condition and well-being of the fetuses, and can allow us to identify cases of placental insufficiency, fetal decompensation, and TAPS. An increased UA PI can indicate increased placental resistance, and negative or reversed end-diastolic flow (AREDF) suggests further fetal deterioration requiring closer surveillance. However, in MC pairs, the flow pattern may also reflect the direction of flow across a large direct artery-to-artery anastomosis, as

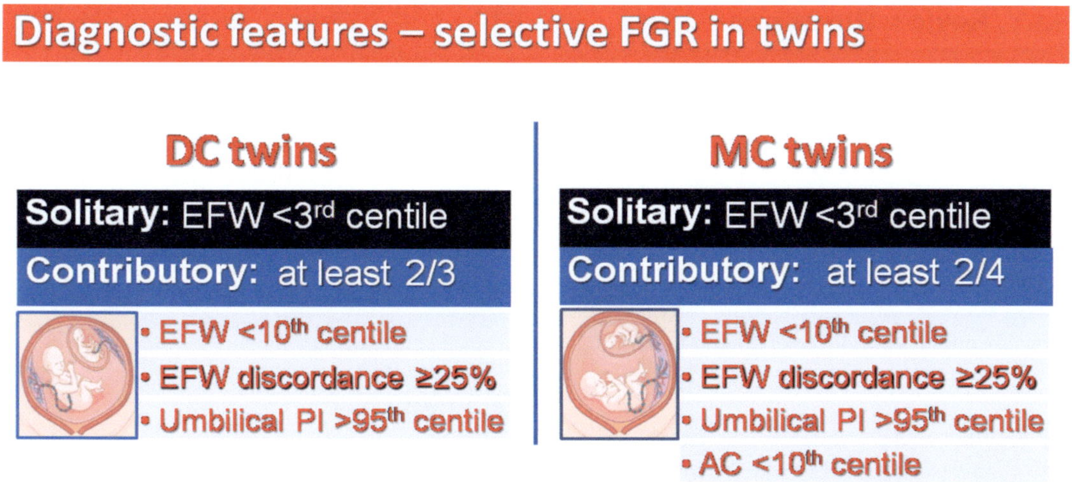

Fig. 9.5 Diagnostic criteria for sFGR as stratified by the recently published Delphi consensus (Khalil 2019) [23] for both dichorionic and monochorionic twins

discussed in ▶ Chap. 10. The MCA can reveal signs of cerebral redistribution, when the fetus is redirecting blood flow to the brain as a coping mechanism (reduced MCA PI). The MCA PSV provides us with information regarding the flow velocity, where a high velocity indicates fetal anaemia, and low velocity polycythaemia. The ductus venosus (DV) is a reflection of fetal cardiac function and a high PI suggests cardiac strain due to the increased placental resistance, and an absent or reversed a-wave usually indicates critical cardiac condition [22–25] for which delivery in the next 24–48 h may be indicated. In MC twins, however, the unstable anastomoses between the fetuses may render this measurement less reliable, and should be interpreted with caution, particularly in the case of type III sFGR. A thorough and accurate assessment of fetal Dopplers is key in assessing fetal condition and making plans for further management.

9.4 Selective Fetal Growth Restriction

SFGR is covered in more detail in ▶ Chap. 14. Discordance in fetal weight is significantly associated with increased perinatal loss [26]. Intrauterine demise of the smaller twin can lead to neurological sequelae and death in the larger twin, as well as preterm labour [7–10]. There have been inconsistencies in the diagnostic criteria for sFGR, but a recent consensus using the Delphi technique has aimed to reach a uniform conclusion [27]. Figure 9.5 outlines the most recently published diagnostic criteria for this condition.

9.5 Conclusion

Twin and higher-order multiple pregnancies have an increased risk of perinatal morbidity and mortality, and therefore require closer ultrasound surveillance. Abdominal palpation and symphysial fundal height measurements are unreliable in this cohort; therefore, these are not recommended. Ultrasound is currently the best surveillance tool for the growth of multiples; however, it is less accurate than that in singletons in detecting growth anomalies. The growth trajectory of multiples is different to that of singletons; therefore, use of singleton growth charts is not recommended as this can lead to overdiagnosis and unnecessary intervention.

9.5.1 Review Questions

1. Describe how the normal growth trajectory differs between twins and singletons?

2. Describe how the normal growth trajectory differs between monochorionic and dichorionic twins?

3. Why is ultrasound more frequently required in multiple pregnancies than in singletons?

4. What is the frequency that monochorionic twins should be monitored by ultrasound?

5. What additional information can fetal Dopplers give us?

6. Apart from monitoring growth velocity, what other conditions can ultrasound diagnose in twin pregnancies?

9.5.2 Multiple-Choice Questions

1. What should be checked at the 24-week scan in monochorionic twins?
   (a) Fetal growth, uterine artery PI, middle cerebral artery PI, deepest vertical pool
   (b) Fetal growth, uterine artery PI, middle cerebral artery PI, deepest vertical pool
   (c) Fetal growth, umbilical artery PI, ductus venosus PI, deepest vertical pool
   (d) Fetal growth, umbilical artery PI, middle cerebral artery PSV, deepest vertical pool

Answer: (d)

2. How often should dichorionic triamniotic triplet pregnancies be monitored?
   (a) Every 4 weeks from 16 weeks
   (b) Every 2 weeks from 16 weeks
   (c) Every 2 weeks from 20 weeks
   (d) Every 4 weeks from 20 weeks

Answer: (b)

3. What 2 pieces of information can be provided by the middle cerebral artery Doppler?
   (a) Uteroplacental insufficiency and twin to twin transfusion syndrome
   (b) Fetal growth restriction and twin to twin transfusion syndrome
   (c) Cerebral redistribution and fetal anaemia
   (d) Fetal cardiac overload and fetal anaemia

Answer: (c)

4. At what point should a referral be considered to a tertiary fetal medicine centre?
   (a) Abdominal circumference <10th centile in one baby
   (b) Uterine artery PI >95th centile, abdominal circumference <10th centile in one baby
   (c) Deepest vertical pool <2 cm, estimated fetal weight <10th centile in one baby
   (d) Estimated fetal weight discordance >25%, estimated fetal weight <10th centile in one baby

Answer: (d)

5. What is the potential benefit of identifying normal twin and triplet growth patterns using twin-specific growth charts?
   (a) To identify abnormal growth earlier
   (b) To prevent overdiagnosis of fetal growth restriction
   (c) To prevent underdiagnosis of fetal growth restriction
   (d) All of the above

Answer: (b)

6. Which fetal Doppler pattern would be the most concerning feature in a dichorionic pair, suggesting fetal decompensation and need for imminent delivery?
   (a) Umbilical artery absent end-diastolic flow
   (b) Umbilical artery reversed end-diastolic flow

(c) Middle cerebral artery PI <5th centile
(d) Ductus venosus absent a-wave
(e) Ductus venosus PI >95th centile

Answer: (d)

References

1. Gielen M, Lindsey PJ, Derom C, Loos RJ, Souren NY, Paulussen AD, Zeegers MP, Derom R, Vlietinck R, Nijhuis JG. Twin-specific intrauterine 'growth' charts based on cross-sectional birthweight data. Twin Res Hum Genet. 2008;11:224–35.
2. Min SJ, Luke B, Min L, Misiunas R, Nugent C, Van de Ven C, Martin D, Gonzalez-Quintero VH, Eardley S, Witter FR, Mauldin JG, Newman RB. Birth weight references for triplets. Am J Obstet Gynecol. 2004;191(3):809–14.
3. American College of Obstetricians and Gynecologists Committee on Practice Bulletins – Obstetrics; Society for Maternal-Fetal Medicine; ACOG Joint Editorial Committee. ACOG Practice Bulletin #56. Multiple gestation: complicated twin, triplet, and high-order multifetal pregnancy. Obstet Gynecol. 2004;104:869–83.
4. National Institute for Health and Clinical Excellence. Twin and triplet pregnancy. NICE clinical guideline 137. London: National Institute for Health and Clinical Excellence; 2019.
5. Morin L, Lim K. Ultrasound in twin pregnancies. J Obstet Gynaecol Can. 2011;33:643–56.
6. D'Antonio F, Odibo AO, Prefumo F, Khalil A, Buca D, Flacco ME, Liberati M, Manzoli L, Acharya G. Weight discordance and perinatal mortality in twin pregnancy: systematic review and meta-analysis. Ultrasound Obstet Gynecol. 2018;52(1):11–23.
7. Townsend R, Khalil A. Twin pregnancy complicated by selective growth restriction. Curr Opin Obstet Gynecol. 2016 Dec;28(6):485–91.
8. Valsky DV, Eixarch E, Martinez JM, Crispi F, Gratacós E. Selective intrauterine growth restriction in monochorionic twins: pathophysiology, diagnostic approach and management dilemmas. Semin Fetal Neonatal Med. 2010;15:342–8.
9. Townsend R, Khalil A. Fetal growth restriction in twins. Best Pract Res Clin Obstet Gynaecol. 2018;49:79–88.
10. Hamilton E, Platt R, Morin L, Usher R, Kramer M. How small is too small in a twin pregnancy? Am J Obstet Gynecol. 1998;179:682–5.
11. Stirrup OT, Khalil A, D'Antonio F, Thilaganathan B. Fetal growth reference ranges in twin pregnancy: analysis of the Southwest Thames Obstetric Research Collaborative (STORK) multiple pregnancy cohort. Ultrasound Obstet Gynecol. 2015;45(3):301–7.
12. Stirrup OT, Khalil A, D'Antonio F, Thilaganathan B. STORK. Patterns of Second and Third Trimester growth and discordance in twin pregnancy: analysis of the Southwest Thames Obstetric Research Collaborative (STORK) multiple pregnancy cohort. Fetal Diagn Ther. 2017;41(2):100–7.
13. Kalafat E, Sebghati M, Thilaganathan B, Khalil A. Southwest Thames Obstetric Research Collaborative (STORK). Predictive accuracy of Southwest Thames Obstetric Research Collaborative (STORK) chorionicity-specific twin growth charts for stillbirth: a validation study. Ultrasound Obstet Gynecol. 2019;53(2):193–9.
14. Alexander G, Kogan M, Martin J, Papiernik E. What are the fetal growth patterns of singletons, twins, and triplets in the United States? Clin Obstet Gynecol. 1998;41(1):115–25.
15. Blickstein I, Jacques D, Keith L. Total and individual triplet birth weights as function of gestational age. Am J Obstet Gynecol. 2002;186:1372–5.
16. Vora NL, Ruthazer R, House M, Chelmow D. Triplet ultrasound growth parameters. Obstet Gynecol. 2006;107(3):694–700.
17. Khalil A, D'Antonio F, Dias T, Cooper D, Thilaganathan B. Southwest Thames Obstetric Research Collaborative (STORK). Ultrasound estimation of birth weight in twin pregnancy: comparison of biometry algorithms in the STORK multiple pregnancy cohort. Ultrasound Obstet Gynecol. 2014;44:210–20.
18. Sklar C, Yaskina M, Ross S, Naud K. Accuracy of prenatal ultrasound in detecting growth abnormalities in triplets: a retrospective cohort study. Twin Res Hum Genet. 2017;20(1):84–9.
19. Warsof SL, Gohari P, Berkowitz RL, Hobbins JC. The estimation of fetal weight by computer-assisted analysis. Am J Obstet Gynecol. 1977;128:881–92.
20. Hadlock FP, Harrist RB, Martinez-Poyer J. In utero analysis of fetal growth: a sonographic weight standard. Radiology. 1991;181:129–33.
21. ISUOG. Practice guidelines: the role of ultrasound in twin pregnancy. Ultrasound Obstet Gynecol. 2016;47:247–63.
22. Mari G, Hanif F. Fetal doppler: umbilical artery, middle cerebral artery, and venous system. Semin Perinatol. 2008;32:253–7.
23. Hoffman C, Galan HL. Assessing the 'at-risk' fetus: Doppler ultrasound. Med Sci Res. 2009;21:161–6.
24. Kaponis A, Harada T, Makrydimas G, Kiyama T, Arata K, Adonakis G, Harada T. The importance of venous doppler velocimetry for evaluation of intrauterine growth restriction. J Ultrasound Med. 2011;30:529–45.
25. Aditya I, Tat V, Sawana A, Mohamed A, Tuffner R, Mondal T. Use of Doppler velocimetry in diagnosis and prognosis of intrauterine growth restric-

tion (IUGR): a review. J Neonatal-Perinatal Med. 2016;9(2):117–26.
26. D'Antonio F, Khalil A, Dias T, Thilaganathan B. Southwest Thames Obstetric Research Collaborative (STORK). Weight discordance and perinatal mortality in twins: analysis of the Southwest Thames Obstetric Research Collaborative (STORK) multiple pregnancy cohort. Ultrasound Obstet Gynecol. 2013;41:643–8.
27. Khalil A, Beune I, Hecher K, Wynia K, Ganzevoort W, Reed K, Lewi L, Oepkes D, Gratacós E, Thilaganathan B, Gordijn SJ. Consensus definition and essential reporting parameters of selective fetal growth restriction in twin pregnancy: a Delphi procedure. Ultrasound Obstet Gynecol. 2019;53:47–54.

Key Reading

D'Antonio F, Khalil A, Dias T, Thilaganathan B. Southwest Thames Obstetric Research Collaborative (STORK). Weight discordance and perinatal mortality in twins: analysis of the Southwest Thames Obstetric Research Collaborative (STORK) multiple pregnancy cohort. Ultrasound Obstet Gynecol. 2013;41:643–8.

ISUOG. Practice guidelines: the role of ultrasound in twin pregnancy. Ultrasound Obstet Gynecol. 2016;47:247–63.

Kalafat E, Sebghati M, Thilaganathan B, Khalil A. Southwest Thames Obstetric Research Collaborative (STORK). Predictive accuracy of Southwest Thames Obstetric Research Collaborative (STORK) chorionicity-specific twin growth charts for stillbirth: a validation study. Ultrasound Obstet Gynecol. 2019;53(2):193–9.

National Institute for Health and Clinical Excellence. Twin and Triplet Pregnancy. NICE clinical guideline 137. London: National Institute for Health and Clinical Excellence; 2019.

Stirrup OT, Khalil A, D'Antonio F, Thilaganathan B. Fetal growth reference ranges in twin pregnancy: analysis of the Southwest Thames Obstetric Research Collaborative (STORK) multiple pregnancy cohort. Ultrasound Obstet Gynecol. 2015;45(3):301–7.

Prenatal Complications in Multiple Pregnancy

Contents

Twin Pregnancies Discordant for Fetal Anomaly

Ann Langedock and Liesbeth Lewi

Contents

Electronic Supplementary Material The online version of this chapter (https://doi.org/10.1007/978-3-030-47652-6_10) contains supplementary material, which is available to authorized users. The videos can be accessed by scanning the related images with the SN More Media App.

A. Khalil et al. (eds.), *Twin and Higher-order Pregnancies*,
https://doi.org/10.1007/978-3-030-47652-6_10

Trailer

Structural anomalies are more common in a twin setting, and usually, only one twin is affected. As such, one expects a structural anomaly in about 1 in 17 dichorionic, 1 in 10 monochorionic, and 1 in 5 monoamniotic twin pregnancies. In contrast, chromosomal anomalies are probably somewhat less common in a twin setting, because aneuploidy is less likely to survive in a twin setting. For the management of a discordant anomaly, it is essential to know the exact chorionicity. In dichorionic pairs, selective reduction is best performed in the first trimester. Therefore, a detailed first-trimester anatomy scan is essential, and a chorionic villous sampling is the preferred diagnostic test for dichorionic twin pregnancies. In monochorionic pairs, selective reduction is to be performed only after 15–16 weeks, and a double amniocentesis is the preferred test for a discordant anomaly in order to diagnose rare heterokaryotypic twins.

Definitions

Discordant anomaly: refers to only one of a twin pair having an anomaly or both having a different anomaly

Heterokaryotypic monozygotic twins: refers to monozygotic twins having a different chromosomal makeup

Learning Objectives

- To understand the incidence and management of discordant structural and chromosomal anomalies in dichorionic and monochorionic twin pregnancies
- To understand the etiology and diagnosis of heterokaryotypic monochorionic twin pregnancies

10.1 Introduction

In a twin setting, the risks, diagnosis, and management of a congenital anomaly are primarily determined by the chorionicity, which should be determined at the time of the first-trimester ultrasound scan (see ▶ Chap. 6). A discordant anomaly refers to the condition where only one of the twins has an anomaly, or more rarely, where both have a different anomaly. In this chapter, we will give an overview of the incidence, diagnosis, and management of discordant structural and chromosomal anomalies in dichorionic and monochorionic twin pregnancies.

10.2 Discordant Structural Anomalies

Structural anomalies are more common in twins than in singletons [1–3]. Despite the more difficult ultrasound scan in twin pregnancies, the detection rate of anomalies is similar to that in singletons [1]. As such, about 27% anomalies are already picked up on the first-trimester scan [4], which is only slightly less than the reported 30% detection rate in singletons [5] (See Section III, ▶ Chap. 9 – O. Kagan). First-trimester detection seems especially relevant for non-lethal anomalies that may result in a severe impairment such as open spina bifida or may threaten the healthy co-twin such as anencephaly (◘ Fig. 10.1, Video 10.1). Nevertheless, certain anomalies such as duodenal atresia or abnormalities of the corpus callosum cannot be detected in the first trimester yet, and detailed second- and third-trimester scans remain mandatory. Preferentially, experienced sonographers per-

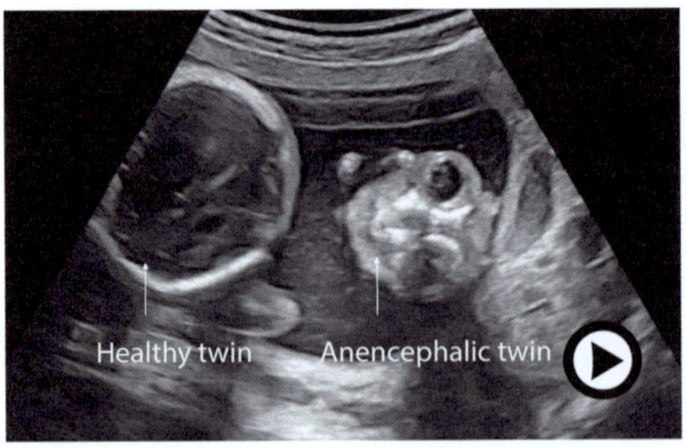

◘ **Fig. 10.1** Sonographic image of discordancy for anencephaly in a monoamniotic twin pair at 19 weeks
Video 10.1 Sonographic image of discordancy for anencephaly in a monoamniotic twin pair at 19 weeks (https://doi.org/10.1007/000-2t6)

form these scans, and sufficient time is foreseen to examine both twins carefully [6].

If a discordant anomaly is diagnosed, an invasive test should be offered, which is best performed in a tertiary care center by the same operator who also performs the reduction and after careful labeling of the twins [7]. Procedure-related loss and inconclusive results after invasive testing are likely to be higher than in singletons. However, in experienced hands, the procedure-related loss is estimated to be low even after double sampling and probably less than 1% [8] (See Section III, ▶ Chap. 8 – O. Kagan).

In a twin setting, the outcome of the anomaly may be worse than in a singleton pregnancy, as twins are born earlier and have a lower birth weight. The low birth weight is especially relevant for cardiac anomalies that require early cardiac intervention, such as in transposition of the great arteries [9] or a critical coarctation of the aorta [10]. Also, the benefit of prenatal intervention (such as thoracic shunting) to improve the outcome of the affected twin must be carefully balanced against the risk of miscarriage and early birth for the healthy twin.

10.2.1 Discordant Structural Anomalies in a Dichorionic Pair

About 90% of dichorionic twins are dizygotic [11], so the chance that at least one has a structural anomaly is twice as high as in singletons since two fetuses are present in one pregnancy. However, being part of a dizygotic twin pair also slightly increases the risk of a structural anomaly. As such, a structural anomaly is found in 3.2% of dizygotic twin fetuses, as compared to 2.4% of singletons [2]. Congenital heart disease is the most common anomaly [12], but there is an increase in almost every organ system [2]. The reason for the rise in structural anomalies in dizygotic twins is currently not well understood. Part may be due to the 10% monozygotic dichorionic twins and the teratogenic effect of the embryonic split. Also, since a significant proportion of dichorionic twins are the result of assisted conception, there is a possible impact of subfertility or its treatment on normal fetal development [2]. In 90% of pregnancies, only one twin is affected. Since a 3.2% of dizygotic twin fetuses have a structural anomaly, one expects to find a structural anomaly in about 1 in 17 dichorionic twin pregnancies.

Selective reduction in a dichorionic setting is performed by the intracardiac injection of potassium chloride or lidocaine under ultrasound guidance using a 22-gauge needle (0.7 mm) (See Section IV, ▶ Chap. 12). In dichorionic twin pregnancies, a detailed first-trimester anatomy scan is of utmost importance to exclude a severe discordant anomaly, since a reduction in the first-trimester carries a lower risk of miscarriage and very preterm birth than a reduction at 20 weeks.

Once we detect a major discordant anomaly, we offer a chorionic villus sampling or, if the diagnosis is made later in pregnancy, an amniocentesis (See Section III, ▶ Chap. 8 – O. Kagan). We usually perform a double sampling, especially in same-sex twins, as 10% of dichorionic pairs are monozygotic, and it seems vital to ascertain that the healthy-looking twin does not have a chromosomal anomaly before a selective reduction is performed. For the sampling of both placentas, we use either a transabdominal or transvaginal sampling or a combination of both. For amniocentesis, we always puncture each sac separately and avoid a septostomy. However, other operators perform a single puncture and septostomy. The disadvantage of septostomy is that preterm rupture of the membranes leads to oligohydramnios in both sacs. Also, septostomy may increase the risk of contamination and inconclusive results.

For second-trimester diagnoses, the amniocentesis and reduction may be referred to after 28 weeks to avoid the risks of miscarriage and extreme preterm birth [13]. The downside of such a late elective reduction is that it is more stressful for parents. Also, since 3–4% of twins are born before 28 weeks [14], an urgent, earlier intervention may be necessary. For conditions expected to be lethal during pregnancy, such as severe Ebstein's anomaly, it may be preferable to manage these expectantly and avoid the procedure-related loss rate of a reduction. Similarly, for conditions expected to result in an early neonatal demise, like in bilateral renal agenesis, it may be preferable not to perform a reduction and to give comfort care after birth.

10.2.2 Discordant Structural Anomalies in a Monochorionic Pair

Even though monochorionic twins are monozygotic and thus genetically identical, in up to 80%, only one is affected [15]. Also, in monochorionic pregnancies, the risk of a structural anomaly per fetus is probably two to three times higher than in singletons, 6.3% compared to 2.4% [2]. As such, one can expect to find a structural anomaly in about 1 in 10 monochorionic diamniotic twin pregnancies. This increased risk of structural anomalies may be related to the early cleavage of the zygote or complications of the shared circulation causing vascular accidents affecting cardiac and neurologic development. Especially congenital heart disease is more prevalent among monochorionic twins, with an estimated sixfold increase as compared to singletons (5.9% versus 0.7%) [16]. After twin-twin transfusion syndrome (TTTS) (See Section V, ▶ Chap. 11 – K. Hecher), 8.7% of twins are born with a congenital heart defect, with right outflow tract obstruction being the most common heart defect mainly affecting the recipient twin (◘ Fig. 10.2, Video 10.2). Also, right ventricular outflow tract obstruction is not unique to TTTS, and it may also affect the larger twin in selective fetal growth restriction, while the smaller twin is at increased risk of coarctation [17] (See Section II, ▶ Chap. 12 A. Khalil). Transfusion imbalances may also explain the higher observed incidence of acquired brain lesions, bowel perforations, and limb amputations in monochorionic twins, which may become apparent only after the second-trimester anomaly scan [18–20] (◘ Fig. 10.3, Videos 10.3 and 10.4). Therefore, a continuous search for these acquired lesions should be performed throughout pregnancy. In monochorionic monoamniotic pairs (See Section V, ▶ Chap. 19 T. Vanmieghem), the risk of a structural anomaly (especially congenital heart disease) is even higher, and an anomaly is expected in about one in five monoamniotic twin pregnancies [21]. Anomalies unique to monochorionic pregnancies are the twin reversed arterial perfusion (TRAP) (See Section V, ▶ Chap. 16) and conjoined twinning (See Section V, ▶ Chap. 20 – A. Johnson).

Once a discordant anomaly is diagnosed, we offer a double amniocentesis and sample both sacs separately, as chromosomal discordances may occur even in a monochorionic and thus monozygotic twin pair (see below). Management is dependent on the severity, the impact on the healthy twin, and the request of the parents. Selective reduction in a monochorionic setting cannot be performed by intrafetal injection as, due to the shared circulation, intrafetal injection may lead to the loss of both twins (See Section IV, ▶ Chap. 12 – L. De Catte). In a monochorionic setting, the circulation of the affected twin must be isolated from that of the healthy twin by intrafetal or cord coagulation, which requires larger access (17 gauge (1.5 mm) to 10 French (3.3 mm)) than the 22-gauge (0.7 mm) needle used in dichorionic twins. Also, since monochorionic twins share the same exocoelomic cavity, the reduction is usually performed only after 15–16 weeks once amnion and chorion have fused. So, in monochorionic twins with a discordant structural anomaly that threatens the well-being of its co-twin like TRAP, a selective reduction can be offered from 15

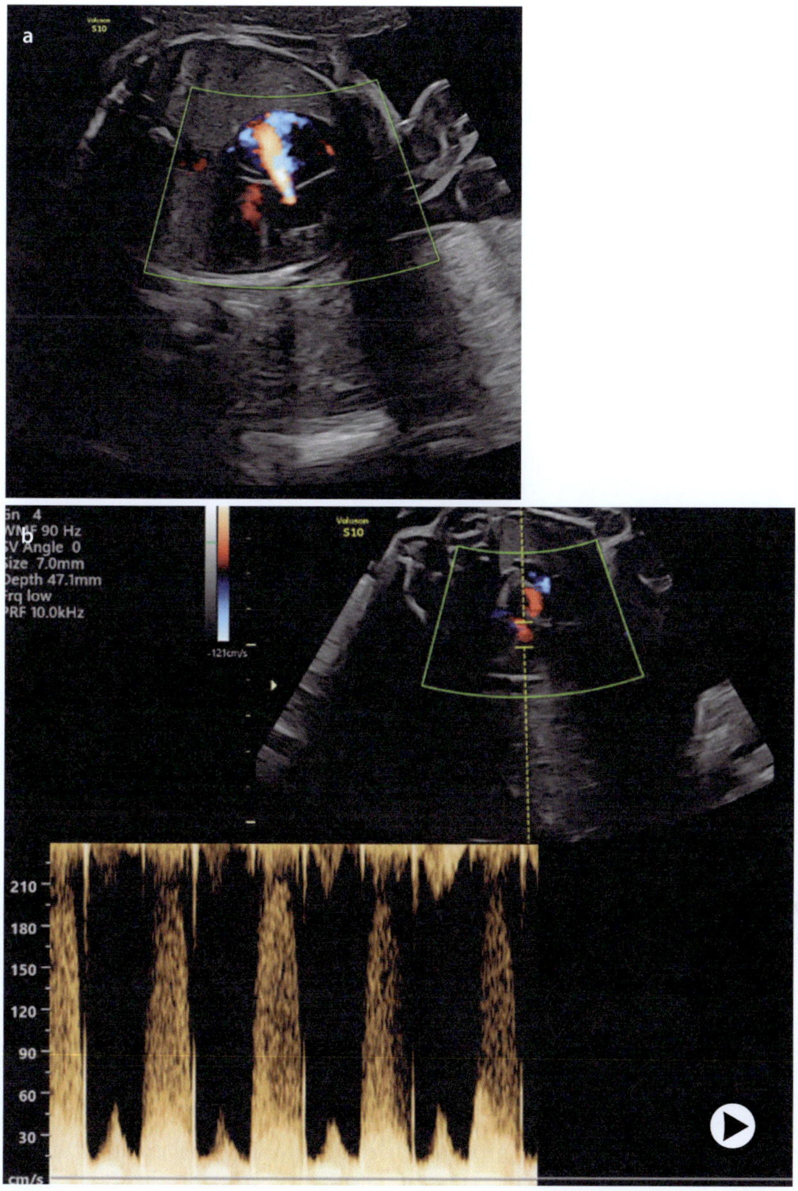

Fig. 10.2 Ultrasound image of tricuspid regurgitation a at 28 weeks in the ex-recipient, 10 weeks after fetoscopic laser surgery for stage 3 twin-twin transfusion syndrome. Prior to surgery, the recipient had a functional pulmonary atresia with reversed flow over the duct and tricuspid regurgitation

Video 10.2 Ultrasound image of tricuspid regurgitation a at 28 weeks in the ex-recipient, 10 weeks after fetoscopic laser surgery for stage 3 twin-twin transfusion syndrome. Prior to surgery, the recipient had a functional pulmonary atresia with reversed flow over the duct and tricuspid regurgitation (https://doi.org/10.1007/000-2t7)

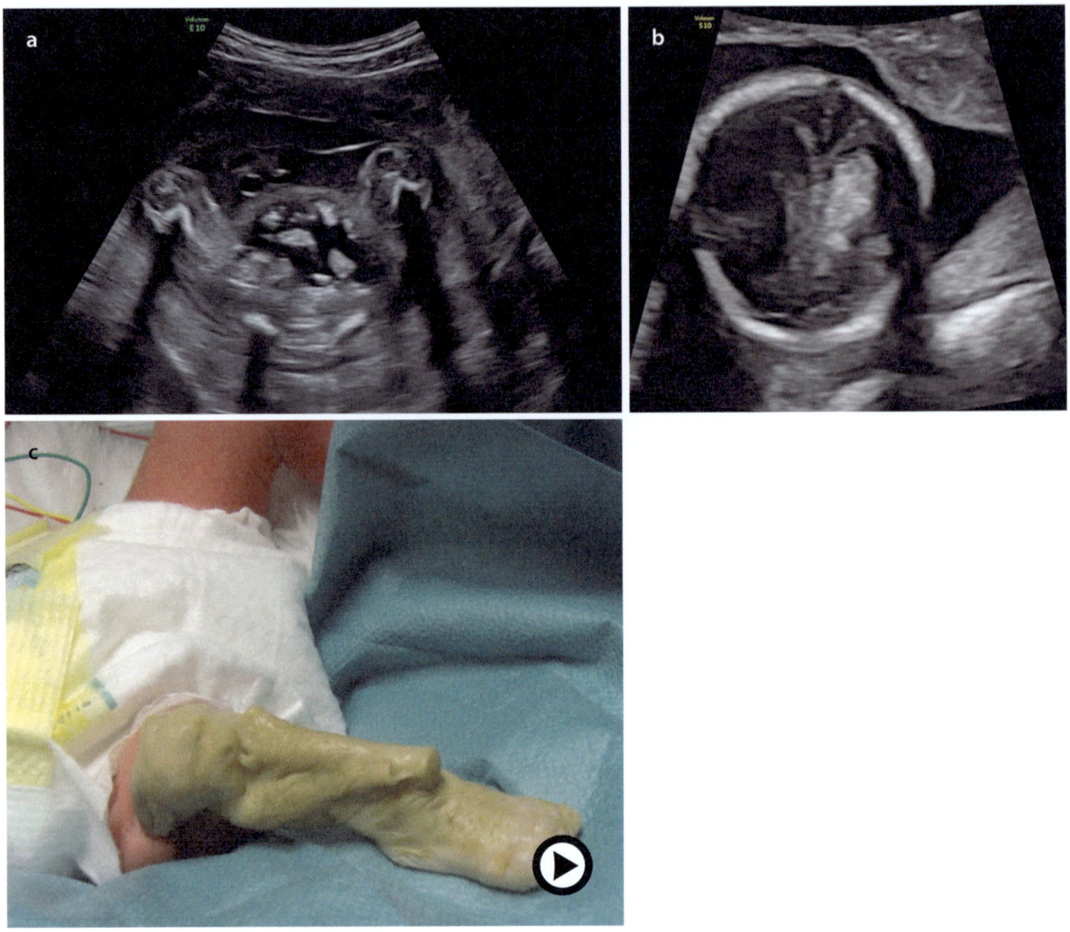

Fig. 10.3 Possible acquired anomalies related to twin-twin transfusion syndrome. **a** Ultrasound image at 23 weeks of bowel necrosis and ascites in donor, 3 weeks after fetoscopic laser surgery at 20 weeks for twin-twin transfusion syndrome stage 4 with postoperative demise of the recipient. **b** Grade 4 intraventricular hemorrhage frontoparietal left in recipient day 1 after fetoscopic laser surgery at 18 weeks for stage 3 twin-twin transfusion syndrome. **c** Image of ischemic leg in recipient twin born at 35 weeks after fetoscopic laser surgery for stage 4 twin-twin transfusion syndrome and twin anemia polycythemia sequence
Video 10.3 Ultrasound image of bowel necrosis and severe ascites in donor twin after fetoscopic laser surgery at 20 weeks for stage 4 twin-twin transfusion syndrome
Video 10.4 Ultrasound image of Grade 4 intraventricular hemorrhage frontoparietal left in recipient day 1 after fetoscopic laser surgery (https://doi.org/10.1007/000-2t8)

to 16 weeks onward. In a dichorionic setting, we preferentially manage conditions that result in an intrauterine demise expectantly to avoid any procedure-related miscarriage and very preterm birth. In monochorionic twins, however, these conditions require an early reduction to avoid the 40% risk of co-twin demise and 25% of acquired brain lesions due to exsanguination of the healthy co-twin [22]. Similarly, as in dichorionic pairs, conditions that are expected to be lethal in the early neonatal period can be managed expectantly in monochorionic twins as well (Fig. 10.4). Also, a late elective reduction at 28–30 weeks is an option for conditions that are non-lethal but associated with severe impairment in countries where this is legally permitted to avoid the procedure-related loss and extreme preterm birth (Figs. 10.5 and 10.6, Video 10.5).

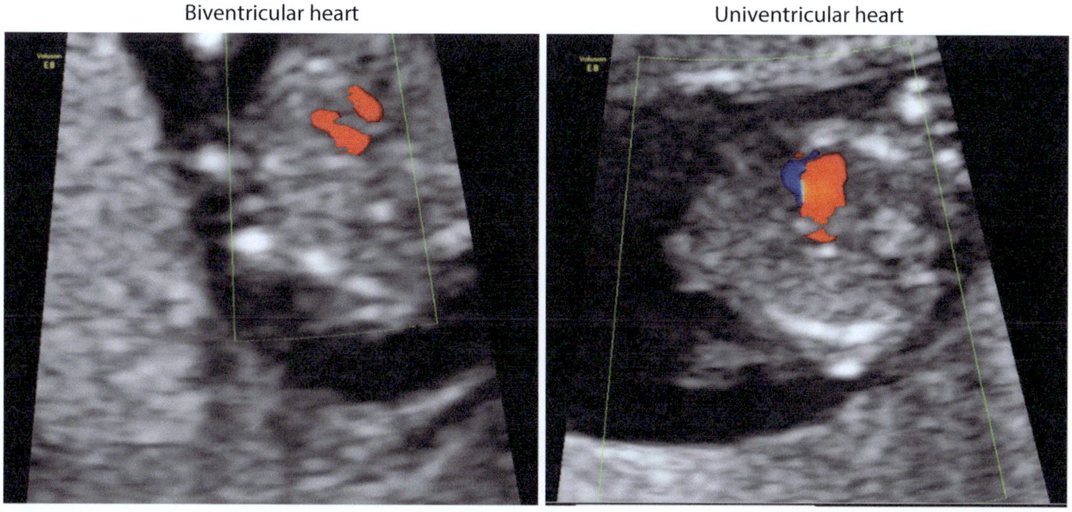

Fig. 10.4 Image of a hypoplastic left heart syndrome in a monochorionic diamniotic twin pregnancy suspected at 12 weeks and confirmed at 16 weeks. Despite the first-trimester diagnosis, the parents opted for comfort care after birth. The patient was induced at 36 weeks and the affected twin passed away 2 days after birth

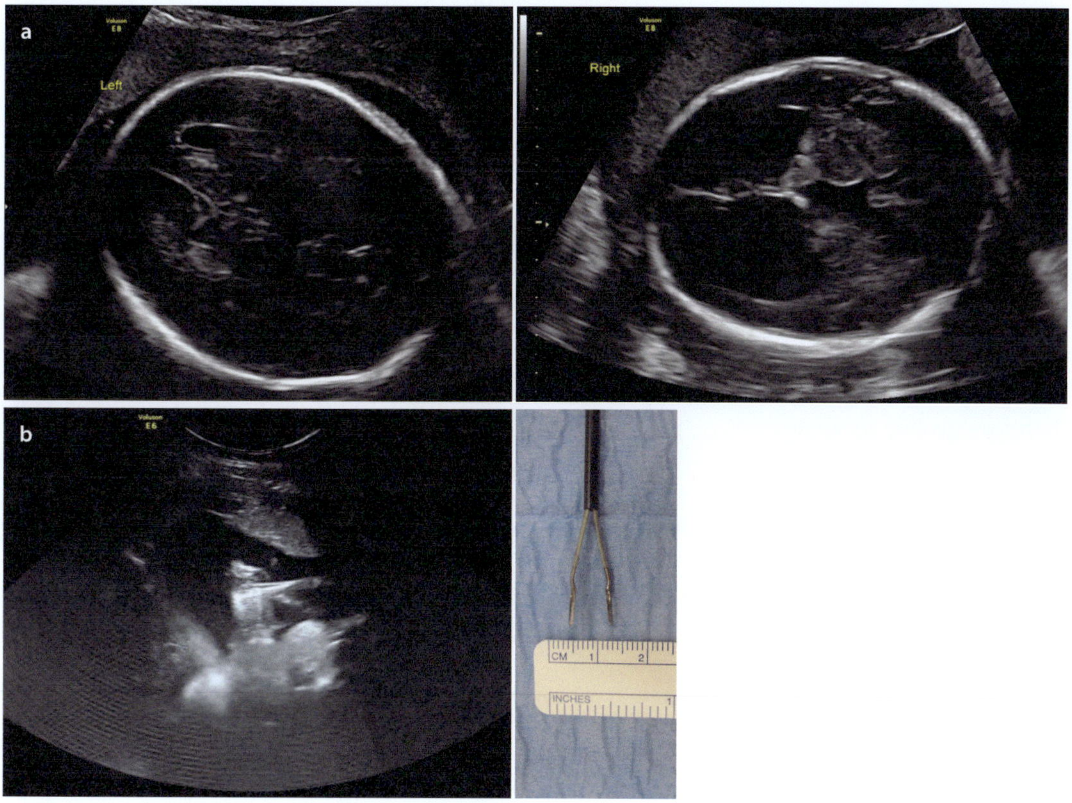

Fig. 10.5 **a** Sonographic image of severe ventriculomegaly in the smaller twin of a monochorionic diamniotic twin pregnancy at 28 weeks. **b** The parents opted for an elective cord occlusion at 29 weeks, which is performed under ultrasound guidance using a bipolar forceps through a 10 French (3.3) cannula

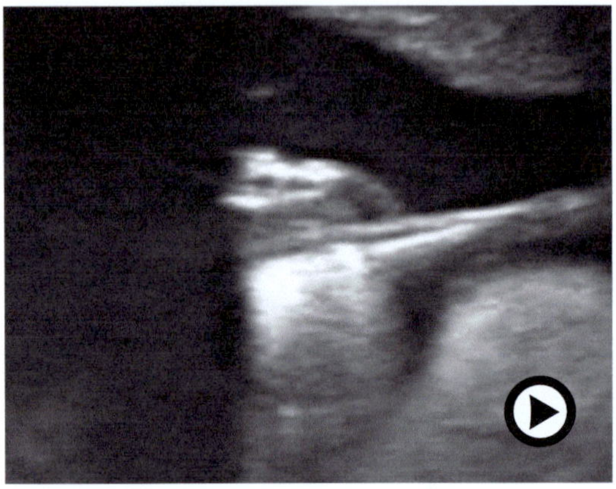

Fig. 10.6 Cord occlusion
Video 10.4 Ultrasound-guided cord coagulation at 28 weeks after amnioinfusion (https://doi.org/10.1007/000-2t9)

10.3 Discordant Chromosomal Anomalies

The most studied aneuploidy in twin pregnancies is trisomy 21 (T21). The maternal age-related risk of a twin having T21 is lower than that of a singleton, as babies with T21 seem less likely to survive a twin setting [23, 24]. When we discuss the option of screening for chromosomal anomalies in a twin setting (See Section III, ► Chap. 8 – O. Kagan), we should also address the possibility of selective reduction should one of the twins be diagnosed with a chromosomal anomaly. Some parents would not consider selective reduction and therefore decline to screen.

10.3.1 Discordant Chromosomal Anomalies in a Dichorionic Pair

Since 90% of dichorionic twins are dizygotic, usually only one twin is affected, and therefore, the risk of one twin having T21 should theoretically be twice the risk of a singleton pregnancy. So, for a 35-year-old mother, the risk is 1 in 250 for a single baby to have T21, but 1 in 125 (twice the singelton risk) that one of her dichorionic twins has T21. However, fetuses with T21 are less likely to survive a dichorionic twin setting, and so the chance of one baby having T21 in a dichorionic setting is 1.34 rather than 2 times the age-related risk [23], and so the risk for a 35-year-old patient having T21 in one of the twins is 1 in 187 rather than 1 in 125. In a dichorionic dizygotic twin, the risk of both having T21 should be extremely low and is calculated by multiplying the adjusted age-related risk (1 in 374 multiplied by 1 in 374).

In dichorionic twins, the combined screening test by maternal age, nuchal translucency, and serum biochemistry adapted to twin chorionicity determines the risk for each individual twin and has a similar detection rate as in singletons (86%) but twice its false-positive rate (10%), as two risks are calculated for each twin separately [25]. Alternatively, noninvasive prenatal testing (NIPT) can be offered, which appears to have similar accuracy as in singleton pregnancies [26].

If a chromosomal anomaly is suspected in one of a dichorionic twin pair, then a chorionic villous sampling is the preferred diagnostic test as it allows for a first-trimester reduction with lower associated risks than a mid-trimester reduction.

10.3.2 Discordant Chromosomal Anomalies in a Monochorionic Pair

T21 is even less common in a monochorionic setting and 0.34 that of a singleton [23]. Because of the monozygocity, however, both are usually affected, and a pregnancy-specific risk is calculated. However, discordances have been reported for all common human aneuploidies [27, 28], but most commonly for Turner syndrome [29] (Fig. 10.7) and increasingly for more subtle chromosomal rearrangements, such as deletions and duplications [30, 31]. The difference in chromosomal makeup between twins of a monochorionic pair is known as hetererokaryotic monochorionic twinning and is only picked up by an amniocentesis of both sacs. Heterokaryotypic monochorionic twins can be mosaic. Here, errors in early mitotic cell division such as nondisjunction and anaphase lagging may give rise to two different cell lines. For example, the

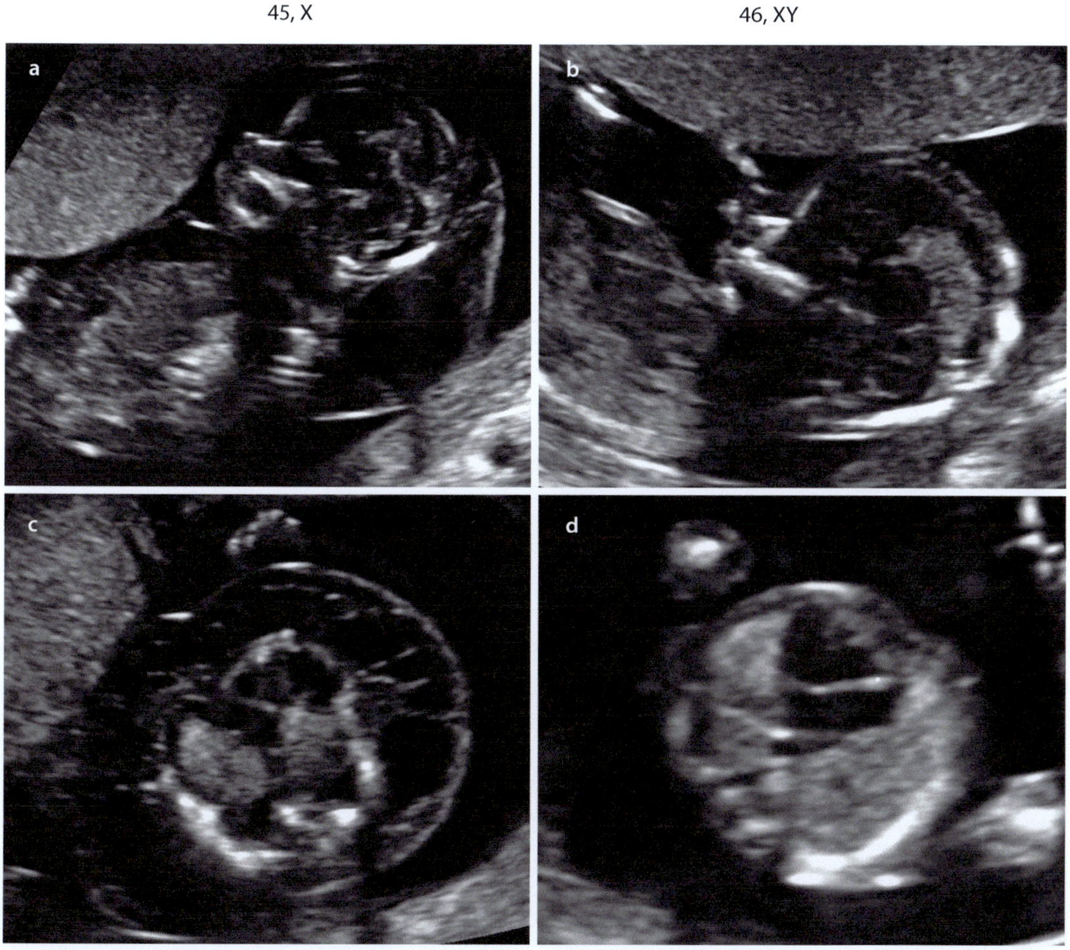

Fig. 10.7 First-trimester sonographic images of a heterokaryotypic monochorionic diamniotic twin pregnancy (45, X; 46, XY), as confirmed at dual amniocentesis. The female with Turner syndrome had a cystic hygroma, generalized subcutaneous edema **a**, and bilateral pleural effusion **b**, whereas the male was structurally normal **c**, **d**

zygote may be a priori trisomic, but the extra chromosome is lost during the early cell divisions. This results in a normal and trisomic cell line, which could trigger a monozygotic cleavage as cells with a different chromosomal constitution will repulse each other. This correction is also known as trisomic rescue, and if the trisomy is maternal in origin and the paternal copy is lost, then the remaining two copies are maternal in origin. This may cause clinically important uniparental disomy in the healthy twin [32]. Uniparental disomy for chromosome 15 is most common, where two maternal copies result in Prader–Willy syndrome. Another explanation for the occurrence of heterokaryotypic monochorionic twinning is chimerism, where there is a fusion of two cell lines from two different conceptions. Chimerism gives rise to the rare dizygotic monochorionic twinning and is probably more common after in vitro fertilization [33].

In monochorionic twins, the combined screening test by maternal age, the average nuchal translucency, and serum biochemistry adapted to twin chorionicity calculates the pregnancy-specific risk for both twins to be affected. The combined test in monochorionic twins has a similar detection rate as in singletons (87%) [25] albeit with slightly higher false-positive rates as in about 1 in 10 monochorionic twin pregnancies the nuchal measurement is increased [34]. Alternatively, noninvasive prenatal testing (NIPT) can be offered, which theoretically should have the same accuracy as in singletons because monochorionic twins are monozygotic.

If a chromosomal anomaly is suspected in only one of a monochorionic twin pair, then a double amniocentesis is the preferred diagnostic test. A chorionic villous sampling of the shared placenta may be normal and may miss the aneuploidy present in one twin. Conversely, the chorionic villous sampling may be abnormal and may miss the presence of a normal twin.

10.4 Conclusion

In a twin setting, it is essential to know whether the twins are monochorionic or dichorionic. Structural anomalies are more common in a twin setting, and usually, only one twin is affected, whereas aneuploidy is probably somewhat less common because fetuses with aneuploidy are less likely to survive a twin setting. The outcome of anomalies that require an early neonatal intervention may be less favorable than in singletons because twins are born early and have a lower birth weight. In dichorionic pairs, selective reduction is best performed in the first trimester and, therefore, chorionic villous sampling is the preferred diagnostic test. In monochorionic pairs, selective reduction is currently only performed after 15–16 weeks, and double amniocentesis is the preferred diagnostic test for a discordant anomaly to diagnose rare heterokaryotypic twins.

10.4.1 Review Questions

1. What is the expected incidence of a structural and chromosomal anomaly for a di- and monochorionic twin pregnancy?

2. What explains the occurrence of heterokaryotypic monochorionic twin pregnancies, and how are they diagnosed?

10.4.2 Multiple-Choice Questions

1. At 12 weeks, you diagnose a dichorionic twin pregnancy. The pregnancy was conceived spontaneously. The patient is 37 years old, and it concerns the first pregnancy. One twin has an increased nuchal translucency of 4.5 mm. The other twin looks structurally normal. What do you tell the patient?
   (a) As a first step, you would offer a noninvasive prenatal test (NIPT) to exclude the presence of a chromosomal anomaly.
   (b) You would offer a chorionic villous sampling to exclude the presence of a chromosomal anomaly.
   (c) You would offer an amniocentesis at 15–16 weeks to exclude the presence of a chromosomal anomaly.
   (d) You would offer a selective reduction as the outcome is likely to be poor.

Answer: (b)

2. At 12 weeks, you diagnose a monochorionic diamniotic twin pregnancy. The pregnancy was conceived spontaneously. The patient is 37 years old, and it concerns the first pregnancy. One twin has an increased nuchal translucency of 4.5 mm. The other twin looks structurally normal. What do you tell the patient?
   (a) As a first step, you would offer a noninvasive prenatal test (NIPT) to exclude the presence of a chromosomal anomaly.
   (b) You would offer a chorionic villous sampling to exclude the presence of a chromosomal anomaly.
   (c) You would offer an amniocentesis at 15–16 weeks to exclude the presence of a chromosomal anomaly.
   (d) You would offer a selective reduction as the outcome is likely to be poor.

Answer: (c)

10

Disclosure Statement

The authors report no conflict of interest.

Financial Support

LL is the recipient of a grant of "Fonds voor Wetenschappelijk Onderzoek" (FWO grant no: 1804718N).

References

1. Boyle B, McConkey R, Garne E, Loane M, Addor M, Bakker BP, Gatt M, Greenlees R, Haeusler M, KlungsØyr K, Latos-Bielenska A, Lelong N, McDonnell R, Métneki J, Mullaney C, Nelen V, O'Mahony M, Pierini RJ, Rissmann A, Tucker D, Wellesley D, Dolk H. Trends in the prevalence, risk and pregnancy outcome of multiple births with congenital anomaly: a registry-based study in 14 European countries 1984–2007. BJOG. 2013;120:707–16.
2. Glinianaia SV, Rankin J, Wright C. Congenital anomalies in twins: a register-based study. Hum Reprod. 2008;23(6):1306–11.
3. Doyle PE, Beral V, Botting B, Wale CJ. Congenital malformations in twins in England and Wales. J Epidemiol Community Health. 1990;45:43–8.
4. D'Antonio F, Familiari A, Thilaganathan B, Papageorghiou A, Manzoli L, Khalil A, Bhide A. Sensitivity of first-trimester ultrasound in the detection of congenital anomalies in twin pregnancies: population study and systematic review. Acta Obstet Gynecol Scand. 2016;95:1359–67.
5. Syngelaki A, Hammami A, Bower S, Zidere V, Akolekar R, Nicolaides KH. Diagnosis of fetal non-chromosomal abnormalities on routine ultrasound examination at 11–13 weeks' gestation. Ultrasound Obstet Gynecol. 2019;54(4):468–76.
6. NICE guideline. Multiple pregnancy: twin and triplet pregnancies Quality standard [QS46] Published date: September 2013. https://www.nice.org.uk/guidance/qs46. Accessed 1st Oct 2019.
7. RCOG Greentop guideline. Amniocentesis and Chorionic Villus Sampling (Green-top Guideline No. 8). https://www.rcog.org.uk/globalassets/documents/guidelines/gtg_8.pdf. Accessed 1st Oct 2019.
8. Salomon LJ, Sotiriadis A, Wulff CB, Odibo A, Akolekar R. Risk of miscarriage following amniocentesis or chorionic villus sampling: systematic review of literature and updated meta-analysis. Ultrasound Obstet Gynecol. 2019;54(4):442–51.
9. Kaneko Y, Tsuchiya K, Yamamoto Y, Yoda H, Yamamoto W, Kobayashi J. Arterial switch in a 1146-gram neonate with transposition of the great arteries and an intramural coronary artery. J Thorac Cardiovasc Surg. 2007;134(4):1064–5.
10. Wirbelauer J, Bauer J, Akintuerk H. Successful surgery and long-term outcome of a critical isthmic coarctation in an extremely preterm infant with a birth weight of 545 g. Pediatr Cardiol. 2009;30(7):1009–11.
11. Derom C, Thiery E, Rutten BPF, et al. The East Flanders Prospective Twin Survey (EFPTS): 55 Years Later [published online ahead of print]. Twin Res Hum Genet. 2019;2019:1–6.
12. Herskind AM, Almind Pedersen D, Christensen K. Increased prevalence of congenital heart defects in monozygotic and dizygotic twins. Circulation. 2013;128(11):1182–8.
13. Shalev J, Meizner I, Rabinerson D, Mashiach R, Hod M, Bar-Chava I, Peleg D, Ben-Rafael Z. Improving pregnancy outcome in twin gestations with one malformed fetus by postponing selective feticide in the third trimester. Fertil Steril. 1999;72(2):257–60.
14. SPE rapport Vlaanderen 2018. https://www.zorg-en-gezondheid.be/jaarrapport-spe-2018-trends-in-geboortes-en-bevallingen-in-vlaanderen. Accessed 1st Oct 2019
15. Couck I, Ponnet S, Deprest J, Devlieger R, De Catte L, Lewi L. The outcome of selective intrauterine growth restriction in monochorionic twin pregnancies at 16, 20 or 30 weeks according to the new consensus definition: a retrospective cohort study. Submitted for UOG.
16. Gijtenbeek M, Shirzada MR, Ten Harkel ADJ, Oepkes D, Haak MC. Congenital heart defects in monochorionic twins: a systematic review and meta-analysis. J Clin Med. 2019;8(6):902.
17. Gijtenbeek M, Haak MC, ten Harkel ADJ, Bokenkamp-Gramann R, Ortibus E, Meynse B, Gewillig M, Lewi L. Critical aortic coarctation in sFGR and the role of coronary stent implantation as bridging therapy for surgery: a case series and systematic review of the literature. Submitted for UOG.
18. Lopriore E, Slaghekke F, Kersbergen KJ, de Vries LS, Drogtrop AP, Middeldorp JM, Oepkes D, Benders MJ. Severe cerebral injury in a recipient with twin anemia-polycythemia sequence. Ultrasound Obstet Gynecol. 2013;41(6):702–6.
19. Tsukimori K, Yumoto Y, Masumoto K, Taguchi T, Kondo H, Sueishi K, Wake N. Ischemic ileal perforation in the donor of monochorionic twins complicated by twin-twin transfusion syndrome. Fetal Diagn Ther. 2009;26(3):173–6.
20. Lopriore E, Lewi L, Oepkes D, Debeer A, Vandenbussche FP, Deprest J, Walther FJ. In utero acquired limb ischemia in monochorionic twins with and without twin-to-twin transfusion syndrome. Prenat Diagn. 2008;28(9):800–4.
21. Van Mieghem T, De Heus R, Lewi L, Klaritsch P, Kollmann M, Baud D, Vial Y, Shah PS, Ranzini AC, Mason L, Raio L, Lachat R, Barrett J, Khorsand V, Windrim R, Ryan G. Prenatal management of monoamniotic twin pregnancies. Obstet Gynecol. 2014;124:498–506.

22. Mackie FL, Rigby A, Morris RK, Kilby MD. Prognosis of the co-twin following spontaneous single intrauterine fetal death in twin pregnancies: a systematic review and meta-analysis. BJOG. 2019;126(5):569–78.
23. Boyle B, Morris JK, McConkey R, Garne E, Loane M, Addor MC, Gatt M, Haeusler M, Latos-Bielenska A, Lelong N, McDonnell R, Mullaney C, O'Mahony M, Dolk H. Prevalence and risk of Down syndrome in monozygotic and dizygotic multiple pregnancies in Europe: implications for prenatal screening. BJOG. 2014;121(7):809–19.
24. Sparks TN, Norton ME, Flessel M, Goldman S, Currier RJ. Observed rate of down syndrome in twin pregnancies. Obstet Gynecol. 2016;128(5):1127–33.
25. Prats P, Rodríguez I, Comas C, Puerto B. Systematic review of screening for trisomy 21 in twin pregnancies in first trimester combining nuchal translucency and biochemical markers: a meta-analysis. Prenat Diagn. 2014;34(11):1077–83.
26. Gil MM, Galeva S, Jani J, Konstantinidou L, Akolekar R, Plana MN, Nicolaides KH. Screening for trisomies by cfDNA testing of maternal blood in twin pregnancy: update of the Fetal Medicine Foundation results and meta-analysis. Ultrasound Obstet Gynecol. 2019;53:734–42.

27. Lewi L, Blickstein I, Van Schoubroeck D, Gloning KP, Casteels M, Brandenburg H, et al. Diagnosis and management of heterokaryotypic monochorionic twins. Am J Med Genet A. 2006;140:272–5.
28. Sepulveda W, Wong AE, Ocaranza M. Heterokaryotypic pregnancy: monozygotic monochorionic twins discordant for trisomy 13. Fetal Diagn Ther. 2010;28:109–13.
29. Bohec C, Douet-Guilbert N, Basinko A, Le Bris MJ, Marcorelles P, Audrézet MP, et al. Difficult diagnosis and management of an heterokaryotypic monochorionic twin pregnancy with discordant fetal sex and 45,X/47,XYY karyotypes. Fetal Pediatr Pathol. 2010;29:424–30.
30. Essaoui M, Nizon M, Beaujard MP, Carrier A, Tantau J, de Blois MC, et al. Monozygotic twins discordant for 18q21.2qter deletion detected by array CGH in amniotic fluid. Eur J Med Genet. 2013;56:502–5.
31. Peng R, Zhou Y, Xie HN, Zheng J, Xie YJ, Yang JB. MCDA twins with discordant malformations: submicroscopic chromosomal anomalies detected by chromosomal microarray analysis and clinical outcomes. Prenat Diagn. 2016;36:766–74.
32. Machin GA. Some causes of genotypic and phenotypic discordance in monozygotic twin pairs. Am J Med Genet. 1996;61:216–28.
33. Souter VL, Kapur RP, Nyholt DR, Skogerboe K, Myerson D, Ton CC, Opheim KE, Easterling TR, Shields LE, Montgomery GW, Glass IA. A report of dizygous monochorionic twins. N Engl J Med. 2003;349(2):154–8.
34. Vandecruys H, Faiola S, Auer M, Sebire N, Nicolaides KH. Screening for trisomy 21 in monochorionic twins by measurement of fetal nuchal translucency thickness. Ultrasound Obstet Gynecol. 2005;25(6):551–3.

Key Reading

Boyle B, McConkey R, Garne E, et al. Trends in the prevalence, risk and pregnancy outcome of multiple births with congenital anomaly: a registry-based study in 14 European countries 1984–2007. BJOG. 2013;120(6):707–16.

Boyle B, Morris JK, McConkey R, Garne E, Loane M, Addor MC, Gatt M, Haeusler M, Latos-Bielenska A, Lelong N, McDonnell R, Mullaney C, O'Mahony M, Dolk H. Prevalence and risk of Down syndrome in monozygotic and dizygotic multiple pregnancies in Europe: implications for prenatal screening. BJOG. 2014;121(7):809–19.

Glinianaia SV, Rankin J, Wright C. Congenital anomalies in twins: a register-based study. Hum Reprod. 2008;23(6):1306–11.

Fetal Reduction/Selective Termination in Uncomplicated Twins and Multiple Pregnancies

Mercede Sebghati, Becky Liu, and Asma Khalil

Contents

Electronic Supplementary Material The online version of this chapter (https://doi.org/10.1007/978-3-030-47652-6_11) contains supplementary material, which is available to authorized users. The videos can be accessed by scanning the related images with the SN More Media App.

A. Khalil et al. (eds.), *Twin and Higher-order Pregnancies*,
https://doi.org/10.1007/978-3-030-47652-6_11

Trailer

The incidence of twin and higher order pregnancies is rising mainly due to increasing maternal age at conception and the resultant widespread use of assisted reproduction techniques. Changes in population demographics have also contributed to the rise. In 2009, 16 women per 1000 giving birth in England and Wales had multiple births, compared with 10 women per 1000 in 1980 [1].

Multiple pregnancies are associated with a high risk of perinatal morbidity and mortality compared with singleton pregnancies. In this chapter, we discuss the associated complications of multiple pregnancies, the risks and benefits of fetal reduction, the techniques used, as well as the ethical dilemma faced by families.

Definitions

Selective fetal reduction: a procedure performed in the first trimester or early second trimester for reducing the total number of fetuses in a multiple pregnancy by one or more.

Selective termination: a procedure in which total fetal number is reduced by directing it at one or more specific fetuses with a known structural anomaly, genetic abnormality, severe selective growth restriction, or advanced twin-to-twin transfusion syndrome.

Bipolar cord coagulation: a procedure to achieve umbilical cord occlusion using bipolar forceps under ultrasound guidance.

Radiofrequency ablation: a procedure where an alternating current in the radiofrequency range is transmitted via tines of a needle, causing tissue heat with subsequent coagulation or tissue necrosis.

Intra-fetal laser ablation: a relatively new technique of selective termination in monochorionic pregnancies, which involves ultrasound-guided laser ablation of the pelvic vessels of one of the monochorionic fetuses.

Learning Objectives

- To understand risks associated with twin and higher order pregnancies
- To discuss evidence-based risks and benefits of fetal reduction
- To discuss methods of fetal reduction in clinical practice and new developments
- To discuss the ethical dilemma faced by clinicians and families

11.1 Introduction

Over the last few decades, the incidence of multiple gestation has risen namely as a result of assisted reproduction techniques, e.g. IVF and use of ovulation induction drugs, although national guidelines [2] on restricting the number of embryos transferred, depending on maternal age and number of IVF cycle, as well as more controlled use of ovulation induction drugs have been implemented in order to reduce the numbers of higher order multiple pregnancies. Despite this, mixed chorionicity higher order multiples have continued to show a relative increase due to gonadotrophin use and embryo splitting [3, 4].

It is well recognised that multiple pregnancies carry a significantly higher risk of preterm birth, perinatal mortality and morbidity, as well as, an increased pregnancy risk of maternal complications such as hypertensive disorders including pre-eclampsia, as well as gestational diabetes and postpartum haemorrhage [5]. Higher order multiple pregnancies present even higher risks than twin pregnancies [6].

Discordant fetal anomalies as well as selective growth restriction in multiple pregnancies can give rise to a clinical dilemma. Monochorionic specific complications such as twin-to-twin transfusion syndrome (TTTS) and twin anaemia polycythaemia sequence (TAPS) can pose added complications to these pregnancies. Compared with singleton pregnancies, multiple pregnancies are associated with an approximately fivefold increased risk of stillbirth and a sevenfold increased risk of neonatal death. These adverse outcomes are primarily due to complications of prematurity [7, 8]. These risks are furthermore increased in higher order multiples, with a third of triplets predicted to deliver before 32 weeks [9], giving rise to cerebral palsy, chronic lung disease, developmental delay and death [7].

Multiple pregnancies are also associated with social and economic implications for the parents, with higher risks of stress, poor quality of life and higher divorce rates observed in parents of multiples [10–12].

Selective fetal reduction is defined as a procedure to reduce the total number of fetuses in a multiple pregnancy by one or more [13]. An earlier systematic review compared the outcomes of trichorionic triplets who were expectantly managed versus those who underwent reduction and found that although the risk of miscarriage was higher in the reduction group (8.1% vs. 4.4%, $p = 0.036$), the rate of preterm labour was significantly lower (10.4% vs. 26.7%, $p < 0.0001$) [14]. It is therefore recommended by the Royal College and the American College of Obstetricians and Gynaecologists, that in all higher order pregnancies, following patient counselling, selective fetal reduction should be discussed [15, 16].

11.2 Selective Fetal Reduction and Selective Termination

Fetal reduction refers to a procedure employed to reduce the total number of fetuses in a multiple pregnancy by terminating one or more fetuses. This procedure aims to improve pregnancy outcomes [17] as well as ameliorate the socio-economic challenges of delivering twin or higher order pregnancies for families. Patient choice may be guided by their socio-economic status, medical history, fertility, parity and fetal well-being. Selective termination applies to those diagnosed with discordant fetal anomalies, or with severe fetal growth restriction, in order to improve the prognosis of the normal fetus [18]. ◘ Table 11.1 outlines the indications for fetal reduction and selective termination.

A Cochrane review published in 2015 concluded that there are no randomised controlled trials to inform the risks and benefits of fetal reduction procedures in multiple pregnancies. It is important to highlight that the current available evidence is drawn from non-randomised studies, which can be associated with the risk of bias [19].

◘ **Table 11.1** Indications for fetal reduction/selective termination

Indications for selective fetal reduction/termination
Uncomplicated higher order multiples
Discordant anomaly or aneuploidy
Advanced twin-to-twin transfusion syndrome (Quintero stage IV)
Severe early onset selective fetal growth restriction
Twin reversed arterial perfusion
Advanced twin anaemia polycythaemia sequence (stage IV)

11.3 Trichorionic Triamniotic (TCTA) Triplets

Triplet pregnancies not only pose the dilemma of expectant management versus selective reduction, but also whether these should be reduced to twins or singletons. A recent systematic review found that fetal reduction in TCTA triplets to twins is associated with a significantly lower risk of preterm birth (17.3% vs. 50.2% in expectant management) without significantly increasing the risk of miscarriage (8.1% vs. 7.4%) [20]. Chaveeva et al. found in a retrospective study that in TCTA triplet pregnancies, the rates of miscarriage and preterm birth in those expectantly managed are approximately 3% and 35%, respectively, compared to a higher rate of miscarriage and lower rate of preterm birth (7.3% and 13.1%) in those reduced to twins. Those reduced to singletons had a further increase in miscarriage rate (11.5%), but a further reduction in preterm birth (8.7%). Therefore, fetal reduction to twins or singletons progressively reduces the rate of preterm birth but also progressively increases the risk of miscarriage [9] (◘ Table 11.2).

Table 11.2 Risk of miscarriage and preterm birth (PTB) following embryo reduction (ER) in triplets according to chorionicity and number of fetuses reduced

	Miscar-riage (%)	PTB <34 weeks (%)
TCTA – Expectant	3	52
TCTA – ER to 2	7	21
TCTA – ER to 1	12	10
DCTA – Expectant	9	67
DCTA – ER to 2	13	31
DCTA - ER to 1	17	9

A meta-analysis comparing the outcomes of 796 triplets that underwent reduction to twins and 899 expectantly managed triplets found that reduction was associated with, delivery at a later gestational age, a 60–70% reduction in early preterm delivery, reduction in neonatal mortality, higher birth weight, lower incidence of hypertensive disorders of pregnancy, lower rates of antenatal hospitalisation and lower rates of Caesarean delivery [21].

11.4 Dichorionic Triamniotic Triplets

Dichorionic triamniotic (DCTA) triplets are complicated by a monochorionic pair, which not only carry extra risks of monochorionic-specific complications, but can give rise to technical challenges during selective reduction/termination. Morlando et al. concluded that conservatively managed DCTA triplets carried a miscarriage risk of 8.9%, and a third suffered from severe preterm delivery. Reduction of the monochorionic pair increased the miscarriage rate to 14.5%, but reduced the preterm delivery rate to 5.5%. Reduction of one of the monochorionic twins and the triplet with the separate placenta yielded a miscarriage and preterm birth rate of 8.8% and 11.8%, and 23.5% and 17.6%, respectively [22]. Chaveeva et al. found that the rate of miscarriage increased with the number of fetuses reduced (9% expectant, 13% reduction to 2, 17% reduction to 1), but the rate of preterm birth decreased with the number of fetuses reduced (67% expectant, 13% reduction to 2, 9% reduction to 1), as demonstrated in Table 11.2 [9].

11.5 Monochorionic Triplets

Monochorionic triamniotic (MCTA) and monochorionic monoamniotic (MCMA) triplets are exceedingly rare. TTTS, TAPS, selective fetal growth restriction, as well as fetal loss often complicate these pregnancies. Due to the rarity of the condition, very limited literature is available for these pregnancies.

One study reported the outcomes of selective fetal reduction in MCTA pregnancies included only 2 pregnancies. Both underwent radiofrequency ablation to two fetuses at 13 weeks gestation, which both resulted in live births at 36 and 38 weeks' gestation [23].

11.6 Twin Pregnancies

Selective reduction/termination can be considered in the presence of obstetric or maternal indications in twins, such as discordant fetal anomaly, severe selective fetal growth restriction, late stage TAPS or TTTS, or severe maternal cardiac disease. Fetal reduction of twins in the absence of obstetric or maternal indications remains controversial; in the presence of maternal request for psychological or social reasons, adequate counselling should be offered regarding the risks and benefits of the procedure [16].

Vieira et al. compared DCDA twin pregnancy outcomes and loss rates in selective reduction to singleton versus expectant management. This concluded that patients who underwent reduction had a higher gestational age at delivery and lower rates of preterm birth and pregnancy complications, without an

Table 11.3 Pregnancy outcomes and loss rates following elective twin pregnancy reduction

	2-1 reduction to singletons ($n = 250$), %	Ongoing twin pregnancies ($n = 601$), %	*P* value
Preterm delivery <37 weeks	17.7	53.7	<0.001
Preterm delivery <34 weeks	7	17	<0.001
Preterm delivery <32 weeks	4.1	8.3	0.03
IUGR	5.4	13.7	0.001
Caesarean delivery	46.8	79.1	<0.001
Pre-eclampsia	4.2	16.8	<0.001
PPROM	5.9	19.4	<0.001
BW <10th centile	15	37.8	<0.001
BW <5th centile	8.6	22.2	<0.001
Total pregnancy loss <24 weeks	4	2.5	0.23
Total pregnancy loss <20 weeks	3.6	1.7	0.09
IUFD >24 weeks	1.2	0.7	0.43

IUGR intrauterine growth restriction, *PPROM* preterm premature rupture of the membranes, *BW* birth weight, *IUFD* intrauterine fetal death

Vieira et al. [24]

increased risk of pregnancy loss. Additionally, the risks of having Caesarean delivery, pre-eclampsia, preterm premature rupture of membranes (PPROM) and low birth weight (less than the fifth and 10th percentiles) were found to be lower in reduced singletons compared to ongoing twins (Table 11.3) [24].

Similarly, Gupta et al. found a decreased rate of preterm birth (10% vs. 43%, $p < 0.001$) and small for gestational age (23% vs. 49%, $p < 0.001$) in those who were reduced to singletons. However, they did not find a difference in preterm birth less than 34 weeks [25].

11.7 Selective Fetal Reduction – The Procedure

Clinicians should be familiar with local and national guidelines and legal requirements, as well as the risks and benefits of selective reduction versus expectant management [16]. Multiple methods have been reported for selective reduction, which is determined by the chorionicity, and the expertise of the clinician. Determining the chorionicity is therefore crucial, and is best established in the first trimester by ultrasound examination.

Fetal reduction is commonly performed at 12–13 weeks' gestation. This will allow time for most spontaneous miscarriages to occur and for first trimester ultrasound to be performed in order to rule out major fetal abnormalities, markers of aneuploidy (such as increased nuchal translucency) and calculate the risk of common chromosomal abnormalities.

An assessment of fetal anatomy of all fetuses is undertaken prior to the procedure, in order to identify obvious structural abnormalities or markers of aneuploidy. Many major and lethal anomalies can be detected by the end of the first trimester [26]; however, some anomalies are only apparent following the second trimester scan. Prenatal testing in the form of amniocentesis or CVS can be performed when a genetic condition is suspected. Correct sampling and labelling of fetuses is paramount, and diagnostic error due to incorrect matching of genetic test results with the fetus or sampling error has been reported in 0.6–0.8% of twins and up to 1.2% of higher order multiple gestations [27].

11.8 Timing of Fetal Reduction

The timing of selective reduction in twin pregnancy influences the risk of miscarriage and/or preterm birth. Fetal reduction in the second trimester carries a higher rate of miscarriage and preterm birth (7% and 14%, respectively), compared to the first trimester. Women who are diagnosed with a fetal anomaly following the second trimester scan can be given the option of a selective reduction in the third trimester, if the law permits, to reduce the risk of losing the entire pregnancy [28]. The pros and cons of each option should be considered (prematurity, loss rate, parental stress, availability of a fetal medicine specialist to perform the procedure in the event of preterm labour, and risk of complications associated with the specific anomaly).

One study compared cases of selective reduction in DCDA pregnancies performed between 15 and 23 weeks of gestation with those performed between 11 and 14 weeks. This study concluded that second trimester reduction of twins is associated with an increased rate of prematurity compared to late first trimester fetal reduction [29].

11.9 The Procedure

Fetuses with features of aneuploidy or those with a significantly smaller crown-rump length (CRL) are preferentially chosen for selective reduction. In the case where all fetuses appear structurally normal, the decision is generally based on the most accessible fetus, which is closest to the anterior abdominal wall or furthest from the cervix.

11.9.1 Intra-thoracic Potassium Chloride

In pregnancies not complicated by monochorionicity, selective feticide is performed by an intra-thoracic or intra-cardiac injection of potassium chloride, under ultrasound guidance. Fetal asystole is usually confirmed within 1 minute of injection. Ultrasound examination is performed after the procedure to confirm the presence of cardiac activity in the remaining fetus/fetuses. This has a 99.5–100% success rate with minimal maternal complications [30]. Following the procedure, a degree of cramping or leaking of amniotic fluid from the sac of the reduced fetus can be expected, however vaginal bleeding is uncommon, and therefore, patients with bleeding should be clinically assessed in view of the potential procedure-related risk of miscarriage.

11.9.2 Selective Reduction in Monochorionic Pregnancies

In monochorionic placenta, there are various vascular anastomoses that may give rise to twin-to-twin transfusion syndrome (TTTS), as well as be responsible for acute inter-fetal transfusions that occur when one twin dies in utero. Neurological injury to the surviving co-twin is believed to occur when it suffers acute severe hypotension when blood is shunted into the dying twin through placental anastomoses. The resulting cerebral hypoperfusion and hypoxia can subsequently cause a spectrum of cerebral injury [31]. In monochorionic pregnancies, therefore, the use of intra-thoracic injection of potassium chloride is contra-indicated.

Other techniques of fetal reduction, which can be performed in monochorionic gestations, are discussed below. Unlike fetal reduction in dichorionic twin pregnancies, selective termination in monochorionic pregnancies requires ablation of blood flow in the umbilical cord to prevent an acute inter-twin transfusion [31].

11.9.2.1 Bipolar Cord Coagulation (BPC)

Ultrasound-guided bipolar cord coagulation is commonly performed, where a 10-F disposable trocar is inserted into the amniotic sac of the targeted fetus. Cord occlusion is achieved using 3 mm bipolar forceps under continuous ultrasound guidance. The umbilical cord is grasped with bipolar forceps and coagulation is performed for 30 seconds at a power setting of 30–50 watts (◘ Fig. 11.1). Cessation of blood flow is confirmed using Colour Doppler after the procedure [32]. The survival rate of

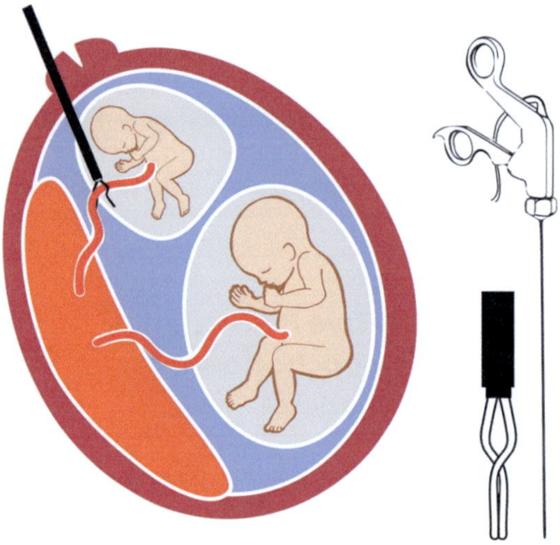

■ **Fig. 11.1** Bipolar cord coagulation using bipolar forceps

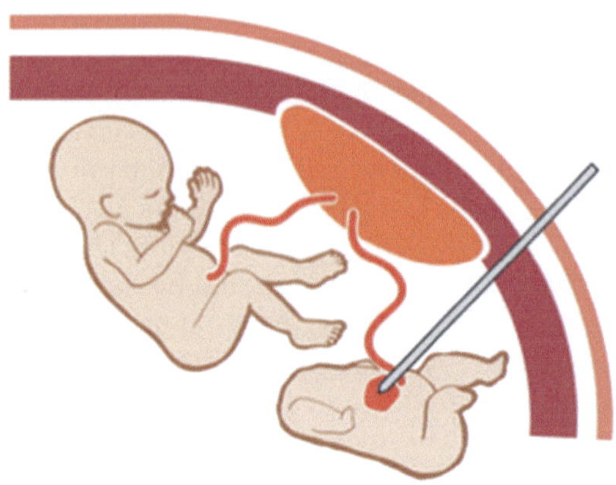

■ **Fig. 11.2** Radiofrequency ablation technique

the co-twin is approximately 80% and the risk of premature rupture of the membranes and preterm birth prior to 32 weeks is 20% [33].

11.9.2.2 Radiofrequency Ablation (RFA)

RFA involves generating changes in alternating current at very high frequencies (200–1200 kHz) between the tines of a needle. As the electrical current alternates in various directions between the tines, tissue ions become agitated as they attempt to align with the electrical field. Frictional heat is then produced, resulting in very high tissue temperatures that cause tissue coagulation and necrosis (■ Fig. 11.2).

A 17-gauge radiofrequency needle is inserted percutaneously under continuous ultrasound guidance into the intra-fetal portion of the umbilical cord. Once the position is confirmed, all three tines are applied and radiofrequency energy is used to generate an average temperature of 110 degrees Celsius in all three tines for 3 minutes [23].

One study compared outcomes of RFA and BPC methods for selective reduction in complicated monochorionic (MC) twin gestations. They concluded that both methods were equal in terms of the overall survival of the remaining twin as well as the rate of adverse perinatal outcome [33].

11.9.2.3 Fetoscopic and Intra-fetal Laser Ablation

Intra-fetal laser is a relatively new technique described in 2014, which has been used in monochorionic pregnancies and involves ultrasound-guided laser ablation of the pelvic vessels of one of the monochorionic fetuses. Following ultrasound assessment, a transverse section of the lower fetal abdomen is obtained and colour flow Doppler is used to visualise the internal iliac arteries and intra-abdominal umbilical vein. Local anaesthesia is administered to the maternal skin, subcutaneous tissues and myometrium. An 18-gauge needle is introduced to the fetal abdomen with the tip being adjacent to the pelvic vessels (■ Fig. 11.3, Video 11.1). A laser fibre is then inserted into the needle and advanced to a couple of millimetres beyond the tip of the needle. Laser coagulation is performed. This will result in hyperechogenicity of tissues in the lower abdomen and cessation of blood flow in the iliac arteries and umbilical vein. Fetal heart activity continues for several minutes. After a period of rest for about 60 minutes, another ultrasound examination is carried out to confirm death of one monochorionic twin and survival of a dichorionic pair [34]. This technique has a co-twin death rate of 46% within 2 weeks following the procedure, likely secondary to bleeding into the placenta of the dead fetus [34].

Fetoscopic laser cord occlusion is used similarly to those for TTTS, where following the insertion of the fetoscope into the

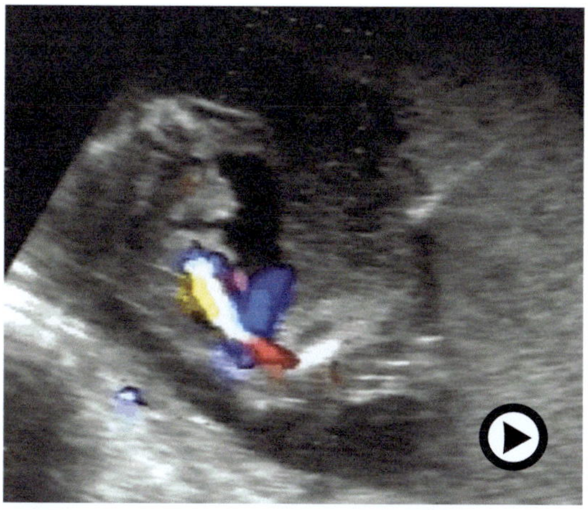

Fig. 11.3 Intra-fetal laser ablation displaying the insertion of the needle into the pelvic vessels
Video 11.1 Intra-fetal laser ablation of TRAP mass (https://doi.org/10.1007/000-2ta)

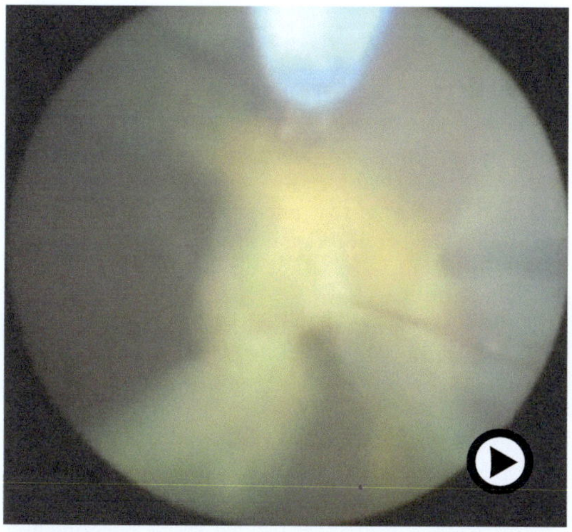

Fig. 11.4 Fetoscopic laser cord occlusion at the site of placental cord insertion, for selective reduction of a twin with severe selective fetal growth restriction
Video 11.2 Fetoscopic laser cord occlusion for a fetus with severe fetal growth restriction (https://doi.org/10.1007/000-2tb)

uterus under local anaesthesia, laser coagulation is used to ablate the umbilical cord of the fetus, until no colour pulsations are seen (Fig. 11.4, Video 11.2).

11.9.3 New Developments

Microwave ablation (MWA) is a novel approach in fetal procedures. Two cases of monochorionic diamniotic twins have been reported in the literature that underwent MWA for selective fetal reduction. MWA was used to deliver energy through a coaxial antenna. The antenna is centred in the abdomen of the abnormal fetus close to the insertion of the umbilical cord and single microwave energy application was delivered. In both cases, MWA was technically easy, and ultrasound evidence of tissue coagulation was seen immediately after the beginning of energy delivery [35].

High intensity focused ultrasound aims to bring a non-invasive technique into fetal therapy. Targeted ultrasound energy is transmitted through the abdominal wall and uterus through a transducer placed on the women's abdomen to cause vessel occlusion. Currently this method is limited to very small numbers of TRAP sequence and TTTS cases, however, due to a high number of incomplete vascular occlusion, it has not yet been proven to be superior to other methods [36].

11.10 Ethics of Patient Counselling

The management of multiple pregnancy is difficult. Non-directive patient counselling should be offered to all women with higher order multiple pregnancies and should include a discussion of the risks unique to the pregnancy as well as the option to continue or reduce the pregnancy, along with likely implications for each option. Resources for providing such counselling can include maternal–fetal medicine specialists, neonatologists, mental health professionals, child development specialists, support groups, and clinicians with procedural expertise in multifetal pregnancy reduction. Informed consent should be obtained by fully discussing risks and benefits associated with any intervention versus risks and benefits of expectant management.

Obstetricians should respect patients' autonomy regarding whether to continue or reduce a multi-fetal pregnancy. Only the patient can weigh the relative importance of the medical, ethical, religious and socioeconomic factors and determine the best course of action for her unique situation [16].

11.10.1 Review Questions

1. What are the indications for selective fetal reduction and at which gestation is it usually performed?

2. What are the rates of miscarriage and preterm birth in expectantly managed TCTA pregnancies?

3. How would you counsel a patient regarding risks and benefits of fetal reduction in TCTA triplets?

4. What are the evidence-based benefits, in terms of pregnancy outcome, of reducing DCDA pregnancies to singleton?

5. Describe possible techniques of fetal reduction in monochorionic and mixed chorionicity pregnancies.

11.10.2 Multiple-Choice Questions

1. When should chorionicity and amnionicity be determined by in multiple pregnancies?
   (a) By 7 + 6 weeks of gestation
   (b) By 12 + 6 weeks of gestation
   (c) By 13 + 6 weeks of gestation
   (d) By 15 + 6 weeks of gestation

2. Which is an indication for counselling and offering patients selective fetal reduction?
   (a) Higher order multiple pregnancy
   (b) Discordant fetal anomaly
   (c) Severe TTTS
   (d) All the above

3. In which of the following use of intrathoracic potassium chloride injection for fetal reduction is appropriate?
   (a) Monochorionic diamniotic twins
   (b) Dichorionic triplets
   (c) Dichorionic diamniotic twins
   (d) None of the above

4. Reduction of multiple fetuses from triplets to twins has been found to be associated with
   (a) Lower risk of miscarriage compared to expectant management
   (b) Delivery at a later gestational age
   (c) Lower birth weight
   (d) None of the above

5. Selective reduction in DCDA twins to singleton has been found to be associated with
   (a) A decreased rate of small for gestational age (birth weight <10th centile)
   (b) A decreased rate of preterm birth <37 weeks of gestation
   (c) A decreased rate of PPROM
   (d) All the above

References

1. National Collaborating Center for Women's and Children's Health (UK). Multiple pregnancy. The management of twin and triplet pregnancies in the antenatal period. Commissioned by the national institute for clinical excellence. London: RCOG Press; 2011.
2. National Institute for Health and Clinical Excellence. Fertility problems: assessment and treatment. NICE Clinical guideline 156. London: National Institute for Health and Clinical Excellence; 2013.
3. Schachter M, Raziel A, Friedler S, Strassburger D, Bern O, Ron-El R. Monozygotic twinning after assisted reproductive techniques: a phenomenon independent of micromanipulation. Hum Reprod. 2001;16:1264–9.
4. Gleicher N, Oleske DM, Tur-Kaspa I, Vidali A, Karande V. Reducing the risk of high order pregnancy after ovarian stimulation with gonadotrophins. N Engl J Med. 2000;343:2–7.
5. Luke B, Brown MB. Contemporary risks of maternal morbidity and adverse outcomes with increasing maternal age and plurality. Fertil Steril. 2007;88(2):283–93.
6. Wen SW, Demissie K, Yang Q, Walker MC. Maternal morbidity and obstetric complications in triplet pregnancies and quadruplet and higher-order multiple pregnancies. Am J Obstet Gynecol. 2004;191(1):254–8.

7. Multifetal gestations: twin, triplet, and higher-order multifetal pregnancies. Practice Bulletin No. 169. American College of Obstetricians and Gynecologists. Obstet Gynecol. 2016;128:e131–46.
8. Scher AI, Petterson B, Blair E, Ellenberg JH, Grether JK, Haan E, et al. The risk of mortality or cerebral palsy in twins: a collaborative population-based study. Pediatr Res. 2002;52:671–81.
9. Chaveeva P, Kosinski P, Puglia D, Poon LC, Nicolaides KH. Trichorionic and dichorionic triplet pregnancies at 10-14 weeks: outcome after embryo reduction compared to expectant management. Fetal Diagn Ther. 2013;34(4):199–205.
10. Glazebrook C, Sheard C, Cox S, Oates M, Ndukwe G. Parenting stress in first-time mothers of twins and triplets conceived after in vitro fertilization. Fertil Steril. 2004;81(3):505–11.
11. Ellison MA, Hotamisligil S, Lee H, Rich-Edwards JW, Pang SC, Hall JE. Psychosocial risks associated with multiple births resulting from assisted reproduction. Fertil Steril. 2005;83:1422–8.
12. Jena AB, Goldman DP, Joyce G. Association between the birth of twins and parental divorce. Obstet Gynecol. 2011;117:892–7.
13. Berkowitz RL, Lynch L. Selective reduction: an unfortunate misnomer. Obstet Gynecol. 1990;75: 873–4.
14. Papageorghiou AT, Avgidou K, Bakoulas V, Sebire NJ, Nicolaides KH. Risks of miscarriage and early preterm birth in trichorionic triplet pregnancies with embryo reduction versus expectant management: new data and systematic review. Hum Reprod. 2006;21:1912–7.
15. Royal College of Obstetricians and Gynaecologists. Management of monochorionic twin pregnancy. Green-top guideline No. 51. London: RCOG; 2016.
16. ACOG Committee Opinion. Multifetal pregnancy reduction. Am Coll Obstet Gynecol. 2017;719
17. Evans MI, Andriole S, Britt DW. Fetal reduction: 25 years' experience. Fetal Diagn Ther. 2014;35:69–82.
18. Yinon Y, Johnson KD, Bryant-Greenwood PK, Kramer RL, Johnson MP, Evans MI. Selective termination and elective reduction in twin pregnancies: 10 years experience at a single centre. Hum Reprod. 1998;13(8):2301–4.
19. Dodd JM, Dowswell T, Crowther CA. Reduction of the number of fetuses for women with a multiple pregnancy. Cochrane Database Syst Rev. 2015;(11):CD003932. https://doi.org/10.1002/14651858.CD003932.pub3.
20. Anthoulakis C, Dagklis T, Mamopoulos A, Athanasiadis A. Risks of miscarriage or preterm delivery in trichorionic and dichorionic triplet pregnancies with embryo reduction versus expectant management: a systematic review and meta-analysis. Hum Reprod. 2017;32:1351.
21. Zipori Y, Haas J, Berger H, Barzilay E. Multifetal pregnancy reduction of triplets to twins compared with non-reduced triplets: a meta-analysis. Reprod Biomed Online. 2017;35(3):296–304.
22. Morlando M, Ferrara L, D'Antonio F, et al. Dichorionic triplet pregnancies: risk of miscarriage and severe preterm delivery with fetal reduction versus expectant management. Outcomes of a cohort study and systematic review. BJOG. 2015;122(8):1053–60. https://doi.org/10.1111/1471-0528.13348.
23. Paramasivam G, Wimalasundera R, Wiechec M, et al. Radiofrequency ablation for selective reduction in complex monochorionic pregnancies. BJOG. 2010;117:1294–8. https://doi.org/10.1111/j.1471-0528.2010.02624.
24. Vieira LA, Warren L, Pan S, et al. Comparing pregnancy outcomes and loss rates in elective twin pregnancy reduction with ongoing twin gestations in a large contemporary cohort. Am J Obstet Gynecol. 2019;221:253.e1.
25. Gupta S, Fox NS, Feinberg J, et al. Outcomes in twin pregnancies reduced to singleton pregnancies compared with ongoing twin pregnancies. Am JObstet Gynecol. 2015;213:580, e1.
26. Bromley B, Shipp TD, Lyons J, Navathe RS, Groszmann Y, Benacerraf BR. Detection of fetal structural anomalies in a basic first-trimester screening program for aneuploidy. J Ultrasound Med. 2014;33(10):1737–45.
27. Eddleman KA, Stone JL, Lynch L, Berkowitz RL. Chorionic villus sampling before multifetal pregnancy reduction. Am J Obstet Gynecol. 2000;183(5):1078–81.
28. Khalil A, Rodgers M, Baschat A, Bhide A, Gratacos E, Hecher K, Kilby MD, Lewi L, Nicolaides KH, Oepkes D, Raine-Fenning N, Reed K, Salomon LJ, Sotiriadis A, Thilaganathan B, Ville Y. ISUOG Practice Guidelines: role of ultrasound in twin pregnancy. Ultrasound Obstet Gynecol. 2016;47:247–63.
29. Zemet R, et al. The earlier the better or the later the better: Optimal timing of fetal reduction from twins to singleton. Am J Obstet Gynecol. 2020;218(1):S94.
30. Sfakianaki AK, Davis KJ, Copel JA, et al. Potassium chloride induced fetal demise – a retrospective cohort study into efficacy and safety. J Ultrasound Med. 2014;33:337–41.
31. Quarello E, Molho M, Ville Y. Incidence, mechanisms, and patterns of fetal cerebral lesions in twin-to-twin transfusion syndrome. J Matern Fetal Neonatal Med. 2007;20:589–97.

32. Yinon Y, Ashwal E, Weisz B, et al. Selective reduction in complicated monochorionic twins: prediction of obstetric outcome and comparison of techniques. Ultrasound Obstet Gynecol. 2015;46:670–7.
33. Roman A, Papanna R, Johnson A, Hassan SS, Moldenhauer J, Molina S, Moise KJ Jr. Selective reduction in complicated monochorionic pregnancies: radiofrequency ablation vs bipolar cord coagulation. Ultrasound Obstet Gynecol. 2010;36:37–41.
34. Chaveeva P, Kosinski P, Birdir C, Orosz L, Nicolaides KH. Embryo reduction in dichorionic triplets to dichorionic twins by intrafetal laser. Fetal Diagn Ther. 2014;35:83–6.
35. Prefumo F, Cabassa P, Fichera A, et al. Preliminary experience with microwave ablation for selective feticide in monochorionic twin pregnancies. Ultrasound Obstet Gynecol. 2013;41(4):470–1.
36. Seo K, Ichizuka K, Okai T, et al. Twin-reversed arterial perfusion sequence using high-intensity focused ultrasound therapy. Ultrasound Obstet Gynecol. 2019;54(1):128–34.

Key Reading

ACOG Committee Opinion. Multifetal pregnancy reduction. The American college of Obstetricians and Gynecologists. 2017;719

Chaveeva P, Kosinski P, Puglia D, Poon LC, Nicolaides KH. Trichorionic and dichorionic triplet pregnancies at 10–14 weeks: outcome after embryo reduction compared to expectant management. Fetal Diagn Ther. 2013;34(4):199–205.

Dodd JM, Dowswell T, Crowther CA. Reduction of the number of fetuses for women with a multiple pregnancy. Cochrane Database Syst Rev. 2015;(11):CD003932. https://doi.org/10.1002/14651858.CD003932.pub3.

Morlando M, Ferrara L, D'Antonio F, et al. Dichorionic triplet pregnancies: risk of miscarriage and severe preterm delivery with fetal reduction versus expectant management. Outcomes of a cohort study and systematic review. BJOG. 2015;122(8):1053–60. https://doi.org/10.1111/1471-0528.13348.

Yinon Y, Ashwal E, Weisz B, et al. Selective reduction in complicated monochorionic twins: prediction of obstetric outcome and comparison of techniques. Ultrasound Obstet Gynecol. 2015;46:670–7.

Risk Assessment and Screening for Preterm Birth in Twin Pregnancy

Amanda Roman, Alexandra Ramirez, Guillermo Gurza, and Vincenzo Berghella

Contents

A. Khalil et al. (eds.), *Twin and Higher-order Pregnancies*,
https://doi.org/10.1007/978-3-030-47652-6_12

Trailer

Twins represent 3.2% of all livebirth. However, they account for 20% of all preterm deliveries, with 60% delivering before 37 weeks, and 10.7% before 32 weeks. Twin pregnancies have five times higher risk of early neonatal and infant death related to prematurity. Monochorionic twins have higher incidence of both indicated and spontaneous preterm delivery compared with dichorionic twins. Transvaginal cervical length before 24 weeks is the best tool to predict preterm birth, independent of other risk factors. Among all the evaluated therapies to decrease or prevent preterm birth in twin pregnancies, only vaginal progesterone in women with transvaginal cervical length <25 mm and physical exam indicated cerclage in women with cervical dilation >1 cm have shown a significant decrease in preterm birth and improvement in neonatal outcomes.

Definitions

Preterm birth is defined as delivery before 37 completed weeks of gestation.

Extremely preterm birth: delivery less than 28 weeks.

Very preterm delivery: delivery between 28 and 32 weeks.

Late preterm birth: delivery from 32 through 36 weeks

History of preterm birth: any previous delivery of a singleton or twin pregnancy delivered before 37 weeks.

Premature preterm rupture of membranes: rupture of the amniotic sac with leaking of amniotic fluid before 37 weeks and before the onset of labor.

Transvaginal cervical length: measured by transvaginal ultrasound between 16 and 24 weeks with empty bladder.

Sludge: dense aggregates of particulate matter in the amniotic sac seen in close proximity to the internal cervical os seen by transvaginal ultrasound. It has imaging characteristics similar to gallbladder sludge.

History-indicated cerclage: cerclage usually performed between 11 and 14 weeks due to the diagnosis of twin pregnancy (unselected) or due to history of preterm delivery.

Ultrasound indicated cerclage: cerclage performed usually between 16 and 24 weeks, due to the finding of short transvaginal cervical length, usually <25 mm, however other cervical length cut off may apply.

Physical exam indicated cerclage: cerclage performed usually between 16 and 25 weeks in women identified with cervical dilation at digital examination or by visual inspection at speculum exam.

Learning Objectives

- To review the incidence of preterm birth in twin pregnancy at different gestational ages
- To evaluate the impact of chorionicity on the incidence of preterm birth
- To evaluate the tools to predict preterm birth in twin pregnancy
- To evaluate and compare the efficacy of different therapies in the prevention of preterm delivery in twin pregnancy (bed rest, progesterone supplementation, pessary, and cerclage)

12.1 Introduction

According to the World Health Organization (WHO) preterm birth (PTB) is defined as delivery before 37 completed weeks of gestation, with extremely PTB defined as occurring at less than 28 weeks, very preterm delivery occurring between 28 and 32 weeks, and moderate to late PTB occurring from 32 through 36 weeks [1]. Worldwide, about 15 millions of babies are born preterm, and PTB accounts for 1 million of neonatal deaths, and an additional 125,000 deaths in children before 5 years of age, representing the leading cause of both neonatal and childhood mortality [2, 3]. Prematurity is associated with increased perinatal morbidity, and long-term neurodevelopmental impairment. Survival and neurological prognosis improve with advancing gestational age.

In the United States, the rate of twin birth in 2018 was 32.6 per 1000 births, but they account for 20% of all PTB, with 60.3% delivering <37 weeks, 19.5% <34 weeks, and 10.7% <32 weeks. Of singleton pregnancies, 8.2% of them deliver <37 weeks, 2.1% <34 weeks, and 1.2% <32 weeks [4]. Twins are also at increased risk for low birth-weight (LBW) and have five times higher risk of early neonatal and infant death and complications related to prematurity and LBW [4–6]. The increased incidence of PTB is probably associated with different pathophysiology of PTB among multiple pregnancies: maternal and fetal complications unique to multiple pregnancy, chorionicity, uterine over distension, cervical insufficiency, as well as intrauterine infection or inflammation, hormonal disorders, placental insufficiency, and uterine hypoxia [7]. Chorionicity also affects the incidence of PTB as they can develop maternal or fetal condition. In a prospective study of 800 dichorionic and 200 monochorionic twin pregnancies, 29% of dichorionic pregnancies delivered before 36 weeks, whereas 34% of the monochorionic twins were born before 34 weeks [8]. It is therefore important to individualize the risk factors associated PTB among asymptomatic and symptomatic twin pregnancies.

12.2 Impact of Chorionicity on the Risk of Preterm Birth

Chorionicity is an important factor associated with the incidence of PTB and perinatal outcomes in twin pregnancies [9]. Monochorionic diamniotic (MCDA) twin pregnancies are at higher risk of PTB associated with maternal and fetal complications compared with dichorionic diamniotic (DCDA) twin pregnancies. In a retrospective cohort including 175 (30.2%) MCDA twin pregnancies and 405 (69.8%) DCDA pregnancies, the incidence of PTB <34 weeks was significantly increased in the MCDA pregnancies: 61 (34.9%) vs. 93 (23.0%), respectively, with aOR 1.80 (1.22–2.65). The increase was seen both for the medically indicated (fetal reasons) PTB: 22 (12.6%) vs. 20 (4.9%) with aOR 2.49 (1.34–5.63) and spontaneous PTB (SPTB): 108 (61.7%) vs. 195 (48.1%) with aOR; 1.74 (1.21–2.49), while maternal indication of PTB was not different: 30 (17.1%) vs. 65 (16.1%) with aOR: 1.05 (0.55–1.70) (Table 12.1) [10].

In a historical cohort of 1407 twin pregnancies comparing MCDA vs. DCDA, the rate of PTB <28 weeks was 11% vs. 7%, and PTB <32 weeks was 26% vs. 18%, respectively [11]. The presence of single IUFD increases the risk of PTB. Among 3013 twin gestations, when compared with twins without fetal loss, the overall risk of PTB at <34 weeks was 66.1% (41/62) vs. 15.5% (457/2948), RR 4.27 (3.5–5.2); PTB <32 weeks 48.4% (30/62) vs. 7.9% (233/2948), RR 6.12 (4.6–8.1); and PTB <28 weeks 19.4% (12/62) vs. 1.6% (46/2948), RR 12.40 (6.9–22.2). However, the risk of PTB in single IUD was not associated with chorionicity [12].

A unique complication of MCDA pregnancies is twin-to-twin transfusion syndrome (TTTS). TTTS complicates about 8–10% of MCDA pregnancies. The prevalence of TTTS is approximately 1–3 per 10,000 births [13]. TTTS contribute highly to the fetal indications of PTB, a systematic review including 26 studies (2699 twin pregnancies) showed that the pooled proportions of PTB <32 weeks' gestation among MCDA pregnancies affected by TTTS classified by Quintero stages were increased as the severity of TTTS progressed [14]. Quintero stage I: two studies (9/34); 27.1 (13.9–42.8) stage II, three studies, (20/47); 42.8 (29.4–56.9) stage III, three studies (32/58); 53.3 (36,1–70.2); and stage IV: three studies (11/18) 59.9 (37.9–80.0). There are also differences in perinatal outcomes according to TTTS treatment modality; a systematic review of MCDA twin pregnancies, (13 studies with 729 women) diagnosed with TTTS before 18 weeks showed that PTB occurred in 74.1% (95% CI 36.9–97.8) of pregnancies managed expectantly, 43.5% (95% CI 26.5–51.3) of those treated with laser and 65.3% (95% CI 45.8–80.7) of those who had amnioreduction [15]. However, data on PTB outcomes were limited by the small sample size of the included studies on both systematic reviews.

Other MCDA-specific complications affecting prematurity rates include selective intrauter-

Table 12.1 Pregnancy outcomes of the monochorionic and dichorionic twin pregnancies

	Monochorionic N = 158 (31.0%)	Dichorionic N = 352 (69.0%)	Crude OR (95% CI)	aOR or MD (95% CI)[a]
GA at delivery (weeks)	34.1 ± 2.9	36.3 ± 3.1	–	−2.20 (−2.76 to −1.64)
PTB <37 weeks	89 (56.3%)	176 (50.0%)	1.29 (1.19–1.88)	1.22 (1.05–1.97)
PTB <34 weeks	56 (35.4%)	80 (22.7%)	1.87 (1.24–2.81)	1.85 (1.09–3.15)
PTB <32 weeks	21 (13.3%)	35 (9.9%)	1.39 (1.22–2.05)	1.35 (1.07–2.47)
PTB <28 weeks	10 (6.3%)	14 (4.0%)	1.63 (1.06–3.12)	1.55 (0.91–4.12)
SPTB <37 weeks	83 (52.5%)	160 (45.5%)	1.22 (1.19–1.74)	1.17 (1.04–1.87)
SPTB <34 weeks	50 (29.7%)	70 (20.5%)	1.87 (1.22–2.85)	1.69 (1.07–3.11)
SPTB <32 weeks	18 (11.4%)	28 (8.0%)	1.49 (1.03–2.78)	1.41 (0.74–2.97)
SPTB <28 weeks	8 (5.1%)	11 (3.1%)	1.65 (0.65–4.19)	1.61 (0.61–4.99)
Indication for delivery				
Maternal indication	26 (16.4%)	45 (12.8%)	1.34 (0.80–2.27)	1.30 (0.67–3.11)
Fetal indication	21 (13.3%)	17 (4.8%)	3.02 (1.55–5.90)	3.00 (1.49–6.03)
Combined	3 (1.9%)	2 (0.6%)	3.39 (0.56–20.47)	3.06 (0.49–23.95)
Planned at term	10 (6.3%)	95 (27.0%)	0.18 (0.09–0.70)	0.35 (0.20–0.76)
Spontaneous onset of labor	98 (62.1%)	193 (54.8%)	1.35 (1.21–1.98)	1.27 (1.15–2.17)

Adapted from Roman et al. [10]
Data presented as mean ± SD or number and percentage
GA Gestational age, *SD* standard deviation, *PTB* preterm birth, *SPTB* spontaneous preterm birth, *OR* odds ratio, *aOR* adjusted odds ratio, *CI* confidence interval, *MD* mean difference
[a]Adjusted for maternal age, body mass index, history of preterm birth, and smoking

ine growth restriction (sIUGR) and twin anemia polycythemia sequence (TAPS). The gestational age at delivery in 134 MCDA twin pregnancies diagnosed with sIUGR between 18 and 26 weeks was 35.4 (16–38) weeks if umbilical artery (UA) Doppler with positive end diastolic flow, and 30.7 (27–40) weeks if persistent absent or reversed end-diastolic flow [16]. In women affected by TAPS, the rate of PPROM was 44.4% in the treated TAPS group versus 18.2% in the non-treated TAPS group and the mean gestational age at delivery was 33.4 ± 3 weeks and 30.4 ± 5.7 weeks, respectively [17].

In summary, monochorionicity is a strong risk factor for PTB compared to dichorionicity in twins due to the inherited unique complications as TTTS, TAPS, single IUFD, and selective IUGR.

12.3 History of Previous Preterm Birth

The incidence of history of PTB and subsequent twin pregnancies is about 10% in most studies [10, 18]. Several retrospective cohorts have shown an increased risk of PTB in twin pregnancy with history of singleton PTB. The preterm prediction study in twins showed an increased risk of recurrent PTB <37 weeks (80% vs. 50%; RR 1.6. 95% CI 1.18–2.17, $p = 0.03$) ($n = 147$). Three retrospective studies in the United States showed as well an increased risk of recurrent PTB <37 weeks in subsequent twin pregnancy (73.9% vs. 44.4%; OR: 3.5, 95% CI 1.4–9.37) [19], recurrent SPTB <35 weeks (37.7% vs. 23.0%; OR 2.0, 95% CI 1.41–2.9, $p < 0.001$) [20], and recurrent PTB <32 weeks (26% vs. 3.5%; OR 9.7, 95% CI 2.95–32.4, $p < 0.001$) when comparing prior PTB with prior term delivery [21]. In a cohort from the Netherlands, the risk of subsequent twin SPTB was significantly higher after previous singleton PTB (56.9% vs. 20.9%; aOR 5.0, 95% CI 3.8–6.6), also the risk was highest after a SPTB singleton delivery 67.3% (aOR 7.8; 95% CI 5.5–11.2) compared with iatrogenic PTB singleton delivery 38.8% (aOR 2.4; 95% CI 1.5–3.8). The risk of subsequent twin PTB was dependent on the gestational age of previous singleton PTB, prior delivery between 22 0/7 and 29 6/7 weeks 71.4% aOR 9.5 (1.8–48.9) was higher than history of delivery between 34 0/7 and 36 6/7 weeks; 65.9%, aOR: 7.3 (5.0–10.6) [22].

12

In summary, history of PTB of a singleton or a twin gestation is an important risk factor for recurrent PTB in subsequent twin pregnancies.

12.4 Cervix Digital Examination

A randomized clinical trial in singleton pregnancy compared cervical examination at every prenatal visit ($n = 2803$) vs. avoidance of cervical examination if possible ($n = 2799$). The median number of cervical examinations was 6 in the experimental group and 1 in the controls. There were no significant difference in PTB <37 weeks between the two groups 6.7% vs. 6.4% [RR 1.05 (0.85–1.29)] [23]. Similar study was done in twin pregnancy with smaller sample size, 89 women attending a Twin Clinic had 7.6 ± 3.2 (mean ± SD) cervical examinations per patient and 288 controls followed up in the high-risk obstetric clinic revealed no significant differences in PTB <37 weeks 77.3% vs. 66.7%, $p = 0.07$ but significantly less PPROM among the patients attending the Twin Clinic (12.4% vs. 23.6%, $p = 0.03$) [24]. Larger studies will be needed to assess this finding.

In summary, routine manual cervical examinations for prediction or prevention of PTB in twin pregnancies cannot be recommended.

12.5 Uterine Activity Evaluation

In 1995, a meta-analysis of six randomized trials involving 260 twin pregnancies compared daily home uterine activity monitor (HUAM) versus abdominal palpation. This study did not find any difference between the incidence of PTB (RR: 1.01; 95% CI: 0.79–1.30; $p = 0.95$) [25]. However, when women with twin pregnancy and cervical dilation >2 cm were evaluated, the incidence of preterm labor was significantly decreased by 56%; RR 0.44 (0.25–0.78, $p = 0.005$). A premature birth prevention program enrolled prospectively 633 singletons and 145 twins to HUAM versus self-identification. This study showed that patients correctly identified only 17.2% of contractions recorded through HUAM by abdominal palpation. This correlation was significantly lower when women with twin pregnancy were compared with singleton pregnancy [26]. There were no differences in preterm labor among 45 women with twin gestations randomized to either daily HUAM and perinatal nursing support or an education group [27].

In 2006, an observational prospective double-blind study enrolled 59 twin and 306 singleton gestations between 22 and 24 weeks. Contraction frequency was recorded with a HUAM from enrollment to delivery or

36–6/7 weeks. The mean uterine contraction frequency was significantly higher in twin gestations than singletons; however, it did not predict SPTB <35 weeks' gestation [28].

In summary, HUAM cannot be recommended for twin pregnancies.

12.6 Cervical Length Measurement in Asymptomatic Women

In 1996, the preterm prediction study evaluated the risk factors for preterm birth in twin gestations [18]. Multiple variables were evaluated in 147 women with twin pregnancy at 24 and 28 weeks including maternal demographics, obstetric history, biochemical markers, and transvaginal ultrasound at 24 and 28 weeks. The transvaginal ultrasound cervical length (TVUCL) ≤25 mm at 24 weeks was the best predictor of SPTB at <32, <35, and <37 weeks. Since then, multiple prospective studies evaluating TVUCL in twins have been published. A systematic review including 16 studies in asymptomatic women with twin pregnancies ($n = 3213$) showed that TVUCL ≤20 mm at 20–24 weeks was the most accurate tool in predicting PTB <32 and <34 weeks of gestation (pooled sensitivities, specificities, and positive and negative likelihood ratios of 39% and 29%, 96% and 97%, 10.1 and 9.0, and 0.64 and 0.74, respectively). A TVUCL ≤25 mm at 20–24 weeks' gestation had a pooled positive likelihood ratio of 9.6 to predict PTB <28 weeks' gestation. The predictive accuracy of TVUCL for PTB was low in symptomatic women. A posterior systematic review identified 21 studies ($n = 2757$) [29]. Despite large variation in gestational age at TVUCL, different cut-off points for cervical length and definitions of PTB, the summary receiver operating characteristic (ROC) curve indicated a good predictive capacity of short cervical length for PTB. Sensitivity and specificity for PTB <34 weeks gestation were 78% and 66%, respectively, for 35 mm, 41% and 87% for 30 mm, 36% and 94% for 25 mm, and 30% and 94% for 20 mm.

A recent individual patient-level meta-analysis evaluated the effect of gestational age and cervical length measurements in the prediction of SPTB in twin pregnancies [30]. A total of 6188 TVUCL measurements were performed on 4409 twin pregnancies in 12 studies. Multinomial logistic regression analysis determined probabilities for birth at ≤28, 28–32, 32–36, and ≥36 weeks as a function of gestational age (GA) at screening and CL measurements. Both GA at screening and TVUCL had a significant and nonlinear effect on GA at birth. The best prediction of PTB ≤28 weeks was provided by screening at ≤18 weeks ($p < 0.001$), whereas the best prediction of birth between 28 and 36 weeks was provided by screening at ≥24 weeks ($p < 0.001$) (Table 12.2).

Table 12.2 The effect of gestational age and cervical length measurements in the prediction of spontaneous preterm birth in twin pregnancies, predicted probability categories

Predicted probability (%) of gestation at sPTB (weeks) Sample size 4409 women					
GA	**TVCL mm**	**≤28 0/7**	**28 1/7 to 32**	**32 1/7 to 36**	**≥36 + 1**
18	5	58.5	34.1	5.9	1.5
	10	51.8	36.8	8.5	2.9
	15	44.5	38.5	11.7	5.3
	20	36.6	38.6	15.6	9.2
	25	28.6	36.7	19.6	15.2
	30	20.9	32.6	23.1	23.4
	35	14.1	27	25.2	33.7
	40	8.9	20.7	25.6	44.8
20	5	53.2	36.4	8.5	1.9
	10	46.1	38.5	11.9	3.5
	15	38.6	39.2	16	6.2
	20	30.8	38.1	20.6	10.5
	25	23.2	35	25	16.8
	30	16.4	30.1	28.5	25.1
	35	10.8	24.1	30.2	35
	40	6.6	18	29.9	45.4

(continued)

Table 12.2 (continued)

Predicted probability (%) of gestation at sPTB (weeks) Sample size 4409 women					
GA	TVCL mm	≤28 0/7	28 1/7 to 32	32 1/7 to 36	≥36 + 1
22	5	47.5	38.2	11.9	2.3
	10	40.2	39.4	16.3	4.2
	15	32.6	38.9	21.3	7.2
	20	25.2	36.6	26.5	11.8
	25	18.3	32.4	31.1	18.1
	30	12.5	27	34.3	26.2
	35	8	21.1	35.4	35.5
	40	4.8	15.4	34.4	45.3
24	5	41.6	39.2	16.4	2.8
	10	34.1	39.3	21.8	4.9
	15	26.8	37.6	27.6	8.1
	20	20	34.1	33.1	12.8
	25	14.1	29.3	37.6	19
	30	9.3	23.7	40.3	26.7
	35	5.8	18	40.7	35.4
	40	3.5	13	39	44.5
26	5	35.4	39.3	22	3.3
	10	28.2	38.1	28.3	5.5
	15	21.4	35.2	34.6	8.8
	20	15.4	30.9	40.3	13.4
	25	10.5	25.7	44.3	19.4
	30	6.8	20.3	46.3	26.6
	35	4.2	15.2	45.9	34.7
	40	2.5	10.9	43.5	43.1

Adapted from Kindinger et al. [30]

Cervical changes are dynamic showing shortening of the cervix and even cervical dilation over time. In singleton pregnancy, TVUCL may present with further shortening as pregnancy progresses; this is the bases of the recommendation of serial TVUCL in women with history of preterm birth [31]. In women without risk for PTB, 30% of women with TVUCL <11 mm had cervical dilation >1 cm at pelvic examination [32]. Serial cervical evaluation has shown different patterns of cervical shortening in twins as well [33], and early rapid cervical length shortening starting at 16 weeks was associated with an incidence of PTB <34 weeks of 44% followed by late onset of shortening starting at 24 weeks with PTB <34 weeks of 20.2%. There are no studies assessing the association of TVUCL with cervical dilation in twins.

In summary, all these studies have established that TVUCL before 24 weeks is the best predictor of PTB in twin pregnancy [18, 34], and the shorter the TVUCL and the earlier GA at presentation, the higher the risk of PTB at any given gestation [30, 34]. While TVUCL is currently the best tool available to screen for PTB in twin pregnancy, independent of other risk factors, ACOG [35] and SMFM still recommend against TVUCL in twins as there are no current proven therapies to offer and TVUCL should be reserved for randomized controlled studies.

12.7 Fetal Fibronectin

The initial reports regarding the role of fetal fibronectin (fFN) in predicting PTB in twin pregnancies were promising [18, 36–38]. However, the overall results were disappointing. A systematic review and meta-analysis published in 2010 included 15 studies (11 in asymptomatic women and 4 in women with symptoms of preterm labor) involving 1221 women with multiple pregnancies) [39]. Among asymptomatic women with multiple or twin pregnancies, the pooled sensitivities, specificities, and positive and negative likelihood ratios for predicting preterm birth <32, <34, and <37 weeks' gestation ranged from 33% to 45%, 80–94%, 2.0–5.5, and 0.68–0.76, respectively. Among women with twin pregnancies and threatened preterm labor, fFN was most accurate in predicting spontaneous PTB within 7 days of testing (pooled sensitivity, specificity, and positive and negative likelihood ratios of 85%, 78%, 3.9, and 0.20, respectively). The systematic review concluded that cervico-vaginal fFN provides moderate to minimal prediction of PTB in women with multiple pregnancies. The test is most accurate in predicting spontaneous preterm birth within 7 days of testing in women with twin pregnancies and threatened preterm labor. The authors of the meta-analysis, however, highlight the high heterogeneity across studies [39]. A combination of TVUCL and fFN was evaluated in a retrospective study in asymptomatic twin pregnancy between 22 and 32 weeks, ($n = 155$) [40]. They found that TVUCL <20 mm and positive fFN had significantly higher positive predictive value than either of the tests alone, and was associated with a 55% risk of birth before 32 weeks. Having either a positive fFN result or a short CL was associated with a higher rate of spontaneous preterm birth than having 2 negative tests, and having both a positive fFN result and a short CL was associated with the highest rates of spontaneous preterm birth at <28, <30, <32, <34, <35, and <37 weeks' gestation.

In summary, cervicovaginal fFN alone has low to moderate accuracy in predicting SPTB in asymptomatic twin gestations. However, the data from the prospective study failed to assess whether the combination of fFN and cervical length are better predictors of PTB than either cervical length or fetal fibronectin alone in asymptomatic women with twin gestations.

12.8 Amniotic Fluid Sludge

Amniotic fluid (AF) sludge was described in 2005, as dense aggregates of particulate matter seen in close proximity to the internal cervical os and have imaging characteristics similar to gallbladder sludge seen by ultrasound. AF sludge has been proposed as an additional ultrasound marker for preterm delivery.

In singletons, the rate of sludge is higher in women with TVUCL <15 mm, <10 mm, and early GA at diagnosis, and was identified as an independent risk factor for early preterm delivery, premature rupture of the membranes (PROM), chorioamnionitis, funisitis, neonatal morbidity, and neonatal mortality in these populations [41]. Similarly, a study including 78 asymptomatic twin pregnancies found that the prevalence of AF sludge was 34.6% (27/78) [42] higher than in singleton pregnancies (22.6%) ($p = 0.02$) [41]. In this study, the presence of AF sludge in twin pregnancies with a short cervix was an independent risk factor for extreme prematurity (<26 weeks: 52.2% vs. 15.6%; $p < 0.01$), histological chorioamnionitis (50.0% vs. 12.8%; $p < 0.01$), and perinatal death (33.3% vs. 3.9%; $p < 0.01$) [42]. This information was confirmed in a larger cohort that included 635 twin pregnancies with TVUCL from 22 0/7 to 25 6/7 weeks [43]. The sludge was present in 61 (9.6%), the risk of PTB <35 weeks in women with sludge was 36.8% versus 16.5% (aOR: 2.11; 95% CI: 1.04–4.27). Sludge constitutes the third marker associated with preterm birth after TVUCL <25 mm and fetal fibronectin. However, sludge was not independently associated with acute inflammation nor funisitis when the placental histology was evaluated [44].

In summary, amniotic fluid sludge is an independent marker of PTB; however, its presence has not been used to select a better candidate in clinical practice.

12.9 Screening for Bacterial Vaginosis

Three prospective studies found no association between the presence of untreated bacterial vaginosis at 24 and 28 weeks of gestation and SPTB at <32, <35, and <37 weeks of gestation [18, 36, 45].

12.10 Prevention of Preterm Birth in Twin Pregnancies

12.10.1 Bed Rest or Limited Physical Activity

Bed rest has been used for long time in the prevention of PTB. However, studies have shown that bed rest could potentially lead to severe psychological and physiological maternal adverse effects [46]. A Cochrane meta-analysis, including six randomized studies, found no decrease in prematurity <34 and <37 weeks in the group of asymptomatic twin pregnancies hospitalized for bed rest. Paradoxically, there was an increase in PTB at <34 weeks (OR: 1.84; 95% CI: 1.01–3.34) [47]. Moreover, decreasing maternal activity or out of work has also been investigated in twin pregnancies. An observational study showed no differences in gestational age at delivery or PTB at different gestational ages [48, 49]. The number of women included in those studies was low and more studies are needed.

In summary, bed rest or modified physical activity in asymptomatic twin pregnancies is not indicated to prevent preterm birth.

12.10.2 Prophylactic Tocolysis

A Cochrane meta-analysis [50] evaluating five randomized trials (344 twin pregnancies) showed that prophylactic oral administration of betamimetics from 20 weeks of gestation in asymptomatic twin pregnant patients did not significantly decrease PPROM, PTB <34, 37 weeks, low birthweight or small-for-gestational age neonates, or neonatal mortality. A maternal death was reported in one trial without a significant difference between the groups.

12.11 Progesterone Supplementation in Asymptomatic Twin Pregnancy

12.11.1 17a-Hydroxyprogesterone Caproate (17-OHPC)

Cochrane review [51] included 5 studies [52–56] where weekly intramuscular progesterone versus no treatment or placebo were administered to women with twin pregnancies after 20 weeks of gestation independent of the obstetrical history or TVUCL. More women delivered at less than 34 weeks' gestation in the IM progesterone group compared with placebo (RR 1.54, 95% CI 1.06–2.26; 399 women; 2 studies; low-quality evidence). There were no clear group differences found in any of the other maternal or infant outcomes: PPROM (RR 1.17, 95% CI 0.84–1.63; 1257 women; 6 studies); PTB <37 weeks (RR 1.05, 95% CI 0.98–1.13; 2010 women; 5 studies high-quality evidence); PTB <28 weeks (RR 1.08, 95% CI 0.75–1.55; 1920 women; 5 studies; moderate-quality evidence) (Table 12.3).

12.11.2 17 OH Progesterone in Twins with Short Cervical Length

Three studies evaluated 17-OHPC in twins with short cervical length; two of them were secondary analysis of previous randomized controlled trials. The study of Durnwald et al. [57] is the secondary analysis of the Maternal Fetal Medicine Unit (MFMU) trial [53]; they analyzed 221 women who had TVUCL done between 16 and 20 weeks. The risk of PTB <35 weeks was increased in women with a TVUCL <25th percentile (<33 mm), (55.8 vs. 36.9%, $p = 0.02$), but the administration of 17-OHPC did not reduce PTB <35 weeks among those women with short cervix (64.3 vs. 45.8%, $p = 0.18$). A secondary analysis from the Netherlands study [58, 59] included 282 of the 671 (42%) women who had two or more cervical length measurements. They concluded that there is a progressive shortening of the cervix during pregnancy, regardless of 17-OHPC use. Senat et al. [54] enrolled 161 twin pregnancies with TVUCL <25 mm and gave them 500 mg of 17-OHPC twice a week versus placebo. There were no differences between the groups from enrollment to delivery, PTB <37 or <34 weeks. However, high dose of 17-OHPC was associated with a significant increase in the rate of PTB <32 weeks. These negative results of 17 OH progesterone in unselected twin pregnancies or those with TVUCL <25 mm were confirmed in 2015 in an individual patient data (IPD) meta-analysis [60] (Table 12.4).

Table 12.3 17 OH Progesterone supplementation in asymptomatic unselected twin pregnancies

Author	Initiation weeks	Preterm birth	RR 95% CI	Infant outcome composite
Hartikainen-Sorri 1980 Finland	28–33 weeks *N* = 77	<37 weeks		No difference
Rouse 2007 MFMU	16–20 to 35 weeks *N* = 659	<35 weeks <34 weeks <32 weeks	1.1 (0.9–1.3) 1.1 (0.8–1.3) 1.2 (0.8–1.7)	RR 1.1 (0.9–1.5)
Briery 2009 USA	20–30 weeks *N* = 30	<35 weeks	P: 0.1	No difference
Combs 2011 USA	16–24 weeks *N* = 238	<34 weeks <32 weeks	1.4 (0.7–2.6) 1.8 (0.6–5.3)	Composite no difference
Lim 2011 Amsterdam	16–20 weeks *N* = 671	<37 weeks <32 weeks	1.1 (0.97–1.28) 1.3 (0.9–2.05)	No difference
Awwad 2015 Lebanon	16–20 to 36 weeks *N* = 288	<37 weeks <32 weeks <28 weeks	1.0 (0.6–1.6) 0.5 (0.3–1.1) 0.5 (0.2–1.3)	VLBW: RR 0.5 (0.3–0.9) composite neonatal morbidity OR 0.53; (0.31–0.90) RDS OR 0.55; (0.31–0.98) ROP OR 0.21;(0.05–0.96) sepsis OR 0.24; (0.10–0.57)
Ward et al 2020	16–20 to 36 weeks History of PTB *N* = 79	SPTB <34 weeks	OR: 1.69; (0.68–4.54)	Composite neonatal morbidity: OR: 0.76; (0.27–2.12)

17 OHP 17 hydroxy progesterone, *RR* relative risk, *CI* confidence interval, *MFMU* Maternal Fetal Medicine Unit, *VLBW* very low birth weight <1500 g, *RDS* respiratory distress syndrome, *ROP* retinopathy of prematurity

12.11.3 17 OH Progesterone in Twins with History of Preterm Birth

A retrospective cohort study evaluated 79 women with twin gestation and prior singleton SPTB between 2005 and 2016 [61]. There were 27 women who received weekly 17 OH progesterone and 52 who did not. There were no significant differences in the risk of SPTB <34, <32, <28, or <24 weeks.

In summary, weekly 17 OH progesterone injection starting during the second trimester do not appear to prevent PTB in asymptomatic unselected twin gestations, twins with short cervical length or with history of singleton preterm birth (◘ Table 12.4).

12.11.4 Vaginal Progesterone in Unselected Twin Pregnancies

A Cochrane review [51] including 6 studies [62–67] evaluated vaginal progesterone or no progesterone/placebo in twin pregnancy. There were no differences in PTB, PPROM, or perinatal mortality: PTB <34 weeks (RR 0.83, 95% CI 0.63–1.09; 1727 women; 6 studies; low-quality evidence), PTB <37 weeks (RR 0.97, 95% CI 0.89–1.06; 1597 women; 6 studies), and PTB <28 weeks (RR 1.22, 95% CI 0.68–2.21; 1569 women; 4 studies). A subgroup analysis evaluating higher or lower weekly dose or gestation age at initiation of the medication (before or after 20 weeks)

Table 12.4 17 OH Progesterone supplementation in asymptomatic twin pregnancies with short cervical length

Author	Initiation weeks	Preterm birth	*P* value or RR 95% CI	Infant outcome composite
Durnwald 2010 MFMU Secondary analysis	16–20 to 35 weeks $N = 220$ <25th% = 35 mm <75th% = 44 mm	<35 weeks TVUCL <25th% <35 weeks TVUCL <75th%	*p*:0.18 *p*:0.85	Not discussed
Lim 2012 Amsterdam Secondary analysis	16–20 weeks until 34 weeks TVUCL ≤10th% history PTB <34 weeks $N = 282$	There is progressive shortening of the cervix during pregnancy, regardless of 17-OHPC use	No difference	No difference
Senat 2013 Paris	24–31 to 36 wks TVUCL ≤25 mm $N = 161$	< 37 weeks < 34 weeks	1.06 (0.75–1.5) 1.67 (0.9–2.9)	No difference

17 OHP 17 hydroxy progesterone, *RR* relative risk, *CI* confidence interval, *MFMU* Maternal Fetal Medicine Unit, *TVUCL* transvaginal ultrasound cervical length, *PTB* preterm birth

12

showed no meaningful differences. Studies not included in the Cochrane review [51] were: Norman et al. [68] with 500 twin pregnancies, using vaginal progesterone gel of 90 mg/day or placebo showed no statistical difference in the prevention of PTB at <28, <32, <34 weeks nor Wood et al 2012 [69], who evaluated 84 women starting vaginal progesterone between 16 and 20.6 weeks until 35 weeks. A recent multicenter randomized controlled trial enrolled 1169 twin pregnancy and compared 600 mg vaginal progesterone daily vs. placebo from 11–14 weeks to 34 weeks [70]. Universal treatment with high dose of vaginal progesterone did not reduce the incidence of spontaneous PTB between 24 0/7 and 33 6/7 weeks' gestation or from enrollment to <34 weeks or other evaluated gestational ages. There was no evidence of interaction between the effects of treatment and chorionicity, parity, method of conception, and adherence (Table 12.5).

12.11.5 Vaginal Progesterone in Twins with Short Cervical Length

Several randomized controlled trials evaluating vaginal progesterone for PTB prevention had included twin pregnancies with short TVUCL [63–66, 71], but these trials have not provided individual data for twin cases in the original publications. The study by El-Rafaie et al. [67] is the only dedicated trial that enrolled women with twin pregnancy and TVUCL 20–25 mm between 20 and 24 weeks, and randomized them to 400 mg of daily vaginal progesterone ($n = 116$) vs. no treatment ($n = 108$). Their results showed a significantly longer gestational age in the study group (34.34 ± 2.23 vs. 33.36 ± 2.72 weeks; $p = 0.007$) and a decreased incidence of PTB <34 weeks (35.3% vs. 52.8%; RR = 0.670; 95% CI = 0.494–0.908; $p = 0.010$) and PTB

Table 12.5 Vaginal progesterone in unselected twins

Author	Initiation weeks	Preterm birth	RR (95% CI)	Infant outcome Composite
Norman 2009 UK	24 weeks $N = 494$	<34 weeks	1.36 (0.9–2)	No difference
Rode 2011 Multicenter	20–24 weeks to 34 weeks $N = 675$	<34 weeks	0.8 (0.5–1.2)	No difference
		<32 weeks	0.8 (0.4–1.3)	No difference
Centigoz 2011 Turkey	24–34 weeks $N = 67$	<37 weeks	3.4 (1.16–10.4)	No difference
		<34 weeks	2.9 (0.7–11.2)	No difference
Wood 2012 Canada	16–20.6–35 weeks $N = 84$	<35 weeks	$p = 0.8$	No difference
Aboulghar 2012 Egypt	IVF/ICSI $N = 78$	<37 weeks	0.73, (0.36–2.0)	No data
Serra 2013 Spain	20–34 weeks $N = 193$	<34 weeks 200 mg	No difference	No difference
		<34 weeks 400 mg	No difference	
Brizot 2016 Brazil	18–20 weeks to 35 weeks $N = 383$	<28 weeks	1.72 (0.5–5.8)	No difference
		<32 weeks	1.34 (0.6–2.8)	
		<34 weeks	1.45 (0.85–2.5)	
		SPTB <34 weeks	1.32 (0.24–2.37)	
		<37 weeks	1.32 (0.85–2.06)	
Rehal 2020 Europe	11–14 weeks to 34 weeks 600 mg $N = 1169$	24 0/7–33 6/7 weeks	1.35 (0.88–2.05)	No difference

RR relative risk, *CI* confidence interval, *PTB* preterm birth, *SPTB* spontaneous preterm birth, *IVF/ICSI* in vitro fertilization/ intracytoplasmatic sperm injection

<32 weeks 12.1 vs. 29.6%; RR = 0.407; 95% CI = 0.230–0.721; $p = 0.002$) in the vaginal progesterone group (Table 12.6). An updated systematic review and individual patient data meta-analysis including 303 women (159 vaginal progesterone and 144 placebo/no treatment) [72] (Fig. 12.1) concluded that vaginal progesterone compared with placebo/no treatment in twin pregnancies with TVUCL <25 mm was associated with a statistically significant reduction in the risk of PTB <33 weeks' gestation (31.4% vs. 43.1%; RR, 0.69 (95% CI, 0.51–0.93); moderate-quality evidence) and also a significant

Table 12.6 Vaginal progesterone in asymptomatic twin pregnancies with short cervical length

Author	Initiation weeks	Preterm birth	RR (95% CI) or OR (95% CI)	Infant outcome composite RR (95% CI)
Fonseca 2007	20–25 TVUCL <15 mm *N* = 24	<34 weeks	OR 0.49 (0.9–2.53)	No data
Klein 2011 Subanalysis	20–24 weeks to 34 weeks TVUCL <30 mm *N* = 47	<34 weeks	OR: 0.6(0.2–2.2)	Composite no difference
		<32 weeks	OR: 1.5(0.4–6.7)	
El-Refaie 2016 Egypt	20–24 weeks to 34 weeks TVUCL 20–25 mm *N* = 224	<34 weeks	RR: 0.67 (0.5–0.9)	VLBW 0.46 (0.3–0.7) RDS 0.6 (0.5–0.8) Mechanical ventilation 0.473 (0.3–0.69) Early neonatal death 0.5 (0.3–0.7)
		<32 weeks	RR:0.4 (0.2–0.7)	
		<28 weeks	RR: 0.37 (0.1–1.9)	
Rehal 2020 Europe	11–14 weeks to 34 weeks 600 mg TVCL <30 mm at 11–14 weeks *N* = 146	24 0/7–33 6/7 weeks	HR: 0.56 (0.2–1.6)	No data
		SPTB <32 weeks	HR 0.23 (0.07–0.69)	

RR relative risk, *CI* confidence interval, *RR* relative risk, *OR* odds ratio, *HR* hazard ratio, *TVUCL* transvaginal ultrasound cervical length, *PTB* preterm birth, *VLBW* very low birth weight <1500 g, *RDS* respiratory distress syndrome

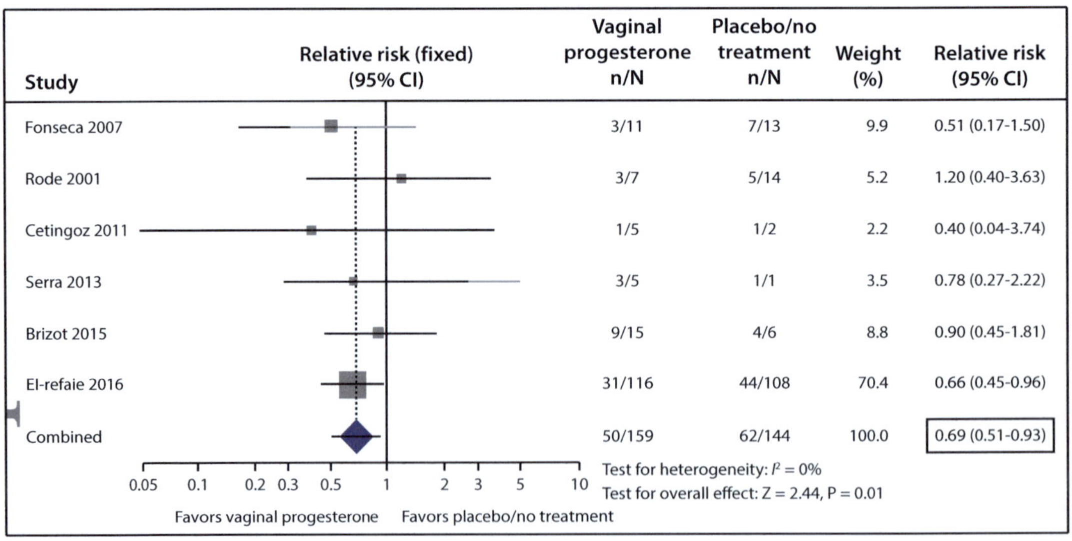

Fig. 12.1 New meta-analysis on vaginal progesterone in twins with short cervical length <25 mm. Forest plot of the effect of vaginal progesterone on the risk of preterm birth <33 weeks' gestation. CI confidence interval. (From Romero et al. [72])

decrease in the risk of PTB <35, <34, <32, and <30 weeks' gestation (RRs ranging from 0.47 to 0.83), decrease in neonatal death (RR,0.53 (95% CI, 0.35–0.81), respiratory distress syndrome (RR, 0.70 (95% CI, 0.56–0.89), composite neonatal morbidity and mortality (RR, 0.61 (95% CI, 0.34–0.98), use of mechanical ventilation (RR, 0.54 (95% CI,0.36–0.81), and birth weight <1500 g (RR, 0.53 (95% CI, 0.35–0.80) (all moderate-quality evidence). The subgroup analysis showed that vaginal progesterone performs better when using 400 mg daily, if TVUCL measures between 10 and 25 mm and in women with no history of PTB. Some limitations are included in the analysis, El-Rafaie et al. [67] provided 74% of the total sample, they enrolled women with a TVUCL 20–25 mm, it was not a placebo control study, and the providers were not blinded for the arm of treatment. All those characteristics of the trial could have added bias in the results. A planned subanalysis of the latest RCT, the study by Rehal et al. [70] evaluated 146 women with twin pregnancy and TVUCL <30 mm at enrollment (11–14 weeks). Women who received 600 mg vaginal progesterone had a significantly lower incidence of spontaneous PTB <32 weeks with a HR 0.23 (0.07–0.69) (◘ Table 12.6).

In summary, vaginal progesterone in unselected twin pregnancies has not shown improvement in PTB or neonatal outcomes. However, a high dose of daily vaginal progesterone (400 mg) in twin pregnancies with TVUCL <25 mm appears promising in the prevention of PTB at different gestational ages and improvement of neonatal outcomes. The results of an ongoing research trial are required before conclusive advice can be provided with regard to the benefits of using vaginal progesterone in women with twin gestation and a short cervix.

12.11.6 Vaginal Pessary

The initial publication evaluating vaginal pessary in twin pregnancy with short TVCL has inspired a lot of research. Seven women with TVUCL <15 mm received vaginal pessary, and 23 were controls; pessary was associated with a significant prolongation of the interval from diagnosis to delivery. The cervical pessary is a silicone ring placed around the cervix; the mechanism of action is to tightly seal the cervical canal, prevent an ascending infection through the mucus plug and, perhaps more importantly, to support the cervix by changing the angle of the cervical canal.

12.11.7 Vaginal Pessary in Unselected Twin Pregnancy

Two randomized trials have addressed the question of effectiveness of vaginal pessary in PTB prevention in unselected twin pregnancies. Liam et al. [73] randomized 808 women (401 in the pessary group; 407 in the control group). The primary outcome, poor perinatal outcome, was not significantly different (RR 0.98, 95% CI 0.69–1.39). There was no significant difference in gestational age at delivery, PTB <37, <32, or <28 weeks. Nicolaides et al. [74] randomized 1180 unselected twin pregnancies to cervical pessary placement (n = 590) from 20 0/ to 24 6/7 weeks' gestation until elective removal or delivery vs. expectant management (590), there were no significant differences in the rates of SPTB <34 weeks (13.6% vs. 12.9%; RR: 1.054, 95% [CI] 0.787–1.413; p = 0.722), perinatal death (2.5% vs. 2.7%; RR 0.908, 95% CI 0.553–1.491; p = 0.702), adverse neonatal outcome (10.0 vs. 9.2%; RR 1.094, 95% CI 0.851–1.407; p = 0.524), or neonatal therapy (17.9% vs. 17.2%; relative risk 1.040, 95% CI 0.871–1.242; p = 0.701) (◘ Table 12.7).

12.11.8 Vaginal Pessary in Twin Pregnancy with Short Cervical Length

Four randomized trials included twin pregnancies and TVUCL results, two were secondary analysis and two were dedicated trials. In Liam et al. [73] the prespecified subgroup of women who had a short cervical length below 25th percentile (<38 mm) at 16–22 weeks of

Table 12.7 Pessary in unselected twin pregnancies

Author	Initiation weeks	Preterm birth	RR (95% CI)	Infant outcome composite RR (95% CI)
Liem 2013 (ProTwin) Nether-lands	12–20 weeks TVUCL (mm) 43·6 (8·1) vs. 44·2 (8·5) *N* = 808	<28 weeks	0·79 (0·50–1·27)	Composite poor perinatal outcome 0·98 (0·69–1·39)
		<32 weeks	0·86 (0·65–1·15)	
		<37 weeks	0·94 (0·87–1·07)	
Nicolaides 2016 UK	20–24 6/7 weeks *N* = 1180	<34 weeks	1.05 (0.78–1.42)	Perinatal death RR 0.9, 95% CI 0.5–1.5 Adverse neonatal outcome RR 1.1, 95% CI 0.8–1.4 Neonatal therapy RR 1.04, 95% CI 0.8–1.2

RR relative risk, *CI* confidence interval, *TVUCL* transvaginal ultrasound cervical length

gestation, the pessary appeared to show efficacy. The rate of adverse neonatal outcomes RR, 0.40 (95% CI 0.19–0.83), neonatal mortality RR, 0.13 (95% CI 0.03–0.60), PTB at <28 weeks RR 0.23 (95% CI 0.06–0.87), and <32 weeks (RR 0.49 (95% CI 0.24–0.97) was significantly lower in the pessary group than in the control group). Goya et al. [75] randomized 137 women with twin pregnant and TVUCL ≤25 mm to receive a cervical pessary or expectant management (1:1 ratio). SPTB <34 weeks of gestation was significantly less frequent in the pessary group than in the expectant management group (11/68 [16.2%] vs. 26/66 [39.4%]; RR, 0.41; 95% CI, 0.22–0.76). No significant differences were observed in the composite neonatal morbidity outcome (8/136 [5.9%] vs. 12/130 [9.1%]; RR, 0.64; 95% CI, 0.27–1.50) or neonatal mortality (none) between the groups. In contrast to Nicolaides et al. [74] posthoc analysis of 214 women with a short cervix (<25 mm) did not show any benefit from the insertion of a cervical pessary. Berghella et al. [76] randomized 46 women with twin pregnancy and TVUCL <30 mm, 23 women to pessary placement, and 23 (50%) to no pessary. TVUCL (16.7 vs. 22.9 mm; p = 0.45) at randomization. There were no significant differences between the pessary and no-pessary groups in the rate of primary outcome, PTB <34 weeks (39% vs. 35%; RR, 1.13 (95% CI, 0.53–2.40), as well as other outcomes, including PTB <37 weeks and < 28 weeks, gestational age at delivery, birth weight, and composite adverse neonatal outcome (Table 12.8).

In summary, treatment with cervical pessary in unselected twin pregnancy has not shown a decrease in PTB at any gestational age. In twin pregnancies with short cervical length, pessary has conflicting results in different large randomized control trials. An ongoing trial by MFMU may elucidate this question.

12.12 Cervical Cerclage

12.12.1 History-Indicated Cerclage in Unselected Twin Pregnancy

Only two RCTs have reported the outcome of cerclage placed in the first or early second trimester for the only indication of being a multiple pregnancies (unselected twin pregnancy) [77, 78]. Both studies have a small sample size. In Dor et al. [77] after induction of ovulation and confirmed twin pregnancy, women received cerclage or no cerclage. PTB

Table 12.8 Pessary in twin pregnancies with short cervical length

Author	Initiation weeks	Preterm birth	RR (95% CI)	Infant outcome composite RR (95% CI)
Liem 2013 Netherlands Subanalysis	<20 weeks TVUCL <38 mm *N* = 133	SPTB <28 weeks	0.23 (0.06–0.87)	Poor neonatal outcomes 0.40 (0.19–0.83). Neonatal mortality 0.13 (0.03–0.60)
		SPTB <32 weeks	0.49 (0.24–0.97)	
		SPTB <37 weeks	0.82 (0.54–1.24)	
Goya 2016 Spain	18–22 weeks TVUCL <25 mm *N* = 134	SPTB <28 weeks	0.43 (0.14–1.33)	No difference
		SPTB <34 weeks	0.41 (0.22–0.76)	
		Any delivery at <34 weeks	0.43 (0.24–0.78)	
Nicolaides 2016 UK	18–24 weeks TVUCL <25 mm *N* = 214	SPTB <34 weeks	1.2 (0.78–1.84)	Adverse neonatal event RR: 1.18 (0.7–2.01)
Berghella 2017	18–24 weeks TVUCL 18-27 mm *N* = 46	PTB <34 weeks	1.13 (0.53–2.4)	No difference
		PTB <28 weeks	1.05 (0.24–4.6)	
		PTB <24 weeks	2.09 (0.15–57.9)	

RR relative risk, *CI* confidence interval, *TVUCL* transvaginal ultrasound cervical length, *PTB* preterm birth, *SPTB* spontaneous preterm birth

<37 weeks was 10 (45.4%) vs. 11 (47.8) and the neonatal death rate was 18.2 vs. 15.2%. The MRC/RCOG [78] Study included 28 women, 12 randomized to cerclage, and 16 to no cerclage. There were no differences in the incidence of PTB <33 or 37 weeks. A large retrospective cohort from a large nationwide database between January 1990 and May 2004 [79] compared 146 (1.8%) women with twin pregnancies that received prophylactic cerclage vs. 8072 women as control group. Patients who received prophylactic cerclage had a significantly higher incidence of PTB < before 32 weeks 56 (19.2%) vs. 1946 (12.1%). No significant difference was seen in the mean gestational age at delivery (◘ Table 12.9).

In summary, history-indicated cerclage based only on the presence of twins should not be recommended.

12.12.2 History-Indicated Cerclage in Twin Pregnancy with History of Preterm Birth

The role of history-indicated cerclage among women with a twin pregnancy and a history of PTB was evaluated in a retrospective study from Israel [80]. Data from 82 women with a twin gestation from 2006 to 2017 were analyzed, first-trimester history-indicated cerclage (n = 41) were matched with those managed expectantly (n = 41). Gestational age at delivery was higher in the cerclage group than in those managed expectantly (median 35 vs. 30 weeks; $p < 0.0001$). Rates of SPTB <24 weeks (2.4% vs. 19.5%; odds ratio (OR), 0.10 (95% CI, 0.01–0.87); $p = 0.03$), PTB <28 weeks (12.2% vs. 34.1%;

Table 12.9 History-indicated cerclage in twin pregnancies

Author	Initiation weeks	Preterm birth	RR (95% CI) or OR (95% CI)	Infant outcome composite
Dor et al. 1982	First trimester	PTD <37 weeks	No difference 10/22 (45.4%) vs. 11/23 (47.8%)	Neonatal death 18.2% vs. 15.2%
MRC/RCOG 1993	First trimester	PTB <33 weeks PTB <37 weeks	There were no difference	
Roman 2013 USA (retro-spective)	First trimester. 146 (1.8%) cerclage vs. 8072 control group	PTB <32 weeks	higher incidence of PTB <32 weeks 56 (19.2%) vs. 1946 (12.1%)	No data
		GA at delivery	No difference	
Rottenst-reich 2019 Israel (retrospec-tive)	History of PTB Cerclage 41 control 41	GA at delivery	(Median 35 vs. 30 weeks; P < 0.0001)	No data
		PTB <24 weeks	2.4% vs. 19.5% OR, 0.10 (95% CI, 0.01–0.87)	
		PTB <28 weeks	12.2% vs. 34.1%; OR, 0.27 (95% CI, 0.09–0.84)	
		PTB <32 weeks	22.0% vs. 56.1%; OR, 0.22 (95% CI, 0.08–0.58)	
		PTB <34weeks	34.1% vs. 82.9%; OR, 0.11 (95% CI, 0.04–0.30) were significantly lower in the cerclage group than in the control group	

RR relative risk, *CI* confidence interval, *TVUCL* transvaginal ultrasound cervical length, *PTB* Preterm birth, *SPTB* spontaneous preterm birth, *GA* gestational age

12

OR, 0.27 (95% CI, 0.09–0.84); $p = 0.03$), PTB <32 weeks (22.0% vs. 56.1%; OR, 0.22 (95% CI, 0.08–0.58); $p = 0.003$) and PTB <34 weeks (34.1% vs. 82.9%; OR, 0.11 (95% CI, 0.04–0.30); $p < 0.0001$) were significantly lower in the cerclage group than in the control group. Additionally, low birth weight, stillbirth, and adverse neonatal outcomes were decreased in the cerclage group (Table 12.9).

In summary, there is limited information to consider if first-trimester cerclage indicated in women with history of preterm birth in twin pregnancy will decrease preterm birth, and more studies are needed in this area.

12.12.3 Ultrasound-Indicated Cerclage in Asymptomatic Twin Pregnancy

Only three RCTs studying the effect of an ultrasound indicated cervical cerclage had included women with twin pregnancy [81–83]. The 49 women with twins identified in the three studies (24 with cerclage and 25 with no cerclage) were analyzed in a systematic review in 2005 [84] and the Cochrane database in 2014 [85] and finally in a dedicated IPD meta-analysis in 2015 [86]. Results from the first meta-analysis suggested that cerclage for asymptomatic twin with a TVUCL <25 mm was associated with an increased risk of PTB at <35 weeks vs. no cerclage (RR: 2.15; 95% CI: 1.15–4.01) [84]. In a new IPD meta-analysis evaluating the initial 49 twin cases, results were adjusted for history of PTB and gestational age at randomization. There were no statistically significant differences in PTB <34 weeks (aOR 1.17, 95% CI 0.23–3.79) or differences in PTB <37, <32, <28, or <24 weeks. Rates of very low birthweight and of respiratory distress syndrome were significantly higher in the cerclage group than in the control group.

Several retrospective case-control studies have been available [87–91]. The largest cohort [88] included 140 women with twin pregnancy and TVUCL ≤25 mm, they were managed with either cerclage (n = 57) or no cerclage (n = 83). After adjusting for GA at presentation, there were no differences in GA at delivery or SPTB <34, <32, <28, or <24 weeks. However, in the subgroup of women with TVUCL ≤15 mm (32 cerclage and 39 no cerclage) the interval between diagnosis to delivery was significantly prolonged by 12.5 ± 4.5 vs. 8.8 ± 4.6 weeks ($p < 0.001$); SPTB <34 weeks was significantly decreased: 16 (50%) vs. 31 (79.5%) (aOR, 0.51; 95% CI, 0.31–0.83) as was admission to neonatal intensive care unit: 38/58 (65.5%) vs. 63/76 (82.9%) (aOR, 0.42; 95% CI, 0.24–0.81) when the cerclage group was compared with the no cerclage group, respectively. Since then, similar results has been published in retrospective cohorts. Houlihan et al. [89] published a retrospective cohort study, including 40 women with dichorionic diamniotic pregnancies with TVUCL <25 mm who were matched with 40 controls. The TVUCL <15 mm was present in 82.5% of all cases. In the cerclage group, SPTB <32 weeks was significantly less frequent (20.0% vs. 50.0%; OR, 0.40 (95% CI, 0.20–0.80)) when compared with controls as well as significantly decreased SPTB <34, 30, and 28 weeks. Adams et al. [90] included 82 women (cerclage: 43 and 39 control) women with twin pregnancy and TVUCL <25 mm; there were no significant differences in rates of PTB or perinatal outcome. However, in the subgroup of women with TVUCL <15 mm (cerclage: 27 and 21 control) PTB <35 weeks and PTB <32 weeks were significantly decreased aRR 0.49 (0.26–0.93) and aRR 0.31 (0.12–0.86), respectively. Han, et al. published a retrospective case-control [91] study of women with twin pregnancy and TVUCL <25 mm (n = 56); among them, 35 women had TVUCL <15 mm. There were no significant differences in the overall or SPTB at <36, 34, or 32 weeks of gestation. All prospective and retrospective studies were evaluated in a systematic review [92]; the meta-analysis demonstrated that cerclage placement was beneficial for reducing PTB <37, <34, and <32 weeks, and the prolongation of pregnancy in twin pregnancies with a TVUCL <15 mm. However, for twin pregnancies with TVUCL 15–25 mm or a normal CL (history of PTB or unselected twin pregnancy), cerclage placement did not seem to be beneficial (◘ Table 12.10).

In summary, there is not enough information to recommend an ultrasound indicated cerclage in asymptomatic twin pregnancy with TVUCL <25 mm. More data are needed in twins with TVUCL <15 mm as the retrospective data is promising. A randomized controlled trial is ongoing on this topic.

12.12.4 Physical Exam-Indicated Cerclage in Twin Pregnancies

Physical exam-indicated cerclage in twins has been evaluated in three retrospective case controls [91, 93, 94]. All three studies were evaluated in a systematic review [92], they included 244 women with twin pregnancy and dilated cervix >1 cm, managed with either cerclage or expectant management. The pooled outcomes showed cerclage placement was associated with a significant prolongation of pregnancy by a mean difference of 6.78 weeks of gestation (95% CI, 5.32–8.24; $p < 0.0001$), significant reduction of PTB rate at <34, <32, <28,

Table 12.10 Ultrasound indicated cerclage in twin pregnancies

Author	Initiation weeks	Preterm birth	RR (95% CI) or OR (95% CI)	Infant outcome composite RR (95% CI) or OR (95% CI)
Roman et al. 2005	TVCL <25 mm 20.8 weeks (15.7–23.6) weeks Cerclage: 19 Control: 12	PTB <37, 34, 32, 30, and 28 weeks	No difference Exp: 34.0 (21.3–38.9) Con: 34.4 (23.1–38.0)	
Saccone, meta-analysis 2015	TVUCL <25 mm 24 (49%) cerclage) 25 (51%) control	PTB <37 weeks PTB <35 weeks PTB <34 weeks PTB <32 weeks PTB <28 weeks PTB <24 weeks	No difference on any outcome	Increased in cerclage group: VLBW (aOR 2.22, 95% CI 1.07–5.73) and RDS (aOR 3.88, 95% CI 1.09–21.03)
Roman 2016 USA	16–24 weeks TVUCL <25 mm. cerclage = 57 control = 83	SPTB <34 weeks SPTB <32 weeks SPTB <28 weeks	There were no difference	No difference
Roman 2016 subanalysis USA	16–24 weeks TVUCL <15 mm cerclage = 32 control = 39	SPTB <34 weeks	0.51 (0.31–0.83)	Admission to NICU: 38/58 (65.5%) vs. 63/76 (82.9%) 0.42 (0.24–0.81)
Houlihan et al. 2016	16–24 TVUCL <25 = 80 TVUCL <15 = 66(82%)	GA at birth (weeks)	36.0 (32.9–37.4) vs. 31.6 (27.1–36.7)	No data
		SPTB <34 weeks	0.26 (0.10–0.67)	
		SPTB <32 weeks	0.22 (0.06–0.83	
		SPTB <28 weeks	0.19 (0.05–0.72)	
Adams et al. 2017	20.8 ± 1.9 weeks TVUCL <25 mm Cerclage: 43 Control: 39	PTB <37, 34, 32, 28, and 24 weeks; neonatal outcomes	GA del: 34.4 ± 4.2 vs. 32.9 ± 5.7 NS No difference PTB or SPTB	TVCL <25 mm No difference in neonatal outcomes
Adams et al. 2017 Subanalysis	TVUCL <15 mm Cerclage: 27 Control: 21	PTB <35 weeks	aRR: 0.49 (0.26–0.93)	TVUCL <15 mm No difference in neonatal outcomes
		PTB <32 weeks	aRR: 0.31 (0.12–0.86)	

12

Table 12.10 (continued)

Author	Initiation weeks	Preterm birth	RR (95% CI) or OR (95% CI)	Infant outcome composite RR (95% CI) or OR (95% CI)
Han, et al. 2019	TVUCL <25 mm = 56 TVUCL <15 mm = 35	SPTB <36 weeks SPTB <34 weeks SPTB <32 weeks	No differences in PTB or SPTB at <36, 34 or 32 weeks of gestation	No separate data

RR relative risk, *CI* confidence interval, *TVUCL* transvaginal ultrasound cervical length, *PTB* preterm birth, *SPTB* spontaneous preterm birth, *GA* gestational age, *NICU* neonatal intensive care unit, *VLBW* very low birth weight <1500 g, *RDS* respiratory distress syndrome

and <24 weeks of gestation by 40% to 65%, and a significant improvement in perinatal outcomes, which included decreased perinatal mortality and composite neonatal morbidity.

A recently published RCT on physical exam-indicated cerclage in twins [95] enrolled 30 women with twin pregnancy and asymptomatic cervical dilation from 1 to 4 cm between 16 0/7 and 23 6/7 weeks in 8 centers. Seventeen women were randomized to a combination of physical exam-indicated cerclage, indomethacin, and antibiotics and 13 were randomized to control (no cerclage or medication). The incidence of SPTB <34 weeks was significantly reduced in the cerclage group: 12/17 (70%) vs. 13/13 (100%) RR: 0.7 [95% CI 0.5–0.96], PTB <32, <28, and <24 weeks were all significantly reduced in the cerclage group by 36%, 52%, and 65%, respectively. The interval from diagnosis to delivery: 8.3 ± 5.8 vs. 2.9 ± 3.0 weeks ($p = 0.02$). Perinatal death was significantly reduced in the cerclage group by 77% (Table 12.11).

In summary, RCT and retrospective studies have shown that physical exam indicated cerclage in twins with dilated cervix >1 cm decreases PTB at all gestational ages and improves perinatal outcome. However, the number of cases in each study is low and results should be interpreted with caution.

12.13 Conclusion

In asymptomatic twin pregnancies, the two best predictive tests for PTB at <28, <32, and <34 weeks of gestation are TVUCL measurement at 20–24 weeks of gestation <20 mm or <25 mm, followed by cervico-vaginal fFN testing. No studies have shown that such detection of a high-risk group has enabled the reduction of PTB risk and improved the health of neonates and mothers. Treatment modalities such as bed rest, limitation of physical activity, prophylactic tocolysis, intramuscular progesterone, history-indicated cerclage, or ultrasound indicated cerclage have not decreased PTB in asymptomatic twin pregnancy.

So far, there are two interventions for the prevention of PTB in twins, evaluated in RCTs. First, a high dose (400 mg) of daily vaginal progesterone in twin pregnancy with TVUCL <25 mm may decrease PTB and improve perinatal outcome. A single RCT showed that physical exam indicated cerclage before 24 weeks might reduce the risk of PTB, perinatal mortality, and improve perinatal outcome. These promising results need to be confirmed in other RCTs before routinely applying their conclusions in clinical practice (Table 12.12).

Table 12.11 Physical exam indicated cerclage in twin pregnancies

Author	Initiation weeks	Preterm birth	RR (95% CI) or OR (95% CI) P value	Infant outcome composite RR (95% CI) or OR (95% CI)
Roman 2016 USA	16–24 weeks Dilated ≥1 cm cerclage = 38 control = 38 Dilated ≥2 cm cerclage = 24 control = 24	GA delivery	31.2 ± 5.6 vs. 24.3 ± 4.2	Perinatal mortality OR 21/76 (27.6) 45/76 (59.2) OR 0.24 (0.11–0.5)
		SPTB <34 weeks	0.06 (0.03–0.34)	
		SPTB <32 weeks	0.08 (0.03–0.34)	
		SPTB <28 weeks	0.05 (0.01–0.21)	
		SPTB <24 weeks	0.17 (0.05–0.54)	
Abasi et al. 2018 Canada	< 25 weeks Dilated >1 cm cerclage = 27 control = 9 Dilated ≥3 cm cerclage = 11 control = 5	Interval (weeks)	7.3 ± 5.5 0.5 ± 0.3 < 0.001	Neonatal survival to discharge Cerclage 70.4% (38/54) Control 55.6% (10/18) ($p = 0.2$). Admission to NICU 27 (65.9%) 10 (100.0%) $p = 0.03$
		GA at birth (weeks)	28.9 ± 6.1 vs. 24.2 ± 2.6 0.03	
		PTB <34 weeks	18 (66.7) 9 (100.0) 0.046	
		PTB <32 weeks	16 (59.3) 9 (100.0) 0.02	
		PTB <28 weeks	16 (59.3) 9 (100.0) 0.02	
		PTB <26 weeks	12 (44.4) 6 (66.7) 0.2	
		PTB <24 weeks	7 (25.9) 4 (44.4) 0.3	
Han, et al. 2019	GA Dilation >1 cm) Cerclage: 54 Control: 17	SPTB <36 weeks	13/17 (76.4%) 26/54 (48.1%) 0.055	No data for subgroups
		SPTB<34 weeks	10/17 (58.8%) 16/54 (29.6%) 43	
		SPTB <32 weeks	7/17 (41.2%) 6/54 (11.1%) 0.01	
Roman et al. 2020 RCT Prospective	16–23 weeks Dilation 1–5 cm Cerclage: 17 Control: 13	GA at delivery (weeks)	29.1 ± 1.7 vs. 22.5 ± 3.9	Overall perinatal mortality[a] RR 0.23 (0.1–0.49)
		interval (weeks)	8.3 ± 5.8 vs. 2.9 ± 3.0 Mean interval 6.9 (2.9–10.9) <0.01	
		SPTB <34 weeks	0.71 (0.52–0.96)	
		SPTB <32 weeks	0.65 (0.46–0.92)	
		SPTB <28 weeks	0.49 (0.26–0.89)	
		SPTB <24 weeks	0.35 (0.16–0.75)	

RR relative risk, *OR* odds ratio, *CI* confidence interval, *PTB* preterm birth, *SPTB* spontaneous preterm birth, *GA* gestational age, *RCT* Randomized controlled trial

[a]Data includes both twin A and B

12

Table 12.12 Therapies for asymptomatic twins

Intervention	Recommendation	Effect	Reference(s)
Activity restriction	Not recommended		[45–48]
Tocolysis Betamimetic	Not recommended		[49]
17 OH Progesterone Caproate			
Unselected	Not recommended		[50–55]
Short cervix	Not recommended		[53, 56, 58]
History of PTB	Not recommended		[60]
Vaginal progesterone			
Unselected	Not recommended		[50, 61, 66–68]
Short cervix	Consider 400 mg in TVUCL <25 mm	Decrease PTB Decrease perinatal mortality and morbidity	[62, 65, 66, 69, 70]
Vaginal pessary			
Unselected	Not recommended		[71, 72]
Short cervix	Conflicting results, not recommended		[71–74]
Cervical cerclage			
HIC	Not recommended		[75–77]
HIC + History PTB	Not recommended		[78]
UIC	Not recommended		[78–88]
PEIC	Consider PEIC in twins with cervical dilation >1 cm	Decreased PTB all GA, decreased perinatal mortality and morbidity	[87–91]

PTB preterm birth, *TVUCL* Transvaginal ultrasound cervical length, *GA* gestational age, *HIC* history indicated cerclage, *UIC* ultrasound indicated cerclage, *PEC* physical exam indicated cerclage

12.13.1 Review Questions

1. Describe the risk of preterm birth in monochorionic twins compared with dichorionic twins.

2. What are the management options for the prevention of preterm birth in twin pregnancy?

3. What are the best predictive test for preterm birth in twin pregnancy?

4. What are the best interventions for the prevention of preterm birth in twins?

12.13.2 Multiple-Choice Questions

1. What is the incidence of preterm birth in twin pregnancies?
   (a) 20%
   (b) 10%
   (c) 60%
   (d) 70%

Answer: (c)

2. What is the neonatal and infant mortality compared with singleton pregnancy?
   (a) Five times higher
   (b) Same
   (c) 20 times higher
   (d) 10 times higher

Answer: (a)

3. What is the best predictor for preterm birth in twin pregnancies?
   (a) Transabdominal cervical length <24 weeks
   (b) Transvaginal cervical length <24 weeks
   (c) Fibronectin
   (d) Cervical elasticity <24 weeks

Answer: (b)

- Bed rest increases risk of preterm birth (True/False): True
- Women correctly identified 50% of the contractions recorded by Home uterine contraction monitoring (True/false): False, only 17%
- What is the incidence of history of preterm birth in twin gestation?
- 10–15%
- What are the complications unique to monochorionic pregnancy?
- TTTS, TAPS, conjoint twin

4. Cervicovaginal fFN alone has high accuracy in predicting spontaneous PTB in asymptomatic twin gestations. (True/False): False, low to moderate.
   - When considering vaginal progesterone supplementation in a woman with twin pregnancy and transvaginal cervical length <24 weeks, the best candidate will be:
   (a) 0–5 mm
   (b) 6–10 mm
   (c) 11–15 mm
   (d) 16–20 mm
   (e) 20–25 mm

Answer: (e)

5. When considering cerclage for preterm birth prevention in twin pregnancy, the evidence suggests that the best candidate will be:
   (a) Presence of sludge
   (b) History of preterm birth
   (c) TVUCL <25 mm
   (d) TVUCL <15 mm
   (e) Cervical dilation >1 cm

Answer: (e)

6. When considering vaginal progesterone for the prevention of preterm birth in women with short cervical length <24 weeks, the best dose is:
   (a) 90 mg
   (b) 100 mg
   (c) 200 mg
   (d) 300 mg
   (e) 400 mg

Answer: (e)

Financial Support No external financial support was received for this study.

References

1. Blencowe H, Cousens S, Oestergaard MZ, Chou D, Moller AB, Narwal R, et al. National, regional, and worldwide estimates of preterm birth rates in the year 2010 with time trends since 1990 for selected countries: a systematic analysis and implications. Lancet. 2012;379(9832):2162–72. PubMed PMID: 22682464.
2. Nour NM. Premature delivery and the millennium development goal. Rev Obstet Gynecol. 2012;5(2):100–5. PubMed PMID: 22866189. Pubmed Central PMCID: 3410509.
3. Liu L, Oza S, Hogan D, Chu Y, Perin J, Zhu J, et al. Global, regional, and national causes of under-5 mortality in 2000–15: an updated systematic analysis with implications for the Sustainable Development Goals. Lancet. 2016;388(10063):3027–35. PubMed PMID: 27839855. Pubmed Central PMCID: 5161777.
4. Martin JA, Hamilton BE, Osterman MJK. Births in the United States, 2018. NCHS Data Brief. 2019;346:1–8. PubMed PMID: 31442195.
5. Martin JA, Hamilton BE, Osterman MJK, Driscoll AK, Drake P. Births: final data for 2017.

Natl Vital Stat Rep. 2018;67(8):1–50. PubMed PMID: 30707672.
6. Matthews TJ, MacDorman MF, Thoma ME. Infant mortality statistics from the 2013 period linked birth/infant death data set. Natl Vital Stat Rep. 2015;64(9):1–30. PubMed PMID: 26270610.
7. Stock S, Norman J. Preterm and term labour in multiple pregnancies. Semin Fetal Neonatal Med. 2010;15(6):336–41. PubMed PMID: 20643592.
8. Breathnach FM, McAuliffe FM, Geary M, Daly S, Higgins JR, Dornan J, et al. Optimum timing for planned delivery of uncomplicated monochorionic and dichorionic twin pregnancies. Obstet Gynecol. 2012;119(1):50–9. PubMed PMID: 22183211.
9. Maruotti GM, Saccone G, Morlando M, Martinelli P. First-trimester ultrasound determination of chorionicity in twin gestations using the lambda sign: a systematic review and meta-analysis. Eur J Obstet Gynecol Reprod Biol. 2016;202:66–70. PubMed PMID: 27180271.
10. Roman A, Saccone G, Dude CM, Ward A, Anastasio H, Dugoff L, et al. Midtrimester transvaginal ultrasound cervical length screening for spontaneous preterm birth in diamniotic twin pregnancies according to chorionicity. Eur J Obstet Gynecol Reprod Biol. 2018;229:57–63. PubMed PMID: 30107361.
11. Hack KE, Derks JB, Elias SG, Franx A, Roos EJ, Voerman SK, et al. Increased perinatal mortality and morbidity in monochorionic versus dichorionic twin pregnancies: clinical implications of a large Dutch cohort study. BJOG. 2008;115(1):58–67. PubMed PMID: 17999692.
12. D'Antonio F, Thilaganathan B, Dias T, Khalil A, Southwest Thames Obstetric Research Collaborative (STORK). Influence of chorionicity and gestational age at single fetal loss on risk of preterm birth in twin pregnancy: analysis of STORK multiple pregnancy cohort. Ultrasound Obstet Gynecol. 2017;50(6):723–7. PubMed PMID: 28150444.
13. Society for Maternal-Fetal Medicine, Simpson LL. Twin-twin transfusion syndrome. Am J Obstet Gynecol. 2013;208(1):3–18. PubMed PMID: 23200164.
14. Mascio DD, Khalil A, D'Amico A, Buca D, Panici PB, Flacco ME, et al. Outcome of twin-twin transfusion syndrome according to the Quintero stage of the disease: a systematic review and meta-analysis. Ultrasound Obstet Gynecol. 2020;56(6):811–20. PubMed PMID: 32330342.
15. D'Antonio F, Benlioglu C, Sileo FG, Thilaganathan B, Papageorghiou A, Bhide A, et al. Perinatal outcomes of twin pregnancies affected by early twin-twin transfusion syndrome: a systematic review and meta-analysis. Acta Obstet Gynecol Scand. 2020;99(9):1121–34. PubMed PMID: 32162305.
16. Gratacos E, Lewi L, Munoz B, Acosta-Rojas R, Hernandez-Andrade E, Martinez JM, et al. A classification system for selective intrauterine growth restriction in monochorionic pregnancies according to umbilical artery Doppler flow in the smaller twin. Ultrasound Obstet Gynecol. 2007;30(1):28–34. PubMed PMID: 17542039.
17. Sananes N, Veujoz M, Severac F, Barthoulot M, Meyer N, Weingertner AS, et al. Evaluation of the utility of in utero treatment of twin anemia-polycythemia sequence. Fetal Diagn Ther. 2015;38(3):170–8. PubMed PMID: 25790745.
18. Goldenberg RL, Iams JD, Miodovnik M, Van Dorsten JP, Thurnau G, Bottoms S, et al. The preterm prediction study: risk factors in twin gestations. National institute of child health and human development maternal-fetal medicine units network. Am J Obstet Gynecol. 1996;175(4 Pt 1):1047–53. PubMed PMID: 8885774.
19. Facco FL, Nash K, Grobman WA. Are women who have had a preterm singleton delivery at increased risk of preterm birth in a subsequent twin pregnancy? Am J Perinatol. 2008;25(10):657–9. PubMed PMID: 18841535.
20. Tarter JG, Khoury A, Barton JR, Jacques DL, Sibai BM. Demographic and obstetric factors influencing pregnancy outcome in twin gestations. Am J Obstet Gynecol. 2002;186(5):910–2. PubMed PMID: 12015510.
21. Fox NS, Stern E, Gupta S, Saltzman DH, Klauser CK, Rebarber A. Preterm birth or small for gestational age in a singleton pregnancy and risk of recurrence in a subsequent twin pregnancy. Obstet Gynecol. 2015;125(4):870–5. PubMed PMID: 25751219.
22. Schaaf JM, Hof MH, Mol BW, Abu-Hanna A, Ravelli AC. Recurrence risk of preterm birth in subsequent twin pregnancy after preterm singleton delivery. BJOG. 2012;119(13):1624–9. PubMed PMID: 23078576.
23. Buekens P, Alexander S, Boutsen M, Blondel B, Kaminski M, Reid M. Randomised controlled trial of routine cervical examinations in pregnancy. European Community Collaborative Study Group on Prenatal Screening. Lancet. 1994;344(8926):841–4. PubMed PMID: 7916399.
24. Bivins HA Jr, Newman RB, Ellings JM, Hulsey TC, Keenan A. Risks of antepartum cervical examination in multifetal gestations. Am J Obstet Gynecol. 1993;169(1):22–5. PubMed PMID: 8333461.
25. Colton T, Kayne HL, Zhang Y, Heeren T. A meta-analysis of home uterine activity monitoring. Am J Obstet Gynecol. 1995;173(5):1499–505. PubMed PMID: 7503191.
26. Beckmann CA, Beckmann CR, Stanziano GJ, Bergauer NK, Martin CB. Accuracy of maternal perception of preterm uterine activity. Am J Obstet Gynecol. 1996;174(2):672–5. PubMed PMID: 8623805.
27. Knuppel RA, Lake MF, Watson DL, Welch RA, Hill WC, Fleming AD, et al. Preventing preterm birth in twin gestation: home uterine activity monitoring and perinatal nursing support. Obstet

Gynecol. 1990;76(1 Suppl):24S–7S. PubMed PMID: 2359575.
28. Newman RB, Iams JD, Das A, Goldenberg RL, Meis P, Moawad A, et al. A prospective masked observational study of uterine contraction frequency in twins. Am J Obstet Gynecol. 2006;195(6):1564–70. PubMed PMID: 16769014.
29. Lim AC, Hegeman MA, Huis In TVMA, Opmeer BC, Bruinse HW, Mol BW. Cervical length measurement for the prediction of preterm birth in multiple pregnancies: a systematic review and bivariate meta-analysis. Ultrasound Obstet Gynecol. 2011;38(1):10–7. PubMed PMID: 21465606.
30. Kindinger LM, Poon LC, Cacciatore S, MacIntyre DA, Fox NS, Schuit E, et al. The effect of gestational age and cervical length measurements in the prediction of spontaneous preterm birth in twin pregnancies: an individual patient level meta-analysis. BJOG. 2016;123(6):877–84. PubMed PMID: 26333191.
31. Berghella V, Roman A, Daskalakis C, Ness A, Baxter JK. Gestational age at cervical length measurement and incidence of preterm birth. Obstet Gynecol. 2007;110(2 Pt 1):311–7. PubMed PMID: 17666605.
32. Boelig RC, Dugoff L, Roman A, Berghella V, Ludmir J. Predicting asymptomatic cervical dilation in pregnant patients with short mid-trimester cervical length: a secondary analysis of a randomized controlled trial. Acta Obstet Gynecol Scand. 2019;98(6):761–8. PubMed PMID: 30681719. Pubmed Central PMCID: 6520180.
33. Melamed N, Pittini A, Hiersch L, Yogev Y, Korzeniewski SS, Romero R, et al. Serial cervical length determination in twin pregnancies reveals 4 distinct patterns with prognostic significance for preterm birth. Am J Obstet Gynecol. 2016;215(4):476, e1–e11. PubMed PMID: 27207277. Pubmed Central PMCID: 5045791.
34. Souka AP, Heath V, Flint S, Sevastopoulou I, Nicolaides KH. Cervical length at 23 weeks in twins in predicting spontaneous preterm delivery. Obstet Gynecol. 1999;94(3):450–4. PubMed PMID: 10472876.
35. American College of Obstetricians and Gynecologists; Society for Maternal-Fetal Medicine. ACOG Practice Bulletin No. 144: multifetal gestations: twin, triplet, and higher-order multifetal pregnancies. Obstet Gynecol. 2014;123(5):1118–32. PubMed PMID: 24785876.
36. Wennerholm UB, Holm B, Mattsby-Baltzer I, Nielsen T, Platz-Christensen J, Sundell G, et al. Fetal fibronectin, endotoxin, bacterial vaginosis and cervical length as predictors of preterm birth and neonatal morbidity in twin pregnancies. Br J Obstet Gynaecol. 1997;104(12):1398–404. PubMed PMID: 9422019.
37. Tolino A, Ronsini S, Zullo F, Pellicano M, Regine V, Nappi C. Fetal fibronectin as a screening test for premature delivery in multiple pregnancies. Int J Gynaecol Obstet. 1996;52(1):3–7. PubMed PMID: 8620985.
38. Oliveira T, de Souza E, Mariani-Neto C, Camano L. Fetal fibronectin as a predictor of preterm delivery in twin gestations. Int J Gynaecol Obstet. 1998;62(2):135–9. PubMed PMID: 9749884.
39. Conde-Agudelo A, Romero R. Cervicovaginal fetal fibronectin for the prediction of spontaneous preterm birth in multiple pregnancies: a systematic review and meta-analysis. J Matern Fetal Neonatal Med. 2010;23(12):1365–76. PubMed PMID: 21067303. Pubmed Central PMCID: 3418880.
40. Fox NS, Saltzman DH, Klauser CK, Peress D, Gutierrez CV, Rebarber A. Prediction of spontaneous preterm birth in asymptomatic twin pregnancies with the use of combined fetal fibronectin and cervical length. Am J Obstet Gynecol. 2009;201(3):313, e1–5. PubMed PMID: 19733285.
41. Vaisbuch E, Romero R, Erez O, Kusanovic JP, Mazaki-Tovi S, Gotsch F, et al. Clinical significance of early (<20 weeks) vs. late (20–24 weeks) detection of sonographic short cervix in asymptomatic women in the mid-trimester. Ultrasound Obstet Gynecol. 2010;36(4):471–81. PubMed PMID: 20503224. Pubmed Central PMCID: 2937193.
42. Boyer A, Cameron L, Munoz-Maldonado Y, Bronsteen R, Comstock CH, Lee W, et al. Clinical significance of amniotic fluid sludge in twin pregnancies with a short cervical length. Am J Obstet Gynecol. 2014;211(5):506, e1–9. PubMed PMID: 24881831.
43. Spiegelman J, Booker W, Gupta S, Lam-Rochlin J, Rebarber A, Saltzman DH, et al. The independent association of a short cervix, positive fetal fibronectin, amniotic fluid sludge, and cervical funneling with spontaneous preterm birth in twin pregnancies. Am J Perinatol. 2016;33(12):1159–64. PubMed PMID: 27434692.
44. Ayodele A, Fox NS, Gupta S, Spiegelman J, Saltzman DH, Booker W, et al. The association between fetal fibronectin, cervical length, and amniotic fluid sludge with histological indicators of placental inflammation in twin gestations. Am J Perinatol. 2018;35(3):242–6. PubMed PMID: 28910845.
45. Ruiz RJ, Fullerton J, Brown CE. The utility of fFN for the prediction of preterm birth in twin gestations. J Obstet Gynecol Neonatal Nurs. 2004;33(4):446–54. PubMed PMID: 15346670.
46. Heaman M, Gupton A. Perceptions of bed rest by women with high-risk pregnancies: a comparison between home and hospital. Birth. 1998;25(4):252–8. PubMed PMID: 9892894.
47. Crowther CA, Han S. Hospitalisation and bed rest for multiple pregnancy. Cochrane Database Syst Rev. 2010;7(7):CD000110. PubMed PMID: 20614420. Pubmed Central PMCID: 7051031.
48. Rydhstrom H. Twin pregnancy and the effects of prophylactic leave of absence on pregnancy duration and birth weight. Acta Obstet Gynecol Scand. 1988;67(1):81–4. PubMed PMID: 3176917.
49. Papiernik E, Richard A, Tafforeau J, Keith L. Social groups and prevention of preterm births

in a population of twin mothers. J Perinat Med. 1996;24(6):669–76. PubMed PMID: 9120751.
50. Yamasmit W, Chaithongwongwatthana S, Tolosa JE, Limpongsanurak S, Pereira L, Lumbiganon P. Prophylactic oral betamimetics for reducing preterm birth in women with a twin pregnancy. Cochrane Database Syst Rev. 2015;8(12):CD004733. PubMed PMID: 26645888.
51. Dodd JM, Grivell RM, CM OB, Dowswell T, Deussen AR. Prenatal administration of progestogens for preventing spontaneous preterm birth in women with a multiple pregnancy. Cochrane Database Syst Rev. 2017;10:CD012024. PubMed PMID: 29086920. Pubmed Central PMCID: 6485912.
52. Rouse DJ, Caritis SN, Peaceman AM, Sciscione A, Thom EA, Spong CY, et al. A trial of 17 alpha-hydroxyprogesterone caproate to prevent prematurity in twins. N Engl J Med. 2007;357(5):454–61. PubMed PMID: 17671253. Epub 2007/08/03. eng.
53. Combs CA, Garite T, Maurel K, Das A, Porto M. 17-hydroxyprogesterone caproate for twin pregnancy: a double-blind, randomized clinical trial. Am J Obstet Gynecol. 2011;204(3):221, e1-8. PubMed PMID: 21376161. Epub 2011/03/08. eng.
54. Senat MV, Porcher R, Winer N, Vayssiere C, Deruelle P, Capelle M, et al. Prevention of preterm delivery by 17 alpha-hydroxyprogesterone caproate in asymptomatic twin pregnancies with a short cervix: a randomized controlled trial. Am J Obstet Gynecol. 2013;208(3):194, e1-8. PubMed PMID: 23433324.
55. Hartikainen-Sorri AL, Kauppila A, Tuimala R. Inefficacy of 17 alpha-hydroxyprogesterone caproate in the prevention of prematurity in twin pregnancy. Obstet Gynecol. 1980;56(6):692–5. PubMed PMID: 7443111.
56. Awwad J, Usta IM, Ghazeeri G, Yacoub N, Succar J, Hayek S, et al. A randomised controlled double-blind clinical trial of 17-hydroxyprogesterone caproate for the prevention of preterm birth in twin gestation (PROGESTWIN): evidence for reduced neonatal morbidity. BJOG. 2015;122(1):71–9. PubMed PMID: 25163819.
57. Durnwald CP, Momirova V, Rouse DJ, Caritis SN, Peaceman AM, Sciscione A, et al. Second trimester cervical length and risk of preterm birth in women with twin gestations treated with 17-alpha hydroxyprogesterone caproate. J Matern Fetal Neonatal Med. 2010;23(12):1360–4. PubMed PMID: 20441408. Pubmed Central PMCID: 2999406. Epub 2010/05/06. eng.
58. Lim AC, Schuit E, Bloemenkamp K, Bernardus RE, Duvekot JJ, Erwich JJ, et al. 17alpha-hydroxyprogesterone caproate for the prevention of adverse neonatal outcome in multiple pregnancies: a randomized controlled trial. Obstet Gynecol. 2011;118(3):513–20. PubMed PMID: 21860279. Epub 2011/08/24. eng.
59. Lim AC, Schuit E, Papatsonis D, van Eyck J, Porath MM, van Oirschot CM, et al. Effect of 17-alpha hydroxyprogesterone caproate on cervical length in twin pregnancies. Ultrasound Obstet Gynecol. 2012;40(4):426–30. PubMed PMID: 23008102. Epub 2012/09/26. eng.
60. Schuit E, Stock S, Rode L, Rouse D, Lim A, Norman J, et al. Effectiveness of progestogens to improve perinatal outcome in twin pregnancies: an individual participant data meta-analysis. BJOG. 2014;122(1):27–37. PubMed PMID: 25145491.
61. Ward A, Greenberg V, Valcarcel B, Boelig RC, Al-Kouatly HB, Berghella V. Intramuscular progesterone in women with twins and prior singleton spontaneous preterm birth. Am J Obstet Gynecol MFM. 2020;2(3):100124. https://doi.org/10.1016/j.ajogmf.2020.100124. Epub 2020 Apr 28. PMID: 33345870
62. Aboulghar MM, Aboulghar MA, Amin YM, Al-Inany HG, Mansour RT, Serour GI. The use of vaginal natural progesterone for prevention of preterm birth in IVF/ICSI pregnancies. Reprod Biomed Online. 2012;25(2):133–8. PubMed PMID: 22695310.
63. Serra V, Perales A, Meseguer J, Parrilla JJ, Lara C, Bellver J, et al. Increased doses of vaginal progesterone for the prevention of preterm birth in twin pregnancies: a randomised controlled double-blind multicentre trial. BJOG. 2013;120(1):50–7. PubMed PMID: 22882759.
64. Rode L, Klein K, Nicolaides KH, Krampl-Bettelheim E, Tabor A. Prevention of preterm delivery in twin gestations (PREDICT): a multicenter, randomized, placebo-controlled trial on the effect of vaginal micronized progesterone. Ultrasound Obstet Gynecol. 2011;38(3):272–80. PubMed PMID: 21739497. Epub 2011/07/09. eng.
65. Cetingoz E, Cam C, Sakalli M, Karateke A, Celik C, Sancak A. Progesterone effects on preterm birth in high-risk pregnancies: a randomized placebo-controlled trial. Arch Gynecol Obstet. 2011;283(3):423–9. PubMed PMID: 20091317.
66. Brizot ML, Hernandez W, Liao AW, Bittar RE, Francisco RPV, Krebs VLJ, et al. Vaginal progesterone for the prevention of preterm birth in twin gestations: a randomized placebo-controlled double-blind study. Am J Obstet Gynecol. 2015;213(1):82, e1-e9. PubMed PMID: 25731690.
67. El-refaie W, Abdelhafez MS, Badawy A. Vaginal progesterone for prevention of preterm labor in asymptomatic twin pregnancies with sonographic short cervix: a randomized clinical trial of efficacy and safety. Arch Gynecol Obstet. 2016;293(1):61–7. PubMed PMID: 26044148.
68. Norman JE, Marlow N, Messow CM, Shennan A, Bennett PR, Thornton S, et al. Vaginal progesterone prophylaxis for preterm birth (the OPPTIMUM study): a multicentre, randomised, double-blind trial. Lancet. 2016;387(10033):2106–16. PubMed PMID: 26921136.
69. Wood S, Ross S, Tang S, Miller L, Sauve R, Brant R. Vaginal progesterone to prevent preterm birth in multiple pregnancy: a randomized controlled trial. J Perinat Med. 2012;40(6):593–9. PubMed PMID: 23093256. Epub 2012/10/25. Eng.

70. Rehal A, Benko Z, De Paco MC, Syngelaki A, Janga D, Cicero S, et al. Early vaginal progesterone versus placebo in twin pregnancies for the prevention of spontaneous preterm birth: a randomized, double-blind trial. Am J Obstet Gynecol. 2020;224(1):86. PubMed PMID: 32598909.
71. Fonseca EB, Celik E, Parra M, Singh M, Nicolaides KH. Progesterone and the risk of preterm birth among women with a short cervix. N Engl J Med. 2007;357(5):462–9. PubMed PMID: 17671254. Epub 2007/08/03. eng.
72. Romero R, Conde-Agudelo A, El-Refaie W, Rode L, Brizot ML, Cetingoz E, et al. Vaginal progesterone decreases preterm birth and neonatal morbidity and mortality in women with a twin gestation and a short cervix: an updated meta-analysis of individual patient data. Ultrasound Obstet Gynecol. 2017;49(3):303–14. PubMed PMID: 28067007.
73. Liem S, Schuit E, Hegeman M, Bais J, de Boer K, Bloemenkamp K, et al. Cervical pessaries for prevention of preterm birth in women with a multiple pregnancy (ProTWIN): a multicentre, open-label randomised controlled trial. Lancet. 2013;382(9901):1341–9. PubMed PMID: 23924878.
74. Nicolaides KH, Syngelaki A, Poon LC, de Paco MC, Plasencia W, Molina FS, et al. Cervical pessary placement for prevention of preterm birth in unselected twin pregnancies: a randomized controlled trial. Am J Obstet Gynecol. 2016;214(1):3, e1–9. PubMed PMID: 26321037.
75. Goya M, de la Calle M, Pratcorona L, Merced C, Rodo C, Munoz B, et al. Cervical pessary to prevent preterm birth in women with twin gestation and sonographic short cervix: a multicenter randomized controlled trial (PECEP-Twins). Am J Obstet Gynecol. 2016;214(2):145–52. PubMed PMID: 26627728.
76. Berghella V, Dugoff L, Ludmir J. Prevention of preterm birth with pessary in twins (PoPPT): a randomized controlled trial. Ultrasound Obstet Gynecol. 2017;49(5):567–72. PubMed PMID: 28170117.
77. Dor J, Shalev J, Mashiach S, Blankstein J, Serr DM. Elective cervical suture of twin pregnancies diagnosed ultrasonically in the first trimester following induced ovulation. Gynecol Obstet Invest. 1982;13(1):55–60. PubMed PMID: 7056503.
78. Final report of the Medical Research Council/Royal College of Obstetricians and Gynaecologists multicentre randomised trial of cervical cerclage. MRC/RCOG working party on cervical cerclage. Br J Obstet Gynaecol. 1993;100(6):516–23. PubMed PMID: 8334085.
79. Roman AS, Saltzman DH, Fox N, Klauser CK, Istwan N, Rhea D, et al. Prophylactic cerclage in the management of twin pregnancies. Am J Perinatol. 2013;30(9):751–4. PubMed PMID: 23303484.
80. Rottenstreich A, Levin G, Kleinstern G, Zigron R, Rottenstreich M, Elchalal U, et al. History-indicated cervical cerclage in management of twin pregnancy. Ultrasound Obstet Gynecol. 2019;54(4):517–23. PubMed PMID: 30549119.
81. Althuisius SM, Dekker GA, Hummel P, Bekedam DJ, van Geijn HP. Final results of the Cervical Incompetence Prevention Randomized Cerclage Trial (CIPRACT): therapeutic cerclage with bed rest versus bed rest alone. Am J Obstet Gynecol. 2001;185(5):1106–12. PubMed PMID: 11717642.
82. Rust OA, Atlas RO, Reed J, van Gaalen J, Balducci J. Revisiting the short cervix detected by transvaginal ultrasound in the second trimester: why cerclage therapy may not help. Am J Obstet Gynecol. 2001;185(5):1098–105. PubMed PMID: 11717641.
83. Berghella V, Odibo AO, Tolosa JE. Cerclage for prevention of preterm birth in women with a short cervix found on transvaginal ultrasound examination: a randomized trial. Am J Obstet Gynecol. 2004;191(4):1311–7. PubMed PMID: 15507959.
84. Berghella V, Odibo AO, To MS, Rust OA, Althuisius SM. Cerclage for short cervix on ultrasonography: meta-analysis of trials using individual patient-level data. Obstet Gynecol. 2005;106(1):181–9. PubMed PMID: 15994635.
85. Rafael TJ, Berghella V, Alfirevic Z. Cervical stitch (cerclage) for preventing preterm birth in multiple pregnancy. Cochrane Database Syst Rev. 2014;9:CD009166. PubMed PMID: 25208049.
86. Saccone G, Rust O, Althuisius S, Roman A, Berghella V. Cerclage for short cervix in twin pregnancies: systematic review and meta-analysis of randomized trials using individual patient-level data. Acta Obstet Gynecol Scand. 2015;94(4):352–8. PubMed PMID: 25644964.
87. Roman AS, Rebarber A, Pereira L, Sfakianaki AK, Mulholland J, Berghella V. The efficacy of sonographically indicated cerclage in multiple gestations. J Ultrasound Med. 2005;24(6):763–8; quiz 70-1. PubMed PMID: 15914680.
88. Roman A, Rochelson B, Fox NS, Hoffman M, Berghella V, Patel V, et al. Efficacy of ultrasound-indicated cerclage in twin pregnancies. Am J Obstet Gynecol. 2015;212(6):788, e1–6. PubMed PMID: 25637840.
89. Houlihan C, Poon LC, Ciarlo M, Kim E, Guzman ER, Nicolaides KH. Cervical cerclage for preterm birth prevention in twin gestation with short cervix: a retrospective cohort study. Ultrasound Obstet Gynecol. 2016;48(6):752–6. PubMed PMID: 26990136.
90. Adams TM, Rafael TJ, Kunzier NB, Mishra S, Calixte R, Vintzileos AM. Does cervical cerclage decrease preterm birth in twin pregnancies with a short cervix? J Matern Fetal Neonatal Med. 2018;31(8):1092–8. PubMed PMID: 28320233.
91. Han MN, O'Donnell BE, Maykin MM, Gonzalez JM, Tabsh K, Gaw SL. The impact of cerclage in twin pregnancies on preterm birth rate

before 32 weeks. J Matern Fetal Neonatal Med. 2019;32(13):2143–51. PubMed PMID: 29363371. Pubmed Central PMCID: 6251764.
92. Li C, Shen J, Hua K. Cercläge for women with twin pregnancies: a systematic review and metaanalysis. Am J Obstet Gynecol. 2019;220(6):543–57, e1. PubMed PMID: 30527942.
93. Roman A, Rochelson B, Martinelli P, Saccone G, Harris K, Zork N, et al. Cerclage in twin pregnancy with dilated cervix between 16 to 24 weeks of gestation: retrospective cohort study. Am J Obstet Gynecol. 2016;215(1):98, e1–e11. PubMed PMID: 26827881.
94. Abbasi N, Barrett J, Melamed N. Outcomes following rescue cerclage in twin pregnancies(). J Matern Fetal Neonatal Med. 2018;31(16):2195–201. PubMed PMID: 28597706.
95. Roman A, Zork N, Haeri S, Schoen CN, Saccone G, Colihan S, Zelig C, Gimovsky AC, Seligman NS, Zullo F, Berghella V. Physical examination-indicated cerclage in twin pregnancy: a randomized controlled trial. Am J Obstet Gynecol. 2020;223(6):902.e1-902.e11. https://doi.org/10.1016/j.ajog.2020.06.047. Epub 2020 Jun 25. PMID: 32592693

Key Reading

Berghella V, Baxter JK, Hendrix NW. Cervical assessment by ultrasound for preventing preterm delivery. Cochrane Database Syst Rev. 2013;1:CD007235. PubMed PMID: 23440813.

Berghella V, Ludmir J, Simonazzi G, Owen J. Transvaginal cervical cerclage: evidence for perioperative management strategies. Am J Obstet Gynecol. 2013;209(3):181–92. PubMed PMID: 23416155.

Blencowe H, Cousens S, Oestergaard MZ, Chou D, Moller AB, Narwal R, et al. National, regional, and worldwide estimates of preterm birth rates in the year 2010 with time trends since 1990 for selected countries: a systematic analysis and implications. Lancet. 2012;379(9832):2162–72. PubMed PMID: 22682464.

Breathnach FM, McAuliffe FM, Geary M, Daly S, Higgins JR, Dornan J, et al. Optimum timing for planned delivery of uncomplicated monochorionic and dichorionic twin pregnancies. Obstet Gynecol. 2012;119(1):50–9. PubMed PMID: 22183211.

Dodd JM, Grivell RM, CM OB, Dowswell T, Deussen AR. Prenatal administration of progestogens for preventing spontaneous preterm birth in women with a multiple pregnancy. Cochrane Database Syst Rev. 2017;10:CD012024. PubMed PMID: 29086920. Pubmed Central PMCID: 6485912.

Frey HA, Klebanoff MA. The epidemiology, etiology, and costs of preterm birth. Semin Fetal Neonatal Med. 2016;21(2):68–73. PubMed PMID: 26794420.

Fuchs F, Senat MV. Multiple gestations and preterm birth. Semin Fetal Neonatal Med. 2016;21(2):113–20. PubMed PMID: 26795885.

Glover AV, Manuck TA. Screening for spontaneous preterm birth and resultant therapies to reduce neonatal morbidity and mortality: a review. Semin Fetal Neonatal Med. 2018;23(2):126–32. PubMed PMID: 29229486. Pubmed Central PMCID: 6381594.

Harrison MS, Goldenberg RL. Global burden of prematurity. Semin Fetal Neonatal Med. 2016;21(2):74–9. PubMed PMID: 26740166.

Koullali B, Oudijk MA, Nijman TA, Mol BW, Pajkrt E. Risk assessment and management to prevent preterm birth. Semin Fetal Neonatal Med. 2016;21(2):80–8. PubMed PMID: 26906339.

Liu L, Oza S, Hogan D, Chu Y, Perin J, Zhu J, et al. Global, regional, and national causes of under-5 mortality in 2000–15: an updated systematic analysis with implications for the Sustainable Development Goals. Lancet. 2016;388(10063):3027–35. PubMed PMID: 27839855. Pubmed Central PMCID: 5161777.

Markham KB, Iams JD. Measuring the cervical length. Clin Obstet Gynecol. 2016;59(2):252–63. PubMed PMID: 27042799.

Martin JA, Hamilton BE, Osterman MJK, Driscoll AK, Drake P. Births: final data for 2017. Natl Vital Stat Rep. 2018;67(8):1–50. PubMed PMID: 30707672.

Martin JA, Hamilton BE, Osterman MJK. Births in the United States, 2018. NCHS Data Brief. 2019;346:1–8. PubMed PMID: 31442195.

Maruotti GM, Saccone G, Morlando M, Martinelli P. First-trimester ultrasound determination of chorionicity in twin gestations using the lambda sign: a systematic review and meta-analysis. Eur J Obstet Gynecol Reprod Biol. 2016;202:66–70. PubMed PMID: 27180271.

Matthews TJ, MacDorman MF, Thoma ME. Infant mortality statistics from the 2013 period linked birth/infant death data set. Natl Vital Stat Rep. 2015;64(9):1–30. PubMed PMID: 26270610.

Nour NM. Premature delivery and the millennium development goal. Rev Obstet Gynecol. 2012;5(2):100–5. PubMed PMID: 22866189. Pubmed Central PMCID: 3410509.

Roman A, Suhag A, Berghella V. Cerclage: indications and patient counseling. Clin Obstet Gynecol. 2016;59(2):264–9. PubMed PMID: 27015230.

Society for Maternal-Fetal Medicine, McIntosh J, Feltovich H, Berghella V, Manuck T. The role of routine cervical length screening in selected high- and low-risk women for preterm birth prevention. Am J Obstet Gynecol. 2016;215(3):B2–7. PubMed PMID: 27133011.

Stock S, Norman J. Preterm and term labour in multiple pregnancies. Semin Fetal Neonatal Med. 2010;15(6):336–41. PubMed PMID: 20643592.

Sykes L, Bennett PR. Efficacy of progesterone for prevention of preterm birth. Best Pract Res Clin Obstet Gynaecol. 2018;52:126–36. PubMed PMID: 30266582.

Wood SL, Owen J. Vaginal cerclage: preoperative, intraoperative, and postoperative management. Clin Obstet Gynecol. 2016;59(2):270–85. PubMed PMID: 26974217.

Fetal Growth Restriction

Becky Liu and Asma Khalil

Contents

Electronic Supplementary Material The online version of this chapter (https://doi.org/10.1007/978-3-030-47652-6_13) contains supplementary material, which is available to authorized users. The videos can be accessed by scanning the related images with the SN More Media App.

A. Khalil et al. (eds.), *Twin and Higher-order Pregnancies*,
https://doi.org/10.1007/978-3-030-47652-6_13

Trailer

Fetal growth restriction (FGR) complicates 19.7% of monochorionic twins and 10.5% of dichorionic twins. It is associated with perinatal mortality, premature delivery, and neurological sequelae and death in the surviving co-twin. Twins show a different pattern of growth to singleton pregnancies; therefore, care should be taken to use twin-specific growth charts to avoid over-diagnosis and unnecessary intervention. To date, its diagnosis has shown inconsistencies amongst clinicians and researchers, but a recent consensus using the Delphi procedure has achieved uniform diagnostic criteria. Close surveillance should be undertaken using ultrasound, and referral to a tertiary unit with relevant expertise should be taken if required. Management of this condition can be difficult, as considerations must be made for the normally grown co-twin; therefore, decisions for delivery must not be made with haste. Risks and benefits of conservative management, prenatal intervention, and early delivery must be carefully assessed, and the parents sensitively counselled, in order to plan the course of action.

Definitions

Fetal growth restriction (FGR): a pathological restriction of the fetus in reaching its full genetic growth potential.

Selective fetal growth restriction (sFGR): in twin pregnancies, when FGR affects at least one twin.

Appropriate for gestational age (AGA): the fetus reaching its full genetic growth potential according to its gestational age.

Fetoscopic surgery: the insertion of a fetoscope into the amniotic sac in order to perform a prenatal intervention.

Selective reduction: the termination of one (or more) fetus(es) in a multiple pregnancy whilst continuing the pregnancy with a live fetus(es).

Intrauterine death (IUD): the death of a fetus in utero.

Preterm delivery: the delivery of babies prior to 37 weeks gestation

Learning Objectives

- To understand the definition of fetal growth restriction in multiple pregnancies.
- To understand the diagnosis and surveillance of these pregnancies
- To understand the risks and outcomes associated with these pregnancies
- To understand the management techniques and their associated complications

13.1 Introduction

Fetal growth restriction (FGR) is defined as a pathological restriction of the fetus in reaching its full genetic growth potential. Selective fetal growth restriction (sFGR) is when this occurs in one twin, while the other twin is appropriate for gestational age (AGA). It is associated with neurological comorbidities, intrauterine and perinatal death, which can in turn lead to preterm birth, and co-twin demise or neurological sequelae for the AGA twin [1, 2]. A higher rate of perinatal mortality is seen in MC than in DC twins (75:1000 vs. 33:1000, respectively), as well as higher neurological comorbidities [3, 4]. This difference may be due to monochorionic specific complications, such as twin-to-twin transfusion syndrome (TTTS) and the different etiology of sFGR [5–7].

In DC twin pregnancies, the normal growth trajectory is similar to that of singletons up to 30 weeks gestation and shows a relative reduction thereafter. In MC twins, the estimated fetal weight (EFW) centile is generally lower than DC twins and singletons throughout the gestations [8]. A discordance in EFW between the twins is significantly associated with perinatal loss [19]. In this chapter, we aim to identify the definitions and classifications for FGR, their outcomes and complications, their diagnosis, and management options.

13.1.1 Etiology

In DC twins, sFGR is typically caused by placental insufficiency of one of the placentas [4]. Conversely in MC twins, it is usually as a result of unequal distribution of blood flow and placental sharing due to placental anastomoses [6]. Pre-eclampsia is therefore more commonly seen in association with sFGR in DC than MC twin pregnancies [9]. Other causes can include discordant fetal anomalies, and intrauterine infections [10, 11]. So far, a link between pre-existing maternal risk factors and sFGR has not been clearly established, and the available literature presents controversial findings [25–29].

13.1.2 Diagnosis

▪ Diagnostic Criteria

The diagnostic criteria for this condition have been inconsistent amongst clinicians and researchers. The International Society of Ultrasound in Obstetrics and Gynecology have recommended that for DC twins, EFW <10th centile for either twin should be used, and for MC twins, EFW <10th centile and an inter-twin weight discordance of >25% should be used to diagnose sFGR [10].

A recent consensus, using the Delphi procedure, aimed to achieve uniform diagnostic criteria and reporting parameters in sFGR twins. This concluded that an EFW <3rd centile alone for one twin should be used to diagnose sFGR. In DC twins, two of the three parameters – EFW <10th centile, EFW discordance of ≥25%, and umbilical artery pulsatility index (UA PI) >95th centile in the smaller twin can also be used for diagnosis. In MC twins, two of the four parameters – EFW <10th centile, AC <10th centile, EFW discordance of ≥25%, and UA PI >95th centile in the smaller twin – have been agreed for the diagnosis of sFGR [12] (◘ Fig. 13.1).

▪ Screening for sFGR

A discrepancy in crown rump length (CRL) in the first trimester screening has been shown to be associated with sFGR. A CRL discordance of ≥7% in the first trimester has a 92% sensitivity and 76% specificity in detecting sFGR [20]. A discordance at this early stage can be associated with other poor outcomes such as pregnancy loss and preterm delivery [11].

DC twins should have ultrasound assessments 4 weekly from 20 weeks, and MC twins 2 weekly from 16 weeks. Head circumference (HC), abdominal circumference (AC), and femur length (FL), as well as UA PI and mid-

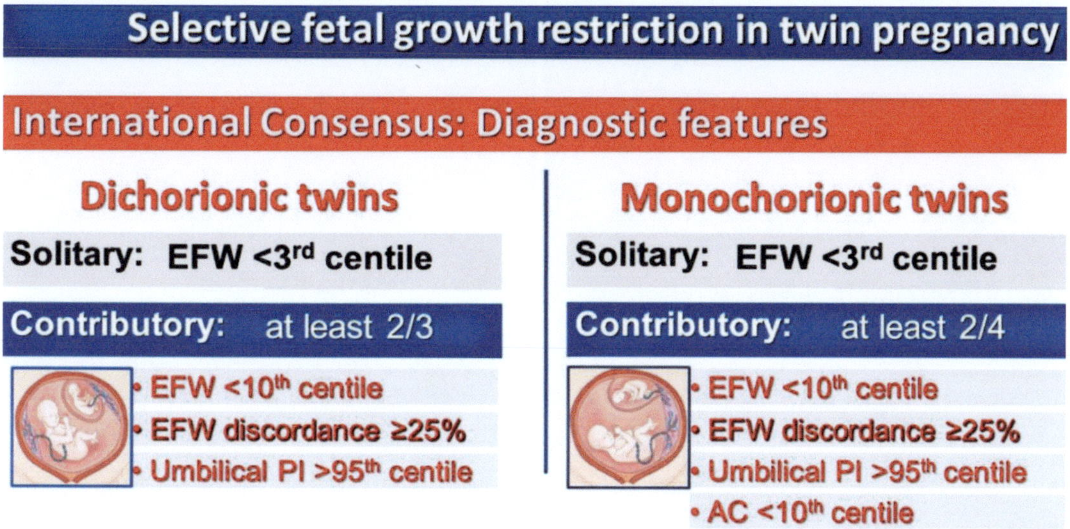

◘ **Fig. 13.1** Diagnostic criteria for sFGR as stratified by the recently published Delphi consensus (Khalil 2019) for both dichorionic and monochorionic twins [12]

dle cerebral artery pulsatility index (MCA PI), and peak systolic velocity (PSV) for MC twins, should be measured at each scan [10]. If the diagnostic criteria above are fulfilled, closer monitoring may be required depending on severity and clinician practice. Detailed ultrasound examinations should also be performed to exclude discordant fetal anomalies, and maternal serum serology taken to check for infection, as well as invasive prenatal testing considered in order to rule out genetic conditions [10]. ◘ Figures 13.2, 13.3, and 13.4 demonstrate ultrasound features of inter-twin size discrepancy in HC and AC measurements.

It is currently common practice to use standardised singleton growth charts to monitor growth in twins. But as the twin growth trajectory is known to be different to that of singletons [8], the usage of singleton growth

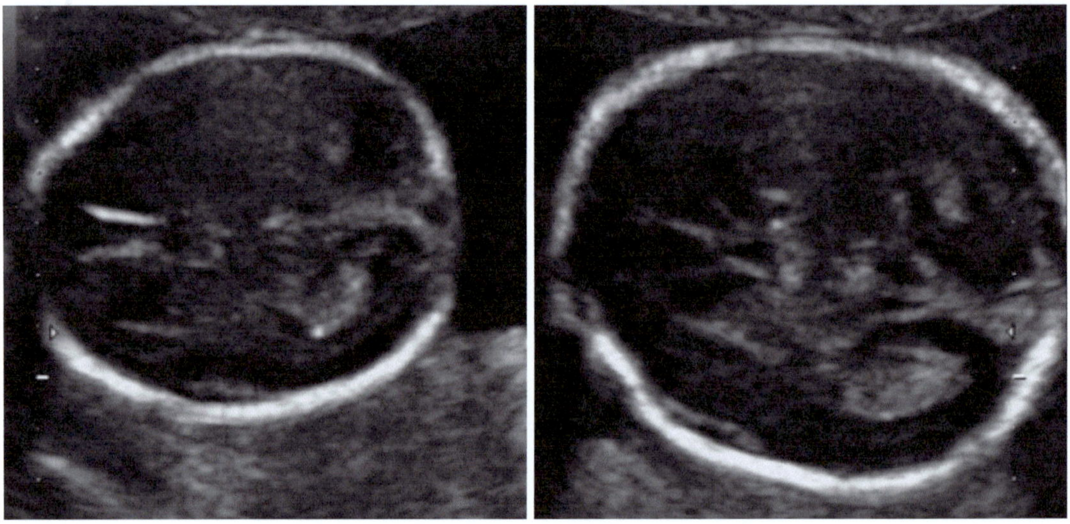

◘ **Fig. 13.2** 2D ultrasound section of the head circumference, displaying a size discordance between twins

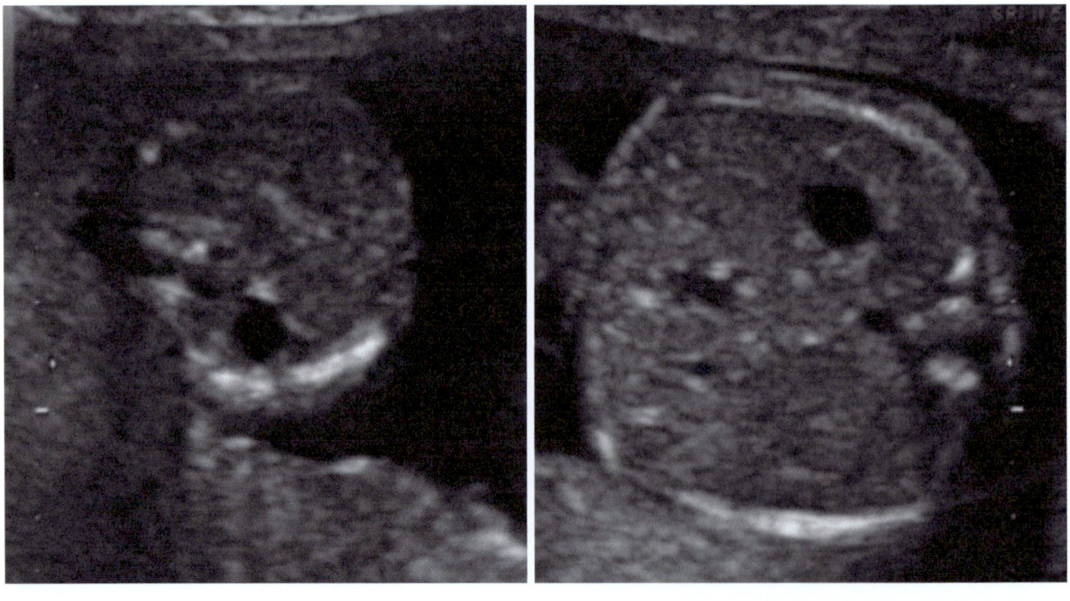

◘ **Fig. 13.3** 2D ultrasound section of the abdominal circumference, displaying a size discordance between twins

charts can lead to over diagnosis of sFGR and unnecessary intervention. Twin-specific growth charts have now been formulated based on twin-specific growth ranges, derived through the analysis of a large cohort of twin pregnancies, which should be used to monitor growth in twin pregnancies [8].

An earlier study showed that in twins where fetuses were classified as FGR according to singleton charts, MC twins were twice as likely to suffer from perinatal death as singletons; however, the outcomes of DC twins were the same as singletons [31]. This may be the reason for the continued use of singleton growth charts in twins, as poor outcomes have been described for small MC twins according to these criteria.

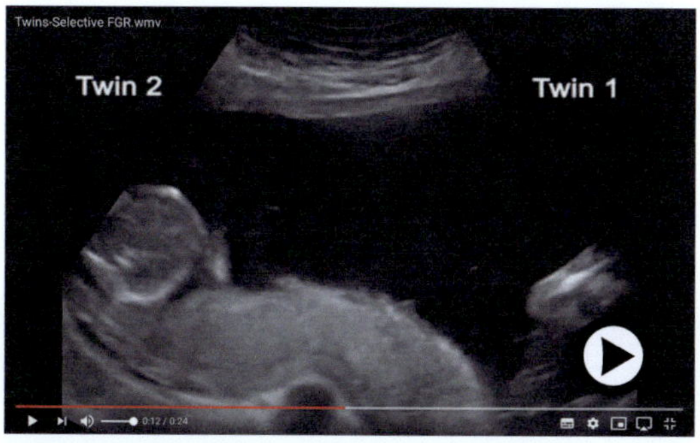

Fig. 13.4 (Twins-Selective FGR): Figure demonstrating the difference in size and amniotic fluid volumes in twins with selective fetal growth restriction (https://doi.org/10.1007/000-2tc)

Classification of sFGR in MC Twins

Gratacós et al. formulated a system to classify sFGR in MC twins. They found that direction and magnitude of blood flow through the different types of placental anastomoses specific to MC twins can give rise to different umbilical artery (UA) Doppler patterns, which in turn, can lead to different clinical evolution and outcomes [4, 13, 14, 18]. These are outlined in Table 13.1. Figure 13.5 displays the different UA Doppler patterns in the different types of sFGR, and Fig. 13.6 demonstrates the bidirectional flow in artery-to-artery anastomosis in type 3 sFGR.

Recent research has looked into the natural history, outcomes according to gestation of onset, and the different diagnostic criteria of sFGR in both MC and DC twins. In MC twins, it was found that early sFGR was slightly more common than late sFGR, with

Table 13.1 Definition, placental anastomoses, perinatal outcomes and overall survival according to Gratacós classification of selective fetal growth restriction (sFGR) in monochorionic (MC) twins [4, 14, 15, 19]

	Type 1	Type 2	Type 3
Definition	Positive UA EDF	Persistent absent or reversed UA EDF	Intermittent absent or reversed UA EDF
Placental anastomoses	Similar to uncomplicated cases	Reduced number large AA anastomoses	Large number of large AA anastomoses (90%), leading to unstable blood sharing and acute TTTS or sudden IUD
Deterioration	Up to 26%	Up to 90%	10.8%
Unexpected IUD	2.6% in small and large twins, 3% double IUD, 2% small twin IUD	0% in small and large twins, 13% double IUD, 10% small twin IUD	15.4% in small twin and 6.2% in large twin, 0% double IUD, and 8% small twin IUD
Overall survival	82–97%	51–58%	77–80%

UA umbilical artery, *EDF* end-diastolic flow, *AA* arterio-arterial, *IUD* intrauterine death, *TTTS* twin-to-twin transfusion syndrome

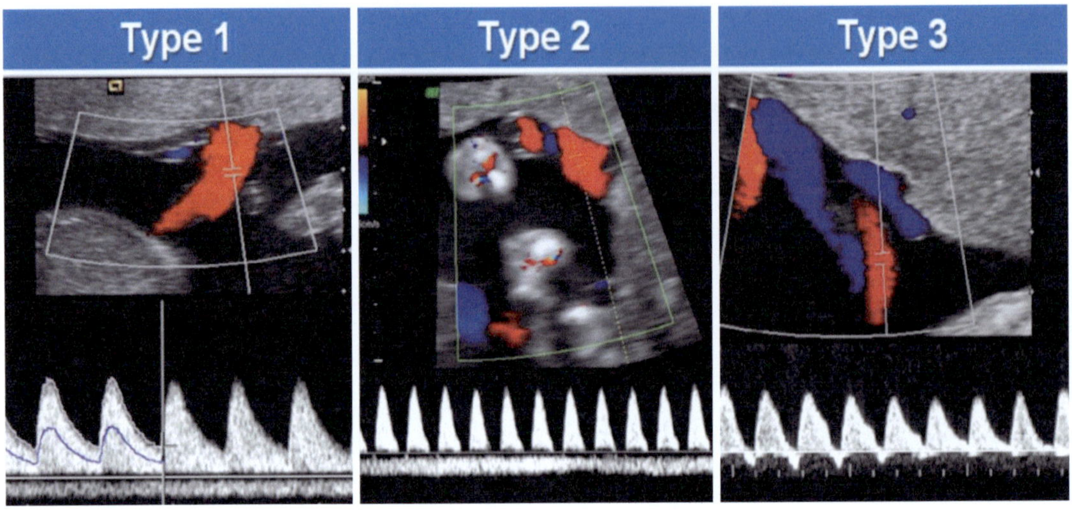

Fig. 13.5 Gratacós classification of selective fetal growth restriction in monochorionic twins. Type 1 displays persistently positive end-diastolic flow in umbilical artery Doppler flow. In type 2, this is persistently absent (or reversed). Type 3 consists of cyclical or intermittently absent or reversed end-diastolic flow

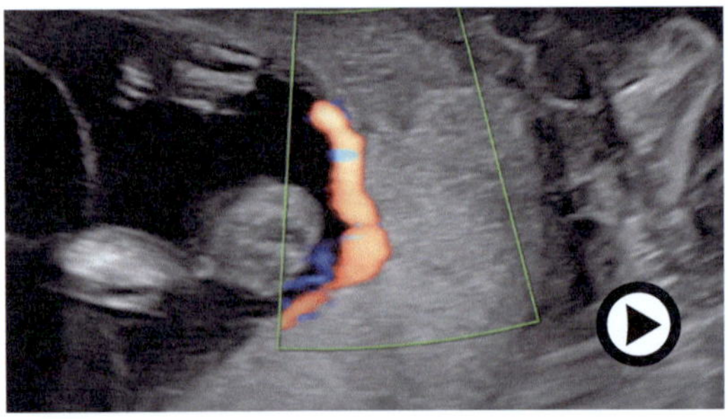

Fig. 13.6 (Clip AA sFGR III): Figure demonstrating the bidirectional flow in artery-to-artery anastomosis in type 2 selective fetal growth restriction (https://doi.org/10.1007/000-2td)

13

worse outcomes [30]. Figure 13.7 demonstrates the incidence of different types of sFGR in early and late sFGR according to Gratacós classification in MC twins. It seems important to mention that large series on unselected monochorionic twin pregnancies are largely missing. The figures in the tables are largely based on retrospective cohort series from tertiary referral centres, so that there may be a selection bias towards more severe cases. In this study, it was found that the different diagnostic criteria gave a varying incidence of sFGR, thereby supporting the use of the standardised international diagnostic criteria.

Superimposed TTTS can be associated with MC twins complicated with sFGR, which may be secondary to the transfusion imbalance that contributed to TTTS. The incidence of this or its correlation with the gestational age at onset of sFGR has previously not been described in the literature. The recent study by Curado et al. found that superimposed TTTS is more prevalent in early sFGR (27%) vs. late sFGR (6%), and that it co-existed in 13% of type I sFGR, 60% of type II sFGR, and none of type III sFGR [30] (as shown in Fig. 13.8).

13.1.3 Management

sFGR in Dichorionic Twins

As the etiology for FGR is the same in DC twins as that of singletons, with separate placentation, the current recommendation is to manage these pregnancies as growth-restricted singletons [10, 11]. Ultrasound to assess growth and Doppler indices should be performed at least twice weekly, or more frequently, depending on the severity [10]. Assessments should be similar to that of singleton pregnancies, where the deterioration of umbilical artery (UA), middle cerebral artery (MCA), and ductus venosus (DV) Dopplers should be monitored carefully. Recent evidence has suggested that the time of deterioration and disease progression in DC twins

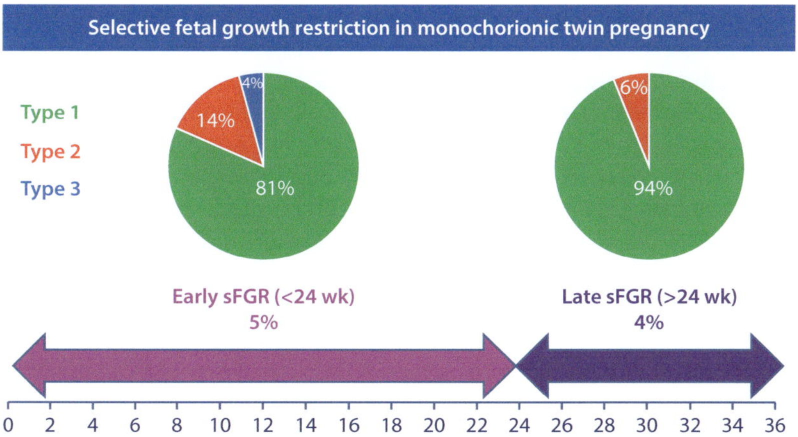

Fig. 13.7 Pie charts demonstrating the incidence of the different types of sFGR according to Gratacós classification in early and late sFGR in monochorionic twins [30]

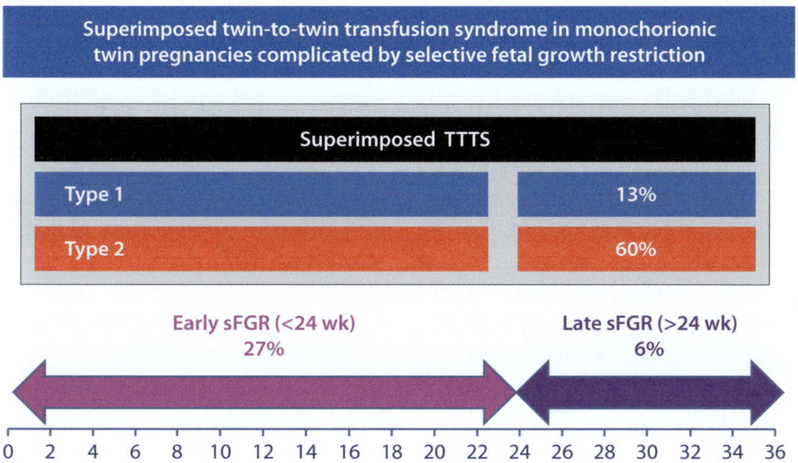

Fig. 13.8 Incidence of superimposed twin-to-transfusion syndrome (TTTS) in different types of sFGR and its prevalence in early and late sFGR in monochorionic twins

may be longer than that of singletons, perhaps due to a delay in delivery to allow more time for growth in the AGA twin [15].

Selective fetocide has a limited role in DC twins, due to the increased risk of preterm labour. A few cases have been reported for its use in severe preterm pre-eclampsia [16]. However, conservative management can lead to intrauterine demise of the sFGR twin, which can in turn lead to preterm delivery in 54%, as well as a 2% risk of neurological damage, and 3% of death in the surviving co-twin [17]. Early delivery may give rise to complications due to prematurity for both the AGA and the FGR twins. Generally, delivery is not recommended prior to 32–34 weeks' gestation. Therefore, these pregnancies require careful monitoring, and the decision for delivery should be made on a risk-benefit assessment for each twin and thorough counselling [10].

sFGR in Monochorionic Twins

Management of MC twin pregnancies can vary according to the Gratacós classification. Ultrasound assessment should be performed to monitor growth two weekly, and to monitor Doppler indices at least weekly [10]. Deterioration of the UA, MCA, and DV Dopplers should be checked to assess disease progression.

Type I sFGR generally has a good prognosis; however, with progression rates reported up to 26% [18], they should continue to receive regular monitoring. Delivery can often take place at 34–36 weeks [4]. Type II sFGR has the worst prognosis, with progression rates up to 90% [13], with an intact survival rate of 33% for both twins [14]. Type III sFGR has a lower rate of progression, but due to the large AA anastomoses, the risk of sudden IUD is higher [13].

In MC twins, single twin demise of the sFGR twin can have drastic consequences for the co-twin, due to the shared placental circulation, it can result in hypoperfusion of the brain and other organs. It has been reported that the surviving co-twin has a 15% risk of IUD, a 26% of neurological morbidity, and a 68% risk of preterm delivery [17]. Therefore, prenatal intervention in the form of fetoscopic surgery are more likely required in sFGR types II and III due to their poor prognosis [4, 11]. According to the International Society of Ultrasound in Obstetrics and Gynecology (ISUOG) guideline, selective fetal reduction might be considered if there is a significant risk of single twin demise before 26 weeks [10]. After 26 weeks, however, the risk of prematurity is lower; therefore, delivery after this gestation can be considered if significant deterioration is evident [4].

13

Recent systematic reviews and meta-analyses of retrospective cohort studies have shown that Type I sFGR have an optimal outcome with conservative management, and that Type II is associated with a higher rate of perinatal morbidity and mortality than Type I, but not significantly different to Type III. Abnormal postnatal brain imaging was more prevalent in Types II and III sFGR, and overall adverse composite outcomes were similar in Types II and III sFGR, and lower in Type I [32]. Selective laser photocoagulation of connecting vessels for Types II and III sFGR revealed a higher mortality, and lower neurological morbidity rate than conservative management. In groups who compared the outcomes of selective reduction with laser treatment, a lower incidence of IUD was found in the larger twin following selective reduction [33]. ◘ Figures 13.9, 13.10, 13.11, 13.12, and 13.13 demonstrate the outcomes following cord occlusion, laser, and expectant managements of MC twins with different types of sFGR. It seems important to mention that the optimal management of sFGR type II-III remains largely uncertain as no randomised control trials exist and retrospective cohort studies are prone to several forms of bias.

▪ Fetoscopic Surgery for sFGR in Monochorionic Twins

Selective laser photocoagulation of connecting vessels (SLPCV) is a procedure commonly used for TTTS. Even though these connecting vessels are not the cause for sFGR, coagula-

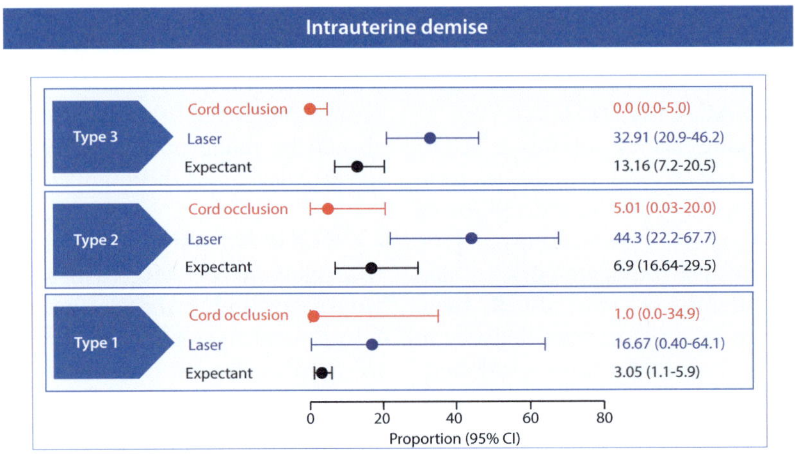

◘ **Fig. 13.9** Demonstration of the proportion of intrauterine demise following cord occlusion (in non-reduced larger twin), laser, and expectant management of MC twins with types 1, 2, and 3 sFGR [33]

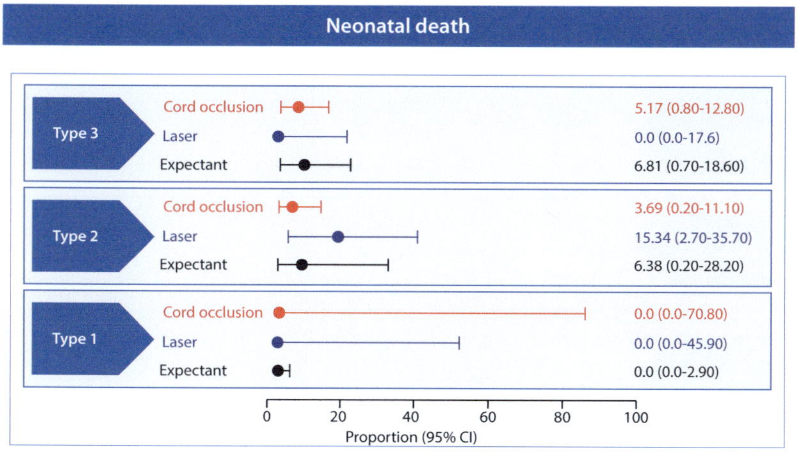

Fig. 13.10 Demonstration of the proportion of neonatal death following cord occlusion (in non-reduced larger twin), laser, and expectant management of MC twins with types 1, 2, and 3 sFGR [33]

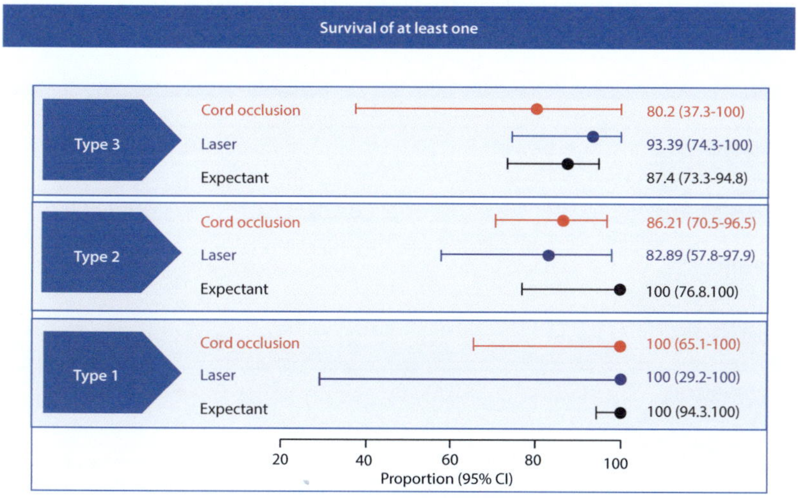

Fig. 13.11 Demonstration of the proportion of survival of at least one twin following cord occlusion (in non-reduced larger twin), laser, and expectant management of MC twins with types 1, 2, and 3 sFGR [33]

tion of these vessels allows separation of the circulations (dichorionisation), allowing protection of the AGA twin in case of co-twin IUD, and may hasten the IUD of the FGR twin, as the protective blood flow from the AGA twin is separated. This technique has an overall survival rate of 53%, and a 72% survival rate of at least one twin. The survival rate of the AGA twin is 68–74% following SLPCV, and the smaller twin 30–39% [21]. This technique is more challenging to perform than for TTTS, due to the normal amniotic fluid volume in the AGA twin (absence of polyhydramnios) [4, 11].

Selective reduction is performed when there is a high risk of single twin demise in the FGR twin prior to 26 weeks. By stopping the blood flow into the FGR twin, it prevents consequences of co-twin demise and neurological sequelae for the AGA twin. Techniques used can include bipolar or laser cord coagulation (Fig. 13.14), radiofrequency ablation (RFA), or interstitial laser coagulation in earlier gestations. This gives a survival rate of 87–93% for the AGA twin, which is higher than that following SLPCV, but given the demise of the FGR twin, the overall survival rate is lower at 44–47% [22–24]. Therefore,

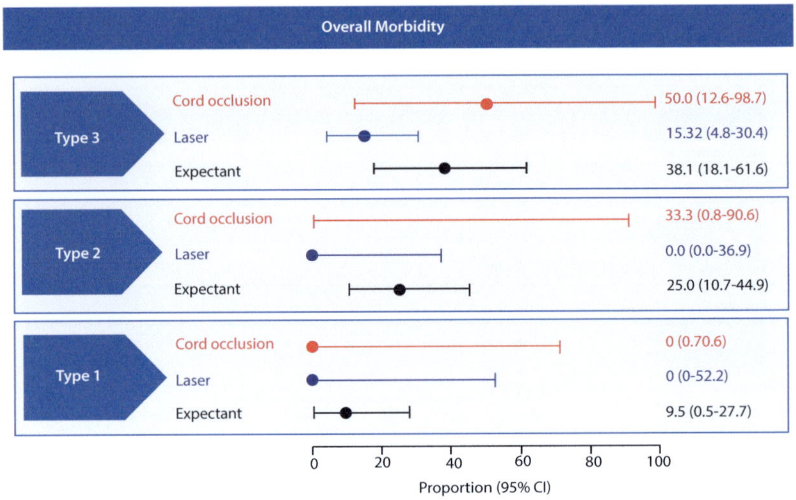

Fig. 13.12 Demonstration of the proportion of the overall neonatal morbidity following cord occlusion (non-reduced larger twin), laser, and expectant management of MC twins with types 1, 2, and 3 sFGR [33]

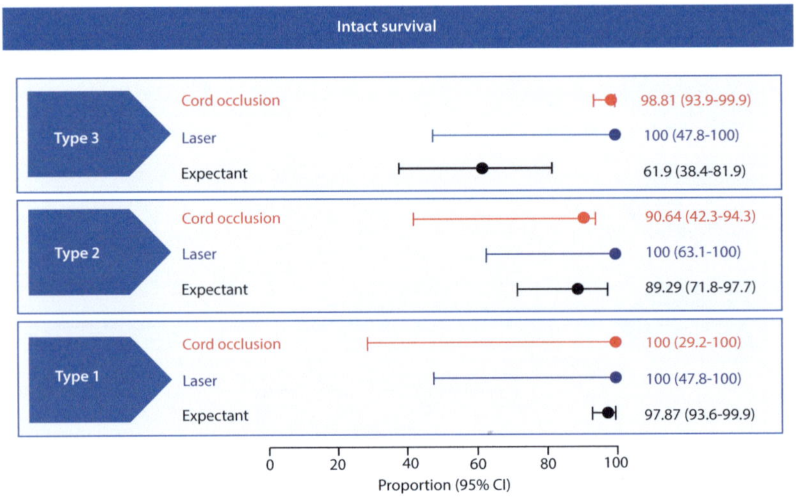

Fig. 13.13 Demonstration of the proportion of intact survival following cord occlusion (non-reduced larger twin), laser, and expectant management of MC twins with types 1, 2, and 3 sFGR [33]

13

this technique gives a higher survival rate for the AGA twin, but SLPCV allows for possible survival of the FGR twin.

Fetoscopic surgery carries a risk of preterm labour, preterm prelabour rupture of membranes, iatrogenic monoamnionicity, and chorioamnionitis. Therefore, consideration should be taken if fetal deterioration is seen after 26 weeks, to balance the risks and benefits of fetoscopic surgery versus preterm delivery.

13.1.4 Triplet Pregnancies

Limited literature is available for FGR in triplet pregnancies. Attempts have been made to

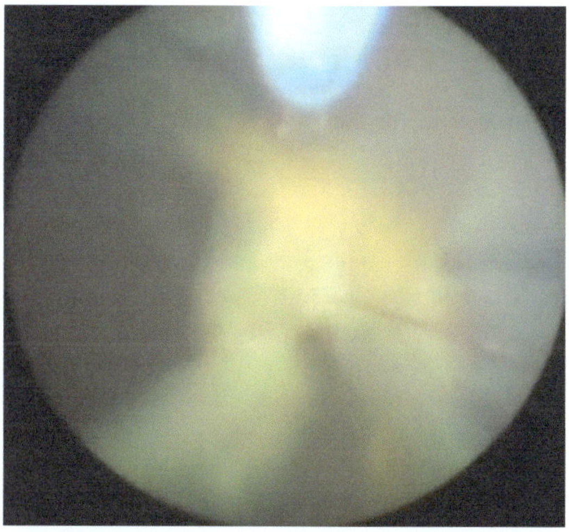

Fig. 13.14 Fetoscopic laser cord occlusion at the site of placental cord insertion, for selective reduction of a twin with severe selective fetal growth restriction

establish normal growth patterns and weight centiles of triplets [34, 35], but currently, singleton growth charts are still being used antenatally to monitor fetal growth. One study found that the incidence of FGR was 13.3% in DC triplets, and 12.3% in trichorionic (TC) triplets [36], whilst an earlier study found this to be as high as 61.8% [37] (defined as birth weight <10th centile). Other observational studies have reported on the incidence of low birthweights in triplets (12.7% TC triplets and 17.4% DC triplets <1000 g, 43% of both groups <1500 g), but this was not adjusted to the gestational age at delivery [38].

In TC triplets, sFGR can be managed in a similar fashion to DC twins. In DC or MC triplets, sFGR in one or more of the monochorionic fetuses can be difficult to manage. Small case series have reported the use of cord occlusion and SLPCV in triplets, where the outcomes were similar to those reported in twin pregnancies (83% survival, 13% long-term comorbidities) [39], but these were not performed for sFGR. Another case series reported the use of SLPCV as a treatment for both sFGR and TTTS in DC and MC triplets. It was found that the overall survival rate was significantly less in DC triplets who underwent SLPCV specifically for sFGR (52.4%) compared to those who received the treatment for TTTS (72.7%) [40].

13.1.5 Conclusion

The management of sFGR poses a clinical conundrum. Conservative management can lead to single twin demise and complications to the surviving co-twin, fetoscopic surgery is associated with a higher mortality of the smaller twin, and early delivery can also expose the AGA twin to significant complications as a result of prematurity. The increased risk of perinatal mortality associated with sFGR requires close monitoring of the condition, whereas over-diagnosis may be minimised using twin-specific growth charts and the most recent diagnostic criteria as proposed by the Delphi consensus. Referral to a tertiary Fetal Medicine centre with adequate levels of expertise is recommended, and patients should be thoroughly counselled regarding the risks and benefits of different management strategies and their outcomes.

13.1.6 Review Questions

1. What is the difference in the etiology of selective fetal growth restriction in monochorionic and dichorionic twins?

2. What is the benefit of designing a uniform diagnostic criterion for selective fetal growth restriction using the Delphi consensus?

3. Describe the differences in umbilical artery end-diastolic flow in the classification of sFGR in monochorionic twins.

4. What is the possible reason that singleton charts are still routinely being used to monitor the growth of twins?

5. What are the options for management in sFGR in monochorionic twins, and what are the differences in outcomes?

6. What are the complications of Type II sFGR in monochorionic twins?

13.1.7 Multiple-Choice Questions

1. What is the incidence of selective fetal growth restriction in dichorionic twins?
   (a) 5.5%
   (b) 10.5%
   (c) 15.5%
   (d) 20.5%
   (e) It depends on the diagnostic criteria used

Answer: (e)

2. Which of the following criteia is not included the diagnosis of selective fetal growth restriction in dichorionic twins?
   (a) Uterine artery PI >95th centile
   (b) Estimated fetal weight <10th centile
   (c) Intertwin estimated fetal weight discordance >25%
   (d) Umbilical artery PI >95th centile

Answer: (a)

3. Which umbilical artery Doppler finding suggests Type III selective fetal growth restriction?
   (a) Persistent absent end-diastolic flow
   (b) Positive end-diastolic flow
   (c) Intermittently reversed end-diastolic flow
   (d) Persistent reversed end-diastolic flow

Answer: (c)

13

4. What is likely the most optimal management in Type I selective fetal growth restriction?
   (a) Conservative
   (b) Selective laser photocoagulation of connecting vessels
   (c) Selective fetocide
   (d) Early delivery

Answer: (a)

5. What is the favourable outcome following selective fetocide compared to selective laser photocoagulation of connecting vessels in treatment of Types II and III fetal growth restriction?
   (a) Reduced neurological comorbidities this does not follow from the text/ figures
   (b) Reduced risk of twin to twin transfusion syndrome
   (c) Reduced stillbirth in co-twin
   (d) Reduced preterm delivery (I would say this is the correct answer 36 weeks vs 32 weeks)

Answer: (d)

6. What is the rate of preterm delivery following the death of one twin in a dichorionic pregnancy?
   (a) 34%
   (b) 44%
   (c) 54%
   (d) 64%

Answer: (c)

7. What is the main concerning risk in Type III selective fetal growth restriction?
   (a) Increased neurological comorbidity (not entirely wrong)
   (b) Increased risk of sudden intrauterine death
   (c) Increased risk of twin to twin transfusion syndrome
   (d) Increased risk of disease progression

Answer: (b)

Patient Testimonials

Stijn and Ruben, Fetal Growth Restriction from a Parent's Perspective

Our little boys, Stijn and Ruben, identical monochorionic twins, were born at 28 weeks and 4 days into the pregnancy. They are now plucky little 5-year-olds. However, my pregnancy and the first year of their life did not proceed in line with what we are usually told or read. Pregnancy diabetes, a difference in growth between the two babies, an emergency caesarean section, premature birth, operations, etc., led to an emotional, fearful period raising many questions.

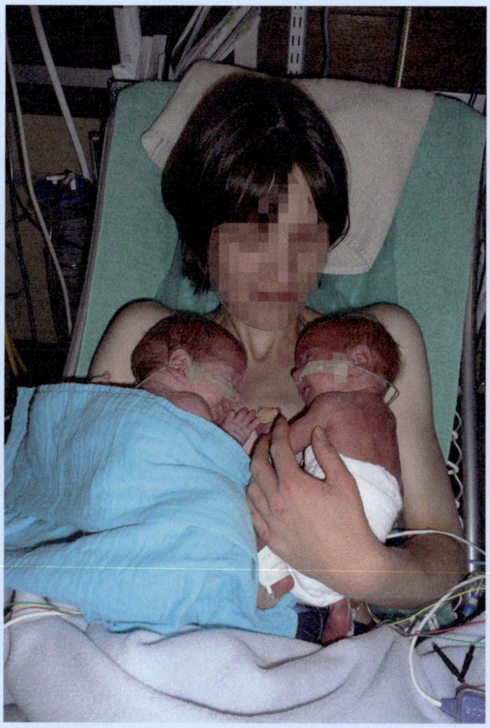

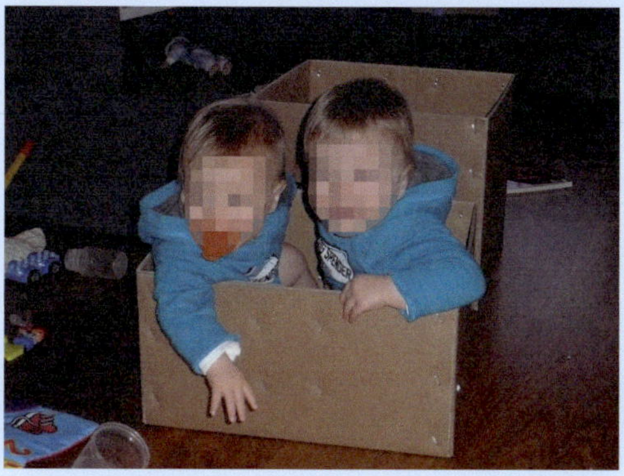

During the first 2 months, everything went well and I encountered no problems. It all started on a night in January when I suffered blood loss. An ultrasound scan revealed that the babies were growing at a different rate and there was doubt as to whether my pregnancy could continue. Because I was being monitored at a fairly small hospital, I was referred to UZ Leuven, which has a team that specialises in monochorionic twins.

My pregnancy was associated with several risks, including twin-to-twin transfusion syndrome between 16 and 26 weeks of pregnancy, discordant growth, or a disorder in one of the babies. It soon became clear after the first examination that it was a case of growth discordance. To monitor the babies as closely as possible and avoid any potential risk, I was monitored with a weekly ultrasound scan. These were always quite worrying moments. Would both hearts still be beating? Would more problems be detected? It makes your pregnancy an emotional and stressful roller coaster. Other women can enjoy their pregnancy and hope it isn't over too soon, but I kept wishing to be another week ahead.

As my pregnancy progressed, we received some more bad news. The brain of the smallest baby wasn't developing as it should. Again, we were given extensive information and were kept up to date. The brain volume was measured at regular intervals and a final estimate would be made at 23 weeks. Would we continue with the pregnancy? Would we decide to keep one baby or give up altogether? Aware that there were quite a few risks, my (mother) heart told me that we would fight this together and not give up. From that moment on, I wanted to name my babies. The biggest baby became Ruben and the smallest one Stijn. This was particularly important to me, because I was safe in the knowledge that our boys had a name, even if something went wrong.

You continue to hope and wait with trepidation. Despite everything and the fact that Stijn's brain was not developing at the same rate, the outlook was still relatively good. When I was 23 weeks pregnant, an assessment was made and fortunately, Stijn's brain had developed satisfactorily to continue the pregnancy.

It became clear that I would be admitted for observation at 28 weeks and have a caesarean section at 32 weeks. Whilst I was in hospital, I was connected to the monitor three times a day. I needed regular glucose tests because of my pregnancy diabetes and had to stick to quite a strict diet.

Sunday 22 May 2011, the fourth day of admission, things suddenly changed apace. The morning graph on the monitor clearly showed there was a problem with Stijn as his heartbeat increased from 80 to 200. There was no other option but to perform a caesarean as soon as possible. Ruben weighed 1.550 kg and Stijn 670 g.

The adrenaline that pumped through my body at the time has awoken a sense of determination in me since the birth of Ruben and Stijn that I was unaware I possessed. Once again, you are confronted with fear about how everything will progress, what the babies' chances are, etc. We were told during the pregnancy that the babies would have to spend some time in the neonatal care unit. Due to the emergency caesarean, my husband and I did not have time to visit this department beforehand, but being a nurse myself, I knew more or less what to expect, e.g. monitors, alarms, drips, etc. Nevertheless, I was now a mother and that initial confrontation was quite difficult and emotional.

13

The first few days were quite challenging. You miss your babies, your emotions are all over the place, you wonder why on earth you had to give birth so prematurely. Aspects that you cannot control yourself and that make you feel powerless. It subsequently became clear that Stijn had been saved before he was born thanks to the twin-to-twin transfusion with Ruben. Without Ruben, Stijn would only have weighed 100 g. That was quite sobering news, we were incredibly lucky.

We received excellent support at the neonatal care unit. We were allowed to see our babies whenever we wanted to. Despite everything that happened, the time went relatively quickly. Ruben and Stijn's condition varied from day to day, small steps forward and sometimes a step backward. New worries and fears presented themselves time and again. Five days after the birth we were told that Stijn suffered from narrowing of the aorta, which was operable but not before he weighed 2.5 kg. A decision was made to insert a temporary stent as soon as he weighed 1 kg. Before that, he was put on medication. After a while, Stijn suffered a pulmonary haemorrhage, but once again he fought his way through. Ruben developed relatively well until they found blood in his stools due to an intestinal infection, which almost resulted in him having a perforated bowel. Fortunately, swift action avoided this. Stijn received a temporary stent on 20th June. It was a particularly high-risk operation with a 50% chance of success, but our little fighter once again pulled through.

Ruben was allowed to come home on 30th July. We obviously had mixed feelings. On the one hand, we were very pleased, but on the other hand, we were sad because we had to leave our other baby behind. Stijn continued to improve but still had to be put in isolation twice when a bacterium was found in his stools. His stent had to be dilated on 6th September. But then … finally!!!! Stijn was allowed to leave hospital on 15th September. My husband and I went to collect him, together with Ruben, a very emotional moment. I had waited so long for this, but finally my family was united! Stijn's operation to treat the narrowing of the aorta went well. Both boys are thriving. During the first 3 years, they were particularly vulnerable and more prone to becoming sick. Now, however, things have much improved.

Because of everything I went through during my pregnancy and the problems affecting Ruben and Stijn after the birth, I have learnt to put things into perspective in life. It was definitely not easy but looking around me, I realised that some people face even greater challenges. We were lucky because our boys were real fighters. It isn't always easy, but despite everything you must not lose faith and continue to hope and believe that it will turn out alright in the end. I always continued to put my faith in Stijn and Ruben and when I see how far they have come, I can only be incredibly happy and more than anything infinitely grateful.

References

1. D'Antonio F, Odibo AO, Prefumo F, Khalil A, Buca D, Flacco ME, Liberati M, Manzoli L, Acharya G. Weight discordance and perinatal mortality in twin pregnancy: systematic review and meta-analysis. Ultrasound Obstet Gynecol. 2018;52(1):11–23.
2. Hillman SC, Morris RK, Kilby MD. Co-twin prognosis after single fetal death: a systematic review and meta-analysis. Obstet Gynecol. 2011;118:928–40.
3. Glinianaia SV, Obeysekera MA, Sturgiss S, Bell R. Stillbirth and neonatal mortality in monochorionic and dichorionic twins: a population-based study. Hum Reprod RCOG, London. 2011;26(9):2549–57.
4. Townsend R, Khalil A. Twin pregnancy complicated by selective growth restriction. Curr Opin Obstet Gynecol. 2016;28(6):485–91.
5. Lewi L, Gucciardo L, van Mieghem T, de Koninck P, Beck V, Medek H, Van Schoubroeck D, Devlieger R, De Catte L, Deprest J. Monochorionic diamniotic twin pregnancies: natural history and risk stratification. Fetal Diagn Ther. 2010;27:121–33.
6. Valsky DV, Eixarch E, Martinez JM, Crispi F, Gratacós E. Selective intrauterine growth restriction in monochorionic twins: pathophysiology, diagnostic approach and management dilemmas. Semin Fetal Neonatal Med. 2010;15:342–8.
7. Inklaar MJ, van Klink JM, Stolk TT, van Zwet EW, Oepkes D, Lopriore E. Cerebral injury in monochorionic twins with selective intrauterine growth restriction: a systematic review. Prenat Diagn. 2014;34:205–13.
8. Stirrup OT, Khalil A, D'Antonio F, Thilaganathan B. Fetal growth reference ranges in twin pregnancy: analysis of the Southwest Thames Obstetric Research Collaborative (STORK) multiple pregnancy cohort. Ultrasound Obstet Gynecol. 2015;45(3):301–7.
9. Wu D, Huang L, He Z, et al. Pre-eclampsia in twin pregnancies: association with selective intrauterine growth restriction. J Matern Fetal Neonatal Med. 2016;29:1967–71.
10. ISUOG. Practice guidelines: the role of ultrasound in twin pregnancy. Ultrasound Obstet Gynecol. 2016;47:247–63.
11. Townsend R, Khalil A. Fetal growth restriction in twins. Best Pract Res Clin Obstet Gynaecol. 2018;49:79–88.
12. Khalil A, Beune I, Hecher K, Wynia K, Ganzevoort W, Reed K, Lewi L, Oepkes D, Gratacós E, Thilaganathan B, Gordijn SJ. Consensus definition and essential reporting parameters of selective fetal growth restriction in twin pregnancy: a Delphi procedure. Ultrasound Obstet Gynecol. 2019;53:47–54.
13. Gratacós E, Lewi L, Munoz M, Acosta-Rojas R, Hernandez-Andrade E, Martinez JM, Carreras E, Deprest J. A classification system for selective intrauterine growth restriction in monochorionic pregnancies according to umbilical artery Doppler flow in the smaller twin. Ultrasound Obstet Gynecol. 2007;30:28–34.
14. Ishii K, Murakoshi T, Takahashi Y, et al. Perinatal outcome of monochorionic twins with selective intrauterine growth restriction and different types of umbilical artery Doppler under expectant management. Fetal Diagn Ther. 2009;26:157–61.
15. Vanlieferinghen S, Anselem O, Le RC, Shen Y, Marcellin L, Goffinet F. Prognostic value of umbilical and cerebral Doppler in fetal growth restriction: comparison of dichorionic twins and singletons. PLoS One. 2015;10(4):e0123067.
16. Audibert F, Salomon LJ, Castaigne-Meary V, et al. Selective termination of a twin pregnancy as a treatment of severe preeclampsia. BJOG. 2003;110:68–9.
17. Hillman SC, Morris RK, Kilby MD. Co-twin prognosis after single fetal death: a systematic review and meta-analysis. Obstet Gynecol. 2011;118:928–40.
18. Rustico MA, Consonni D, Lanna M, et al. Selective intrauterine growth restriction in monochorionic twins: changing patterns in umbilical artery Doppler flow and outcomes. Ultrasound Obstet Gynecol. 2017;49(3):387–93.
19. D'Antonio F, Khalil A, Dias T, Thilaganathan B. Southwest Thames Obstetric Research Collaborative (STORK). Weight discordance and perinatal mortality in twins: analysis of the Southwest Thames Obstetric Research Collaborative (STORK) multiple pregnancy cohort. Ultrasound Obstet Gynecol. 2013;41:643–8.
20. Memmo A, Dias T, Mahsud-Dornan S, Papageorghiou AT, Bhide A, Thilaganathan B. Prediction of selective fetal growth restriction and twin-to-twin transfusion syndrome in monochorionic twins. BJOG. 2012;119(4):417–21.
21. Peeva G, Bower S, Orosz L, Chaveeva P, Akolekar R, Nicolaides KH. Endoscopic placental laser coagulation for monochorionic diamniotic twins with type II selective fetal growth restriction. Fetal Diagn Ther. 2015;38(2):86–93.
22. Bebbington MW, Danzer E, Moldenhauer J, Khalek N, Johnson MP. Radiofrequency ablation vs bipolar umbilical cord coagulation in the management of complicated monochorionic pregnancies. Ultrasound Obstet Gynecol. 2012;40(3):319–24.
23. Chalouhi GE, Marangoni MA, Quibel T, Deloison B, Benzina N, Essaoui M, et al. Active management of selective intrauterine growth restriction with abnormal Doppler in monochorionic diamniotic twin pregnancies diagnosed in the second trimester of pregnancy. Prenat Diagn. 2013;33(2):109–15.
24. Parra-Cordero M, Bennasar M, Martínez JM, Eixarch E, Torres X, Gratacós E. Cord occlusion

in monochorionic twins with early selective intrauterine growth restriction and abnormal umbilical artery doppler: a consecutive series of 90 cases. Fetal Diagn Ther. 2016;39(3):186–91.
25. Vasario E, Borgarello V, Bossotti C, Libanori E, Biolcati M, Arduino S, Spinelli R, Delle Piane L, Revelli A, Todros T. IVF twins have similar obstetric and neonatal outcome as spontaneously conceived twins: a prospective follow-up study. Reprod Biomed Online. 2010;21(3):422–8.
26. Geisler ME, O'Mahony A, Meaney S, Waterstone JJ, O'Donoghue K. Obstetric and perinatal 254 outcomes of twin pregnancies conceived following IVF/ICSI treatment compared with 255 spontaneously conceived twin pregnancies. Eur J Obstet Gynecol Reprod Biol. 2014;78-83(256):181.
27. Moini A, Shiva M, Arabipoor A, Hosseini R, Chehrazi M, Sadeghi M. Obstetric and neonatal outcomes of twin pregnancies conceived by assisted reproductive technology compared with twin pregnancies conceived spontaneously: a prospective follow-up study. Eur J Obstet Gynecol Reprod Biol. 2012;165(1):29–32.
28. Qin JB, Wang H, Sheng X, Xie Q, Gao S. Assisted reproductive technology and risk of adverse obstetric outcomes in dichorionic twin pregnancies: a systematic review and meta-analysis. Fertil Steril. 2016;105(5):1180–92.
29. Gerber RS, Fields JC, Barberio AL, Bodenlos K, Fox NS. Outcomes of twin pregnancies in women 45 years of age or older. Obstet Gynecol. 2017;129(5):827–30.
30. Curado J, Sileo F, Bhide A, Thilaganathan B, Khalil A. Early and late selective fetal growth restriction in monochorionic diamniotic twin pregnancies: natural history and diagnostic criteria. Ultrasound Obstet Gynecol. 2019; https://doi.org/10.1002/uog.20849. [Epub ahead of print]
31. Hamilton E, Platt R, Morin L, Usher R, Kramer M. How small is too small in a twin pregnancy? Am J Obstet Gynecol. 1998;179:682–5.
32. Buca D, Pagani G, Rizzo G, Familiari A, Flacco ME, Manzoli L, Liberati M, Fanfani F, Scambia G, D'Antonio F. Outcome of monochorionic twin pregnancy with selective intrauterine growth restriction according to umbilical artery Doppler flow pattern of smaller twin: a systematic review and meta-analysis. Ultrasound Obstet Gynecol. 2017;50(5):559–68.
33. Townsend R, D'Antonio F, Sileo FG, Kumbay H, Thilaganathan B, Khalil A. Perinatal outcome of monochorionic twin pregnancy complicated by selective fetal growth restriction according to management: systematic review and meta-analysis. Ultrasound Obstet Gynecol. 2019;53(1):36–46.
34. Min SJ, Luke B, Min L, Misiunas R, Nugent C, Van de Ven C, Martin D, Gonzalez-Quintero VH, Eardley S, Witter FR, Mauldin JG, Newman RB. Birth weight references for triplets. Am J Obstet Gynecol. 2004;191(3):809–14.
35. Vora NL, Ruthazer R, House M, Chelmow D. Triplet ultrasound growth parameters. Obstet Gynecol. 2006;107(3):694–700.
36. Spencer J, Ingardia C, Nold C, Borgida A, Herson V, Egan J. Perinatal and neonatal outcomes of triplet gestations based on placental chorionicity. Am J Perinatol. 2009;26(08):587–90.
37. Boulot P, Hedon B, Pelliccia G, Sarda P, Montoya F, Mares P, Humeau C, Arnal F, Laffargue F, Viala JL. Favourable outcome in 33 triplet pregnancies managed between 1985-1990. Eur J Obstet Gynecol Reprod Bio. 1992;43(2):123–9.
38. Simões T, Queiros A, Gonçalves MR, Periquito I, Silva P, Blickstein I. Perinatal outcome of dichorionic-triamniotic as compared to trichorionic triplets. J Perinat Med. 2016;44(8):875–9.
39. Schoubroeck D, Lewi L, Ryan G, Carreras E, Jani J, Higueras T, Deprest J, Gratacos E. Fetoscopic surgery in triplet pregnancies: a multicenter case series. Am J Obstet Gynecol. 2004;191(5):1529–32.
40. Peeva G, Chaveeva P, Gil Guevara E, Akolekar R, Nicolaides KH. Endoscopic placental laser coagulation in dichorionic and monochorionic triplet pregnancies. Fetal Diagn Ther. 2016;40:174–80.

Key Reading

Gratacós E, Lewi L, Munoz M, Acosta-Rojas R, Hernandez-Andrade E, Martinez JM, Carreras E, Deprest J. A classification system for selective intrauterine growth restriction in monochorionic pregnancies according to umbilical artery Doppler flow in the smaller twin. Ultrasound Obstet Gynecol. 2007;30:28–34.
ISUOG. Practice guidelines: the role of ultrasound in twin pregnancy. Ultrasound Obstet Gynecol. 2016;47:247–63.
Khalil A, Beune I, Hecher K, Wynia K, Ganzevoort W, Reed K, Lewi L, Oepkes D, Gratacós E, Thilaganathan B, Gordijn SJ. Consensus definition and essential reporting parameters of selective fetal growth restriction in twin pregnancy: a Delphi procedure. Ultrasound Obstet Gynecol. 2019;53:47–54.
Townsend R, Khalil A. Twin pregnancy complicated by selective growth restriction. Curr Opin Obstet Gynecol. 2016;28(6):485–91.
Townsend R, Khalil A. Fetal growth restriction in twins. Best Pract Res Clin Obstet Gynaecol. 2018;49:79–88.

Fetal Demise in Twins: Single and Double Fetal Loss

L. R. I. Gurney, R. K. Morris, J. L. Gibson, and M. D. Kilby

Contents

A. Khalil et al. (eds.), *Twin and Higher-order Pregnancies*,
https://doi.org/10.1007/978-3-030-47652-6_14

Trailer

Approximately 1 in 60 pregnancies are multiple pregnancies and almost 98% are twins. Multiple pregnancy incidence across the UK and worldwide is increasing due to uptake of assisted reproduction techniques and changing childbirth demographics, with women deferring pregnancy until an age when multiple pregnancy occurs more frequently.

Twin pregnancies face greater risk of stillbirth and neonatal death than singleton pregnancies. Monochorionic twin pregnancies, comprising approximately 20% of twin pregnancies, have a risk of stillbirth up to five times that of singletons. The UK confidential enquiry data over 15 years indicates an overall declining trend in rates of stillbirth for monochorionic and dichorionic twin pregnancies. Improved outcomes possibly reflect the establishment of national guidelines for multiple pregnancy management.

A single twin demise presents significant risks for surviving co-twins. The main determinant for co-twin morbidity and mortality is the chorionicity of the pregnancy. Monochorionic twin pregnancies face increased risks of single fetal loss due to the unique complications of twin to twin transfusion syndrome (TTTS), early-onset severe selective growth restriction (sGR) and twin anaemia polycythaemia sequence (TAPS), arising from the conjoining of the fetal circulations by placental anastomoses within the shared placenta. Furthermore, following single twin demise, shared inter-fetal circulations predispose surviving monochorionic co-twins to increased risks of death or neurological disability.

This chapter evaluates single and double fetal loss in twin pregnancies, examining difficulties posed in collecting accurate data on such losses. It describes causes of twin demise, discussing challenges faced by both surviving co-twins and clinicians responsible for further management.

Definitions

Early Single Twin Demise

Loss of a twin before 12 weeks of gestation may be referred to as "vanishing twin syndrome". It occurs when an early first trimester diagnosis of twin pregnancy has been made via ultrasound and subsequent ultrasound assessment demonstrates a single viable fetus. The non-viable embryo may become incorporated into placental membranes and may not be identified, inevitably leading to a proportion of such pregnancies being mis-classified as singleton gestations. Such a situation makes recording the rates of first trimester twin loss difficult, although it is suggested that these early pregnancy loss rates may be as high as 29% [1]. There is a lack of evidence to inform the risk of adverse outcome to the surviving twin, but early co-twin loss does not seem to be associated with subsequent morbidity in surviving infants, irrespective of the chorionicity of the pregnancy.

Twin Demise from Second Trimester Onwards

A single twin demise in the second or third trimester of a pregnancy (for either mono- or dichorionic twins) is considered differently to earlier loss as such an event carries with it an increased risk of late miscarriage, stillbirth, preterm birth and morbidity for the surviving twin. Monochorionic pregnancies have the highest risk of adverse co-twin loss or morbidity due to the conjoined fetal circulations.

Learning Objectives

- Understand the challenges in defining rates of single and double twin stillbirth in national surveillance and the importance of national guidelines in reducing these rates.

- Understand the aetiology of sIUFD or double twin pregnancy loss.
- Understand the risks posed to the surviving co-twin.
- Understand the determinants and pathophysiology of risks to the surviving co-twin.
- Develop an understanding of the management strategies for both di- and monochorionic twin pregnancies once sIUFD has occurred.

14.1 Defining Rates and Analysing Trends of Fetal Loss in Twins

The UK MBRRACE perinatal mortality report published in October 2019 reported the UK stillbirth (after 24 weeks) and infant death surveillance data from 2014 to 2017. These data demonstrated a slight increase in the number of twin stillbirths from 6.16/1000 total births (live and stillbirths) to 6.99/1000 total births from the previous report [2]. Note that the total number of individual fetal losses is divided by the total number of live born neonates to allow appropriate comparison with the stillbirth rate in singleton pregnancies (3 per 1000 live births). Although the recent slight rise in fetal loss rate in multiple pregnancy is disappointing, it comes on the background of an apparent significant drop in the UK twin stillbirth rate since 2014 from 11.07/1000, and a trend of progressive reduction in UK twin stillbirth rates over the last 15 years [3]. Accurate data on the rate of stillbirths in twins divided by chorionicity are less readily available due to the lack of accurate capture within national databases regarding the total number of live born monochorionic or dichorionic twin neonates. National stillbirth rates in dichorionic and monochorionic twin pregnancies can however be estimated by knowledge of the total number of live born neonates from twin pregnancies, and assuming 80% of these are dichorionic. Utilising data from UK MBRRACE perinatal reports between 2016 and 2018, it has been estimated the stillbirth rates fell from 27 to 19 per 1000 total births in monochorionic twins, and from 5 to 3 per 1000 total births in dichorionic twins [3].

These national reports not only demonstrate the data for stillbirths but now also the data on fetal losses after 22 weeks. However, complications of twin pregnancies, particularly of monochorionic twin pregnancies such as TTTS and severe sGR, may present early in the second trimester and be associated with spontaneous or iatrogenic fetal demise at gestations earlier than 22 weeks. Thus, these pregnancy losses will not be recorded by national registries [3].

In the current published format, the UK MBRRACE perinatal mortality reports do not present data on the number of twin pregnancies that suffered single or double fetal loss. The majority are single fetal losses. The importance of such statistical information will hopefully be realised by a "deep dive" analysis of twin fetal losses currently being performed by MBRRACE-UK for the 2018 cohort of losses.

Despite limitations, the analysis of stillbirth rates in twin pregnancies is encouraging, suggesting improved outcomes that may reflect a greater awareness and implementation of evidence-based clinical interventions. National and international guidelines for multiple pregnancy help health care professionals plan effective delivery of maternity care, and a key element of guidance is the establishment of multidisciplinary multiple pregnancy clinics and the targeted use of obstetric ultrasound for fetal surveillance and screening. Such intensive surveillance and timely management of pregnancy complications had resulted in steady decline in stillbirth in dichorionic twin pregnancies so that the rate of loss per fetus now compares favourably to that seen in singleton pregnancies. Stillbirth rates have fallen also in monochorionic pregnancies, but the shared fetoplacental circulations continue to predispose these pregnancies to a significant risk of adverse outcomes despite intensive surveillance and targeted interventions for complications.

14.2 Aetiology of Fetal Loss in Twin Pregnancy

There are many causes of single or double fetal loss during a multiple pregnancy. They can be broadly divided into those affecting the mother, causes affecting one or both fetuses, those specifically related to the chorionic and amniotic status of the pregnancy and iatrogenic causes.

14.2.1 Causes Affecting the Mother

Pregnancy-related maternal conditions such as hypertensive disorders and gestational diabetes have a higher incidence in multiple pregnancy compared to singleton pregnancies [4, 5], and these conditions are associated with an increased risk of stillbirth. Several maternal pre-existing diseases are associated with increased risk of fetal loss in singleton pregnancies with such risks amplified in multiple pregnancy. Conditions including antiphospholipid syndrome, autoimmune conditions such as systemic lupus erythematosus and cardiac and renal disease may place a fetus at particular risk of stillbirth, and such pregnancies must be intensively monitored and managed by expert multidisciplinary clinical teams [6, 7].

14.2.2 Causes Affecting the Fetus

14.2.2.1 Chromosomal Anomaly

The process of spontaneous twinning does not appear to be associated with an increased risk of chromosome anomalies in embryos. The majority of dichorionic twin pregnancies are however dizygotic, and therefore as each embryo is associated with its own aneuploidy risk, the overall pregnancy is at nearly two-fold risk of carrying at least one fetus with a chromosome anomaly. Monochorionic twin pregnancies have a similar risk to singleton pregnancies of common trisomies, but, if affected, the pregnancy will contain two identical, karyotypically anomalous fetuses. Discordant fetal chromosome complements can occur rarely in monochorionic twin pregnancies and arise from post-mitotic mutations or loss of genetic material. A population-based study investigating registry data from North-East England provides one of the largest data sets on the prevalence of chromosome anomalies in twin pregnancies [8]. The cohort was limited due to the low incidence of chromosome anomalies; however, extrapolation from the data presented supports the assumptions described above and suggests 72 per 10,000 dichorionic pregnancies are affected by a fetal chromosome anomaly (40 per 10,000 fetuses), 49 per 10,000 monochorionic pregnancies are affected by fetal chromosome anomalies (usually of both fetuses = 74 per 10,000 fetuses). The rates compare to a prevalence of fetal chromosome anomalies in 44 per 10,000 in singleton pregnancies.

Lethal fetal autosomal trisomy may be associated with spontaneous single twin demise in dichorionic pregnancies and double loss in monochorionic pregnancies. Rare discordant fetal chromosome anomalies in monochorionic pregnancies (heterokaryotypic monozygotism, most commonly monosomy X) carry a risk of loss to both fetuses.

For twin pregnancies undergoing combined first trimester screening, there is a greater false-positive rate for twins compared with singleton pregnancies [9], which can lead to an increased likelihood of being offered prenatal invasive testing. The risks of pregnancy loss following invasive testing is increased for twins with overall pregnancy loss rates as high as 3.8% following chorionic villus sampling and 3.1% following amniocentesis for twin pregnancies compared with rates of 0.5–1% for singletons [10]. If aneuploidy discordance occurs in twin pregnancies and selective fetal reduction is performed, this can pose a risk of loss for the unaffected twin.

14.2.2.2 Structural Abnormalities

Structural abnormalities, particularly cardiac problems, are more common in twin pregnancy than in singleton pregnancy [8]. This is largely related to the greater incidence of abnormalities in monozygotic twin pregnancies due to problems that can occur during embryonic cleavage, thus leading to an increased risk of midline defects such as cardiac abnormalities, holoprosencephaly and neural tube defects [8]. Monochorionic pregnancies are therefore at highest risk but as up to 10% of dichorionic twins may be monozygotic; therefore, UK guidelines recommend extended views of fetal heart anatomy during 18-22 anomaly scan for all multiple pregnancies [11]. Structural abnormalities, discordant or concordant, increase the risk of fetal loss in twin pregnancy both due to the anomaly itself, and iatrogenically via prenatal investigation and/or selective twin reduction or termination of the whole twin pregnancy.

14.2.2.3 Infection

Congenital fetal infection is associated with pregnancy losses. Transplacental infections such as cytomegalovirus or parvovirus B19 are recognised causes of stillbirth [12]. Although these infections are not known to be increased in twin pregnancies compared to singletons, they are likely to affect both fetuses increasing the chance of the pregnancy suffering a least one fetal loss. Furthermore, a surviving co-twin may be at additional risk should an initial fetal loss occur.

The rate of preterm, prelabour rupture of membranes (PPROM) in twin pregnancies may be as high as 11% versus a singleton rate of 3–4% [13]. This can expose the pregnancy to ascending bacterial infection including Group B Streptococcus, *E. coli* or Enterococcus with the potential to place either twin at risk of preterm birth, stillbirth or early neonatal death.

14.2.3 Causes Related to Chorionicity or Amnionicity

Monochorionic diamniotic (MCDA) pregnancies constitute approximately 20% of twin pregnancies and can have up to five-fold increased risk of single or double fetal loss compared to both singleton and dichorionic pregnancies [14]. This can be explained by the presence of a communicating placental circulation from which may develop the conditions of TTTS, TAPS and selective fetal growth restriction.

TTTS occurs in up to 15% of MCDA twin pregnancies and arises from an unbalanced, unidirectional arterio-venous anastomosis resulting in a net transfer of blood from a donor to recipient twin. The donor twin becomes hypovolaemic, with a decrease in cardiac output and an increase in peripheral vascular resistance leading to hypoxia and acidosis. On ultrasound examination this twin will have oligohydramnios, may be growth restricted with an empty bladder and at late stages will develop abnormal Doppler waveforms prior to death. The recipient twin will become hypervolaemic, will have associated polyhydramnios, a large bladder and may show signs of high-output cardiac failure with abnormal Doppler waveforms prior to death. In the UK, national guidance suggests that fortnightly ultrasound screening for TTTS in monochorionic twin pregnancy which should begin at 16 weeks. When diagnosed TTTS should be classified according to the Quintero staging system. If TTTS is diagnosed prior to 26 weeks gestation at Quintero stages 2 and above, the recommended treatment is fetoscopic laser ablation (FLA) using the SOLOMON technique [15]. When compared to serial amnioreduction, FLA leads to a significant increase in survival and neurologically intact survival at 6 years of age (RR 1.57 95% CI: 1.05–2.34) [16].

TAPS is defined by a significant discordance in haemoglobin levels between twins without substantial differences in amniotic fluid volume. It is presumed to occur from a low volume "slow" transfusion of blood from a donor to recipient fetus via miniscule artery-vein anastomoses. It affects 2% of all MCDA pregnancies, but this figure may increase up to 13% following FLA [17]. Current UK recommendations advise serial ultrasonographic monitoring with middle cerebral artery peak systolic velocity (MCA-PSV) for high-risk monochorionic twin pregnancies such as those affected by TTTS or sGR [11]. Twin pregnancies with this condition will be at increased risk of stillbirth; however, there is little evidence from prospective cohort studies regarding outcomes and optimal management in this situation [18].

Selective growth restriction (sGR) is defined as a condition whereby one fetus is growth restricted, defined as <10th centile for estimated fetal weight (EFW), and there is an inter-twin growth discordance is >25% [19]. At these thresholds, there is an associated significant risk of subsequent in utero demise of the growth-restricted fetus. This is usually due to placental dysfunction. However, there is also the possibility of non-placentally mediated pathology predisposing to pregnancy loss, such as infection (CMV, toxoplasmosis) or discordant chromosomal abnormality. In monochorionic pregnancies, severe sGR can be a reflection of unequal placental sharing of blood flow between twins: a phenomenon which can be classified according to the pattern of end-diastolic waveform in the umbilical artery Doppler velocimetry [20]. Type 1-sGR has positive end-diastolic flow and a 90% survival rate; for type 2-sGR, there is absent or reversed end-diastolic flow (AREDF), which is associated with a 29% risk of stillbirth for either twin. Type 3-sGR is defined by a cyclical/intermittent pattern of AREDF, which is more unpredictable and associated with a 10–20% risk of intrauterine death of the smaller fetus. A number of management approaches exist for monochorionic twins with sGR including conservative management, early delivery, FLA or selective cord ablation of the smaller twin [21]; however, existing evidence is yet to evince the most appropriate management strategy and therefore a tailored approach should be taken for individual pregnancies.

Monochorionic monoamniotic (MCMA) twin pregnancies are rare, constituting 5% of all monochorionic pregnancies but <1% of all twin pregnancies. They have a very high fetal and perinatal loss rate of 50% prior to 16 weeks gestation, secondary to fetal abnormality or spontaneous miscarriage; however, loss rates at later gestations have fallen from 40% to 10–15% largely due to an increased awareness that such cases need to be managed in specialist centres and delivered at an optimal preterm gestation. All MCMA twin pregnancies will have a degree of cord entanglement; therefore, this is not a prognostic factor for fetal loss. Due to large placental arterio-arterial anastomosis between the two fetal circulation, rates of TTTS are low (5%). MCMA twins are at increased risk of fetal loss from 34 weeks gestation, and therefore delivery is indicated between 32 and 33 + 6 weeks of pregnancy: with caesarean section mandated due to the increased risk of cord accident with descent of the first twin through the pelvis during vaginal birth [22].

14.2.4 Iatrogenic Causes

The main iatrogenic cause of fetal loss in twin pregnancies is selective feticide performed in cases of discordant anomaly [22]. The method of feticide will depend on the chorionicity of the pregnancy. Ultrasound guided injection of an abortifactant (e.g. potassium chloride) into the fetal circulation of the affected twin is the technically most straightforward method but is only appropriate for dichorionic pregnancies. This is associated with a risk of co-twin loss of approximately 5–7%.

Due to the shared feto-placental circulation, vascular occlusive procedures such as ultrasound-guided intra-fetal laser, radiofrequency ablation or the use of bipolar cord coagulation are required for selective fetal termination in monochorionic pregnancies [11]. These are all technically advanced invasive procedures and associated with a significant risk of co-twin demise. The rates of co-twin loss vary between studied cohorts but appear be at least 12%. Such procedures are more difficult to perform with advancing gestation, and this correspondingly increases the risk of associated co-twin demise.

Fetoscopic laser therapy for TTTS offers the possibility of improved survival for one or both affected twins; however, there remains a chance of single (20–25%) or double (10–15%) fetal loss from which there is likely to be an iatrogenic contribution from the risk of procedure itself [16].

14.3 Determinants of Co-twin Prognosis

In cases of single fetal loss, the co-twin may be at risk from the same condition(s) that led to the initial death of the first twin. In addition to this, the key determinants that affect the prognosis of the remaining co-twin are the chorionicity of pregnancy and the gestation at the time of initial twin loss.

A recent systematic review and meta-analysis analysed prognosis of the co-twin after single intrauterine fetal death (sIUFD) (Table 14.1). In this study, pregnancies were stratified according to chorionicity to allow for separate analysis of mono- and dichorionic twin pregnancies [14]. Early prenatal diagnosis of TTTS and intervention in the form of FLA can influence overall fetal and perinatal loss rate results either through improved survival of both twins, or early loss of one or both twins [3]. Therefore, to avoid confounding factors relating to FLA, pregnancies that had undergone such interventions were removed from analysis in this study [14]. Following a single intrauterine twin death, there was an approximately two-fold increased risk for co-twin death in monochorionic compared to dichorionic pregnancy (41% vs. 22.4%). The rates of neonatal deaths were also increased for monochorionic pregnancies, although this result was not statistically significant (27.8% vs. 21.2%). Of other outcomes studied, including preterm birth, abnormal antenatal brain fMRI, neurodevelopmental comorbidity, preterm birth and abnormal postnatal brain imaging, only abnormal postnatal brain imaging demonstrated significantly different rates between groups, with monochorionic pregnancies being more at risk (OR 5.41, 95% CI 1.03–28.58) [14, 23].

Table 14.1 Adverse outcomes affecting surviving co-twin following single intra-uterine fetal death

Adverse outcome in co-twin	Monochorionic event rate	Dichorionic event rate	Odds ratio [95% CI] comparing MC vs. DC
Co-twin intra-uterine fetal death	41.0% [95% CI 33.7, 49.9] 32 studies, 379 pregnancies	22.4% [95% CI 16.2, 30.9] 20 studies, 255 pregnancies	**2.06 [95% CI 1.14, 3.71] $P = 0.016$, 19 studies, 441 pregnancies**
Preterm birth	58.5% [95% CI 48.2, 70.9] 20 studies, 202 pregnancies	53.7% [95% CI 40.8, 70.6] 12 studies, 107 pregnancies	1.42 [95% CI 0.67, 2.99] $P = 0.356$,10 studies 167 pregnancies
Abnormal antenatal brain fMRI	20.0% [95% CI 12.8, 31.1] six studies, 116 pregnancies	NP	NP
Abnormal postnatal brain imaging	43.0% [95% CI 32.8, 56.3] 12 studies, 140 pregnancies	21.2% [95% CI 10.6, 42.4] 7 studies, 75 pregnancies	**5.41 [95% CI 1.03, 28.58 $P = 0.047$, 7 studies, 142 pregnancies**
Neuro-developmental comorbidity	28.5% [95% CI 19.0, 42.7] 13 studies, 103 pregnancies	10% [95% CI 3.9, 27.7] 8 studies, 62 pregnancies	3.06 [95% CI 0.88, 10.61] $P = 0.08$, 8 studies, 129 pregnancies
Neonatal death	27.9% [95% CI 21.1, 36.9] 18 studies, 206 pregnancies	21.2% [95% CI 14.5, 31.2] 12 studies, 130 pregnancies	1.95 [95% CI 1.00, 3.79] $P = 0.051$, 11 studies, 232 pregnancies

Adapted from Mackie et al. [14]

Table includes the monochorionic and dichorionic event rates and comparative odds ratios for the following outcomes: co-twin death, preterm birth (less than 34 weeks), abnormal fetal brain MRI, other abnormal fetal brain imaging, neuro-developmental morbidity and neonatal death

14

This study also demonstrated that for monochorionic twins, when the single intrauterine fetal death occurred less than 28 weeks, there was a significantly increased rate of co-twin fetal intrauterine death (OR 2.31, 95% CI 1.02–5.25) or co-twin neonatal death (OR 2.84, 95% CI 1.14–20.47) compared to twin gestations where the single intrauterine fetal death occurred after 28 weeks gestation.

Thus, outcomes are worse for monochorionic compared to dichorionic pregnancies, and a worse prognosis can be predicted should the initial intrauterine death occur prior to 28 weeks.

14.4 Pathophysiology of Sequelae of Single Twin Demise in Monochorionic Pregnancies

In monochorionic pregnancies, there are two proposed mechanisms to explain the risk of increased morbidity and mortality for the surviving co-twin following single twin demise. These are acute transfusion (exsanguination) from the surviving co-twin to the demised twin leading to hypoperfusion, anaemia and acute tissue acidosis, or the risk of transchorionic embolization and coagulopathy.

14.4.1 Acute Transfusion from Surviving Co-twin

The "transfusional" hypothesis was first proposed by Fusi et al. [24]. The demise of the initial twin leads to a comparative fall in the vascular pressure on the side of the chorionic unit supplying the demised twin compared to the area supplying the surviving twin. Due to the presence of arterial-arterial (AA) and venous-venous (VV) anastomosis within the shared placenta, an acute transfusion occurs from the survivor to the demised twin. This leads to hypoperfusion, hypotension and fetal anaemia in the surviving twin, with subsequent tissue hypoxia and acidosis causing damage to the most metabolically active fetal tissues.

Evidence to support this hypothesis arises from a study examining the results of fetal blood sampling that occurred less than 24 hours before and then 24 hours after a single twin death in a series of 8 twins. The authors found that the majority of the pregnancies had no signs of anaemia prior to the twin demise, but that following the death samples taken from surviving twins all demonstrated significant anaemia [25].

14.4.2 Transchorionic Embolization

Transchorionic embolization describes the passage of thromboembolic material through vascular anastomosis in the placenta from the demised to the surviving twin following single intrauterine twin death in monochorionic pregnancies. Such material is thought to cause disseminated intravascular coagulation (DIC) and widespread damage to sensitive tissues within the surviving twin. Thrombo-occlusive disease has been noted in surviving twins either through MRI radiological investigation or at post-mortem [26]. However, many of these findings are thought to be secondary in nature and, currently the "transfusional" hypothesis remains the predominant theory to explain the increased morbidity and mortality that affects the monochorionic co-twin following single twin demise.

14.5 Pregnancy Associated Risks Following Single IU Fetal Death

14.5.1 Risk of Preterm Birth

The background risk of preterm birth is significantly higher for twin pregnancies compared with singleton pregnancies. Following single IU fetal death, there is an additional increased risk of early delivery for the remaining co-twin. The risk of preterm birth between 24 + 0 and 34 + 0 weeks gestation is defined in systematic review as non-significantly increased for monochorionic (58.5%) compared with dichorionic (53.7%) pregnancies [14]. The authors attempted to sub-analyse the relative proportions of spontaneous versus iatrogenic preterm birth from the data available. The data were limited but indicated that iatrogenic preterm birth appeared to occur more commonly in monochorionic pregnancies. This suggests a lower threshold for intervention and therefore an increased risk of delivery planning at an earlier gestational age in these pregnancies.

14.5.2 Risk of Maternal Infection, Hypertensive Disorders or Disseminated Intravascular Coagulation (DIC)

Maternal sepsis is a recognised sequelae following stillbirth in singleton pregnancies [27], and there are UK national guidelines regarding maternal management following late singleton stillbirth [12]. Studies reporting maternal outcomes in cases of single twin demise do not demonstrate an increased risk of maternal infection, but an increase in hypertensive disorders in pregnancy can be observed when compared to viable twin pregnancy controls [28, 29].

There is a small body of evidence to suggest that mothers of singleton pregnancies may be at risk of low serum fibrinogen levels or DIC following stillbirth [30]. This risk appears to increase with time following fetal loss by up to 10% after 4 weeks, but it does not appear to correlate with the degree of fetal maceration [30, 31]. There is no published evidence to suggest an increased risk of DIC for a mother of a twin pregnancy complicated by a single fetal loss.

14.5.3 Monochorionic Pregnancies: Risk of Co-twin Neurological Morbidity Following sIUFD

Due to the shared vasculature within the placental unit and the pathophysiological mechanisms described elsewhere in this chapter, monochorionic twins are at a unique risk of brain injury following in utero demise of a co-twin. This is evidenced by an increased incidence of macroscopic lesions and by an increased risk of neurodevelopmental morbidity.

Recent systematic review and meta-analysis of co-twin data for monochorionic pregnancies complicated by sIUFD demonstrated abnormal antenatal brain imaging in 20% of survivors [14]. A large multicentre retrospective observational study examined prenatal in utero magnetic resonance imaging (iuMRI) from monochorionic co-twin survivors with the aim of classifying the types of brain injury that occur [32]. Of 484 consecutive cases of sIUFD whereby iuMRI had been performed, the authors analysed 42 (9.7%) cases whereby abnormal brain imaging, other than simple ventriculomegaly, had been identified. For those with abnormal imaging, 22 pregnancies (52%) were complicated by TTTS of which 14 had undergone fetoscopic laser therapy and 4 cases had undergone selective termination of pregnancy. The median gestational age of sIUFD was 21 weeks and the median age at imaging was 23 weeks, with a median demise to imaging interval of 3 weeks. Cases were classified according to two broad groups: focal and non-focal brain abnormality. These groups were subdivided into haemorrhagic or non-haemorrhagic (focal), and periventricular leukomalacia, generalised encephalomalacia, posterior encephalomalacia or bilateral para-sagittal and peri-sylvian abnormality (non-focal). The study demonstrated that most brain imaging abnormalities occurred within the cerebral hemispheres, with a predominance towards non-focal lesions. Such non-focal brain abnormalities are more likely to have been produced via an acute transfusional mechanism, supporting the current view that this is the most likely pathophysiological mechanism of co-twin injury following sIUFD in monochorionic pregnancies [24]. Interestingly, the authors also noted a significantly greater proportion of pregnancies complicated by TTTS or that had undergone FLA had had focal lesions on brain imaging, leading to the speculative theory that thromboembolic events may contribute to brain injuries in these pregnancies.

Existing literature suggests that co-twin survivors of sIUFD are at significantly increased risk of neurodevelopmental abnormalities when compared to viable twin pregnancy controls. In cases of sIUFD, surviving twins are at greater risk of subsequent cerebral palsy (CP) than pregnancies where both twins survive, with an odds ratio for risk of CP of 6.3 (95% CI: 3.1–12.8) [33]. Again, chorionicity appears to be a key determinant of risk: epidemiological studies reviewing the rates of cerebral palsy for survivors in pregnancies affected by single twin demise, using same or different sex twin as a surrogate means of determining chorionicity, found a rate of CP of 106 per 1000 for same sex twins compared with 26 per 1000 for different sex twins [34].

More recent data from systematic review and meta-analysis reports event rates for neuro-developmental abnormality of 28.5% for monochorionic twins and 10% for dichorionic twins following sIUFD [14]. However, such figures must be viewed in the context of the high risk of premature birth for twin pregnancies in general and following IUFD, as prematurity can predispose towards or cause secondary neurological disability.

The incidence of non-febrile seizures is also increased for surviving twins of pregnancies complicated by sIUFD (5% for sIUFD compared with 0.8% where both twins survive), although studies examining differences in IQ as a measure of intellectual impairment have not demonstrated differences between co-twin survivors and viable twin controls [35].

A major risk factor for sIUFD monochorionic twins is TTTS. The treatment modality for this condition will influence the subsequent risk of neurological abnormality in surviving fetuses. Serial amnioreduction carries a higher risk (14–26%) of neuro-developmental delay in surviving neonates than fetoscopic laser therapy (4–18%). In pregnancies that have undergone FLA as treatment for TTTS, there appears to be no difference in the incidence of neuro-developmental deficiency (14–16%) in infants that are born twins or singleton survivors [36]. This suggests that closure of the vascular anastomoses protects co-twins from acute hypovolaemic sequelae associated with sIUFD. A similar moderation of risk is also proposed when sIUFD occurs following selective fetal reduction by cord occlusion in comparison to spontaneous demise. However, studies examining the use of FLA to treat type 3 sIUGR found that such treatment significantly increases the risk of fetal demise in the growth-restricted twin, and although laser treatment is protective of co-twin death in the surviving twin, there is presently insufficient data to determine overall rates of neurological abnormality in survivors [21].

14.5.4 Risk to Other Organ Systems in Monochorionic Pregnancies

Although neurological abnormality is the commonest and most well-described sequelae for surviving monochorionic co-twins in cases of sIUFD, other injuries that have been described include renal cortical necrosis, small bowel atresia, aplasia cutis and terminal limb infarction [26].

14.6 Pregnancy Management Following sIUFD

As with prognosis, the management of sIUFD is highly dependent on chorionicity and gestation. There remains a lack of a strong evidence base to guide clinicians in cases of sIUFD in multiple pregnancy, with recommendations being largely based on case reports, case studies and expert opinion. An approach to the management of such pregnancies, as suggested by the authors, is outlined in Fig. 14.1.

For multiple pregnancies complicated by sIUFD in the first trimester, there is minimal evidence to support significant ongoing risk to the remaining co-twin in mono- or dichorionic pregnancies other than an increased risk of miscarriage to the whole pregnancy; therefore, a conservative approach throughout the remaining natural pregnancy duration is warranted. For pregnancies complicated by

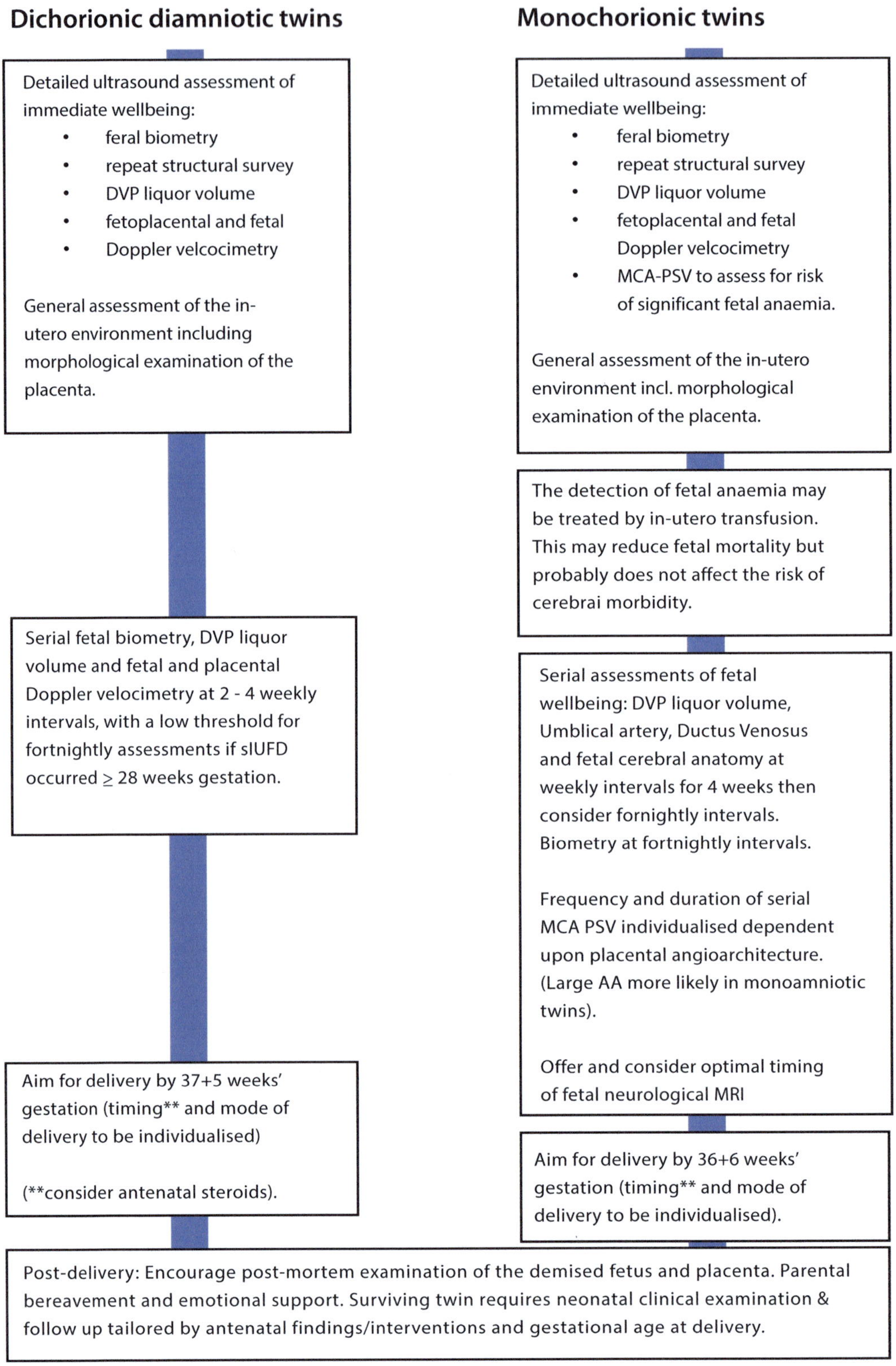

Fig. 14.1 Authors' suggested management approach for co-twin survivors in cases of single in utero fetal demise for both dichorionic and monochorionic pregnancies

sIUFD in the second and third trimester, subsequent management must be dictated by the chorionicity of the pregnancy.

14.6.1 Dichorionic Pregnancies

As fetuses of dichorionic twin pregnancies do not share a circulation, there is not an increased risk of antenatal neurological damage to the surviving co-twin. Thus, the most prominent risk faced by such pregnancies is preterm birth. Mothers should be sensitively counselled about the benefits and harms of iatrogenic preterm delivery. Although there are limited outcome data available for preterm twin pregnancies, it is recognised that for singleton pregnancies moderate to late preterm deliveries (32–36 weeks) can exhibit developmental delay at 2 years age when compared to full-term controls, and prior to 32 weeks there is an increased risk of both short- and long-term mortality from prematurity [37]. Therefore, in the absence of any evidence of in utero fetal compromise a sensible aim is to prolong the pregnancy to as near as possible 37 weeks gestation.

Regular surveillance of such pregnancies with ultrasonography to assess fetal growth, liquor volume and umbilical artery Doppler should be performed to ensure ongoing conservative management is of benefit to the developing fetus. This will additionally play a valuable role to support maternal psychological wellbeing.

Once sIUFD has been confirmed, rhesus-negative mothers should have a Keilhauer test taken, and an appropriate volume of anti-D administered to minimise risk of allo-immunisation. The mother should have close surveillance for hypertensive disorders of pregnancy and due to the increased risk of spontaneous preterm birth should be educated about the signs and symptoms of preterm labour and advised to present early for assessment if any concerns. Ideally the ongoing monitoring of her pregnancy should be provided though a dedicated specialised day care facility, allowing the mother to be cared for by a named multidisciplinary team to whom she can promptly self-refer with ease if she has any concerns such as reduced fetal movements.

The indication for other interventions, such as antenatal steroids to aid fetal lung maturity or magnesium sulphate for fetal neuroprotection, should be based on a critical assessment of optimal benefit and reduced potential harm. Thus, they are not indicated prophylactically following sIUFD but should be considered when preterm labour is suspected or preterm delivery is planned.

Vaginal delivery is not contraindicated in twin pregnancies where sIUFD has occurred and decisions regarding mode of delivery can be individualised in discussion with the woman once the above considerations have been taken into account. Although evidence is not available in the literature, if the demised twin is presenting, then there is the potential for intrapartum dystocia or obstruction to occur and delivery by caesarean section is typically preferred.

14.6.2 Monochorionic Pregnancies

In addition to the risks of preterm delivery, surviving co-twins of a monochorionic pregnancy complicated by sIUFD are at increased risk of stillbirth and neurological insult. Due to the complex nature of decision-making involving such pregnancies, referral to a specialist centre for further discussion, surveillance and management is recommended. The initial key clinical consideration is whether to manage such pregnancies conservatively or opt for immediate delivery. If conservative management is indicated, then further considerations include the intensity of antenatal fetal surveillance, whether it is beneficial to screen and treat the surviving fetus for anaemia, and how long to aim to prolong the pregnancy.

14.6.2.1 Prompt Delivery Versus Conservative Management in Monochorionic Pregnancies

Although it is known that the prognosis of the co-twin is adversely affected in monochorionic compared to dichorionic twin pregnan-

Study	Year	MC co-twin IUFD	MC no co-twin IUFD	DC co-twin IUFD	DC no co-twin IUFD	OR	(95%CI)
Cherouny	1989	0	8	0	4	0.50	(0.01, 30.16)
Fusi	1990	0	7	1	7	0.50	(0.01, 17.45)
Gaucherand	1994	0	6	0	2	0.33	(0.00, 23.00)
Ishimatsu	1994	0	12	0	3	0.25	(0.00, 15.37)
Kilby	1994	0	2	0	13	6.50	(0.10, 430.48)
Santema	1995	2	11	0	16	5.82	(0.24, 141.69)
Tordjeman	1996	0	2	0	8	4.00	(0.06, 270.79)
Sebire	1997	12	3	4	8	8.00	(1.40, 45.76)
Krayenbuhl	1998	0	12	0	7	0.58	(0.01, 32.79)
Axt	1999	0	4	0	2	0.50	(0.01,35.82)
Petersen	1999	0	4	0	6	1.50	(0.02, 92.25)
Bajoria	1999	13	37	1	41	14.41	(1.80, 115.53)
Malinowski	2000	0	1	0	5	5.00	(0.06, 436.52)
Malinowski	2003	0	3	0	9	3.00	(0.05, 186.90)
Baghdadi	2003	1	0	2	10	10.00	(0.24, 412.14)
Chelli	2009	0	9	1	18	1.00	(0.03, 32.71)
Mahony	2011	5	6	2	9	3.75	(0.54,26.04)
McPherson	2012	11	17	19	30	1.02	(0.39, 2.65)
Deveer	2013	0	9	0	16	1.78	(0.03, 97.46)
Overall (I^2 = 0.0%)						**2.06**	**(1.14, 3.71)**

NOTE: Weights are from random effects analysis

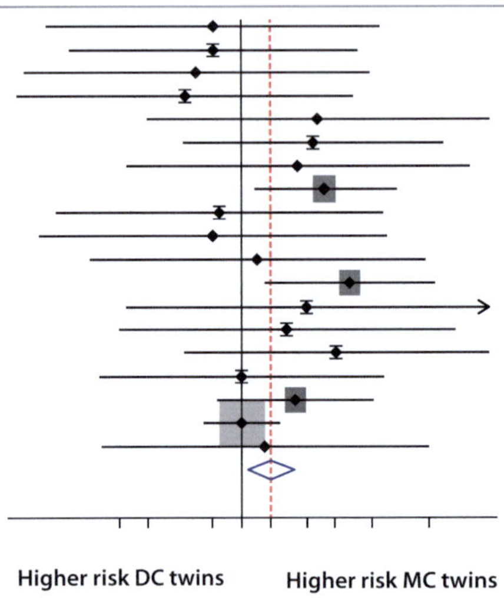

Fig. 14.2 Forest plot demonstrating risk of fetal demise for surviving co-twins following single in utero fetal death with comparison of monochorionic and dichorionic pregnancies. (Adapted from Mackie et al. [14])

cies following sIUFD (Table 14.1, Fig. 14.2), there is little evidence to guide the obstetrician as to whether immediate delivery is of benefit or harm. As discussed previously, there is a 41% risk of co-twin demise, and the precise timing of subsequent co-twin demise will rest on many factors that cannot be generalised to prognosticate for individual cases. However, a number of themes exist: cotwin demise appears more likely within a short time (within 7 days) of sIUFD, large placental vascular anastomoses predispose to adverse outcome (presumed in monoamniotic fetuses), and, although there is not a clear evidence base, detailed ultrasound assessment of the wellbeing of the surviving co-twin is the only available indicator as to whether the fetus is at imminent risk of loss.

In addition, little is known about the timing of neurological insult in monochorionic surviving co-twins following an acute transfusion response, and it is possible that subsequent co-twin end-organ damage may occur immediately following single twin demise. Therefore, immediate delivery may not have any value in reducing the risk of neurodevelopmental delay in surviving co-twins, even at advanced gestations.

The decision for immediate delivery versus conservative management upon diagnosis of sIUFD therefore rests on gestational age, presumed surviving fetal condition, maternal wellbeing and the obstetric lack of equipoise regarding the ongoing risk of in utero demise compared to the iatrogenic preterm delivery risks of neonatal mortality and morbidity.

14.6.2.2 Surviving Co-twin Immediate Assessment and Ongoing Monitoring in Monochorionic Pregnancies

Following diagnosis, sIUFD surviving monochorionic co-twins should have an urgent assessment of general fetal wellbeing to comprise biometry, liquor volume, umbilical artery and ductus venosus Doppler, and assessment for the risk of severe fetal anaemia via middle cerebral artery Doppler.

14.6.2.3 Assessment and Treatment of Fetal Anaemia

A case series of 20 monochorionic pregnancies complicated by sIUFD whereby middle cerebral artery peak systolic velocity (MCA-PSV) Doppler studies were performed on co-twin survivors, both before and after in utero fetal blood sampling and intrauterine transfusion (IUT), have demonstrated a strong correlation between MCA-PSV and pre- and post-transfusion haemoglobin concentration [38]. In a further case series reporting on pregnancy outcomes following IUT, all non-anaemic babies achieved normal outcomes, anaemic babies receiving intrauterine transfusion demonstrated improved survival but up to 30% of these babies had subsequent neurological abnormalities [39]. Surveillance of MCA PSV can therefore be recommended for surviving co-twins of monochorionic pregnancies complicated by sIUFD, from within 24 hours after sIUFD. Fetal blood sampling and delivery of IUT may be offered on the basis of abnormal MCA-PSV; however, it should be discussed with parents that although the evidence supports improved survival, it may not alter the neurological prognosis of these co-twins.

14.6.2.4 Ongoing Monitoring in Monochorionic Pregnancies

Regular fetal ultrasound should be performed to assess fetal growth, liquor volume and Doppler assessment of fetal wellbeing. Although there is no evidence to guide the frequency of these ultrasound assessments, weekly assessments are suggested by the authors for at least the first 4 weeks following sIUFD, and then, if reassuring, may be spaced to fortnightly intervals. Maternal anxieties must however be taken into consideration.

Previous literature has recommended weekly ultrasound assessment of the fetal brain to examine for signs of injury, a series of 121 MC pregnancies with sIUFD identified that 6 (4.9%) of pregnancies developed abnormal features on fetal brain ultrasound within 1–2 weeks of co-twin death [40]. The increased availability of intrauterine fetal brain MRI means that fetal brain ultrasound surveillance regimes can be tailored according to gestation of pregnancy, availability of resources and patient preferences as described below.

14.6.2.5 iuMRI of Fetal Brain

In cases of sIUFD for monochorionic twins, MRI has been demonstrated to identify 33% more brain lesions than can be demonstrated by fetal brain ultrasound alone [41]. The largest multicentre study examining antenatal iuMRI fetal brain changes in MC pregnancies following sIUFD demonstrated ventriculomegaly as the only intracranial finding in 3.4%, and other abnormalities in 9.7% of surviving twins [32]. Previously, it was suggested that surviving twin imaging should not be performed until 3 weeks following the death of the first twin to allow for the development of cavitating lesions. More recent evidence supports an assessment of brain damage to be performed with higher resolution single-shot fast-spin-echo T2-weighted MRI sequences from 7 days after fetal demise [32]; however, this may not be readily available.

If sIUFD occurred at an early gestation such that the original MRI was performed prior to 28 weeks and was normal, then consideration can be given to further MRI later in pregnancy to pick up neuronal migration disorders that may have been acquired [32]. If a brain lesion that may lead to neurodevelopmental morbidity is confirmed radiologically, the option of terminating the pregnancy should be discussed with the parents in a non-judgemental fashion.

14.6.3 Maternal Surveillance, Timing and Mode of Delivery in Monochorionic Pregnancies

As with sIUFD complicating dichorionic pregnancies, the mother should have assessment of fetal maternal haemorrhage and appropriate anti-D prophylaxis if Rhesus negative. Regular surveillance for an increased risk of hypertensive disorders, and counselling regarding the signs and symptoms of preterm labour should also occur.

Uncomplicated monochorionic twin pregnancies are advised to be delivered prior to

37 weeks gestation due to the accepted risks of stillbirth thereafter [42], but in a pregnancy already complicated by sIUFD, delivery is likely to be justified earlier, the precise timing individualised by the complex interplay of both obstetric and maternal concerns. Due to an increased risk of planned delivery by 34 weeks gestation, these pregnancies will have an increased likelihood of delivery by Caesarean section.

14.7 Post Delivery

Parents should be encouraged to consider the benefits of post-mortem and placental histology to investigate or help confirm the cause of single or double in utero death. Surviving neonates should be assessed for the need for neonatal and paediatric follow-up. Infants delivered preterm and those with known abnormal antenatal neurological findings should have specialised neuro-developmental follow-up. Parents should be offered a postnatal follow-up with a senior obstetrician, ideally the clinician managing their case prenatally. This discussion should cover what occurred during the pregnancy, review the results of any investigations, discuss any implications for future pregnancies and ensure that parents are managing emotionally and have multidisciplinary support in place. Loss of a twin is a devastating emotional experience for parents, and a couple can be at high risk of pre- and post-natal depression or pre-clinical emotional disturbance [43]. An awareness of previous risk factors and alerting parents to the presence of support and counselling services is important, and referral to peri-natal mental health services is necessary if depression has occurred.

14.8 Conclusion

The intrauterine death of one of the twins is an emotionally devastating event for parents. In addition to the careful counselling and management of the pregnancy from a perspective of fetal loss, there are special considerations with regard to the optimal management of the surviving co-twin. The management approach is largely dependent upon the chorionicity and gestation of the pregnancy, and a clinician must take these and other factors into account to apply an individualised plan for optimal surveillance, safe delivery and follow-up.

14.8.1 Review Questions

1. Describe the current UK trends in twin stillbirth rates and outline where potential limitations for data collection and analysis may occur.
2. List the recognised maternal and fetal factors predisposing to stillbirth in multiple pregnancy.
3. Describe how causes related to chorionicity or amnionicity contribute to stillbirth in multiple pregnancy.
4. Outline the proposed mechanisms used to explain the demise of co-twins following single twin demise monochorionic pregnancies.
5. Describe the variety of brain injuries seen to occur following single twin demise in monochorionic pregnancy.
6. Discuss an approach to management of co-twin survivors following single twin demise in
   (a) Dichorionic twin pregnancy
   (b) Monochorionic twin pregnancy

14.8.2 Multiple-Choice Questions

1. The UK twin stillbirth rate in 2017 was:
   (a) 11.74 per 1000 births.
   (b) 7.84 per 1000 births.
   (c) 6.16 per 1000 births.
   (d) 6.99 per 1000 births.
   (e) 6.51 per 1000 births.

Answer: (d)

2. Data regarding twin stillbirth rates included for UK surveillance reports may be influenced by the following factors:
   (a) Only twin losses from 20 weeks onwards are counted.
   (b) Some UK centres do not collect data.
   (c) Early surveillance and intervention for monochorionic twin pregnancies may influence later twin outcomes.
   (d) There is improved adherence to national guidance.
   (e) Losses are variably classified as stillbirths or miscarriages.

Answer: (c)

3. Regarding causes of fetal loss in twin pregnancy:
   (a) Risks of chromosomal anomaly are increased for mono- compared to dichorionic pregnancy.
   (b) Infectious causes of twin loss are increased in twin pregnancy compared to singletons.
   (c) Monoamniotic twin pregnancies have a loss rate of 40% in late gestations.
   (d) Fetoscopic laser ablation for twin-to-twin transfusion syndrome can be a cause of iatrogenic fetal loss.
   (e) Fetoscopic laser ablation as treatment for type 3 s-FGR has been clearly demonstrated to reduce single twin losses.

Answer: (d)

4. Regarding the risks to the surviving co-twin in cases of single in utero fetal demise:
   (a) Risks of subsequent preterm birth are 40% for dichorionic and 55% for monochorionic pregnancies.
   (b) Abnormal fetal brain MRI imaging may occur in up to 20% of dichorionic pregnancies.
   (c) Where subsequent lesions of the fetal brain occur in monochorionic pregnancies, they are more likely to be focal than diffuse.
   (d) Renal cortical necrosis is the most well described sequalae for monochorionic twin survivors.
   (e) Rates of neurodevelopmental abnormality may be as high as 28.5% for monochorionic twin survivors.

Answer: (e)

5. Regarding the management of twin pregnancies complicated by single in utero twin demise:
   (a) The optimal gestation for delivery of a surviving monochorionic twin is 34 weeks.
   (b) Urgent chorionicity assessment should be made if this has not already been defined.
   (c) Immediate delivery for the surviving co-twin is associated with reduced rates of cerebral palsy.
   (d) In utero fetal brain MRI may pick up to 50% more brain lesions than fetal brain ultrasound alone.
   (e) Post-mortem should be offered to parents only in selected circumstances.

Answer: (b)

Patient Testimonials

Fred and Magnus – Single Fetal Loss from a Parent's Perspective

14 June 2018. The house is a sea of blue, yellow and orange with all this birthday bunting and balloons. Magnus turns five today! While we're handing out chocolate cake and fruit juice to his class, Magnus is getting hugs from his friends. It's great to see how big he's growing. He also gets a big kiss on the cheek from his teacher.

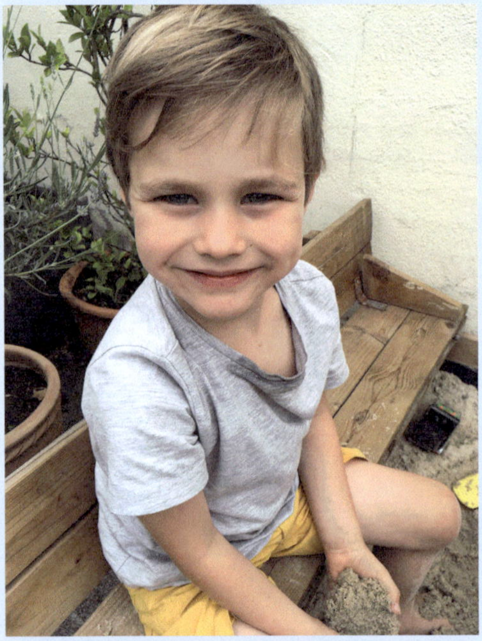

Magnus has brought in a book to show his classmates the pictures of his birth. Pictures of a tiny baby with red skin, full of wires and tubes in an incubator, with sunglasses to protect him from the light… His teacher looks surprised. She didn't know that Magnus was born so prematurely. When it comes to intelligence and coordination, she always thought he was completely normal, if not a little mature for his age, emotionally speaking. Secretly, I'm relieved that everything seems to be going well and we've not had any major issues.

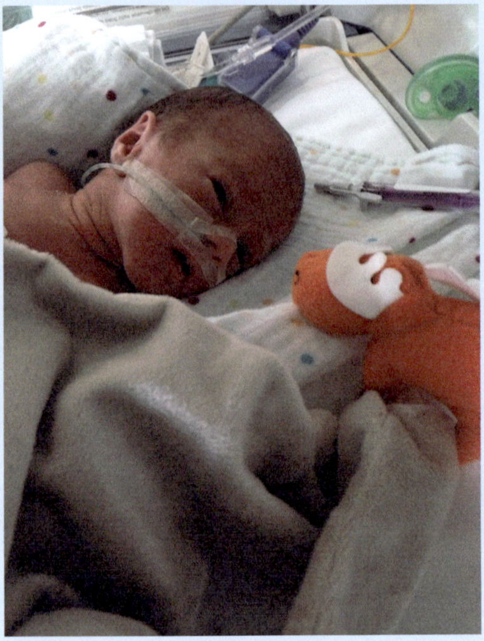

Magnus also tells his friends about Fred, his little brother who was in the tummy with him, but who passed away and is now a star up in the sky. He's telling the story in an easy and relaxed manner as if he's talking about the most normal thing in the world. When I look at him, I fill with pride, because he's had to fight hard, but he's turned into a big, smart, charming and honest child.

30 May 2013. I've been pregnant for 28 weeks with our twins. Until recently, my pregnancy was going smoothly, but over the last week or so, I'm finding it a bit trickier. I feel nauseous and bloated. The gynaecologist in Antwerp said I need to rest and take it easy for a while. It's a Friday afternoon, and David and I have just been to start our gift list. We've waited a long time to do so, because we were told several times in no uncertain terms that being pregnant with identical twins is always risky, especially in the first part of the term up to 26 weeks. Now that we've got past that milestone, it feels like a minor victory. After we're back from the shops, David sets off for

14

Brussels Airport. He's planned a trip with some of his friends before our twins will be taking up all of our energy and time. I'm due for my monthly check-up at the university hospital, so I set off as well. Even getting in and out of the car is getting a lot more difficult. My belly feels like a balloon that's about to burst.

At the university hospital, I'm examined by one of the assistants. He seems surprised at what he finds and immediately calls his supervisor. The latter is in no doubt: despite being in an advanced stage of my pregnancy, this is a clear case of twin-to-twin transfusion syndrome. Of course, the news comes as a shock to me. The only thing I can think of is what they told us at the information day: if you've got TTTS, doctors can perform laser surgery and there is a good chance that everything will be alright. Or that's how I remember it, at least. The doctor says that she'd like to perform laser surgery as soon as possible because both of my babies are severely ill and that I should ask David to come back from his holiday. Luckily, he isn't on the plane yet, so as soon as I tell him the news, he promises to hurry down to the hospital. I can tell from his voice that he's not overly worried either. It feels like we're both holding on to the hope that everything will be ok in the end, and that neither of us has realised just how serious the situation is.

With laser surgery, everything has to move quickly. I find myself in a sterile room with two doctors busy working on my belly. Suddenly, one of the doctors looks up in shock and says she's unable to detect any heartbeat in the donor baby, our tiny Fred.

For a moment, I'm left hoping I misheard her – perhaps I didn't want to hear her – but straightaway, she confirms my worst fear: that one of our babies suddenly passed away, and that she's shocked herself because this has never happened before.

I start crying and beg the doctor to tell David the news because I can't do it myself. I simply can't tell him that one of our babies has died. I think that somehow, I feel responsible: after all, it was me who was carrying them. Surely, I should have felt something earlier if they weren't doing well? Why did I not come to the sooner?

That same moment, David arrives at the hospital and runs through the corridors of the maternity ward, full of hope and saying hello to the nurses he encounters along the way. Afterwards, he said that he could already see it in their faces; in the way they didn't really make eye contact because they knew what he was about to find out.

As soon as the doctor tells him about Fred, David collapses. It breaks my heart to see him this way. The next few days are just awful. We need to process the biggest shock of our lives, but it feels unreal because I still look exactly the same and I'm still pregnant. Every now and then, we manage to forget for a while, but then it all hits us again. It's over. We are no longer having twins.

David returns to work 2 days later; he needs something to occupy his mind and the business he works for gives him exactly that.

I stay at the hospital because Magnus is still alive and needs constant monitoring as he's very sick. Aside from the regular check-ups, my days are filled with crying, falling asleep from pure exhaustion, waking up again and crying some more at all the well-wishes we've received. The room is full of flowers sent by friends, family and colleagues. I don't want to see anyone right now, apart from David and my mother. David is driving back and forth to the university hospital all the time. I keep thinking he must feel lonely on those trips.

Soon, the first of a series of hurtful situations occurs, such as a new person on the ward who is complaining all day just because the doctors have told her to lie flat, and concerned family members who want to remove the twin-things from our house to make things more bearable for me. But above all, there's love: in messages, in e-mails, from the doctor who came to see me late at night because I asked her to and from all the nurses on the ward.

The doctor says it would be good for me to go home, to see friends and to talk about what happened. But that's the last thing I want. I feel safe in these hospital surroundings, and

I'm terrified of losing Magnus as well without sensing that anything is wrong – yet again. But then, the doctors notice that the surgery has caused some membranes to detach that could choke Magnus' umbilical cord without me ever noticing. So, I end up staying in hospital after all. The tension starts to become unbearable: I really don't want to lose another baby inside me. I want to give birth. However, the doctors are adamant that I should wait until I'm 30 weeks in, to give Magnus the best chance of recovery from the transfusion syndrome. A few days before I reach week 30, it looks like the membranes are closing in around Magnus' umbilical cord, and the doctors decide to schedule a caesarean.

I give birth to a tiny, tiny baby. Magnus is perfect and starts crying immediately. The midwife briefly holds him to my face, but I have no idea what I should be feeling towards that little human. There's still too much sadness. Magnus is taken away immediately and placed in an incubator in the neonatal intensive care unit, on oxygen. David stays with him. He's extremely proud of his son.

Then, I give birth to a dead baby. Fred passed away 2 weeks ago and it's clear to see: his head is totally misshapen, but his hands and feet are perfect. I don't have the courage to hold him; something I regret to this day as I don't have a single photograph of my second son. What follows next is 54 days of travelling back and forth to the hospital. I stay with Magnus as much as possible, from early in the morning until late at night. The clockwork functioning of the neonatal intensive care unit is what I've started to rely on now, together with the love and sympathy of my sister who's a nurse on the unit where Magnus is being looked after. I pump breast milk, I help care for Magnus where I can, I give him hugs, and I don't give up.

In the meantime, Fred is cremated. David and I both say goodbye to him for the final time, and we wait on a bench outside until his ashes are ready to take home. The days are quiet and long.

More difficult moments follow: the certificate that suddenly confirms everything in black and white, the family composition document that no longer includes Fred (yes madam, because he passed away, right?), people close to you asking whether you'd like a second child (I already had two), people around you making it through their pregnancy without a care in the world (or so it seems, anyway) and sharing their great news with everyone who will listen.

In August, Magnus is finally ready to come home. We're both over the moon, but it's also difficult to say goodbye to the cocoon of safety offered by the hospital for the second time. We arrive at home with a baby who cries all the time and who we don't understand. Now, I know that he was crying for my attention; my full and undivided attention. Because at the time, my heart was still heavy with our loss. I spend more time thinking about Fred than about Magnus, and he can sense that. He's crying for me to put him first. I start to feel less and less sure of what I'm doing as a mother. For over 6 weeks, machines and nurses did something that I couldn't do as a mum, and something that should be the most ordinary thing in the world: care for my son. Once Magnus is home, I need to rediscover my maternal instinct, and I struggle to do so. It's a very unhappy period for both me and Magnus.

I get pregnant again soon. The doctor told me that a new pregnancy would offer comfort; that new life would bring happiness, and that's exactly what happens.

When Oscar is born, I suddenly realise what it's like to give birth without any worries and to feel nothing but love straightaway. At the same time, I still feel it's all very unfair, and I'm angry about what me, Magnus and David had to go through. It's only at that moment that I'm able to close the chapter of my first pregnancy.

We're 5 years on now, and I still hope from the bottom of my heart that Magnus is able to deal with it all now and in the future as well as I've been able to. Later, when he's older, I want to apologise to him once again for the difficult start we had and explain to him that I couldn't have done anything differently.

Magnus and Oscar are the best of friends, and I'm extremely happy with my beautiful family. That might sound like a cliché, but I really am. At the end of May every year, we pause to think about what happened and David and I go out for a meal or on a trip. The sadness is easing, but it will always be there, somewhere in the background.

Recently, friends of ours lost a baby early in their pregnancy. With our experience, we were able to support them through every step of the grieving process and they really appreciated that. It was good to see that everything we've been through wasn't for nothing.

References

1. Shek NW, Hillman SC, Kilby MD. Single-twin demise: pregnancy outcome. Best Pract Res Clin Obstet Gynaecol. 2014;28(2):249–63.
2. MBBRACE-UK. Perinatal mortality surveillance report. 2019. https://www.npeu.ox.ac.uk/mbrrace-uk/reports.
3. Kilby MD, Gibson JL, Ville Y. Falling perinatal mortality in twins in the UK: organisational success or chance? BJOG. 2019;126(3):341–7.
4. Hiersch L, Berger H, Okby R, Ray JG, Geary M, McDonald SD, et al. Incidence and risk factors for gestational diabetes mellitus in twin versus singleton pregnancies. Arch Gynecol Obstet. 2018;298(3):579–87.
5. Sibai BM, Hauth J, Caritis S, Lindheimer MD, MacPherson C, Klebanoff M, et al. Hypertensive disorders in twin versus singleton gestations. Am J Obstet Gynecol. 2000;182(4):938–42.
6. Antovic A, Sennström M, Bremme K, Svenungsson E. Obstetric antiphospholipid syndrome. Lupus Sci Med. 2018;5(1):e000197.
7. Smyth A, Oliveira GHM, Lahr BD, Bailey KR, Norby SM, Garovic VD. A systematic review and meta-analysis of pregnancy outcomes in patients with systemic lupus erythematosus and lupus nephritis. Clin J Am Soc Nephrol. 2010;5(11):2060–8.
8. Glinianaia SV, Rankin J, Wright C. Congenital anomalies in twins: a register-based study. Hum Reprod. 2008;23(6):1306 11.
9. Audibert F, Gagnon A, Genetics Committee of the Society of Obstetricians, Gynaecologists of Canada, Prenatal Diagnosis Committee of the Canadian College of Medical Geneticists. Prenatal screening for and diagnosis of aneuploidy in twin pregnancies. J Obstet Gynaecol Can. 2011;33(7):754–67.
10. Agarwal K, Alfirevic Z. Pregnancy loss after chorionic villus sampling and genetic amniocentesis in twin pregnancies: a systematic review. Ultrasound Obstet Gynecol. 2012;40(2):128–34.
11. RCOG. Management of monochorionic twin pregnancy: green-top guideline no. 51. BJOG. 2017;124(1):e1–e45.
12. RCOG. Late intrauterine fetal death and stillbirth: green top guideline no. 55. BJOG. 2010;124(1):e1–e33.
13. Pakrashi T, Defranco EA. The relative proportion of preterm births complicated by premature rupture of membranes in multifetal gestations: a population-based study. Am J Perinatol. 2013; 30(1):69–74.
14. Mackie FL, Rigby A, Morris RK, Kilby MD. Prognosis of the co-twin following spontaneous single intrauterine fetal death in twin pregnancies: a systematic review and meta-analysis. BJOG. 2019;126(5):569–78.
15. Lopriore E, Slaghekke F, Middeldorp JM, Klumper FJ, Oepkes D, Vandenbussche FP. Residual anastomoses in twin-to-twin transfusion syndrome treated with selective fetoscopic laser surgery: localization, size, and consequences. Am J Obstet Gynecol. 2009;201(1):66.e1–4.
16. Roberts D, Neilson JP, Kilby MD, Gates S. Interventions for the treatment of twin-twin transfusion syndrome. Cochrane Database Syst Rev. 2014;(1):CD002073.
17. Robyr R, Lewi L, Salomon LJ, Yamamoto M, Bernard JP, Deprest J, et al. Prevalence and management of late fetal complications following successful selective laser coagulation of chorionic plate anastomoses in twin-to-twin transfusion syndrome. Am J Obstet Gynecol. 2006;194(3):796–803.
18. Slaghekke F, Kist WJ, Oepkes D, Pasman SA, Middeldorp JM, Klumper FJ, et al. Twin anemia-polycythemia sequence: diagnostic criteria, classification, perinatal management and outcome. Fetal Diagn Ther. 2010;27(4):181–90.
19. Sueters M, Oepkes D. Diagnosis of twin-to-twin transfusion syndrome, selective fetal growth restriction, twin anaemia-polycythaemia sequence, and twin reversed arterial perfusion sequence. Best Pract Res Clin Obstet Gynaecol. 2014;28(2):215–26.
20. Gratacos E, Lewi L, Munoz B, Acosta-Rojas R, Hernandez-Andrade E, Martinez JM, et al. A classification system for selective intrauterine growth restriction in monochorionic pregnancies according to umbilical artery Doppler flow in the

smaller twin. Ultrasound Obstet Gynecol. 2007;30(1):28–34.
21. Gratacos E, Antolin E, Lewi L, Martinez JM, Hernandez-Andrade E, Acosta-Rojas R, et al. Monochorionic twins with selective intrauterine growth restriction and intermittent absent or reversed end-diastolic flow (type III): feasibility and perinatal outcome of fetoscopic placental laser coagulation. Ultrasound Obstet Gynecol. 2008;31(6):669–75.
22. Khalil A, Rodgers M, Baschat A, Bhide A, Gratacos E, Hecher K, et al. ISUOG practice guidelines: role of ultrasound in twin pregnancy. Ultrasound Obstet Gynecol. 2016;47(2):247–63.
23. Hillman SC, Morris RK, Kilby MD. Co-twin prognosis after single fetal death: a systematic review and meta-analysis. Obstet Gynecol. 2011;118(4):928–40.
24. Fusi L, McParland P, Fisk N, Nicolini U, Wigglesworth J. Acute twin-twin transfusion: a possible mechanism for brain-damaged survivors after intrauterine death of a monochorionic twin. Obstet Gynecol. 1991;78(3 Pt 2):517–20.
25. Nicolini U, Pisoni MP, Cela E, Roberts A. Fetal blood sampling immediately before and within 24 hours of death in monochorionic twin pregnancies complicated by single intrauterine death. Am J Obstet Gynecol. 1998;179(3 Pt 1):800–3.
26. Hillman SC, Morris RK, Kilby MD. Single twin demise: consequence for survivors. Semin Fetal Neonatal Med. 2010;15(6):319–26.
27. Jamal S, Agarwal S. IUFD incidence, causes and complications: a retrospective study done at a tertiary care centre in greater Noida, India. Int J Reprod Contracept Obstet Gynecol. 2017;6(12):5483–7.
28. Kilby MD, Govind A, O'Brien PM. Outcome of twin pregnancies complicated by a single intrauterine death: a comparison with viable twin pregnancies. Obstet Gynecol. 1994;84(1):107–9.
29. Santema JG, Swaak AM, Wallenburg HC. Expectant management of twin pregnancy with single fetal death. Br J Obstet Gynaecol. 1995;102(1):26–30.
30. Parasnis H, Raje B, Hinduja IN. Relevance of plasma fibrinogen estimation in obstetric complications. J Postgrad Med. 1992;38(4):183–5.
31. Muin DA, Haslacher H, Koller V, Kiss H, Scharrer A, Farr A. Impact of fetal maceration grade on risk of maternal disseminated intravascular coagulation after intrauterine fetal death – a retrospective cohort study. Sci Rep. 2018;8(1):12742.
32. Conte G, Righini A, Griffiths PD, Rustico M, Lanna M, Mackie FL, et al. Brain-injured survivors of monochorionic twin pregnancies complicated by single intrauterine death: MR findings in a multicenter study. Radiology. 2018; 288(2):582–90.
33. Bonellie SR, Currie D, Chalmers J. Comparison of risk factors for cerebral palsy in twins and singletons. Dev Med Child Neurol. 2005;47(9):587–91.
34. Pharoah PO, Adi Y. Consequences of in-utero death in a twin pregnancy. Lancet. 2000;355(9215):1597–602.
35. Nelson KB, Ellenberg JH. Childhood neurological disorders in twins. Paediatr Perinat Epidemiol. 1995;9(2):135–45.
36. Graef C, Ellenrieder B, Hecher K, Hackeloer BJ, Huber A, Bartmann P. Long-term neurodevelopmental outcome of 167 children after intrauterine laser treatment for severe twin-twin transfusion syndrome. Am J Obstet Gynecol. 2006;194(2):303–8.
37. Cheong JL, Doyle LW, Burnett AC, Lee KJ, Walsh JM, Potter CR, et al. Association between moderate and late preterm birth and neurodevelopment and social-emotional development at age 2 years. JAMA Pediatr. 2017;171(4):e164805.
38. Senat MV, Loizeau S, Couderc S, Bernard JP, Ville Y. The value of middle cerebral artery peak systolic velocity in the diagnosis of fetal anemia after intrauterine death of one monochorionic twin. Am J Obstet Gynecol. 2003;189(5):1320–4.
39. Tanawattanacharoen S, Taylor MJ, Letsky EA, Cox PM, Cowan FM, Fisk NM. Intrauterine rescue transfusion in monochorionic multiple pregnancies with recent single intrauterine death. Prenat Diagn. 2001;21(4):274–8.
40. O'Donoghue K, Rutherford MA, Engineer N, Wimalasundera RC, Cowan FM, Fisk NM. Transfusional fetal complications after single intrauterine death in monochorionic multiple pregnancy are reduced but not prevented by vascular occlusion. BJOG. 2009;116(6):804–12.
41. Jelin AC, Norton ME, Bartha AI, Fick AL, Glenn OA. Intracranial magnetic resonance imaging findings in the surviving fetus after spontaneous monochorionic cotwin demise. Am J Obstet Gynecol. 2008;199(4):398.e1–5.
42. Cheong-See F, Schuit E, Arroyo-Manzano D, Khalil A, Barrett J, Joseph KS, et al. Prospective risk of stillbirth and neonatal complications in twin pregnancies: systematic review and meta-analysis. BMJ. 2016;354:i4353.
43. Druguet M, Nuno L, Rodo C, Arevalo S, Carreras E, Gomez-Benito J. Emotional effect of the loss of one or both fetuses in a monochorionic twin pregnancy. J Obstet Gynecol Neonatal Nurs. 2018;47(2):137–45.

Key Reading

Conte G, Righini A, Griffiths PD, Rustico M, Lanna M, Mackie FL, et al. Brain-injured survivors of monochorionic twin pregnancies complicated by single intrauterine death: MR findings in a multicenter study. Radiology. 2018;288(2):582–90.

Glinianaia SV, Rankin J, Wright C. Congenital anomalies in twins: a register-based study. Hum Reprod. 2008;23(6):1306–11.

Kilby MD, Gibson JL, Ville Y. Falling perinatal mortality in twins in the UK: organisational success or chance? BJOG. 2019;126(3):341–7.

Mackie FL, Rigby A, Morris RK, Kilby MD. Prognosis of the co-twin following spontaneous single intrauterine fetal death in twin pregnancies: a systematic review and meta-analysis. BJOG. 2019;126(5):569–78.

Complications Unique to Monochorionic Twin Pregnancies

Contents

Twin-Twin Transfusion Syndrome

Christian Bamberg and Kurt Hecher

Contents

Electronic Supplementary Material The online version of this chapter (https://doi.org/10.1007/978-3-030-47652-6_15) contains supplementary material, which is available to authorized users. The videos can be accessed by scanning the related images with the SN More Media App.

A. Khalil et al. (eds.), *Twin and Higher-order Pregnancies*,
https://doi.org/10.1007/978-3-030-47652-6_15

Trailer

Twin-twin transfusion syndrome (TTTS) is a severe complication that affects 10–15% of monochorionic multiple pregnancies. It is caused by an imbalanced blood flow through communicating placental vessels on the chorionic surface between the donor and recipient twin circulations. Regarding treatment, evidence demonstrates that fetoscopic laser ablation is superior to serial amnioreductions in terms of survival and neurological outcome for stage II to stage IV TTTS. However, the optimal management of stage I TTTS remains controversial. It is well established that all chorionic plate anastomoses should be closed by laser. Compared to the selective laser method, the Solomon technique yields a significant reduction of recurrent TTTS and post-laser twin anemia-polycythemia sequence (TAPS). Over the past 25 years, survival rates after fetoscopic laser surgery have significantly increased. High-volume centers report up to 70% double survival, and >90% survival of at least one twin after laser treatment of TTTS. About 10% of laser surgery survivors exhibit long-term neurodevelopmental delay. In this chapter, we discuss TTTS pathophysiology, diagnosis, and optimal treatment, as well as long-term outcomes after laser intervention.

Definitions

Monochorionicity: Sharing of a single placenta. Almost all cases have vascular anastomoses between the fetal umbilical circulations, which is the prerequisite for the development of TTTS.

Twin-twin transfusion syndrome: A severe complication of monchorionic twins with imbalanced blood flow between the two twins (donor to recipient). Fetoscopic laser surgery is the treatment of choice.

Quintero staging:

Stage	Poly-/oligohy-dram-nios	Non-visible blad-der in donor	Severely abnormal Doppler findings in umbilical artery and/or ductus venosus	Hydrops
I	+	–	–	–
II	+	+	–	–
III	+	+	+	–
IV	+	+	+	+

Solomon technique: Represents modification of fetoscopic laser surgery. After coagulation of all visible anastomoses, a thin laser line is drawn along the vascular equator from one edge of the placenta to the other one.

Learning Objectives

- Women carrying an MC pregnancy should be informed about the clinical symptoms of TTTS: rapid increase of uterine size, preterm contractions, and back pain.
- Every MC twin pregnancy should be monitored by ultrasound fortnightly for timely TTTS diagnosis.
- Amniotic fluid discordance is the basic ultrasound criteria for TTTS.
- Fetoscopic laser surgery is the first-line treatment for severe TTTS, as it shows evidence-based effectiveness and addresses the underlying cause.
- Centralization of intrauterine surgery is recommended since laser surgery at high-volume fetal medicine centers yields the highest survival rates.
- The Solomon technique is a promising method, but larger studies regarding complications and long-term follow-up are needed.

15

15.1 Introduction

Twin-twin transfusion syndrome (TTTS) is a serious complication that occurs in approximately 10–15% of monochorionic (MC) multiple pregnancies. MC twins share a single placenta, which almost always exhibits vascular anastomoses on the chorionic surface (◘ Fig. 15.1). This connection between fetal umbilical circulations is the fundamental prerequisite for the development of TTTS, which is essentially a chronic blood transfusion from the donor twin to the recipient twin. There are three different types of anastomoses: arterio-venous, arterio-arterial, and veno-venous. The type, number, and diameter of these anastomoses determine the risk profile for TTTS development [1]. TTTS usually occurs between the 16th and 26th completed gestational week [2]. Among MC placentas, arterio-arterial anastomoses with bidirectional blood flow between the two cord insertions are reportedly significantly less frequent in TTTS cases (47%) compared to uncomplicated MC pregnancies (96%) [3]. Furthermore, compared to uncomplicated MC pregnancies, the artery-to-artery connections in TTTS placentas exhibit a significantly thinner median diameter and more central location. These findings emphasize the unique role of MC placentation in TTTS development. In this chapter, the authors discuss TTTS pathophysiology, diagnosis, and optimal treatment, as well as long-term outcome after laser intervention, inspired by our previously published review [4].

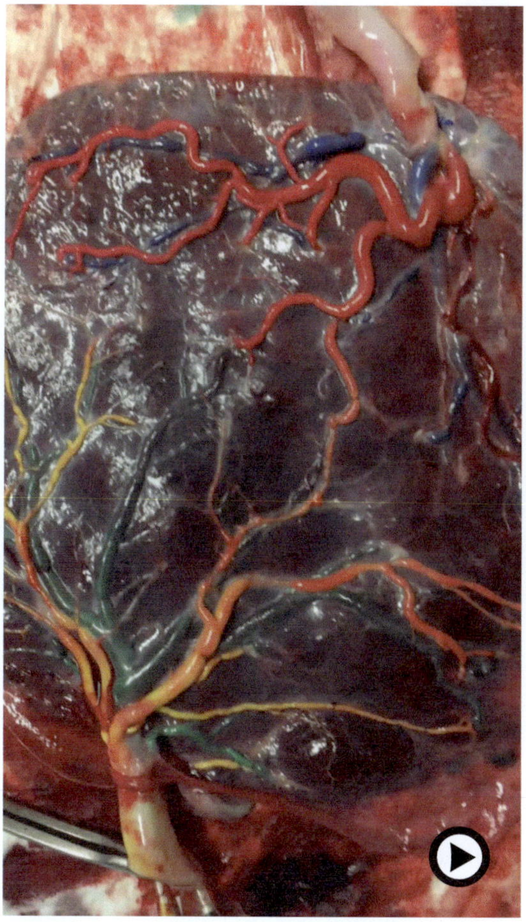

◘ **Fig. 15.1** Colour-dye-stained monochorionic twin placenta after an umcomplicated pregnancy course. Red and yellow dye was used to stain the arteries, and blue and green dye was used to stain the veins (https://doi.org/10.1007/000-2te)

15.2 Diagnosis of TTTS

From a practical point of view, symptoms of TTTS may include sudden maternal abdominal swelling disproportionate to the gestational age, combined with abdominal discomfort, back pain, tense uterus, and contractions. These symptoms are caused by the increased amount of amniotic fluid in the recipient twin's sac. Healthcare providers should inform mothers about these symptoms and should immediately perform an ultrasound examination if they are reported. TTTS is generally diagnosed by sonography, and all MC pregnancies should be screened by ultrasound biweekly starting at a gestational age of 16 weeks [5]. Delayed detection is associated with worse perinatal outcome of TTTS. The main sonographic finding in cases of TTTS is a wide discordance in the amount of fluid between amniotic sacs. The recipient fetus exhibits a polyuric polyhydramnios, defined as a deepest vertical pocket of >8 cm before 20 weeks and of >10 cm after 20 weeks of gestation. In contrast, the donor fetus displays oligo- or anhydramnios, with a deepest vertical pocket of <2 cm, and becomes stuck to the uterine wall or placenta due to the recipient twin's polyhydramnios (◘ Fig. 15.2).

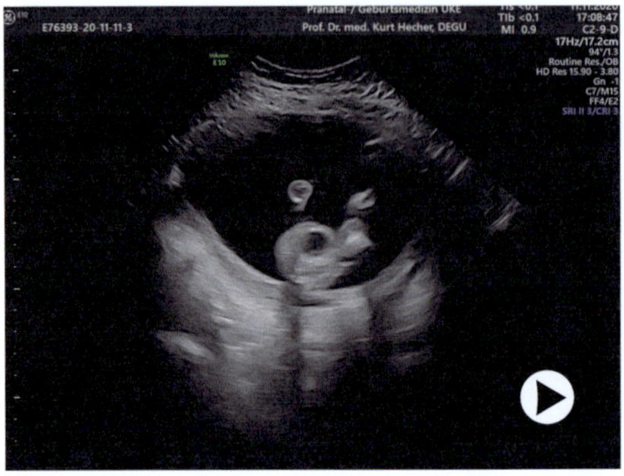

Fig. 15.2 Ultrasound image of a pregnancy with twin-twin transfusion syndrome stage II at 17 weeks of gestation. the donor is stuck to the right, whereas there is polyhydramnios in the recipient on the left (https://doi.org/10.1007/000-2tf)

There are several pitfalls in amniotic fluid evaluation. Sometimes the donor fetus may be wrapped within its membranes and free floating in the polyhydramnios of the recipient twin (cocoon sign). Additionally, the single largest vertical pocket should be measured free from fetal extremities or umbilical cord and may vary in relation to uterus tone. The probe should be gently positioned on the maternal abdomen, perpendicular to the longitudinal axis of the uterus and without tilting. The above-mentioned amniotic fluid cut-off values were defined by the Eurofoetus group. In the USA, most fetal medicine specialists use a cutoff of 8 cm regardless of gestational age. Khalil recently suggested a modification of the diagnostic criteria for TTTS prior to 18 weeks of gestation [6]. Based on a recent investigation of the amniotic fluid volume in MC twins from the first trimester until delivery, a deepest vertical pocket of >6 cm may be a more sensitive cut-off value than >8 cm before 18 weeks of gestation [7]. The researchers found that from 16 to 17 weeks of gestation, a deepest vertical pocket of >6 cm represented the 90th centile, while >7 cm the 97.5th centile. However, it must be noted that in cases with an anterior placenta and a deepest pool of <8 cm, complete laser coagulation along the entire vascular equator may be difficult to perform or non-feasible.

Importantly, TTTS may be superimposed with selective intrauterine growth restriction (sIUGR) or anemia in the donor twin and polycythemia in the recipient twin. First-trimester prenatal ultrasound criteria can be used to estimate the risk of TTTS development—including inter-twin discordance of crown rump length >10%, nuchal translucency over the 95th centile in one or both fetuses, and abnormal ductus venosus flow velocity waveforms—however, these parameters show poor positive predictive values [8, 9]. Focusing on the umbilical coiling index in TTTS cases, we have performed a prospective study using three-dimensional ultrasound with color Doppler imaging of the umbilical cord in untreated TTTS cases [10]. On the day of laser surgery, the coiling index could be quantified in 65 recipients and 56 donors, and the mean coiling index was significantly higher in recipient twins than in donors. This discordance of umbilical cord coiling in TTTS may reflect the recipient's hypervolemia and the donor's hypovolemia. Further investigation is required to evaluate whether inter-twin first trimester coiling index discordance may be useful as an early TTTS predictor.

15.3 Classification and Staging of TTTS

TTTS staging is most frequently performed according to Quintero [11]. Briefly, at all stages, polyhydramnios is present in the recipient and oligo/anhydramnios in the donor. The donor's bladder is visible at stage I and cannot be seen at stage II. Stage III is characterized by critical abnormal Doppler findings, including absent or reversed end-diastolic flow in the umbilical artery and negative A-wave in the ductus venosus. In stage IV, one or both twins become hydropic. The Quintero staging system was developed for a heterogeneous and dynamic clinical entity, which remains the most frequently used system due to its simplicity.

The Quintero staging system also has a variety of limitations. For instance, a donor twin with a visible bladder may have abnormal Doppler findings, and a recipient twin can show signs of heart failure even at an early TTTS stage. Wohlmuth and coworkers reviewed the fetal cardiovascular hemodynamics in TTTS [12], showing that up to 70% of recipients show echocardiographic signs of anatomical or functional cardiac compromise, while donor twins typically exhibit normal cardiac parameters. The Quintero staging system does not represent the chronological order of deterioration in all cases—for example, intrauterine fetal demise may occur at stage I. Moreover, in some cases with rapid progression, the donor twin may exhibit bladder filling even though the recipient is hydropic.

Regarding the distinguishing factor of a filled bladder of the donor twin, its visualization often depends on the duration of examination [13]. Small bladder filling without dynamic changes indicates an absence of voiding due to an inadequate blood supply to the fetal kidneys [14]. This particular aspect of TTTS stage I pregnancies will be addressed in the following chapter.

15.4 Natural History and Treatment of TTTS

Untreated TTTS pregnancies carry an 80–90% risk of perinatal mortality due to intrauterine fetal death, miscarriage, or extremely preterm delivery [15]. The results of a systematic review and meta-analysis revealed a 27% incidence of progression from stage I to more advanced stages. At stage I, many fetal surgeons offer expectant management and close surveillance to avoid unnecessary interventions. The pooled overall survival was 79% with expectant treatment, 77% with amnioreduction, 68% with laser treatment following progression, and 84% with laser treatment as the first-line choice [16].

A multicenter RCT was conducted to compare expectant management versus immediate laser surgery for stage I cases [17]. Women diagnosed with TTTS between 16+0 and 26+6 weeks of gestation were randomly assigned to primary laser treatment or conservative management, with weekly ultrasound follow-up. In the conservative management group, laser treatment was performed in cases that progressed to stage II or higher, in which severe maternal discomfort occurred due to polyhydramnios or in cases that exhibited cervical shortening to <15 mm. The primary outcome was overall intact survival at 6 months after birth. Recently, this study was prematurely completed after 117 inclusions. Intact survival was seen in 84 of 109 (77%) expectant cases and in 89 of 114 (78%) immediate surgery cases ($p = 0.88$). In patients followed expectantly, 41% remained stable with a dual intact survival of 86%, whereas it was 78% and 71% following immediate or rescue surgery, respectively, although these differences were not statistically significant. The authors could not identify any meaningful predictors of progression.

15.5 Fetoscopic Laser Surgery Versus Serial Amnioreduction

Evidence clearly shows that in severe TTTS cases, fetoscopic laser coagulation of placental vascular anastomoses is superior to serial amniodrainages. Senat and coworkers conducted a multicenter RCT comparing fetoscopic laser therapy with serial amnioreductions in cases of TTTS between 15 and 26 weeks of gestation. Compared to serial amnioreductions, fetoscopic laser therapy resulted in higher survival of at least one twin, higher gestational age at delivery, and better neurological outcomes at all stages, likely because laser therapy addresses the cause of TTTS [18, 19].

The goal of fetoscopic laser intervention is to ablate all inter-twin connections. However, this raises the question of whether all connecting vessels can be identified by eye [20]. After standard fetoscopic laser treatment, up to 33% of placentas exhibited residual anastomoses [21]. Therefore, a modified laser method called the Solomon technique was introduced. In this method, anastomoses are identified and coagulated, and then a laser line is drawn from one placenta margin to the other, with the aim of ablating the entire vascular equator and minimizing the risk of residual anastomoses (◘ Fig. 15.3). A multicenter European RCT compared the conventional selective laser method ($n = 135$) with the Solomon technique ($n = 139$) [22]. The results

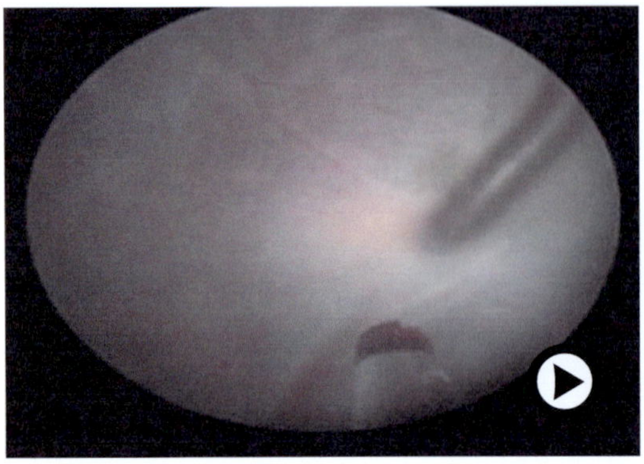

Fig. 15.3 Fetoscopic images of laser coagulation of the vascular anastomoses of twin-twin transfusion syndrome followed by drawing a laser line from one placental margin to the other, with the aim of ablating the entire vascular equator and minimizing the risk of residual anastomoses (Solomon technique) (https://doi.org/10.1007/000-2tg)

showed that the Solomon technique was associated with significant reductions of recurrent TTTS (1% vs 7%) and post-laser twin anemia-polycythemia sequence (TAPS) (3% vs 16%), while the two groups did not significantly differ in perinatal mortality or severe neonatal morbidity. The authors recommended that fetal surgeons should consider applying the Solomon technique in the absence of any identifiable adverse complication. A secondary analysis of the trial revealed a significant reduction ($p = 0.04$) of residual anastomoses with the Solomon technique (19%; 14/74) compared to the standard method (34%; 26/77) [23]. Within the subgroup of cases in which the surgeon reported that laser surgery was complete, an even larger reduction of residual anastomoses was found: 12% in the Solomon group compared to 32% in the standard group ($p < 0.01$). However, despite the significant reduction with the Solomon technique, residual anastomoses are still present, necessitating careful ultrasound follow-up.

Although the procedure time was identical between Solomon treatment and standard laser treatment, the total amount of laser energy used was approximately twofold higher with Solomon treatment (9275 J vs 4933 J; $p < 0.0001$). This prompts concerns about whether it is warranted to expose the healthy placental tissue between anastomoses and laser treatment, resulting in an increased extent of placental injury [24]. A retrospective study compared 287 cases treated with selective laser coagulation to 86 cases treated after introduction of the Solomon procedure [25]. Perinatal survival was significantly higher after Solomon treatment compared to that after the selective procedure (77% vs 54%, $p < 0.001$). However, the Solomon treatment group showed a significantly increased risk of placental abruption compared with the selective group (14% vs 3%, OR 13.5, 95% CI 3.7–49.2). The authors concluded that this may have been due to the more extensive tissue damage of the thinner areas at the placenta edges with the Solomon procedure. At our center, we apply a partial Solomon technique in which we coagulate an area of neighboring anastomoses along the vascular equator, to avoid unnecessarily damaging placental tissue in areas where there are no detectable vessels at all.

Irrespective of the utilized laser technique, the procedure should be performed under local anesthesia. The fetoscope should enter the sac of the recipient under ultrasound guidance, ideally directed perpendicular to the longitudinal axis of the donor and between both cord insertions. With this setup, it is very likely that the entire vascular equator can be visualized. After identifying the inter-twin membrane with crossing anastomotic vessels (placental mapping), the inter-twin communications will be closed using an Nd:YAG or a diode laser. At the end of the procedure, amniotic fluid should be drained until achieving a normal fluid level (5–6 cm).

Some evidence suggests that laser treatment in TTTS at a gestational age of <16 weeks or >26 weeks is feasible and safe and may improve perinatal outcome [26, 27]. However, only 2.5% of all TTTS patients are affected before 16 weeks of gestation. In such cases, the perinatal outcome after conventional laser therapy is comparable to that between 16 and 26 weeks; there is an increased risk of PPROM within 1 week after laser treatment and a hypothetical chance of spontaneous regression. The prevalence of TTTS after a gestational age of 26 weeks is

4–8%. In such cases, laser therapy can lead to delayed delivery and recovery of both twins in utero and a trend of better neonatal outcome. The fetal surgeon must be prepared for the possible presence of turbid amniotic fluid and the increased difficulty of coagulating larger placental vessels in cases treated after 26 weeks [28].

15.6 Complications of Fetoscopic TTTS Treatment

Fetoscopic laser treatment is an invasive procedure with several non-negligible risks. One complication of selective laser photocoagulation for TTTS treatment is postoperative membrane separation, which has been associated with an increased risk of preterm rupture of membranes and consequently with a higher risk of preterm delivery before 32 weeks [29]. Using an optimal point of entry for the fetoscope is very important for systematically examining the placental surface along the entire length of the inter-twin membrane but may be challenging in cases with an extensive anterior placenta. Chmait et al. recently demonstrated that trocar insertion, particularly in the lateral lower uterine segment, was associated with an increased risk of preterm rupture of membranes within 21 days after the procedure [30]. Research has been focused on the prevention of complications, such as iatrogenic preterm rupture of membranes, and consequent miscarriage and preterm birth, which are also complications of TTTS itself. To date, iatrogenic fetal membranes damage seems to be the "Achilles heel" of operative fetoscopy.

Fetoscopy performed by an experienced specialist is considered safe for the mother. In a multicenter review of maternal complications following fetoscopic laser photocoagulation for TTTS, the total rate of adverse events was 5.4% and the total rate of severe complications was 1.0% [31]. Recently, Sacco et al. summarized the outcome of 9403 fetoscopic surgery patients and reported a ~2% rate of severe maternal complications and a ~4% rate of minor complications [32].

15.7 Outcomes After Laser Treatment for TTTS

15.7.1 Perinatal Survival

In 2015, a systematic review was published that included 25 years of fetoscopic laser coagulation for TTTS [33]. The authors summarized the outcomes of 3868 women from 34 studies and highlighted the large variations in caseloads and outcomes among different fetal medicine centers. Over the time period, the mean survival of both twins significantly increased from 35% to 65%, and the mean survival of at least one twin significantly increased from 70% to 88%. For the entire series, the mean gestational age at birth was 32.4 ± 1.3 weeks.

We recently published the largest single-center experience with laser coagulation [34]. Our analysis included the perinatal outcomes of 1020 consecutive pregnancies with severe mid-gestational TTTS and had a follow-up rate of nearly 100% (1019/1020). During the study period (January 1995 to March 2013), the yearly caseload more than doubled from 43 to 91 patients. The rate of fetal survival of both twins significantly increased from 50% in the first group of 200 cases to 69.5% in the last group of 220 cases ($p = 0.018$) and reached a plateau after 600 procedures. The rate of at least one twin surviving showed a non-significant trend of increase from 80.5% to 91.8% ($p = 0.072$). The mean gestational age at delivery with at least one liveborn was 33.7 ± 3.2 weeks. The introduction of 30° scopes with a special mechanism to deflect the laser fiber for anterior placentas occurred in 2001, after which the double-survival rate was independent from placental location.

Furthermore, from a prognostic point of view and based on our own results, it seems reasonable to summarize cases as stage I/II and III/IV [35]. The double survival rate was significantly higher (75% vs 62%) at stages I and II vs stages III and IV in our most recent study group.

We concluded that double survival rates were improved by the concentration of laser treatment at national and international specialized high-volume fetal medicine centers. This success was attributed to technical developments and the provision of hands-on training supervised by an experienced team. These results are in agreement with the findings of Stirnemann and colleagues [36], who presented the follow-up of 1017/1092 cases (93%) following TTTS treatment with percutaneous fetoscopic laser between 2000 and 2016. They reported 84% overall survival of at least one twin and 53% survival of both twins. During their study period, the rate of dual survival increased from 42% to 66%, highlighting the improvement in perinatal outcomes. They found that a gestational age of <17 weeks at the time of surgery was a significant risk factor for PPROM.

15.7.2 Neurodevelopment

Another important aspect of TTTS is neurodevelopmental follow-up among survivors after fetoscopic laser surgery. Approximately 2% of such patients exhibit fetal brain lesions (equally distributed between donors and recipients), which may be ischemic or hemorrhagic [37]. Significant risk factors include recurrent TTTS and post-laser TAPS following incomplete laser surgery. Schou et al. investigated children at 2 years of age after fetoscopic laser surgery for TTTS [38]. Among 86 children, 9 (10.5%) exhibited severe neurodevelopment impairment, such as cerebral palsy, bilateral blindness and/or deafness, and severe cognition and/or motor delay. Importantly, follow-up studies of TTTS cases treated with laser surgery have reported varying rates of cerebral palsy and neurodevelopment impairment, possibly due to differences in methodology, heterogeneity within small case series, and lack of uniform criteria regarding outcome. A review of 13 studies reported a 6.1% prevalence of cerebral palsy and a 9.8% prevalence of neurodevelopmental impairment [39]. Preterm delivery was an independent risk factor for neurodevelopmental impairment after laser treatment [40]. Other important risk factors included increased gestational age at intervention, higher Quintero stage, perinatal severe cerebral injury, and low birthweight [41, 42].

15.7.3 Cardiovascular System

Congenital heart defects are more frequent among twins with TTTS compared to uncomplicated MC twins and singletons. Cohort studies have examined the prevalence of heart disease in children after laser therapy for TTTS. Herberg and coworkers analyzed 62 survivors at the age of 10 years and found that 6 (9.7%) exhibited structural heart defects [43]. The main finding was pulmonary stenosis, which was detected in five cases, including both former recipient and donor twins. We recently published a detailed review of long-term outcomes for MC twins after laser therapy for TTTS, which includes neurodevelopmental and cardiovascular outcomes, growth, renal function, and ischemic events [44].

15.8 TTTS in Monoamniotic Twins and Triplets

TTTS rarely develops in monoamniotic twin pregnancies (6% prevalence) [45] due to the abundant anastomoses between the two placental shares and the close umbilical cord insertions. Monoamniotic TTTS cases exhibit polyhydramnios in the common amniotic sac. In such cases, the donor twin exhibits absent or tiny fetal bladder filling, while the recipient twin displays an oversized urinary bladder.

Monochorionic triplets may also develop TTTS, and such cases should be treated with laser intervention. Among triplet pregnancies, 75% are dichorionic triamniotic. In monochorionic diamniotic or triamniotic

15

triplet pregnancies, the number of donors and recipients varies depending on the placental architecture. The fetal surgeon may enter two sacs to have access to all anastomoses. A dichorionic sac should not be touched during laser surgery.

We retrospectively analyzed the outcomes of 20 triplet pregnancies (16 dichorionic triamniotic and 4 monochorionic triamniotic pregnancies) with severe TTTS that were treated at our center [46]. Fetoscopy was performed in 18 cases, at a median gestational age of 19.7 weeks. Cesarean delivery was performed in all cases, at a median gestational age of 31.9 weeks. The overall perinatal survival rate was 65%. Survival of at least one fetus was achieved in 83% of cases, survival of at least two fetuses in 72%, and survival of all three triplets in 39%.

D'Antonio and coworkers summarized the perinatal outcomes of triplets after laser treatment for TTTS. Their analysis included eight studies and a total of 126 triplet pregnancies (104 dichorionic triamniotic and 22 monochorionic triamniotic pregnancies) [47]. In general, these pregnancies carried high risks of fetal and perinatal loss, and preterm birth. The perinatal outcomes are summarized in ◘ Table 15.1.

15.9 Conclusion

In conclusion, TTTS occurs due to unbalanced blood shunting between MC multiples across placental vascular connections. The treatment of choice is fetoscopic laser coagulation of the anastomoses. Some evidence suggests that laser interventions for TTTS at a gestational age of <16 weeks and >26 weeks are feasible and may improve outcome. For stage I TTTS, some fetal medical centers offer conservative management with close surveillance, but laser treatment is recommended for women with a short cervix, discomfort, and increasing polyhydramnios. Perinatal survival has significantly improved over the past 25 years, since the introduction of fetoscopic laser surgery for TTTS. High-volume centers can achieve 70% double twin survival and >90% survival of at least one twin after fetoscopic laser treatment. For these success rates, laser therapy should be offered in specialized fetal medicine centers that perform at least 20 procedures per surgeon annually. We have demonstrated that centralization of TTTS laser treatment improved the learning curve, reduced complications, and improved the survival rates of both twins. There remains a need for prospective registration and standardized long-term outcome studies.

◘ Table 15.1 Pooled proportions of the perinatal outcomes modified from [47]

	Dichorionic triamniotic		Monochorionic triamniotic	
	Pregnancies (*n*/*N*)	**Pooled proportion (%)**	**Pregnancies (*n*/*N*)**	**Pooled proportion (%)**
PTB < 28 weeks	7/48	16.9	8/22	37.1
PTB < 32 weeks	24/48	50	16/22	69.5
Perinatal survival of at least one triplet	99/104	94.1	19/22	83.2
Perinatal survival of at least two triplets	83/103	80.2	15/22	61.9
Perinatal survival of all three triplets	52/102	51	11/22	48.7

PTB Preterm birth

15.9.1 Review Questions

1. Why is TTTS not a complication in dichorionic twins?

2. What is the benefit of laser surgery in TTTS and quantify the perinatal survival rates (at least one twin, double) in high-volume fetal therapy centers?

3. What are the options for management in TTTS stage I?

4. What are the long-term complications of monochorionic twins after TTTS laser treatment?

15.9.2 Multiple-Choice Questions

1. The Solomon method represents a new laser technique in TTTS treatment. Which statement is correct?
   1. This new technique is developed only for posterior placentas.
   2. A randomized controlled trial showed a significant reduction in perinatal mortality using the Solomon technique in comparison to the standard selective laser method.
   3. After coagulation of all vascular anastomoses, a thin laser line from one edge to the other edge of the placenta is drawn.
   4. There was no association between Solomon technique and placental abruption described.
   5. Recurrent TTTS and post-laser TAPS are absent following the Solomon technique.

Answer to question 1

1. F
2. F
3. T
4. F
5. F

Explanations to question 1

1. The Solomon technique can be used for anterior and posterior placentas. Successful laser coagulation in TTTS depends on appropriate visualization of the chorionic connecting vessels. In case of an extensive anterior placenta, there may be no adequate view. However, all described laser techniques have to deal with this problem.
2. 4 + 5 are correct statements. The Solomon trial showed a significant reduction of TAPS and recurrent TTTS without differences in survival rates. It has been mentioned that the trial was underpowered to find a significant difference in perinatal mortality.
3. Correct statement: this represents exactly the description of the Solomon technique. The rationale of this method is coagulation of the whole vascular equator (including tiny anastomoses that might not be visualized).
4. Some authors passed the critical comment that the surgeons should prevent unnecessary sacrifice of placental tissue during laser treatment. Indeed, very recently, the Solomon technique was associated with a higher risk of placental abruption.

2. In evaluating MC twin pregnancies with TTTS and research in this filed, one of the following statements is wrong.
   1. TTTS occurs in approximately 10% of all MC twin pregnancies and represents a severe complication.
   2. Fetoscopic laser treatment is the first-line treatment in Quintero stages II–IV.
   3. High-volume fetal medicine centers are able to achieve 70% double twin survival and at least one surviving twin in 90% of the cases after fetoscopic laser treatment.
   4. Quintero stage I TTTS progress in the vast majority of cases and am-

nioreduction are evidence-based therapies.

Answer to question 2

1. T
2. T
3. T
4. F

Explanations to question 2

1. Whereas intertwine anastomoses are found in all MC placentas, TTTS occurs only in 10% of MC pregnancies. The risk suffering from TTTS depends on the type, number, and diameter of the anastomoses. However, TTTS is definitely a severe complication in MC twinings.
2. In an RCT, Senat and coworkers compared serial amnioreduction vs fetoscopic laser surgery in stage II–IV TTTS cases and found improved neonatal survival, increased gestational age at delivery, and better neurodevelopment after laser treatment. Therefore laser surgery has become the first-line choice.
3. High-volume fetal medicine centers have improved the outcome in the last 25 years in terms of neonatal survival rate after laser surgery. In fact there is growing evidence that centralization and at least 20–30 procedures per surgeon annually are needed to maintain high quality.
4. Stage I cases do not necessarily progress to more advances stages, and some of them are stable or regress, actually. To date there is no evidence that amnioreduction is better than laser treatment or expectant management in these cases.

3. Women carrying an MC pregnancy should be informed about some important points. One of the following sentences is not true.
    1. If the mother-to-be detects a remarkable and rapid increase of her belly, a TTTS may be the reason.
    2. Every MC pregnancy should be evaluated at least once every 2 weeks by ultrasound starting after 16 weeks of gestation.
    3. TTTS is common in monoamniotic twin pregnancies.
    4. Prematurity is still a serious complication following TTTS laser treatment and around 10% of surviving twins show severe neurodevelopment impairment in long-term follow-up studies.
    5. The mean gestational age at delivery after TTTS laser is 32–34 weeks of gestation.

Answer to question 3

1. T
2. T
3. F
4. T
5. T

Explanations to question 3

1. Women pregnant with MC twins should be specially instructed to seek medical attention when they feel a rapid increase in uterine size and a tensed belly. This represents the polyhydramnios of the recipient twin.
2. TTTS occurs between 16 and 26 weeks of gestation in most cases. It makes sense that prenatal ultrasound should be performed at least every 2 weeks and amniotic fluid assessment is indicated.
3. Monoamniotic twins are rare and they will infrequently develop a TTTS. The cord insertions are close together and sufficient anastomoses between the two circulations are present.
4. 4 + 5 Prematurity seems the major risk factor for neurodevelopmental impairment in survivors after TTTS laser treatment. The mean gestational age at delivery following TTTS laser surgery is 32–34 weeks.

Patient Testimonials

Cyriel and Pol – A Twin-to-Twin Transfusion Story from a Parent's Perspective

"Pregnant? Congratulations! Would you like to book your first ultrasound?"

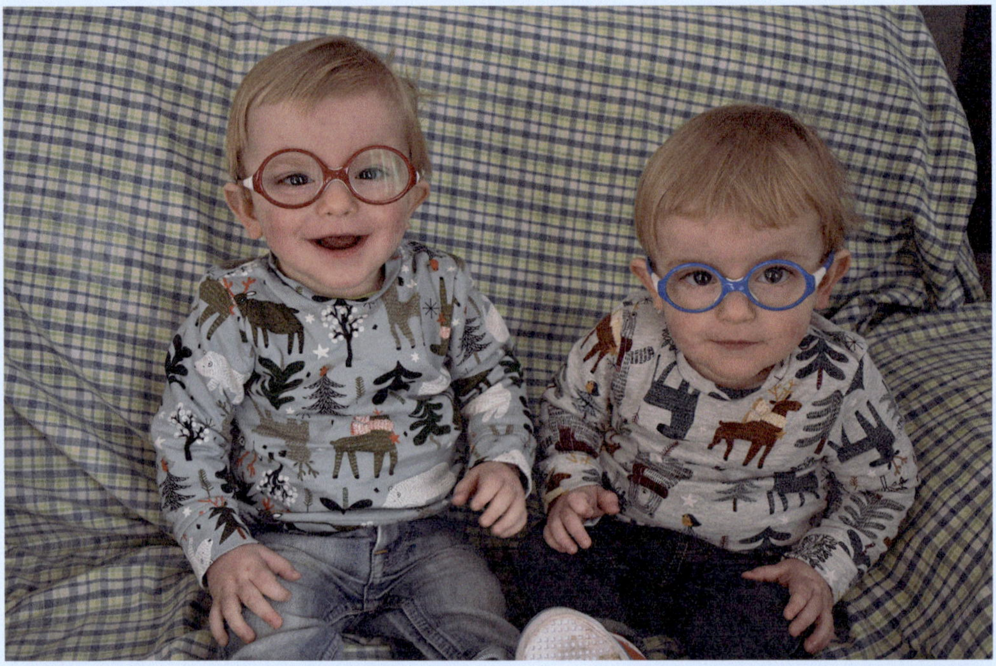

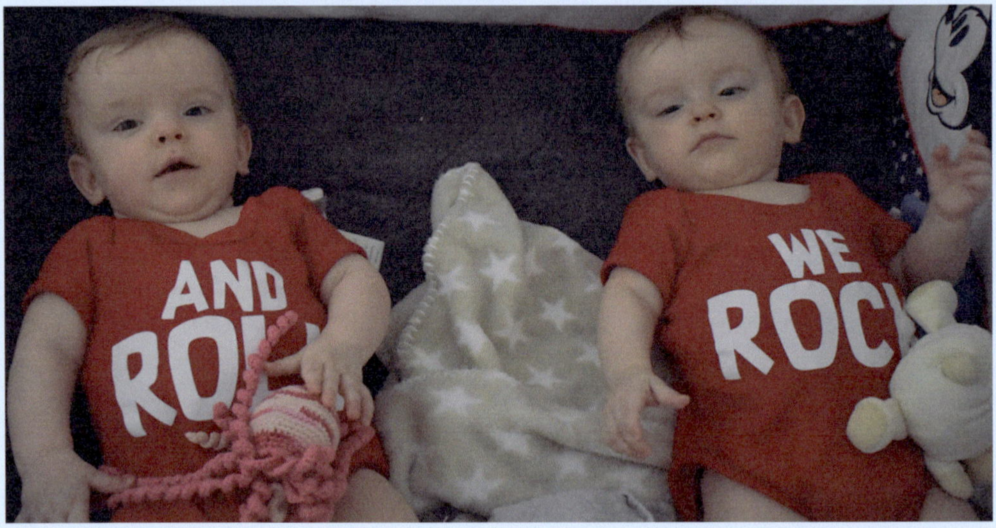

The main thing you want to hear during that first ultrasound is that your baby is exactly where it should be and that its heart is beating... "Can you see that too?," the midwife asked the student sitting in during the scan. "Yeah, there are two babies, right?" ...and the other thing is whether you're having just one baby or more, of course!

That photo is actually the most beautiful ultrasound photo we've got. The first in a long line where they both still managed to fit in a single image.

15

Later on, the photos became a little less idyllic. For most other couples, every ultrasound is a happy reunion with their baby (or babies), but for us, every ultrasound was a moment where we held our breath and hoped for positive news.

That's because at 16 weeks, an amniotic fluid imbalance was detected. Finally, you're starting to feel relieved that you're feeling less nauseous, and you build up the confidence to tell everyone that you're pregnant—and then this kind of news dampens your enthusiasm. According to the statistics, there's an even higher chance than during the first 3 months that you'll lose at least one of your babies. That's followed by a series of situations in which you, as parents, have to make heart-wrenching choices, with statistics on the chances and outcomes of each option being the only thing to rely on. As long as our babies were healthy and we didn't see them suffering, we kept choosing them both.

Pol and Cyriel received successful laser surgery. Even at that time, we knew exactly who was who – they both had their own story. After 2 weeks, and against all expectations, it was donor Pol, and not recipient Cyriel, who presented us with a dilemma. His heart was still able to circulate blood, but its right ventricle had stopped working.

This wasn't a problem as long as I kept supplying him with oxygen as a mother, but he would struggle to survive in the great big world outside of my womb.

Once again, we had to prepare ourselves for a tough choice: we could either allow Pol to grow in my womb until the end of my pregnancy, with an increased chance of complications for Cyriel, or we could let Pol go to give Cyriel the best chance at life.

Pol was still in good health at that time, and we couldn't face giving up a healthy baby. As a parent, you keep talking to your child, explaining to them their heart needs to beat just a little differently... you never lose faith in the strength of your own children.

And our faith was repaid during the next ultrasound: Pol's right ventricle had fixed itself. His blood was flowing just as it should, and everything seemed to be stabilizing. In addition, his amniotic sac, which had become detached during the surgery, had reattached itself. Finally, we were faced with an "ordinary" pregnancy: just what we needed! But it didn't last long. At 24 weeks, recipient Cyriel's waters broke. He was in the amniotic sac through which the surgery was performed. The chance that the babies would be born right at that moment rose enormously. Yet another dilemma presented itself. What if the babies were to be born now? Would you like us to help them make it through? Luckily, we received excellent guidance on every choice we were faced with.

The next few weeks were very tense, and the rest of my pregnancy played out full-time at the hospital. At 28 weeks, Pol's waters broke as well. They certainly knew how to keep things exciting, our little rascals! Still, they were able to top up their own amniotic fluid independently, and they kept swimming around without a care in the world.

At 33 weeks, the tension got too much. Blood in the amniotic fluid isn't too much of a problem in itself, but at 33 weeks, the time came to relieve me from my motherly role as the only person responsible for the well-being of my babies. The twins were born at 33 weeks and 2 days. We received the best possible care from the awesome team in the neonatal unit. But honestly speaking, their premature birth was the least of our worries. Our most difficult weeks were already well behind us at that point. Of course, we spent as much time with them as we could, because we had been a team for such a long time, and as the saying goes, "never change a winning team!" We're still a team today, and we hope to remain a team for many, many years to come.

References

1. Benirschke K, Masliah E. The placenta in multiple pregnancy: outstanding issues. Reprod Fertil Dev. 2001;13:615–22.
2. Lewi L, Jani J, Blickstein I, Huber A, Gucciardo L, Van Mieghem T, Done E, Boes AS, Hecher K, Gratacos E, Lewi P, Deprest J. The outcome of monochorionic diamniotic twin gestations in the era of invasive fetal therapy: a prospective cohort study. Am J Obstet Gynecol. 2008;199:514 e1-8.
3. Zhao DP, de Villiers SF, Slaghekke F, Walther FJ, Middeldorp JM, Oepkes D, Lopriore E. Prevalence, size, number and localization of vascular anastomoses in monochorionic placentas. Placenta. 2013;34:589–93.
4. Bamberg C, Hecher K. Update on twin-to-twin transfusion syndrome. Best Pract Res Clin Obstet Gynaecol. 2019;58:55–65.
5. Khalil A, Rodgers M, Baschat A, Bhide A, Gratacos E, Hecher K, Kilby MD, Lewi L, Nicolaides KH, Oepkes D, Raine-Fenning N, Reed K, Salomon LJ, Sotiriadis A, Thilaganathan B, Ville Y. ISUOG practice guidelines: role of ultrasound in twin pregnancy. Ultrasound Obstet Gynecol. 2016;47:247–63.
6. Khalil A. Modified diagnostic criteria for twin-to-twin transfusion syndrome prior to 18 weeks' gestation: time to change? Ultrasound Obstet Gynecol. 2017;49:804–5.
7. Dekoninck P, Deprest J, Lewi P, Richter J, Galjaard S, Van Keirsbilck J, Van Calsteren K, Lewi L. Gestational age-specific reference ranges for amniotic fluid assessment in monochorionic diamniotic twin pregnancies. Ultrasound Obstet Gynecol. 2013;41:649–52.
8. Mackie FL, Hall MJ, Morris RK, Kilby MD. Early prognostic factors of outcomes in monochorionic twin pregnancy: systematic review and meta-analysis. Am J Obstet Gynecol. 2018;219:436–46.
9. Stagnati V, Zanardini C, Fichera A, Pagani G, Quintero RA, Bellocco R, Prefumo F. Early prediction of twin-to-twin transfusion syndrome: systematic review and meta-analysis. Ultrasound Obstet Gynecol. 2017;49:573–82.
10. Bamberg C, Diemert A, Glosemeyer P, Tavares de Sousa M, Hecher K. Discordance of umbilical coiling index between recipients and donors in twin-twin transfusion syndrome. Placenta. 2019;76:19–22.
11. Quintero RA, Morales WJ, Allen MH, Bornick PW, Johnson PK, Kruger M. Staging of twin-twin transfusion syndrome. J Perinatol. 1999;19:550–5.
12. Wohlmuth C, Gardiner HM, Diehl W, Hecher K. Fetal cardiovascular hemodynamics in twin-twin transfusion syndrome. Acta Obstet Gynecol Scand. 2016;95:664–71.
13. Ville Y. Twin-to-twin transfusion syndrome: time to forget the Quintero staging system? Ultrasound Obstet Gynecol. 2007;30:924–7.
14. Yamamoto M, Essaoui M, Nasr B, Malek N, Takahashi Y, Moreira de Sa R, Ville Y. Three-dimensional sonographic assessment of fetal urine production before and after laser surgery in twin-to-twin transfusion syndrome. Ultrasound Obstet Gynecol. 2007;30:972–6.
15. Berghella V, Kaufmann M. Natural history of twin-twin transfusion syndrome. J Reprod Med. 2001;46:480–4.
16. Khalil A, Cooper E, Townsend R, Thilaganathan B. Evolution of stage 1 Twin-to-Twin Transfusion Syndrome (TTTS): systematic review and meta-analysis. Twin Res Hum Genet. 2016;19:207–16.
17. Stirnemann J, Slaghekke F, Khalek N, Winer N, Johnson A, Lewi L, et al. Intrauterine fetoscopic laser surgery versus expectant management in stage 1 twin-to-twin transfusion syndrome: an international randomized trial. Am J Obstet Gynecol. 2021;224(5):528 e1–e12.
18. Salomon LJ, Ortqvist L, Aegerter P, Bussieres L, Staracci S, Stirnemann JJ, Essaoui M, Bernard JP, Ville Y. Long-term developmental follow-up of infants who participated in a randomized clinical trial of amniocentesis vs laser photocoagulation for the treatment of twin-to-twin transfusion syndrome. Am J Obstet Gynecol. 2010;203: 444 e1-7.
19. Senat MV, Deprest J, Boulvain M, Paupe A, Winer N, Ville Y. Endoscopic laser surgery versus serial amnioreduction for severe twin-to-twin transfusion syndrome. N Engl J Med. 2004;351:136–44.
20. Lewi L, Jani J, Cannie M, Robyr R, Ville Y, Hecher K, Gratacos E, Vandecruys H, Vandecaveye V, Dymarkowski S, Deprest J. Intertwin anastomoses in monochorionic placentas after fetoscopic laser coagulation for twin-to-twin transfusion syndrome: is there more than meets the eye? Am J Obstet Gynecol. 2006;194:790–5.
21. Lopriore E, Middeldorp JM, Oepkes D, Kanhai HH, Walther FJ, Vandenbussche FP. Twin anemia-polycythemia sequence in two monochorionic twin pairs without oligo-polyhydramnios sequence. Placenta. 2007;28:47–51.
22. Slaghekke F, Lopriore E, Lewi L, Middeldorp JM, van Zwet EW, Weingertner AS, Klumper FJ, DeKoninck P, Devlieger R, Kilby MD, Rustico MA, Deprest J, Favre R, Oepkes D. Fetoscopic laser coagulation of the vascular equator versus selective coagulation for twin-to-twin transfusion syndrome: an open-label randomised controlled trial. Lancet. 2014;383:2144–51.
23. Slaghekke F, Lewi L, Middeldorp JM, Weingertner AS, Klumper FJ, Dekoninck P, Devlieger R, Lanna MM, Deprest J, Favre R, Oepkes D, Lopriore E. Residual anastomoses in twin-twin transfusion syndrome after laser: the Solomon randomized trial. Am J Obstet Gynecol. 2014;211:285 e1-7.
24. Quintero RA, Kontopoulos E, Chmait RH. Laser treatment of twin-to-twin transfusion syndrome. Twin Res Hum Genet. 2016;19:197–206.

25. Lanna MM, Faiola S, Consonni D, Rustico MA. Increased risk of placental abruption after Solomon laser treatment of twin-twin transfusion syndrome. Placenta. 2017;53:54–6.
26. Baud D, Windrim R, Keunen J, Kelly EN, Shah P, van Mieghem T, Seaward PG, Ryan G. Fetoscopic laser therapy for twin-twin transfusion syndrome before 17 and after 26 weeks' gestation. Am J Obstet Gynecol. 2013;208:197 e1-7.
27. Valsky DV, Eixarch E, Martinez-Crespo JM, Acosta ER, Lewi L, Deprest J, Gratacos E. Fetoscopic laser surgery for twin-to-twin transfusion syndrome after 26 weeks of gestation. Fetal Diagn Ther. 2012;31:30–4.
28. Baud D, Windrim R, Keunen J, Ryan G. Fetoscopic laser therapy for twin-twin transfusion syndrome: beyond current gestational age limits. Am J Perinatol. 2014;31(Suppl 1):S19–24.
29. De Zoysa MY, Chon AH, Korst LM, Llanes A, Chmait RH. Membrane separation and perinatal outcomes after laser treatment for twin-twin transfusion syndrome. Fetal Diagn Ther. 2020;47:307–14.
30. Chmait RH, Chon AH, Korst LM, Llanes A, Kontopoulos EV, Quintero RA. Risks of preterm premature rupture of membranes and preterm birth post fetoscopy based on location of trocar insertion site. Am J Perinatol. 2018;35:801–8.
31. Merz W, Tchatcheva K, Gembruch U, Kohl T. Maternal complications of fetoscopic laser photocoagulation (FLP) for treatment of twin-twin transfusion syndrome (TTTS). J Perinat Med. 2010;38:439–43.
32. Sacco A, Van der Veeken L, Bagshaw E, Ferguson C, Van Mieghem T, David AL, Deprest J. Maternal complications following open and fetoscopic fetal surgery: a systematic review and meta-analysis. Prenat Diagn. 2019;39:251–68.
33. Akkermans J, Peeters SH, Klumper FJ, Lopriore E, Middeldorp JM, Oepkes D. Twenty-five years of fetoscopic laser coagulation in twin-twin transfusion syndrome: a systematic review. Fetal Diagn Ther. 2015;38:241–53.
34. Diehl W, Diemert A, Grasso D, Sehner S, Wegscheider K, Hecher K. Fetoscopic laser coagulation in 1020 pregnancies with twin-twin transfusion syndrome demonstrates improvement in double-twin survival rate. Ultrasound Obstet Gynecol. 2017;50:728–35.
35. Bamberg C, Diehl W, Diemert A, Sehner S, Hecher K. Neither the differentiation between twin-twin transfusion syndrome stages I and II nor III and IV makes a difference regarding the probability of double survival after laser therapy. Ultrasound Obstet Gynecol. 2020 Sep 22. https://doi.org/10.1002/uog.23131.
36. Stirnemann J, Djaafri F, Kim A, Mediouni I, Bussieres L, Spaggiari E, Veluppillai C, Lapillonne A, Kermorvant E, Magny JF, Colmant C, Ville Y. Preterm premature rupture of membranes is a collateral effect of improvement in perinatal outcomes following fetoscopic coagulation of chorionic vessels for twin-twin transfusion syndrome: a retrospective observational study of 1092 cases. BJOG. 2018;125:1154–62.
37. Stirnemann J, Chalouhi G, Essaoui M, Bahi-Buisson N, Sonigo P, Millischer AE, Lapillonne A, Guigue V, Salomon LJ, Ville Y. Fetal brain imaging following laser surgery in twin-to-twin surgery. BJOG. 2018;125:1186–91.
38. Schou KV, Lando AV, Ekelund CK, Jensen LN, Jorgensen C, Norgaard LN, Rode L, Sogaard K, Tabor A, Sundberg K. Long-term neurodevelopmental outcome of monochorionic twins after laser therapy or umbilical cord occlusion for twin-twin transfusion syndrome. Fetal Diagn Ther. 2019;46:20–7.
39. van Klink JM, Koopman HM, Rijken M, Middeldorp JM, Oepkes D, Lopriore E. Long-term neurodevelopmental outcome in survivors of twin-to-twin transfusion syndrome. Twin Res Hum Genet. 2016;19:255–61.
40. Lenclen R, Paupe A, Ciarlo G, Couderc S, Castela F, Ortqvist L, Ville Y. Neonatal outcome in preterm monochorionic twins with twin-to-twin transfusion syndrome after intrauterine treatment with amnioreduction or fetoscopic laser surgery: comparison with dichorionic twins. Am J Obstet Gynecol. 2007;196:450 e1-7.
41. Lopriore E, Ortibus E, Acosta-Rojas R, Le Cessie S, Middeldorp JM, Oepkes D, Gratacos E, Vandenbussche FP, Deprest J, Walther FJ, Lewi L. Risk factors for neurodevelopment impairment in twin-twin transfusion syndrome treated with fetoscopic laser surgery. Obstet Gynecol. 2009;113:361–6.
42. van Klink JM, Koopman HM, van Zwet EW, Middeldorp JM, Walther FJ, Oepkes D, Lopriore E. Improvement in neurodevelopmental outcome in survivors of twin-twin transfusion syndrome treated with laser surgery. Am J Obstet Gynecol. 2014;210:540 e1-7.
43. Herberg U, Bolay J, Graeve P, Hecher K, Bartmann P, Breuer J. Intertwin cardiac status at 10-year follow-up after intrauterine laser coagulation therapy of severe twin-twin transfusion syndrome: comparison of donor, recipient and normal values. Arch Dis Child Fetal Neonatal Ed. 2014;99:F380–5.
44. Hecher K, Gardiner HM, Diemert A, Bartmann P. Long-term outcomes for monochorionic twins after laser therapy in twin-to-twin transfusion syndrome. Lancet Child Adolesc Health. 2018;2:525–35.
45. Baxi LV, Walsh CA. Monoamniotic twins in contemporary practice: a single-center study of perinatal outcomes. J Matern Fetal Neonatal Med. 2010;23:506–10.
46. Diemert A, Diehl W, Huber A, Glosemeyer P, Hecher K. Laser therapy of twin-to-twin transfusion syndrome in triplet pregnancies. Ultrasound Obstet Gynecol. 2010;35:71–4.

47. D'Antonio F, Thilaganathan B, Toms J, Manzoli L, Bhide A, Papageorghiou A, Khalil A. Perinatal outcome after fetoscopic laser surgery for twin-to-twin transfusion syndrome in triplet pregnancies. BJOG. 2016;123:328–36.

Key Reading

Lewi L, Jani J, Blickstein I, Huber A, Gucciardo L, Van Mieghem T, Done E, Boes AS, Hecher K, Gratacos E, Lewi P, Deprest J. The outcome of monochorionic diamniotic twin gestations in the era of invasive fetal therapy: a prospective cohort study. Am J Obstet Gynecol. 2008;199:514 e1–8.

Khalil A, Rodgers M, Baschat A, Bhide A, Gratacos E, Hecher K, Kilby MD, Lewi L, Nicolaides KH, Oepkes D, Raine-Fenning N, Reed K, Salomon LJ, Sotiriadis A, Thilaganathan B, Ville Y. ISUOG Practice Guidelines: role of ultrasound in twin pregnancy. Ultrasound Obstet Gynecol. 2016;47:247–63.

Senat MV, Deprest J, Boulvain M, Paupe A, Winer N, Ville Y. Endoscopic laser surgery versus serial amnioreduction for severe twin-to-twin transfusion syndrome. N Engl J Med. 2004;351:136–44.

Slaghekke F, Lopriore E, Lewi L, Middeldorp JM, van Zwet EW, Weingertner AS, Klumper FJ, DeKoninck P, Devlieger R, Kilby MD, Rustico MA, Deprest J, Favre R, Oepkes D. Fetoscopic laser coagulation of the vascular equator versus selective coagulation for twin-to-twin transfusion syndrome: an open-label randomised controlled trial. Lancet. 2014;383:2144–51.

Diehl W, Diemert A, Grasso D, Sehner S, Wegscheider K, Hecher K. Fetoscopic laser coagulation in 1020 pregnancies with twin-twin transfusion syndrome demonstrates improvement in double-twin survival rate. Ultrasound Obstet Gynecol. 2017;50:728–35.

Lopriore E, Ortibus E, Acosta-Rojas R, Le Cessie S, Middeldorp JM, Oepkes D, Gratacos E, Vandenbussche FP, Deprest J, Walther FJ, Lewi L. Risk factors for neurodevelopment impairment in twin-twin transfusion syndrome treated with fetoscopic laser surgery. Obstet Gynecol. 2009;113:361–6.

Hecher K, Gardiner HM, Diemert A, Bartmann P. Long-term outcomes for monochorionic twins after laser therapy in twin-to-twin transfusion syndrome. Lancet Child Adolesc Health. 2018;2: 525–35.

Twin Anemia Polycythemia Sequence

L. S. A. Tollenaar and Enrico Lopriore

Contents

Electronic Supplementary Material The online version of this chapter (https://doi.org/10.1007/978-3-030-47652-6_16) contains supplementary material, which is available to authorized users. The videos can be accessed by scanning the related images with the SN More Media App.

A. Khalil et al. (eds.), *Twin and Higher-order Pregnancies*,
https://doi.org/10.1007/978-3-030-47652-6_16

Trailer

Twin anemia polycythemia sequence (TAPS) is a chronic form of unbalanced feto-fetal transfusion in monochorionic twin pregnancies, leading to anemia in the donor and polycythemia in the TAPS recipient. TAPS can occur spontaneously in up to 5% of monochorionic twin pregnancies or can develop after incomplete laser for twin-twin transfusion syndrome due to the presence of minuscule residual anastomoses. Spontaneous TAPS can develop throughout the entire second and third trimesters. The majority of post-laser TAPS cases is detected within 4 weeks after laser surgery for TTTS, but the condition can manifest up until 17 weeks after treatment. Antenatal diagnosis for TAPS is based on middle cerebral artery – peak systolic velocity showing an increased measure in the donor, combined with a decreased measure in the recipient. Treatment options for TAPS include expectant management, preterm delivery, intrauterine blood transfusion (IUT) with or without a partial exchange transfusion (PET), fetoscopic laser surgery, and selective feticide. The best treatment option for TAPS is unknown. Spontaneous fetal demise occurs in 5–11% of TAPS twins and significantly more often in TAPS donors (8–18%) than in recipients (2–5%). Long-term neurodevelopmental impairment is seen in 9% of TAPS twins and is higher in TAPS donors (18%) than in recipients (3%).

Learning Objectives

After reading this chapter, the reader should be able to:

- Understand the pathophysiology of TAPS and how it can be distinguished from TTTS
- Explain how TAPS can be diagnosed antenatally
- Summarize the additional ultrasound markers in TAPS
- Elaborate on the different management options for TAPS
- Differentiate between TAPS and acute peripartum TTTS, based on hematological and placental characteristics
- Describe the perinatal and long-term outcome and potential differences between donor and recipient

16.1 Introduction

Twin anemia polycythemia sequence (TAPS) is a severe complication in monochorionic twin pregnancies caused by unbalanced feto-fetal transfusion through placental anastomoses leading to large hemoglobin discordances [1]. In contrast to twin-twin transfusion syndrome, TAPS develops in the absence of twin oligohydramnios polyhydramnios sequence (TOPS). The classical picture of TAPS at birth is the combination of a pale anemic neonate and a plethoric polycythemic neonate (◘ Fig. 16.1). There are two types of TAPS: spontaneous and post-laser TAPS. Spontaneous TAPS occurs in up to 5% of monochorionic twin pregnancies [2, 3]. Post-laser TAPS can develop in 2–16% of TTTS twins treated with laser surgery as the results of residual anastomoses [4, 5]. Robyr et al. were the first to describe post-laser TAPS when they described 12 cases with anemia and polycythemia after laser surgery [4]. Shortly thereafter, Lopriore et al. reported the same condition to occur spontaneously in monochorionic twins that showed no signs of TOPS antenatally [1]. To clearly demarcate this new form of unbalanced feto-fetal transfusion, the term "twin anemia polycythemia sequence" was introduced, as well as its acronym "TAPS."

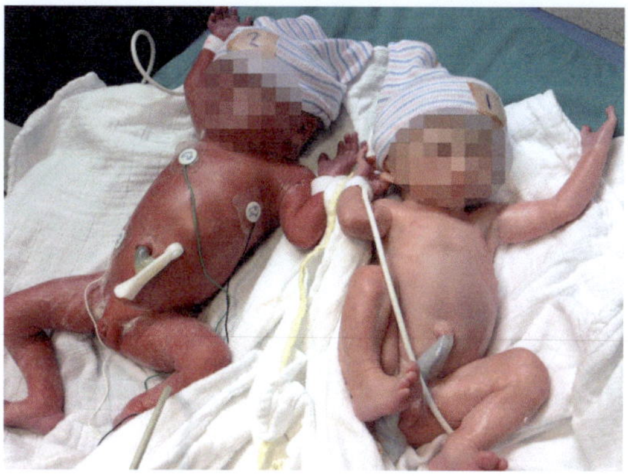

◘ **Fig. 16.1** Spontaneous TAPS twins at birth. On the right hand side is the plethoric polycythemic recipient and on the left hand side the pale anemic donor

16.2 Pathogenesis

16.2.1 Placental Characteristics

TAPS results from slow and chronic unbalanced feto-fetal transfusion through minuscule placental anastomoses, gradually leading to highly discordant hemoglobin levels, causing the donor twin to become anemic and the recipient twin to become polycythemic [1]. Compared to uncomplicated monochorionic placentas, anastomoses in TAPS are more scarce and almost always minuscule (diameter <1 mm) (◘ Fig. 16.2). The majority of TAPS placentas show only arterio-venous (AV) anastomoses, which allow unidirectional feto-fetal blood flow [6, 7]. Arterio-arterial (AA) anastomoses are considered to protect against the development of TTTS or TAPS because of their bidirectional nature, enabling inter-twin equilibration of blood volumes. In line, AA anastomoses are reported in only 19% of spontaneous TAPS and 8% of post-laser TAPS placentas [6, 7]. Veno-venous (VV) anastomoses are even more rare in TAPS placentas and are detected in 7%. Spontaneous TAPS placentas differ from post-laser TAPS placentas. Spontaneous TAPS placentas have a higher total number of anastomoses compared to post-laser TAPS placentas (median of 3 vs. 1, respectively), and anastomoses are located across the entire vascular equator of the placenta [8]. Residual anastomoses in post-laser TAPS placentas are more often found at the margin of the placenta.

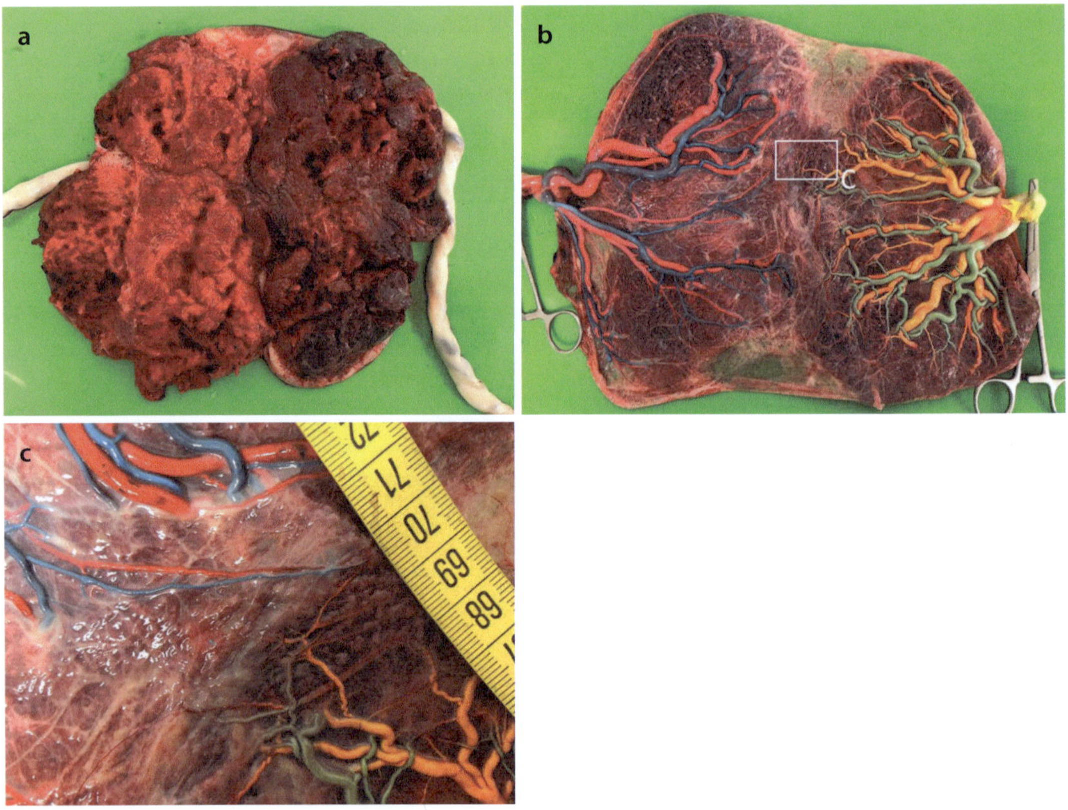

◘ **Fig. 16.2** Placenta from a spontaneous TAPS twin. **a** The maternal side of the placenta, demonstrating a striking color difference with a pale placental share for the anemic donor and a plethoric share for the polycythemic recipient. **b** Fetal side of the placenta injected with color dye. The placental share of the donor is injected with blue (arteries) and red (veins) and the placental share of the recipient is injected with green (arteries) and yellow (veins). **c** A minuscule arterio-venous anastomosis responsible for TAPS

16.2.2 TAPS Versus TTTS

The absence of TOPS is an essential element in the diagnosis of TAPS. The presence of TOPS is only pathognomonic for TTTS. The mechanism that prevents the donor from developing an oligohydramnios and the recipient from a polyhydramnios is not clear. The most probable hypothesis is that the chronic character of the feto-fetal transfusion allows more time for a hemodynamic compensatory mechanism to take place. Furthermore, TTTS results from large unbalanced feto-fetal transfusion with rapid deterioration, combined with unbalanced hormonal regulation [9]. TTTS donors show high renin levels, likely as results of renal hypoperfusion, and recipients do not have renin protein, due to downregulation caused by hypervolemia. In TAPS, this hormonal discordance is not described.

Although TTTS and TAPS have been described as to separate entities, there seems to be an area of overlap between the two conditions. Approximately 8–19% of TTTS twins show signs of fetal anemia in the donor and fetal polycythemia in the recipient twin before laser treatment [10–12]. Placentas from the twins with TTTS and anemia polycythemia showed fewer anastomoses, had a later time of onset, and a more favorable neonatal and long-term outcome compared to twins with TTTS alone [12].

16.2.3 Post-laser TAPS

The first studies on post-laser TAPS showed that it was mostly the former TTTS donor that became the polycythemic TAPS recipient and the former TTTS recipient that became the anemic TAPS donor [4, 13, 14]. However, recent results of a large international TAPS registry show that reversal of donor-recipient role in post-laser TAPS occurred less frequently than previously thought. From a total of 164 post-laser TAPS cases, 55% changed donor-recipient role when post-laser TAPS developed and 45% did not change donor-recipient role [6].

16.2.4 TAPS and Fetal Growth Restriction

Severe fetal growth restriction (FGR; birth weight < p3) is present in 29% of spontaneous TAPS twins and in 23% of post-laser TAPS twins [6, 7]. In spontaneous TAPS, severe FGR occurs more frequently in donors than in recipients (49% vs. 12%) [7]. In post-laser TAPS, this difference between donor and recipient is not observed, probably due to the fact that a large part of post-laser TAPS donors have previously been TTTS recipients, which in their turn are often the larger twin [6]. Although the donor is usually the smaller infant, it often has a paradoxically larger placental share compared to its recipient co-twin [15]. This finding is only reported in TAPS twins and not in twins with isolated selective FGR or TTTS [16]. FGR in TAPS therefore appears to be determined by inter-twin blood transfusion rather than unequal placental sharing. Besides low levels of erythrocytes, TAPS donors also show decreased albumin and total protein measures, which might contribute to a deteriorated fetal growth [17, 18].

16.3 Antenatal Diagnosis

16.3.1 MCA-PSV Doppler Measurements

The antenatal diagnosis of TAPS is based on discordant middle cerebral artery peak systolic velocity (MCA-PSV) Doppler measurements, with an increased measure in the TAPS donor, suggestive of anemia, combined with a decreased measure in the recipient, suggestive of polycythemia. MCA-PSV criteria for TAPS have been changed over the years. First, cut-off values of MCA-PSV > 1.5 Multiples of the Median (MoM) in the donor combined with MCA-PSV < 0.8 MoM in the recipient were proposed for the antenatal detection of the condition [4]. Thereafter, a more conservative approach was adopted with regard to the cut-off level for the recipient, and <1.0

Table 16.1 Antenatal classification system for TAPS

TAPS stage	Findings at Doppler ultrasound examination
Stage 1	A delta MCA-PSV > 0.5 MoM Without other signs of fetal compromise[a]
Stage 2	A delta MCA-PSV > 0.7 MoM Without other signs of fetal compromise[a]
Stage 3	As stage 1 or 2, with cardiac compromise of the donor, defined critically abnormal flow
Stage 4	Hydrops in the donor
Stage 5	Intra-uterine demise of one or both fetuses preceded by TAPS

[a]Critically abnormal Doppler is defined as absent or reversed end-diastolic flow in the umbilical artery, pulsatile flow in the umbilical vein, increased pulsatility index, or reversed flow in the ductus venosus.

MoM was introduced to detect fetal polycythemia in TAPS [19]. Three recent cohort studies show that an inter-twin difference (or delta) MCA-PSV > 0.5 MoM might be more sensitive to detect TAPS than the use of strict cut-off levels, and the classification system for TAPS was subsequently updated with a delta MCA-PSV > 0.5 MoM for stage 1 and >0.7 MoM for stage 2 (Table 16.1) [20–22]. In a recent Delphi investigation, a selection of perinatologists and neonatologists agreed on the use of ≥1.5 MoM for the donor and MCA-PSV ≤ 0.8 MoM for the recipient or a delta MCA-PSV > 1.0 MoM to identify TAPS [23]. What is the best diagnostic criterion still remains a subject of debate. Due to the low incidence of TAPS, studies investigating the diagnostic accuracy of MCA-PSV criteria are based on small numbers and generally retrospective, thereby limiting generalizability and reliability of the proposed diagnostic values. Large prospective studies investigating MCA-PSV Doppler in the general monochorionic twin population are urgently needed to create a consensus on the matter, to increase antenatal detection rate, and ultimately to improve outcome in TAPS twins.

16

16.3.2 Additional Ultrasound Findings

Although discordant MCA-PSV values are essential elements of the diagnosis of TAPS, additional ultrasound markers have also been reported in TAPS. The placenta in TAPS can appear dichotomous on sonographic examination with a hyperechogenic (enlarged) placental share for the donor and a hypoechogenic (flattened) placental share for the recipient (Figs. 16.3a and 16.4) [24]. Moreover, donors can present with cardiomegaly as a sign of cardiac remodulation to the chronic anemic environment [25]. Lastly, a so-called "starry sky liver" has been detected in recipients, an observation that is based on the hyperechogenic congested portal venules and diminished liver parenchyma, thereby mimicking a starry sky (Fig. 16.3b) [26]. A recent study shows that placental dichotomy is seen in 44% of TAPS twins, that 70% of donors present with cardiomegaly, and that a starry sky liver is observed in 66% of recipients [25]. A total of 86% of TAPS twins presented with at least one of these ultrasound markers. The prevalence of these findings increased with incrementing TAPS stage, suggesting that they might be related to the severity of the disease.

16.4 Antenatal Management

Treatment options for TAPS include expectant management, preterm delivery, intrauterine blood transfusion (IUT) in the donor with or without a partial exchange transfusion (PET) in the recipient, fetoscopic laser coagulation of the placental anastomoses, and selective feticide.

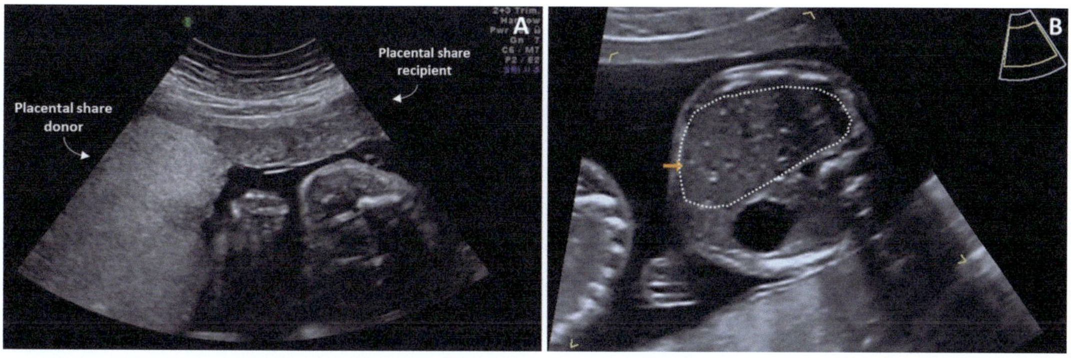

Fig. 16.3 **a** Sonographic image of placental dichotomy, with an enlarged hyperechogenic placental share for the TAPS donor and a flattened hypo-echogenic placental share for the TAPS recipient. **b** Starry sky liver in a TAPS recipient

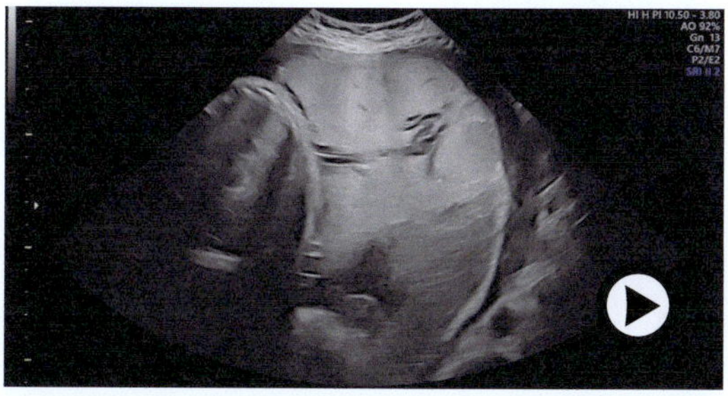

Fig. 16.4 Sonographic image of placental dichotomy in a spontaneous TAPS case at 32 weeks. The upper part from the donor twin is enlarged and hyperechogenic and the lower part from the recipient is flattened and hypo-echogenic. At birth, there were only tiny unidirectional arteriovenous anastomoses, mostly from the anemic donor to the polycythemic recipient. (Courtesy from the twin clinic UZ Leuven, Belgium) (https://doi.org/10.1007/000-2th)

16.4.1 Expectant Management

With expectant management, no intrauterine intervention is performed, but twins are monitored more intensively with ultrasound Doppler. The benefit of expectant management is that the pregnancy will not be at risk for intervention-related complications, while allowing the condition to resolve spontaneously. Spontaneous resolution has been reported before and might occur after thrombosis of the responsible AV anastomosis, or reequilibration of blood flow through the few small AV/VA anastomoses [27]. Results of the TAPS Registry demonstrate that spontaneous resolution is seen in 16% of TAPS twins managed expectantly [28].

16.4.2 Preterm Delivery

In some cases of TAPS, it is more preferable to deliver the twins and treat TAPS at the NICU than continuing the pregnancy and extending exposure to chronic fetal anemia and polycythemia. A preterm delivery is of course only feasible after viability is achieved and preferably takes place after administration of steroids and magnesium sulfate to promote fetal lung and brain maturation. The results of the TAPS Registry show that TAPS twins treated with preterm delivery were diagnosed at a later gestational age with a milder form of TAPS (mostly stage 1) [28].

16.4.3 IUT (with or Without PET)

In case of severe anemia in the donor, an IUT can be considered. Treatment with IUT can be performed intravascularly into the umbilical cord, intrahepatically into the umbilical vein, or indirectly into the peritoneal cavity. An intraperitoneal IUT might have benefits, as it allows for a slower absorption of blood cells into the circulation of the anemic fetus [29]. A possible side effect of IUT is further deterioration of the polycythemia-hyperviscosity syndrome in the TAPS recipient, which might result in skin necrosis or limb ischemia [4]. Therefore, in cases with signs of severe fetal polycythemia in the recipient, an intrauterine PET can be considered (Fig. 16.5). With a PET, the recipient's blood is replaced with

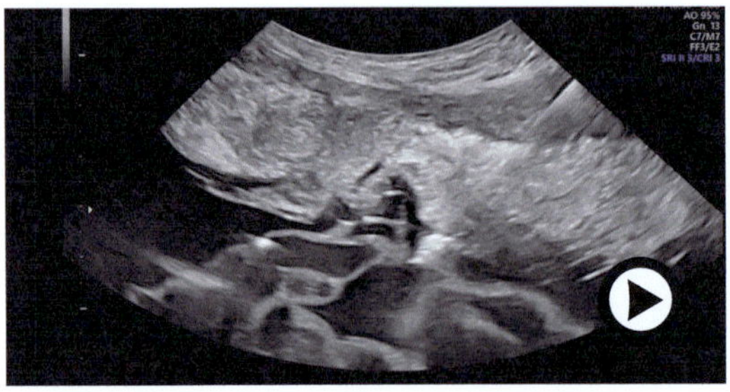

Fig. 16.5 Sonographic images of a transfusion of the anemic donor (Hemoglobin 6 g/dL) and an exchange transfusion of the polycythemic recipient (Hemoglobin 21 g/dL) at 29 weeks as a treatment for post-laser TAPS. (Courtesy from the twin clinic UZ Leuven, Belgium) (https://doi.org/10.1007/000-2tj)

saline repeatedly, aiming to decrease its viscosity. Although the added value of PET has been supported by a computational model and several case reports, IUT was only combined with PET in 21% of the cases collected in the TAPS Registry [28, 30–32]. Treatment with IUT (± PET) is not a definitive treatment and only a temporary solution and, therefore, reintervention might be required. Time between interventions is reported to be approximately 2 weeks, but it varies between 1 and 3 weeks depending on the progressiveness of TAPS [28]. In TAPS, IUT (± PET) is mostly performed after viable gestation and the majority of cases receive only one intervention, followed by preterm delivery. However, reintervention up to four to six times has also been described.

16.4.4 Laser Surgery

The only definitive treatment for TAPS is fetoscopic laser surgery of the vascular anastomoses at the placental surface. Laser surgery has shown to drastically decrease mortality and morbidity in TTTS [33]; however, in TAPS, the procedure might be technically challenging due to the absence of TOPS and size of the anastomoses, resulting in reduced accessibility and visibility of the vascular equator. TOPS can be artificially created with amniodrainage of one sac and amnioinfusion in the other sac, but this requires more needle insertions and might increase the risk of PPROM. Confirming technical limitations, the recurrence rate of TAPS is 15%, which is higher than the recurrence rate of TTTS, or the rate of post-laser TAPS after laser for TTTS [28, 34]. Residual anastomoses are found in 19% of the color-dye injected TAPS placentas that were treated with laser surgery [28]. This rate is comparable with the residual anastomosis rate in TTTS [35]. However, in contrast to TTTS, residual anastomoses after laser for TAPS always result in recurrence of the disease [28]. To increase likelihood of coagulation of all minuscule anastomoses, even the ones that can't be visualized, the Solomon technique might be of added value [35]. The rate of PPROM in laser for TAPS is 37% and comparable with the PPROM rate in TTTS cases that have been treated with laser [28, 36].

16.4.5 Selective Feticide

Selective feticide can be an option in cases of severe early-onset TAPS, or on request of the parents, and is aimed at sacrificing one fetus to increase the chances of healthy survival for the co-twin. In TAPS, it is commonly the donor twin in which the selective feticide is performed (in 87%) [28]. Selective feticide does not guarantee a complication-free survival for the co-twin, as perinatal mortality and severe neonatal morbidity occur in 7% in 25% of co-twins, respectively.

16.4.6 Best Treatment Option

There is currently no consensus on the best treatment for TAPS. Results of the TAPS Registry show that treatment choices differ considerably among fetal therapy centers; some centers only perform laser surgery and selective feticide and other centers refrain from any in-utero intervention and treat their TAPS cases mostly expectantly or with preterm delivery [37]. When outcome is compared between expectant management, preterm delivery, IUT (± PET), laser surgery, and selective feticide for 370 TAPS cases, there is no difference in perinatal mortality between treatment groups [28]. This confirmed results from previous smaller studies [38, 39]. Severe neonatal morbidity was significantly higher in cases treated with IUT (± PET) or with preterm delivery [28]. Pregnancy was best prolonged in twins that were managed expectantly, treated with laser surgery or with selective feticide. As treatment groups were not comparable at baseline and differed considerably in terms of type of TAPS, gestational age at diagnosis, and antenatal TAPS stage, it is likely that outcome is heavily biased. Therefore, the true effect of management of TAPS can only be properly investigated when TAPS cases are randomized between treatment groups, when stratification for risk factors is applied, and when long-term consequences are taken into account. Recently, the TAPS trial, an international multicenter open-label RCT comparing laser surgery to standard care (expectant management, IUT (± PET), preterm delivery) has started recruiting patients [40].

16.5 Postnatal Diagnosis

As approximately 40–63% of TAPS twins are not detected antenatally and only diagnosed after birth, postnatal diagnostic criteria for TAPS have also been proposed [8, 19]. To be identified as TAPS, there needs to be an inter-twin hemoglobin difference >8 g/dL [41]. However, TAPS is not the only condition that presents with discordant hemoglobin levels at birth. Acute peripartum TTTS, the rare form of the well-known chronic TTTS that is believed to develop during labor, presents with a pale and plethoric twin pair as well [42]. As the two conditions require a different therapeutic neonatal approach, distinction at birth is vital. To differentiate between TAPS and acute peripartum TTTS, two additional criteria have been proposed. The first is a reticulocyte count ratio (‰) >1.7 [41]. In TAPS, there is a high reticulocyte count (‰) in the donor twin, as a result of increased erythropoiesis due to chronic anemia. In acute peripartum TTTS, the rapid feto-fetal blood flow has not allowed the TAPS donor to adapt and, therefore, reticulocyte values will be normal. The second criterion for the postnatal diagnosis of TAPS is the presence of only minuscule placental anastomoses (diameter <1 mm), detected through color dye injection [1]. The pathogenesis of acute peripartum TTTS is based on large placental AA or VV anastomoses with low resistance, allowing a large volume of blood to flow directly from donor to recipient [42]. To indicate the severity of TAPS postnatally, a postnatal classification system, based on magnitude of the inter-twin hemoglobin difference, has been proposed (Table 16.2). Since reticulocytes are not always measured and placental injection is a complex and time-consuming procedure, an additional criterion has been proposed. In analogy with the neonatal presentation of TAPS, the maternal side of the placenta shows a striking color difference, with a pale placental share for the TAPS donor and a plethoric placental share for the TAPS recipient [43]. In acute peripartum TTTS, this color difference on the maternal side of the placenta is not observed [44].

Table 16.2 Postnatal classification system for TAPS

TAPS stage	Inter-twin hemoglobin difference (g/dL)
Stage 1	>8.0
Stage 2	>11.0
Stage 3	>14.0
Stage 4	>17.0
Stage 5	>20.0

16.6 Short- and Long-Term Outcomes

16.6.1 Perinatal Mortality

In the TAPS Registry cohort, spontaneous fetal demise occurred in 5% of spontaneous TAPS twins and in 11% of post-laser TAPS twins [6, 7]. Donor twins have increased risk of fetal demise compared to recipient twins, both in spontaneous (8% vs 2%, respectively) and post-laser TAPS (18% vs. 5% respectively). Neonatal mortality occurs in 10% of post-laser TAPS infants, and significantly more often in post-laser TAPS donors (15%) than in recipients (6%). In spontaneous TAPS, the rate of neonatal mortality is lower (4%), and comparable for donors (6%) and recipients (3%). Aside from donor status, risk factors for perinatal mortality are high antenatal TAPS stage and gestational age at birth.

16.6.2 Neonatal Morbidity

Neonatal outcome in TAPS may vary between isolated large inter-twin hemoglobin differences to severe neonatal morbidity, including severe cerebral injury [32, 45]. Hematological complications are frequently seen in TAPS, requiring a blood transfusion in the donor twin and a PET in the recipient twin. Aside from low erythrocyte levels, donor twins may also demonstrate low levels of albumin and total protein [17]. Moreover, donor twins may be diagnosed with leukopenia at birth and seem to have an increased risk for early-onset neonatal sepsis compared to recipient twins [46]. This suggests that not only erythrocytes are transported through the minuscule anastomoses in TAPS, but also that albumin, protein, and leukocytes might be unequally distributed between the two fetuses. Chronic transfusion in TAPS might also lead to short-term renal dysfunction in TAPS donors, probably as the result of chronic renal hypoperfusion [47]. TAPS recipients may develop polycythemia-hyperviscosity syndrome, which can lead to necrosis of the skin and (multiple) limb ischemia [4]. Although this has been described in a few case reports, limb ischemia was not reported in a cohort of 413 TAPS cases in the TAPS Registry and should therefore be considered a rare complication in TAPS [6, 7]. In addition, recipients may be diagnosed with thrombocytopenia at birth, particularly in case of severe polycythemia-hyperviscosity [41, 48]. Chronic anemia or polycythemia might also result in severe cerebral injury, which is reported to occur in 4% of spontaneous TAPS twins and in 10% of post-laser TAPS twins and with similar rates for donors and recipients for both types of TAPS [6, 7]. Severe neonatal morbidity occurs in 32–39% of TAPS twins, with no differences between donors and recipients. The risk for severe neonatal morbidity in TAPS strongly depends on the degree of prematurity, and also the severity of TAPS antenatally plays an important role in neonatal health.

16.6.3 Long-Term Outcome

Due to the low incidence of the condition, large long-term outcome studies in TAPS are scarce and data is based on uncontrolled cohort studies. In post-laser TAPS, severe neurodevelopmental impairment (NDI) was observed in 9% and was comparable with the rate of impairment in TTTS twins treated with laser surgery [14]. The rate of NDI was comparable for post-laser-TAPS donors and recipients. Risk factors for NDI in post-laser TAPS survivors were low gestational age at birth and treatment with IUT (± PET).

In a recent study on long-term outcome in spontaneous TAPS, severe NDI was detected in 9% of survivors and was higher in donors (18%) than in recipients (3%) [49]. Overall, donors showed higher rates of mild cognitive impairment (35% vs. 18%) and lower rates of NDI-free survival (45% vs. 80%) than recipients. Additionally, a surprisingly high rate of bilateral deafness (15%) was observed in TAPS donors and in 0% of recipients. Deafness was in all donors based on auditory neuropathy spectrum disorder. The exact cause for the high rate of deafness in donor twins is not entirely clear. Importantly, this finding is not observed in TTTS twins or children that suffered from chronic fetal anemia based on erythrocyte alloimmunization [50, 51]. Furthermore, the prevalence of deafness in TAPS donors is higher compared to the prevalence of deafness in NICU infants (1–3%) [52]. Aside from severe anemia, NDI was strongly depending on gestational age at birth, once again illustrating the profound impact of prematurity on lifelong outcome.

16.6.4 Conclusion

TAPS is a severe condition that can occur in monochorionic twin pregnancies as a result of chronic unbalanced transfusion through minuscule placental anastomoses. To date, TAPS has been thought to be a relatively benign form of feto-fetal transfusion, but results of recent studies show that perinatal and long-term outcomes are poor, especially in donor twins. These findings stress the need for increased awareness by clinicians concerning the severity of TAPS. Adaptation of guidelines to ensure early diagnosis is needed, as well as prospective, well-controlled studies to determine the most optimal diagnostic criteria and management strategy.

16.6.5 Essay Questions

? *Question 1:* A 35-year-old woman, G2P1, is diagnosed with TAPS stage 1 at 28 weeks of gestation. The twins are managed expectantly. At 32 + 5, TAPS progressed to stage 2, upon which an elective cesarean section is planned.

? Describe what you expect to observe with regard to:
- Clinical presentation of the infants
- Hemoglobin difference
- Reticulocyte count
- Placental characteristics

16.6.6 Multiple Choice Questions

? 1. The pathogenesis of TAPS is based on:
   (a) A rapid transfusion a blood through large arterio-venous placental anastomoses during delivery
   (b) A chronic transfusion of blood trough minuscule arterio-venous placental anastomoses
   (c) A rapid transfusion of blood through large arterio-arterial placental anastomoses during delivery
   (d) A chronic transfusion of blood through minuscule arterio-arterial placental anastomoses

✓ Answers: (b)

? 2. Postnatal diagnosis of TAPS is based on:
   (a) An inter-twin hemoglobin difference >8 g/dL, a reticulocyte count ratio <1.7, and the presence of only minuscule placental anastomoses on color-dye examination
   (b) An inter-twin hemoglobin difference >8 g/dL, a reticulocyte count ratio >1.7, and the presence of a large placental anastomoses on color-dye examination
   (c) An inter-twin hemoglobin difference >8 g/dL, a reticulocyte count ratio <1.7, and the presence of a large color difference on the maternal side of the placenta
   (d) An inter-twin hemoglobin difference >8 g/dL, a reticulocyte count ratio >1.7, and the presence of only minuscule placental anastomoses on color-dye examination

✓ Answers: (d)

? 3. Which of the following is true?
   I Laser surgery and treatment with IUT (with or without PET) are the only two definitive treatment options for TAPS.
   II TAPS donors often present with a starry-sky liver (indicating severe anemia) on ultrasound.
   III TAPS donors are at increased risk of fetal demise compared to recipient twins.
   IV Placental anastomoses in TAPS are usually large (diameter >1.0 mm).
   (a) Only III is true.
   (b) II and III are true.
   (c) I and II are true.
   (d) All are false.

✓ Answers: (a)

Patient Testimonials

Mara and Kyra: Twin Anemia Polycythemia Sequence from a Parent's Perspective

After much soul searching, my husband and I decided to try for a third and final baby.

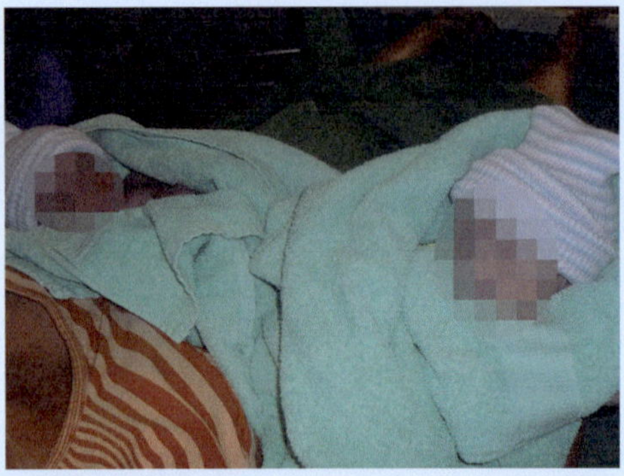

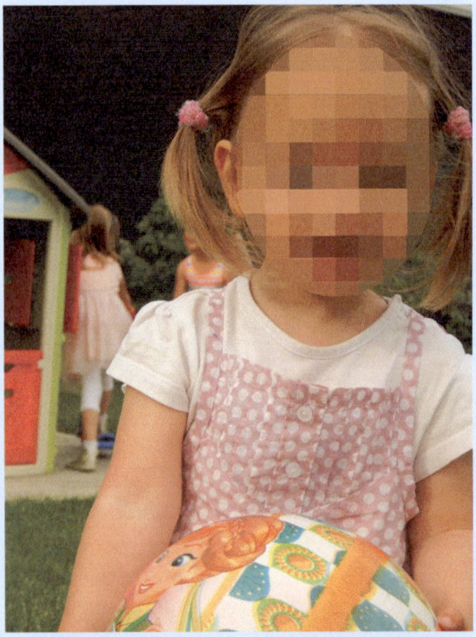

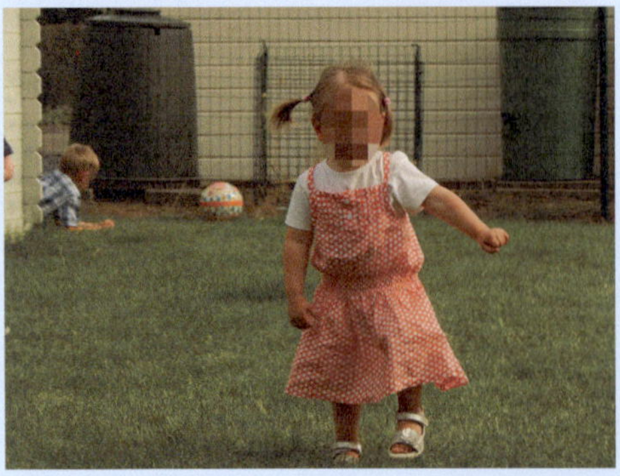

To our great amazement, I became pregnant immediately. This was followed by another shock at the first checkup: I was carrying not one but two babies. The gynecologist felt that it would be better to keep this to ourselves for the time being, because of the risk of something going wrong with one or both babies. It was a quite a difficult time – first a huge surprise to be expecting twins but at the same time fear that something might go wrong.

The second checkup at 12 weeks provided good news though. Both hearts were beating nicely and everything seemed to be fine. There now followed a period of disbelief and great happiness. Similar to most couples expecting twins, we totally had not expected this.

When the pregnancy reached 20 weeks, we attended the twin clinic in a tertiary care center for an extensive checkup. Our gynecologist had recommended this as the unit is highly experienced in twin pregnancies. A long and comprehensive ultrasound scan was performed, which confirmed that we were expecting identical twin girls. And the fact that they were doing extremely well and no problems had been found was the icing on the cake. We were advised, however, to have another extensive checkup at 30 weeks.

During this 30-week examination, it was noted that the exchange of blood via the placenta was not evenly distributed, resulting in one baby receiving too little blood and the other baby too much blood. It was referred to as twin anemia polycythemia sequence or TAPS. Although it was bad news for both girls, it particularly affected little Mara, who received too little blood and was less mobile than her sister. We had to return 2 days later to check how things were developing. Suddenly our babies' condition had changed from normal to potentially life-threatening. Fortunately, we received excellent support from the twin births team, who assured us that the babies would be very carefully monitored and interventions would be made in good time if necessary. After two nail-biting days, it appeared that, although not stable, the situation was not alarming. Once again, we had to wait for another 2 days for the next extensive examination.

This showed that Mara, the baby receiving insufficient blood, was gradually deteriorating and it was decided that admission to hospital was necessary to successfully monitor the situation. While in hospital, it was decided to administer a blood transfusion for Mara. However, on the day of the planned transfusion she was doing very poorly. Her heartbeat regularly disappeared and she was virtually immobile. I received an injection to promote lung development and preparations were made for the blood transfusion and, in case things went wrong, an emergency caesarean. I was on my own in the hospital at the time because it was my other daughter's birthday. Everyone was at home celebrating, or trying to at any rate. It was without doubt one of the most difficult days of my life. Very soon after the blood transfusion, it became clear that it had helped, Mara's heart improved and she was more mobile.

We were told that the girls would still need to be regularly examined to check that Kyra did not receive too much blood. Until then our main concern had been Mara, but now it appeared that Kyra was equally at risk, because an excess blood supply could lead to a stroke. We consequently had to attend a checkup every 2 days. Each additional day in the womb was a bonus. During the first checkup after the blood transfusion, it became clear that the blood was indeed reaching Kyra quite quickly. Eventually, a week after the blood transfusion, it was decided that the girls should be born at 32 weeks of gestation.

We discussed what would be the best option: induction or a caesarean. Because I preferred to have a "natural birth" and this option would also be better for the babies, we opted for induction. I was given an epidural to ensure that an emergency caesarean could be performed immediately if necessary.

The delivery went very quickly, Mara and Kyra were born just a couple of minutes apart. I was allowed to have both girls with me for a short time, but soon they had to be transferred to the neonatal intensive care unit. My husband accompanied them and there I was, on my own and very emotional. It was such a strange day. Until then I had not been certain that everything would be ok with the girls. It wasn't until I was on my own in the delivery room that I realized how lucky we had been.

I then experienced an extremely emotional period as I was on the maternity ward, but my babies were not with me. I visited them as much as possible and tried to enjoy the delight of these two little wonder babies. In the end, Mara had fewer problems after the birth than Kyra, who did struggle a bit. It was a strange feeling for me because it had always been the other way around before they were born.

Eventually, both girls spent 2 weeks at the neonatal intensive care unit and 3 weeks at the neonatal care unit, before we were allowed to take them home. Again an emotional and very challenging period, but we are immensely grateful for the support and assistance we received from everyone at the hospital.

Now, almost 2 years later, our two fragile premature babies have grown into sturdy little toddlers with no physical or mental problems. We want to relate our story to emphasize how important effective monitoring is. Without the additional examination at 30 weeks, the outcome would probably not have been the same for us. We will always be grateful to the twin clinic for their care and dedication to our girls.

References

1. Lopriore E, Middeldorp JM, Oepkes D, Kanhai HH, Walther FJ, Vandenbussche FP. Twin anemia-polycythemia sequence in two monochorionic twin pairs without oligo-polyhydramnios sequence. Placenta. 2007;28(1):47–51.
2. Lewi L, Jani J, Blickstein I, Huber A, Gucciardo L, Van Mieghem T, et al. The outcome of monochorionic diamniotic twin gestations in the era of invasive fetal therapy: a prospective cohort study. Am J Obstet Gynecol. 2008;199(5):514 e1-8.
3. Yokouchi T, Murakoshi T, Mishima T, Yano H, Ohashi M, Suzuki T, et al. Incidence of spontaneous twin anemia-polycythemia sequence in monochorionic-diamniotic twin pregnancies: single-center prospective study. J Obstet Gynaecol Res. 2015;41(6):857–60.
4. Robyr R, Lewi L, Salomon LJ, Yamamoto M, Bernard JP, Deprest J, et al. Prevalence and management of late fetal complications following successful selective laser coagulation of chorionic plate anastomoses in twin-to-twin transfusion syndrome. Am J Obstet Gynecol. 2006;194(3):796–803.
5. Slaghekke F, Lewi L, Middeldorp JM, Weingertner AS, Klumper FJ, Dekoninck P, et al. Residual anastomoses in twin-twin transfusion syndrome after laser: the Solomon randomized trial. Am J Obstet Gynecol. 2014;211(3):285 e1-7.
6. Tollenaar LSA, Lopriore E, Faiola S, Stirnemann J, Lewi L, Weingertner AS, et al. Post-laser twin anemia polycythemia sequence: management and outcome in a large international cohort of 164 cases. Ultrasound Obstet Gynecol. 2019;9: 1759.
7. Tollenaar LSA, Slaghekke F, Lewi L, Colmant C, Lanna MM, Weingertner AS, et al. Spontaneous twin anemia polycythemia sequence: management and outcome in a large international cohort of 249 cases. Ultrasound Obstet Gynecol. 2019; In preparation
8. de Villiers SF, Slaghekke F, Middeldorp JM, Walther FJ, Oepkes D, Lopriore E. Placental characteristics in monochorionic twins with spontaneous versus post-laser twin anemia-polycythemia sequence. Placenta. 2013;34(5):456–9.
9. Mahieu-Caputo D, Dommergues M, Delezoide AL, Lacoste M, Cai Y, Narcy F, et al. Twin-to-twin transfusion syndrome. Role of the fetal renin-angiotensin system. Am J Pathol. 2000;156(2):629–36.
10. Van Winden KR, Quintero RA, Kontopoulos EV, Korst LM, Llanes A, Chmait RH. Pre-operative twin anemia/polycythemia in the setting of Twin-Twin Transfusion Syndrome (TTTS). Fetal Diagn Ther. 2015;37(4):274–80.
11. Donepudi R, Papanna R, Snowise S, Johnson A, Bebbington M, Moise KJ Jr. Does anemia-polycythemia complicating twin-twin transfusion syndrome affect outcome after fetoscopic laser surgery? Ultrasound Obstet Gynecol. 2016;47(3): 340–4.
12. Tollenaar LSA, Slaghekke F, van Klink JMM, Groene SG, Middeldorp JM, Haak MC, et al. Twin-twin transfusion syndrome with anemia-polycythemia: prevalence, characteristics, and outcome. J Clin Med. 2019;8(8):1129.
13. Lewi L, Jani J, Cannie M, Robyr R, Ville Y, Hecher K, et al. Intertwin anastomoses in monochorionic placentas after fetoscopic laser coagulation for twin-to-twin transfusion syndrome: is there more than meets the eye? Am J Obstet Gynecol. 2006;194(3):790–5.
14. Slaghekke F, van Klink JM, Koopman HM, Middeldorp JM, Oepkes D, Lopriore E. Neurodevelopmental outcome in twin anemia-polycythemia sequence after laser surgery for twin-twin transfusion syndrome. Ultrasound Obstet Gynecol. 2014;44(3):316–21.
15. Zhao D, Slaghekke F, Middeldorp JM, Duan T, Oepkes D, Lopriore E. Placental share and hemoglobin level in relation to birth weight in twin anemia-polycythemia sequence. Placenta. 2014;35(12):1070–4.
16. Groene SG, Tollenaar LSA, van Klink JMM, Haak MC, Klumper F, Middeldorp JM, et al. Twin-twin transfusion syndrome with and without selective fetal growth restriction prior to fetoscopic laser surgery: short and long-term outcome. J Clin Med. 2019;8(7):969.
17. Verbeek L, Slaghekke F, Hulzebos CV, Oepkes D, Walther FJ, Lopriore E. Hypoalbuminemia in donors with twin anemia-polycythemia sequence: a matched case-control study. Fetal Diagn Ther. 2013;33(4):241–5.
18. Groene SG, Tollenaar LSA, Slaghekke F, Middeldorp JM, Haak M, Oepkes D, et al. Placental characteristics in monochorionic twins with selective intrauterine growth restriction in relation to the umbilical artery Doppler classification. Placenta. 2018;71:1–5.
19. Slaghekke F, Kist WJ, Oepkes D, Pasman SA, Middeldorp JM, Klumper FJ, et al. Twin anemia-polycythemia sequence: diagnostic criteria, classification, perinatal management and outcome. Fetal Diagn Ther. 2010;27(4):181–90.
20. Tollenaar LS, Lopriore E, Middeldorp JM, Haak MC, Klumper FJ, Oepkes D, Slaghekke F. Improved antenatal prediction of twin anemia polycythemia sequence by delta middle cerebral artery peak systolic velocity – a new antenatal classification system. Ultrasound Obstet Gynecol. 2018;53:788.
21. Tavares de Sousa M, Fonseca A, Hecher K. Role of fetal intertwin difference in middle cerebral artery peak systolic velocity in predicting neonatal twin anemia-polycythemia sequence. Ultrasound Obstet Gynecol. 2019;53(6):794–7.
22. Fishel-Bartal M, Weisz B, Mazaki-Tovi S, Ashwal E, Chayen B, Lipitz S, et al. Can middle cerebral

artery peak systolic velocity predict polycythemia in monochorionic-diamniotic twins? Evidence from a prospective cohort study. Ultrasound Obstet Gynecol. 2016;48(4):470–5.
23. Khalil A, Gordijn S, Ganzevoort W, Thilaganathan B, Johnson A, Baschat A, et al. Consensus diagnostic criteria and monitoring of twin anemia polycythemia sequence: a Delphi procedure. Ultrasound Obstet Gynecol. 2019;56:388.
24. Stritzke A, Thomas S, Somerset D. Placental dichotomy: a hint in twin anemia polycythemia sequence. J Obstet Gynaecol Can. 2014;36(12):1097–100.
25. Tollenaar LSA, Lopriore E, Middeldorp JM, Klumper F, Haak MC, Oepkes D, et al. Prevalence of placental dichotomy, cardiomegaly and starry-sky liver on antenatal ultrasound in twin anemia polycythemia sequence. Ultrasound Obstet Gynecol. 2019;56:395.
26. Soundararajan LP, Howe DT. Starry sky liver in twin anemia-polycythemia sequence. Ultrasound Obstet Gynecol. 2014;43(5):597–9.
27. Lopriore E, Hecher K, Vandenbussche FP, van den Wijngaard JP, Klumper FJ, Oepkes D. Fetoscopic laser treatment of twin-to-twin transfusion syndrome followed by severe twin anemia-polycythemia sequence with spontaneous resolution. Am J Obstet Gynecol. 2008;198(2):e4–7.
28. Tollenaar LSA, Slaghekke F, Lewi L, Ville Y, Lanna MM, Weingertner AS, et al. Treatment and outcome in 370 cases with spontaneous and post-laser twin anemia polycythemia sequence managed in 17 different fetal therapy centers. Ultrasound Obstet Gynecol. 2019;56:378.
29. Herway C, Johnson A, Moise K, Moise KJ Jr. Fetal intraperitoneal transfusion for iatrogenic twin anemia-polycythemia sequence after laser therapy. Ultrasound Obstet Gynecol. 2009;33(5):592–4.
30. Slaghekke F, van den Wijngaard JP, Akkermans J, van Gemert MJ, Middeldorp JM, Klumper FJ, et al. Intrauterine transfusion combined with partial exchange transfusion for twin anemia polycythemia sequence: modeling a novel technique. Placenta. 2015;36(5):599–602.
31. Bahtiyar MO, Ekmekci E, Demirel E, Irani RA, Copel JA. In utero partial exchange transfusion combined with in utero blood transfusion for prenatal management of twin anemia-polycythemia sequence. Fetal Diagn Ther. 2018;45:28.
32. Genova L, Slaghekke F, Klumper FJ, Middeldorp JM, Steggerda SJ, Oepkes D, et al. Management of twin anemia-polycythemia sequence using intrauterine blood transfusion for the donor and partial exchange transfusion for the recipient. Fetal Diagn Ther. 2013;34(2):121–6.
33. Senat MV, Deprest J, Boulvain M, Paupe A, Winer N, Ville Y. Endoscopic laser surgery versus serial amnioreduction for severe twin-to-twin transfusion syndrome. N Engl J Med. 2004;351(2):136–44.
34. Slaghekke F, Lopriore E, Lewi L, Middeldorp JM, van Zwet EW, Weingertner AS, et al. Fetoscopic laser coagulation of the vascular equator versus selective coagulation for twin-to-twin transfusion syndrome: an open-label randomised controlled trial. Lancet. 2014;383(9935):2144–51.
35. Slaghekke F, Lewi L, Middeldorp JM, Weingertner AS, Klumper FJ, Dekoninck P, et al. Residual anastomoses in twin-twin transfusion syndrome after laser: the Solomon randomized trial. Am J Obstet Gynecol. 2014;211(3):285 e1-7.
36. Slaghekke F, Lopriore E, Lewi L, Middeldorp JM, van Zwet EW, Weingertner AS, et al. Fetoscopic laser coagulation of the vascular equator versus selective coagulation for twin-to-twin transfusion syndrome: an open-label randomised controlled trial. Lancet. 2014;383(9935):2144–51.
37. Hill KM, Masoudian P, Fung-Kee-Fung K, El Demellawy D. Intrauterine interventions for the treatment of twin anemia-polycythemia sequence: a systematic review. J Obstet Gynaecol Can. 2019;41(7):981–91.
38. Sananes N, Veujoz M, Severac F, Barthoulot M, Meyer N, Weingertner AS, et al. Evaluation of the utility of in utero treatment of twin anemia-polycythemia sequence. Fetal Diagn Ther. 2015;38(3):170–8.
39. Slaghekke F, Favre R, Peeters SH, Middeldorp JM, Weingertner AS, van Zwet EW, et al. Laser surgery as a management option for twin anemia-polycythemia sequence. Ultrasound Obstet Gynecol. 2014;44(3):304–10.
40. The TAPS Trial: fetoscopic laser surgery for twin anemia polycythemia sequence - a multicenter open-label randomized controlled trial https://www.trialregister.nl/trial/6879: Netherlands Trial Register 2019.
41. Lopriore E, Slaghekke F, Oepkes D, Middeldorp JM, Vandenbussche FP, Walther FJ. Hematological characteristics in neonates with twin anemia-polycythemia sequence (TAPS). Prenat Diagn. 2010;30(3):251–5.
42. Lopriore E, Holtkamp N, Sueters M, Middeldorp JM, Walther FJ, Oepkes D. Acute peripartum twin-twin transfusion syndrome: incidence, risk factors, placental characteristics and neonatal outcome. J Obstet Gynaecol Res. 2014;40(1):18–24.
43. Tollenaar LS, Zhao DP, Middeldorp JM, Slaghekke F, Oepkes D, Lopriore E. Color difference in placentas with twin anemia-polycythemia sequence: an additional diagnostic criterion? Fetal Diagn Ther. 2016;40(2):123–7.
44. Tollenaar LSA, Zhao DP, Middeldorp JM, Oepkes D, Slaghekke F, Lopriore E. Can color difference on the maternal side of the placenta distinguish between acute peripartum twin-twin transfusion syndrome and twin anemia-polycythemia sequence? Placenta. 2017;57:189–93.
45. Lopriore E, Slaghekke F, Kersbergen KJ, de Vries LS, Drogtrop AP, Middeldorp JM, et al. Severe cerebral injury in a recipient with twin anemia-polycythemia sequence. Ultrasound Obstet Gynecol. 2013;41(6):702–6.

46. Visser GL, Tollenaar LSA, Bekker V, Te Pas AB, Lankester AC, Oepkes D, et al. Leukocyte counts and other hematological values in twin-twin transfusion syndrome and twin anemia-polycythemia sequence. Fetal Diagn Ther. 2019:1–6.
47. Verbeek L, Slaghekke F, Favre R, Vieujoz M, Cavigioli F, Lista G, et al. Short-term postnatal renal function in twin anemia-polycythemia sequence. Fetal Diagn Ther. 2016;39(3):192–7.
48. Sarkar S, Rosenkrantz TS. Neonatal polycythemia and hyperviscosity. Semin Fetal Neonatal Med. 2008;13(4):248–55.
49. Tollenaar LSA, Lopriore E, Slaghekke F, Oepkes D, Middeldorp JM, Haak MC, et al. High risk of long-term impairment in donor twins with spontaneous twin anemia polycythemia sequence. Ultrasound Obstet Gynecol. 2019
50. Lindenburg IT, Smits-Wintjens VE, van Klink JM, Verduin E, van Kamp IL, Walther FJ, et al. Long-term neurodevelopmental outcome after intrauterine transfusion for hemolytic disease of the fetus/newborn: the LOTUS study. Am J Obstet Gynecol. 2012;206(2):141 e1-8.
51. Spruijt MS, Lopriore E, Tan R, Slaghekke F, Klumper F, Middeldorp JM, et al. Long-term neurodevelopmental outcome in twin-to-twin transfusion syndrome: is there still room for improvement? J Clin Med. 2019;8(8):1226.
52. Hille ET, van Straaten HI, Verkerk PH, Dutch NNHSWG. Prevalence and independent risk factors for hearing loss in NICU infants. Acta Paediatr. 2007;96(8):1155–8.

Key Reading

Tollenaar LS, Slaghekke F, Middeldorp JM, Klumper FJ, Haak MC, Oepkes D, Lopriore E. Twin anemia polycythemia sequence: current views on pathogenesis, diagnostic criteria, perinatal management, and outcome. Twin Res Hum Genet. 2016;19(3):222–33.

Tollenaar LSA, Lopriore E, Middeldorp JM, Haak MC, Klumper FJ, Oepkes D, Slaghekke F. Improved prediction of twin anemia-polycythemia sequence by delta middle cerebral artery peak systolic velocity: new antenatal classification system. Ultrasound Obstet Gynecol. 2019;53(6):788–93.

Tollenaar LSA, Lopriore E, Slaghekke F, Oepkes D, Middeldorp JM, Haak MC, Klumper FJCM, Tan RNGB, Rijken M, Van Klink JMM. High risk of long-term neurodevelopmental impairment in donor twins with spontaneous twin anemia-polycythemia sequence. Ultrasound Obstet Gynecol. 2020;55(1):39–46.

16

Twin Reversed Arterial Perfusion Sequence

Liesbeth Lewi

Contents

Electronic Supplementary Material The online version of this chapter (https://doi.org/10.1007/978-3-030-47652-6_17) contains supplementary material, which is available to authorized users. The videos can be accessed by scanning the related images with the SN More Media App.

A. Khalil et al. (eds.), *Twin and Higher-order Pregnancies*,
https://doi.org/10.1007/978-3-030-47652-6_17

Trailer

Twin reversed arterial perfusion (TRAP) sequence is an unusual anomaly that only occurs in monochorionic multiple pregnancies. If one twin dies in the early embryonic period, its body may continue to grow, thanks to a reversed perfusion through an artery-to-artery anastomosis by its surviving co-twin. This parasitism puts the healthy survivor at risk of high-output cardiac and demise. In this chapter, we provide up-to-date information on the pathophysiology, diagnosis, and management of this rare anomaly.

Definitions

Twin reversed arterial perfusion (TRAP) sequence: an anomaly unique to monochorionic multiple pregnancies in which an early embryonic demise of one twin leads to a reversed perfusion by the surviving pump twin through a large artery-to-artery anastomosis.

Holoacardia: when the heart is absent.

Hemiacardia: when there is a rudimentary heart with some functional activity.

Acephalus: the most common presentation in which there is still a reasonable development of the lower limbs whereas the head is absent and the upper limbs are only partially developed.

Acormus: the rarest form in which only the head is present.

Anceps: when the entire body is reasonably well preserved.

Amorphus: which is the least differentiated form presenting as a shapeless mass of tissue.

Learning Objectives

- To understand the pathophysiology, diagnostic features, and management of TRAP
- To know the natural history and the different in utero interventions to arrest the reversed blood flow

17.1 Introduction

Twin reversed arterial perfusion (TRAP) sequence is a rare anomaly unique to monochorionic multiple pregnancies. A nonviable fetus becomes a parasite perfused through the vascular anastomoses on the surface of the monochorionic placenta. This parasitism strains the heart of the host, leading to heart failure and polyhydramnios-related preterm birth [1]. Based on estimates at the time of birth, an incidence of 1 in 100 monochorionic twins or 1 in 35,000 pregnancies is quoted [2, 3]. However, with the introduction of the first-trimester ultrasound scan, likely, more TRAP cases are now detected that would go unnoticed at birth, and an incidence of 1 in 40 monochorionic twins or 1 in 15,000 pregnancies is probably more accurate [4]. Monoamniotic pregnancies are at higher risk of TRAP (See Section V, ► Chap. 19, T. Vanmieghem). However, since most monochorionic twins are diamniotic, two-thirds of the TRAP cases are diagnosed in a diamniotic setting [5]. This chapter aims to give an up-to-date overview of the pathophysiology, diagnosis, and management of TRAP.

17.2 Pathophysiology

TRAP arises if there is an early embryonic demise in a monochorionic multiple pregnancy. In a dichorionic pregnancy, such an early demise leads to a "vanishing twin syndrome," whereas in a monochorionic pregnancy, the demised twin may continue to grow, thanks to the blood supply by the vascular anastomoses. Through an artery-to-artery anastomosis, deoxygenated blood flows from the healthy "pump" twin in a reversed direction into the cord of its demised "acardiac" co-twin – hence the name twin reversed arterial perfusion sequence. Severely deoxygenated blood returns to the pump through a vein-to-vein anastomosis (◘ Fig. 17.1). In this way, the blood flow bypasses the placenta, and the acardiac twin thus lacks functional placental

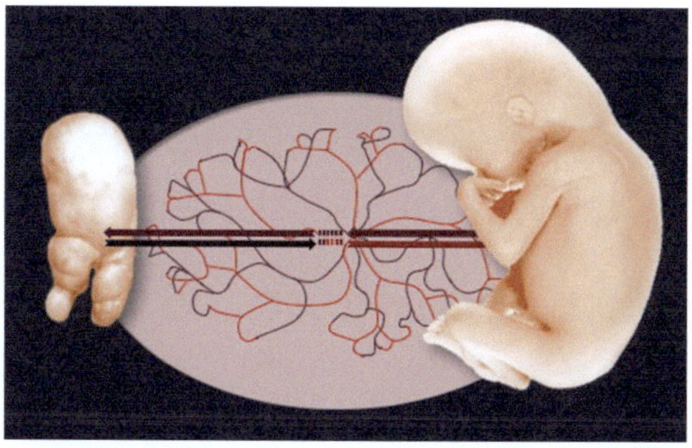

Fig. 17.1 In twin reversed arterial perfusion (TRAP) sequence, deoxygenated blood flows from a structurally normal pump twin through an artery-to-artery anastomosis in a reversed direction to a severely abnormal demised co-twin (brown arrow). Oxygen-depleted blood (black arrow) then circulates back to the pump twin through a vein-to-vein anastomosis, causing hypoxemia in the only viable fetus in this twin pregnancy

territory. The parasitic acardiac twin threatens the well-being of the pump twin in two critical ways. First, the perfusion of the acardiac twin may lead to high-output heart failure and polyhydramnios [6]. Second, severely deoxygenated blood is circulated back to the pump twin to a vein-to-vein anastomosis, further reducing the oxygen level and leading to hypoxemia [7].

17.3 Diagnosis

TRAP should be diagnosed at the time of the first-trimester scan between 11 and 14 weeks. Typically, there is one normal and one grossly abnormal twin in a monochorionic twin pregnancy. Usually, the acardiac twin does not show a heartbeat and has marked cystic subcutaneous edema [8] (Fig. 17.2). The features of the acardiac twin are extremely variable and depend on the timing of the demise and the direction of the reversed flow. Typically, poorly oxygenated arterial blood enters the acardiac through the umbilical and iliac vessels to preferentially supply its caudal body parts. As the blood becomes progressively more deoxygenated as it travels upward, this results in an atrophy of the upper limbs and head. Therefore, most acardiac twins still have a reasonable development of the lower limbs and pelvis, but no thoracic organs and head, and often also no upper limbs. This form is known as acardiacus acephalus. The rarest presentation is when there is only a development of the head: the acephalus acormus. When most body parts are present, we speak of acardiacus anceps, whereas acardiacus amorphus refers to a shapeless mass of tissue without any recognizable parts (Fig. 17.3) [9]. Usually, the heart is absent (holoacardiacus), but sometimes a rudimentary heart (hemiacardiacus) is present, albeit with slow heart rhythm and weak output.

Pathognomonic for TRAP sequence is the demonstration by Doppler examination of the reversed cord blood flow, which is toward rather than away from the acardiac twin (Fig. 17.4, Video 17.1). Of note is that two-thirds of acardiac twins have a single umbilical artery [10]. Sometimes, the cord of the acardiac may not insert on the placental surface but originate directly from the pump's cord.

The differential diagnosis should be made with an early spontaneous demise without reversed transfusion (Fig. 17.5) by using Doppler ultrasound to ascertain the absence of reversed flow in the cord and body of the demised twin. Also, it is good practice to review the patient after 1 week to confirm the absence of flow, which may only be visible intermittently. Other diagnoses to consider are a placental teratoma or chorioangioma (Fig. 17.6). Both conditions may also cause congestive heart failure, but the acardiac twin usually has a separate, though often rudimentary, cord, and is covered by normal skin.

Treatment will vary according to whether the acardiac and pump twin share a single amniotic sac or not, so it is essential to determine the amnionicity correctly (See Section III, ► Chap. 6, Vanoppen M Determining Chorionicity and Amnionicity). In the first trimester, the acardiac sac still contains amniotic fluid due to diffusion from the maternal compartment even in the absence of kidneys, and the biamniotic septum will be visible in

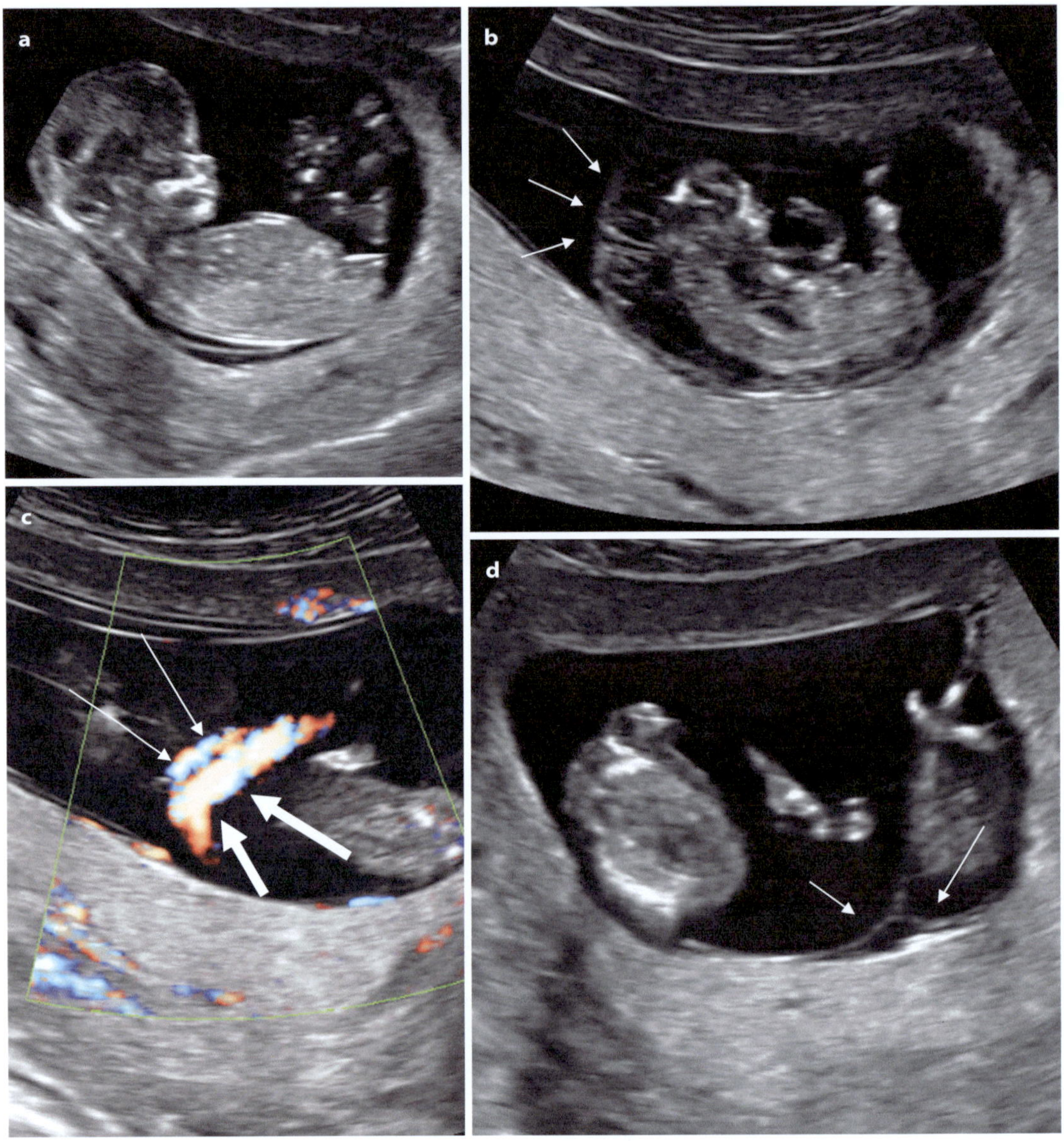

Fig. 17.2 Sonographic image of the typical presentation of twin reversed arterial perfusions sequence in a monochorionic diamniotic twin pregnancy at 12 weeks. **a** Structurally normal pump twin; **b** acardiac twin with typical cystic edema (arrows); **c** the thin cord of the acardiac twin (thin arrows) originates directly from the thicker cord of the pump twin (thick arrows); **d** the empty lambda sign (arrows) suggests a diamniotic pregnancy

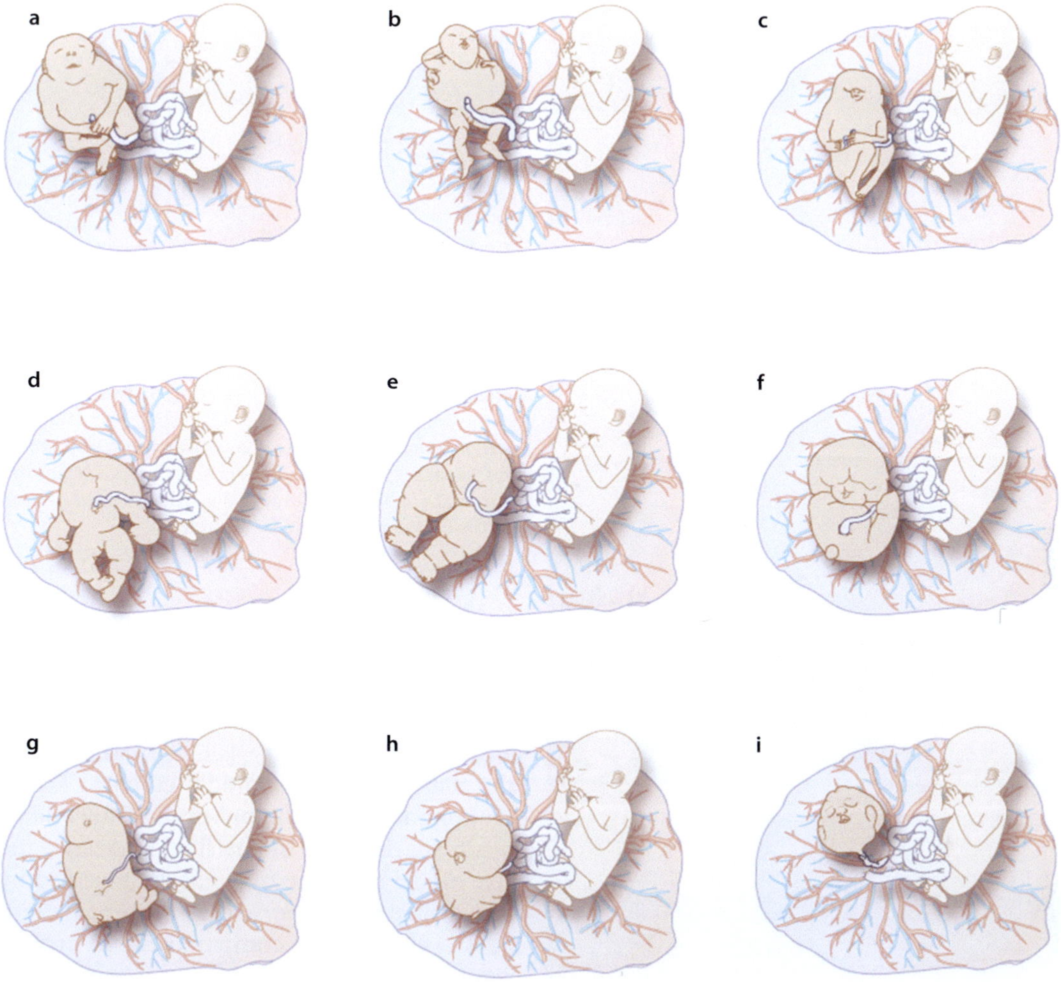

Fig. 17.3 Graphic representation of the different presentations of the acardiac twin. **a–c** Acardiacus anceps when most body parts are preserved; **d**, **e** acardiacus acephalus when the head is absent, whereas the lower limbs are reasonably well developed; **f–h** acardiacus amorphus when there are no recognizable structures; **i** acardiacus acormus when only the head is developed

a diamniotic pregnancy. In the second trimester, the septum may no longer be visible if the acardiac lacks functional kidneys. However, in a diamniotic pregnancy, the acardiac is stuck, whereas in a monoamniotic setting, the acardiac twin moves freely in the shared amniotic sac.

As mentioned above, in the second trimester, it may be useful to look for high-output cardiac failure, such as tricuspid

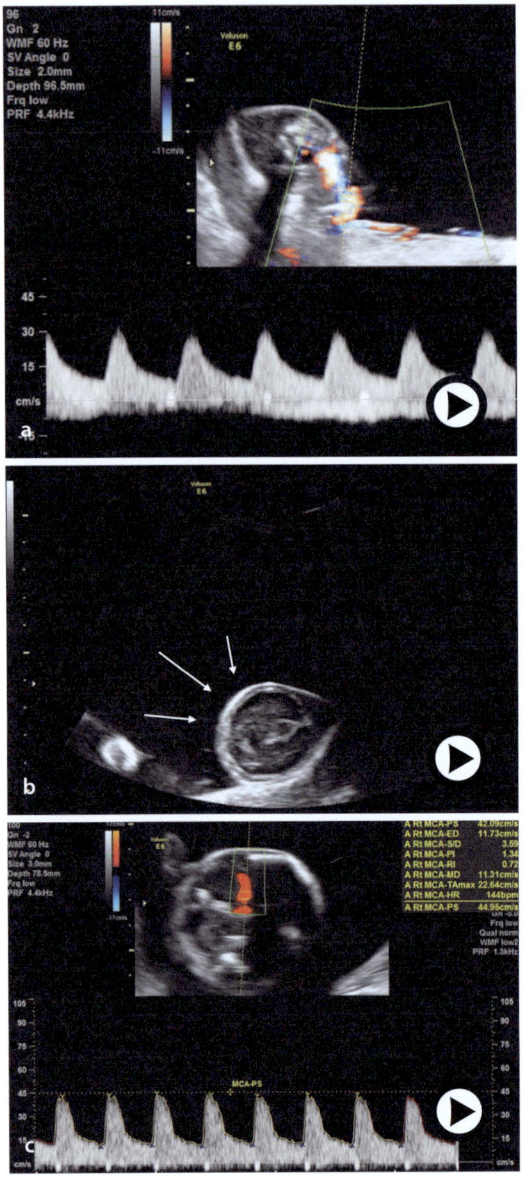

■ **Fig. 17.4** **a** Color and pulsed wave Doppler demonstrating the reversed blood flow in an acadiacus acormus diagnosed at 23 weeks. **b** The acardiacus consisted of a head with rudimentary brain (arrows) stuck to the posterior uterine wall. **c** The pump had brain sparing and an elevated peak-systolic velocity of the middle cerebral artery suggestive of anemia

Video 17.1 Acardiacus acormus at 23 weeks presenting with polyhydramnios, anemia, and cardiac hypertrophy in the pump twin (https://doi.org/10.1007/000-2tk) (https://doi.org/10.1007/000-2tm) (https://doi.org/10.1007/000-2tn)

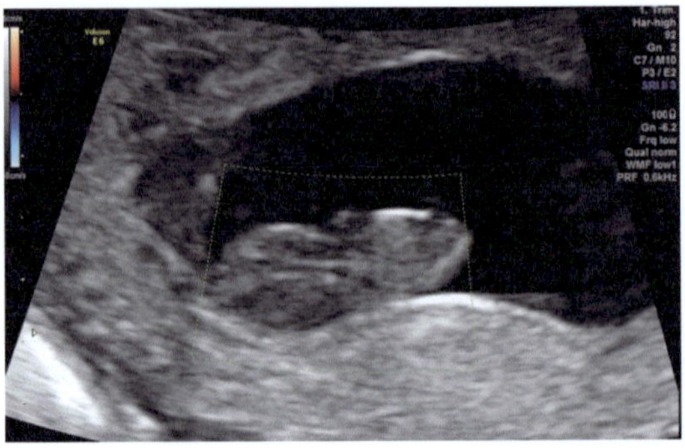

■ **Fig. 17.5** Sonographic image at 12 weeks of a single demise of one twin of a monochorionic twin pair with crown-rump length of 9 weeks. Color Doppler could not demonstrate any flow and the typical cystic subcutaneous edema is absent. Follow-up scan 1 week later confirmed the absence of flow, and a twin reversed arterial perfusion sequence could be excluded

regurgitation, abnormal ductus venosus blood flow, a pulsatile umbilical vein, and polyhydramnios. Also, low resistance in the umbilical artery of the acardiac suggests high vascularity [11–13], whereas in the pump twin, the middle cerebral artery Doppler indicates the presence of anemia or brain sparing [7]. In the first trimester, the size of the acardiac twin can be assessed by measuring the upper pole to rump length (URL) that can be compared to the crown-rump length (CRL) of the pump twin by calculation of the URL/CRL ratio [14]. In the second trimester, the weight of the acardiac twin can be calculated by using the equation of the prolate ellipsoid ($V = \pi/6 \times$ longitudinal $\times$ transverse $\times$ anterior-posterior diameter) in cm^3 or gram [15].

17.4 Natural History

Due to high-output cardiac failure and polyhydramnios-related very preterm birth, the risk of perinatal death for the pump twin is about 35–55%, and birth is, on average, around 30 weeks [6, 10]. Several factors pre-

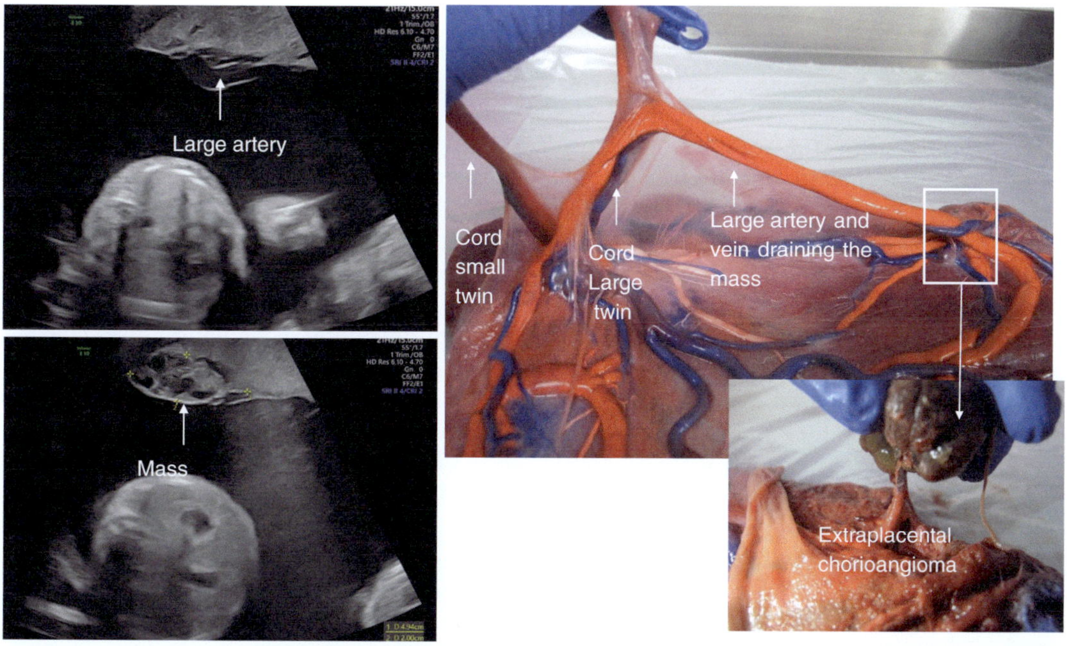

Fig. 17.6 Sonographic image of a monochorionic diamniotic twin pregnancy at 25 weeks with selective growth restriction type 3. **a** On the placenta, a large artery originating from the larger twin to supply a placental mass was seen on ultrasound scan **b**. The differential diagnosis was a monochorionic diamniotic triplet pregnancy with an acardiac twin embedded in the placenta or a chorio-angioma. **c** The placenta after birth showing a large artery and vein supplying a placental mass. The cord from the growth restricted twin inserted next to the cord of the appropriately growing twin **d**. Histology demonstrated an extraplacental chorio-angioma in a monochorionic diamniotic twin pregnancy

dict a poor prognosis, such as an acardiac to the pump size ratio of more than 50% [16] or an increase in absolute size, signs of cardiac failure (tricuspid regurgitation, abnormal ductus venosus, a pulsatile umbilical vein, polyhydramnios), and a high vascularity of the acardiac mass as evidenced by a low resistance in its umbilical artery blood flow [11–13].

The 35–55% perinatal mortality is based on TRAP diagnosed at the time of the second-trimester anomaly scan [6, 10]. Looking from the first trimester, however, about one in three pump twins dies between the first trimester and the 16–18 weeks evaluation. In about one in five cases, the reversed blood flow stops spontaneously, but only 40% of pump twins ultimately survive. Differences in nuchal translucency or crown-rump length do not predict subsequent pump twin demise [16].

17.5 Management

In TRAP sequence, the pump is the only viable twin. Parents must be counseled about the options of conservative management, in-utero intervention to arrest the reversed blood flow, or termination of the entire pregnancy.

In Europe, most centers offer a prophylactic in utero intervention to arrest the reversed perfusion if still present in the early second trimester [16]. There are several reasons to offer treatment once amnion and chorion are fused. First, the prognostic features like the acardiac's size have not been properly validated in prospective series, and their accuracy remains mostly unknown. As such, sudden pump twin demise may occur in the absence of any of these features. Also, these variables were identified in postnatal series or cohorts of mid-trimester TRAP, and their predictive value in the early second trimester is uncertain. Second, it may be more difficult to arrest the reversed flow later in pregnancy. Third, there is concern that long-standing hypoxemia adversely affects the pump twin's neurodevelopment [7]. As such, there was a developmental delay in 3 of 4 infants who underwent an in utero intervention for cardiac decompensation in TRAP after 23 weeks, whereas all of the 15 infants treated before 23 weeks showed a normal development [17].

In the United States, most centers only offer in utero treatment once the acardiac to pump weight ratio exceeds 50% or if the acardiac mass grows rapidly, if the resistance in the acardiac's umbilical artery is lower than that of its pump twin, or if the pump twin shows signs of heart failure or anemia. This more cautious approach aims to avoid unnecessary in utero intervention. In the absence of poor prognostic features, they follow TRAP cases with a weekly follow-up scan until blood flow to the acardiac twin has stopped, or the relative weight of the acardiac twin has declined or remained constant for two consecutive scans. Insufficient data are available on the number of cases that eventually undergo in utero surgery with such initial expectant management and on the long-term neurodevelopmental outcome of surviving pump twins [7].

While awaiting further refinement of the noninvasive high-intensity focused ultrasound [18], the currently preferred techniques to arrest the reversed flow in TRAP are percutaneous interventions with coagulation of the acardiac's cord, the intrafetal vessels, or the vascular anastomoses (See Section IV, ▶ Chap. 12, see chapter on selective reduction). Ideally, the surgeon adapts the approach to the individual requirements of each case. As such, in a monoamniotic setting, cord coagulation and transection [19] are the preferred techniques to avoid late pump twin demise due to cord entanglement [15]. In a diamniotic pregnancy, intrafetal coagulation is also less indicated if the acardiac's sac is not accessible, as puncture of the intertwin septum will create an iatrogenic monoamniotic pregnancy with a similar risk of remote pump demise due to cord entanglement [17]. If the acardiac's sac is inaccessible, coagulation of the anastomoses through the sac of the pump twin may be a safer option [20]. In most other settings, intrafetal coagulation is the most commonly used technique in TRAP.

With intrafetal coagulation, we place a 20-gauge (0.8 mm) to 15-gauge (1.45 mm) (G) needle into the abdomen or pelvis of the acardiac twin near the target vessels under ultrasound guidance. We stop the reversed flow using laser [21], radiofrequency (RFA) [15] (Video 17.2), or microwave coagulation [22]. No studies compare the efficacy of the different energy sources, but laser is most commonly used for interventions at 16–18 weeks through a 20–18 G needle (0.8–1 mm), whereas RFA may be more effective at later gestational ages by using a 17 G (1.14 mm) needle. Microwave ablation is a relatively new technique that uses a 15 G (1.45 mm) needle. Microwave ablation does not carry the risk of maternal burns reported of RFA and is probably more suitable for the coagulation of large vessels than RFA ablation [22].

Fetoscopic laser coagulation of the cord and anastomosing vessels through a 7 (2.3 mm) to 10 (3.3 mm) trocar is similar to the technique used for TTTS (See Section 11.5, ▶ Chap. 11, K. Hecher) (Video 17.3). As mentioned above, cord coagulation with transection is the preferred treatment in monoamniotic pregnancies. Even if the flow stopped spontaneously, transection of the cord prevents the unexpected demise of the pump twin due to entanglement (◘ Fig. 17.7, Video 17.2). Coagulation of the anastomosing vessels through the sac of the pump twin is probably the best option when the acardiac's sac is only accessible through septostomy. Ultrasound-guided coagulation using a bipolar forceps is not so commonly used for TRAP anymore, except in a monoamniotic setting before transection, when the cord is too thick to achieve occlusion with laser (Video 17.4). Often the cord of the acardiac twin is very short or originates directly from the pump's

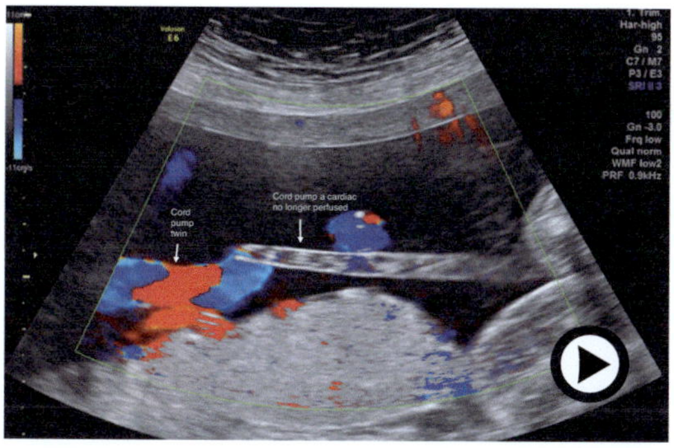

Fig. 17.7 Ultrasound image twin of cord entanglement of a twin reversed arterial perfusion sequence at 18 weeks in a monoamniotic twin pregnancy. The reversed flow had stopped spontaneously, but because of the cord entanglement and the significant risk of unexpected pump twin demise, a cord transection was performed using fetoscopic laser surgery. First, the cord was coagulated using a bipolar forceps under ultrasound guidance to facilitate the cord transection (Video 17.2)

Video 17.2 Ultrasound image twin of cord entanglement of a twin reversed arterial perfusion sequence at 18 weeks in a monoamniotic twin pregnancy. The reversed flow had stopped spontaneously, but because of the cord entanglement and the significant risk of unexpected pump twin demise, a cord transection was performed using fetoscopic laser surgery. First, the cord was coagulated using a bipolar forceps under ultrasound guidance to facilitate the cord transection (Video 17.2) (https://doi.org/10.1007/000-2tp)

cord, which makes it challenging to grasp the cord under ultrasound guidance. Although there are no randomized studies, the current practice is to perform intrafetal coagulation in a diamniotic pregnancy if there is a direct access target sac. TRAP in higher-order monochorionic pregnancies poses a challenging situation for in utero intervention, such as in a triplet pregnancy with one pump and two acardiac triplets [23] or with one acardiac and one pump and one “draining” triplet.

After an in utero intervention, the survival rate for the pump twin is between 75% and 90% [15–17; 20–22]. The pump twin remains at risk of intrauterine demise, miscarriage, and extreme preterm birth with subsequent neonatal demise. The average gestational age birth is between 34 and 36 weeks, and the risk of very preterm birth is between 10% and 20% [15–17; 20–22]. Insufficient data are available on the long-term development of pump twin survivors. After an in-utero intervention, we always offer magnetic resonance imaging of the fetal brain around 28–30 weeks to exclude antenatally acquired brain lesions. As mentioned above, no randomized studies exist to compare the different techniques, and the choice is best adapted to the specifics of each case. Nevertheless, intrafetal coagulation, as a needle-based technique, may carry a lower risk of iatrogenic membrane rupture compared with laser or bipolar cord coagulation [24]. Also, there seems to be an inverse relationship between the gestational age at surgery and the timing of birth, with earlier interventions delivering at later gestational ages [21].

Some centers [14, 21, 25] already offer intrafetal coagulation in the first trimester, given the 33% risk of pump twin demise between the first-trimester diagnosis and the planned intervention at 16–18 weeks [16]. However, since monochorionic twins share the same exocoelomic cavity, a first-trimester intervention may increase the miscarriage risk. The question of whether to intervene in the first (12–14 weeks) or early second (16–19 weeks) trimester is currently the subject of the multicenter randomized TRAPIST study (TRAP Intervention STudy NCT02621645).

17.6 Conclusion

TRAP sequence is the most unusual human malformation that only affects monochorionic pregnancies as it requires a reversed transfusion through vascular anastomoses from the healthy pump twin toward its demised acardiac twin. The acardiac twin has neither a functional heart nor any placental territory but continues to grow, thanks to the reversed blood supply. This parasitic situation carries a high risk of cardiac failure and loss. An intervention to arrest the reversed flow can be offered either prophylactically or once there are poor prognostic signs. Survival after in utero surgery is around 80% with an average gestation at birth of 36 weeks but still a very preterm birth rate of 10–20%. Better data are needed that document the best timing of the intervention and the impact of TRAP and its treatment on the long-term neurodevelopment of the pump twin.

17.6.1 Review Questions

1. Why does twin reversed arterial perfusion sequence only occur in monochorionic multiple pregnancies?

2. What are the diagnostic features of twin reversed arterial perfusion sequence?

3. In what circumstances is intrafetal coagulation not the preferred surgical technique?

17.6.2 Multiple-Choice Questions

1. Which of the following statements about TRAP is correct?
   (a) Oxygenated blood travels in a reversed direction from the pump toward the acardiac twin.
   (b) Most acardiac twins present as a shapeless mass without any recognizable features.
   (c) The presence of cardiac activity in the severely malformed twin excludes TRAP sequence.
   (d) The acardiac twin lacks functional placental territory.

Answer: (d)

2. What is the best treatment of TRAP in a monoamniotic twin pregnancy?
   (a) Coagulation of the vascular anastomoses that supply the acardiac twin.
   (b) Intrafetal coagulation of the feeding vessels in the acardiac mass.
   (c) Occlusion and transection of the acardiac's cord.
   (d) Expectant management as the risk of postoperative rupture of the membranes is too high.

Answer: (c)

Disclosure Statement

The author reports no conflict of interest.

Financial Support

LL is the recipient of a grant of "Fonds voor Wetenschappelijk Onderzoek" (FWO grant no: 1804718N).

References

1. Van Allen MI, Smith DW, Shepard TH. Twin reversed arterial perfusion (TRAP) sequence: a study of 14 twin pregnancies with acardius. Semin Perinatol. 1983;7:285–93.
2. Napolitani FD, Schreiber I. The acardiac monster. A review of the world literature and presentation of two cases. Am J Obstet Gynecol. 1960;80:582–9.
3. James WH. A note on the epidemiology of acardiac monsters. Teratology. 1977;16:211–6.
4. van Gemert MJ, van den Wijngaard JP, Vandenbussche FP. Twin reversed arterial perfusion sequence is more common than generally accepted. Birth Defects Res A Clin Mol Teratol. 2015;103:641–3.
5. Benirschke K, Kaufmann P. Pathology of the human placenta. 2nd ed. New York: Springer; 1995. p. 702–10.
6. Moore TR, Gale S, Benirschke K. Perinatal outcome of forty-nine pregnancies complicated by acardiac twinning. Am J Obstet Gynecol. 1990;163:907–12.
7. Peyvandi S, Feldstein VA, Hirose S, Rand L, Brook MM, Moon-Grady AJ. Twin-reversed arterial perfusion sequence associated with decreased fetal cerebral vascular impedance. Ultrasound Obstet Gynecol. 2015;45:447–51.
8. Sepulveda WH, Quiroz VH, Giuliano A, Henriquez R. Prenatal ultrasonographic diagnosis of acardiac twin. J Perinat Med. 1993;21:241–6.
9. Wong AE, Sepulveda W. Acardiac anomaly: current issues in prenatal assessment and treatment. Prenat Diagn. 2005;25:796–806.
10. Healey MG. Acardia: predictive risk factors for the co-twin's survival. Teratology. 1994;50:205–13.
11. Sherer DM, Armstrong B, Shah YG, Metlay LA, Woods JR. Prenatal sonographic diagnosis, Doppler velocimetric umbilical cord studies, and subsequent management of an acardiac twin pregnancy. Obstet Gynecol. 1989;74:472–5.
12. Brassard M, Fouron JC, Leduc L, Grignon A, Proulx F. Prognostic markers in twin pregnan-

cies with an acardiac fetus. Obstet Gynecol. 1999;94:409–14.
13. Dashe JS, Fernandez CO, Twickler DM. Utility of Doppler velocimetry in predicting outcome in twin reversed-arterial perfusion sequence. Am J Obstet Gynecol. 2001;185:135–9.
14. Roethlisberger M, Strizek B, Gottschalk I, Mallmann MR, Geipel A, Gembruch U, Berg C. First-trimester intervention in twin reversed arterial perfusion sequence: does size matter? Ultrasound Obstet Gynecol. 2017;50:40–4.
15. Lee H, Bebbington M, Crombleholme TM, North American Fetal Therapy Network. The North American Fetal Therapy Network Registry data on outcomes of radiofrequency ablation for twin-reversed arterial perfusion sequence. Fetal Diagn Ther. 2013;3:224–9.
16. Lewi L, Valencia C, Gonzalez E, Deprest J, Nicolaides KH. The outcome of twin reversed arterial perfusion sequence diagnosed in the first trimester. Am J Obstet Gynecol. 2010;203:213, e1–4.
17. Lewi L, Gratacos E, Ortibus E, Van Schoubroeck D, Carreras E, Higueras T, et al. Pregnancy and infant outcome of 80 consecutive cord coagulations in complicated monochorionic multiple pregnancies. Am J Obstet Gynecol. 2006;194:782–9.
18. Seo K, Ichizuka K, Okai T, Dohi S, Nakamura M, Hasegawa J, Matsuoka R, Yoshizawa S, Umemura SI, Nagatsuka M, Sekizawa A. Treatment of twin-reversed arterial perfusion sequence using high-intensity focused ultrasound. Ultrasound Obstet Gynecol. 2019;54:128–34.
19. Molina FS, Gomez LF, Gonzalía DA, Fresneda MD, Padilla MC, Lewi L. Cord transection in monoamniotic twins: use of a 1000-micron fiber with conical tip. Ultrasound Obstet Gynecol. 2014;44:116–8.
20. Hecher K, Lewi L, Gratacos E, Huber A, Ville Y, Deprest J. Twin reversed arterial perfusion: fetoscopic laser coagulation of placental anastomoses or the umbilical cord. Ultrasound Obstet Gynecol. 2006;28:688–91.
21. Chaveeva P, Poon LC, Sotiriadis A, Kosinski P, Nicolaides KH. Optimal method and timing of intrauterine intervention in twin reversed arterial perfusion sequence: case study and meta-analysis. Fetal Diagn Ther. 2014;35:267–79.
22. Stephenson CD, Temming LA, Pollack R, Iannitti DA. Microwave ablation for twin-reversed arterial perfusion sequence: a novel application of technology. Fetal Diagn Ther. 2015;38:35–40.
23. Smet M, Smet D, DeKoninck P, De Catte L, Deprest J, Devlieger R. Prenatal surgery in a triplet pregnancy complicated by a double twin reversed arterial perfusion (TRAP) sequence. Case Rep Perinatal Med. 2012;1:83–6.
24. Tan TY, Sepulveda W. Acardiac twin: a systematic review of minimally invasive treatment modalities. Ultrasound Obstet Gynecol. 2003;22:409–19.
25. Tavares de Sousa M, Glosemeyer P, Diemert A, Bamberg C, Hecher K. First-trimester intervention in twin reversed arterial perfusion sequence. Ultrasound Obstet Gynecol. 2020;55(1):47–9. https://doi.org/10.1002/uog.20860.

Key Reading

Chaveeva P, Poon LC, Sotiriadis A, Kosinski P, Nicolaides KH. Optimal method and timing of intrauterine intervention in twin reversed arterial perfusion sequence: case study and meta-analysis. Fetal Diagn Ther. 2014;35:267–79.

Lewi L, Valencia C, Gonzalez E, Deprest J, Nicolaides KH. The outcome of twin reversed arterial perfusion sequence diagnosed in the first trimester. Am J Obstet Gynecol. 2010;203:213, e1–4.

Monochorionic Monoamniotic Twin Pregnancy

Noa Gilad, Vagisha Pruthi, Shiri Shinar, Johannes Keunen, Greg Ryan, and Tim Van Mieghem

Contents

Electronic Supplementary Material The online version of this chapter (https://doi.org/10.1007/978-3-030-47652-6_18) contains supplementary material, which is available to authorized users. The videos can be accessed by scanning the related images with the SN More Media App.

A. Khalil et al. (eds.), *Twin and Higher-order Pregnancies*,
https://doi.org/10.1007/978-3-030-47652-6_18

Trailer

Monochorionic monoamniotic multiple pregnancies are characterized by the presence of multiple fetuses sharing a single placenta and a single amniotic cavity. Early diagnosis of chorionicity and amnionicity is critical as complication rates are significantly higher in monoamniotic twins than in diamniotic twins. Although the perinatal mortality of monoamniotic twins has significantly decreased compared to the extremely high rates that were reported previously, survival of unselected monoamniotic twin pregnancies is still only ~70%, and this is mainly related to fetal anomalies and termination of pregnancy, twin-twin transfusion syndrome, selective intrauterine growth restriction, and cord-related complications. In uncomplicated monoamniotic twins however, after viability, fetal mortality should be less than 5% with close surveillance, which can either be in an inpatient or outpatient setting. Elective delivery by cesarean section is recommended around 33 weeks gestation.

Definition and Epidemiology

Monochorionic monoamniotic multiple pregnancies are characterized by the presence of multiple fetuses sharing a single placenta and a single amniotic cavity. The overall incidence of monoamniotic twin pregnancies is 8 per 100,000 pregnancies [1] (multiples and singletons combined), and they make up about 1% of all twin pregnancies and 5% of all monochorionic twins [2]. Monoamniotic twins are the result of the late splitting of a single embryo between day 8 and 13 days after fertilization and are more common after assisted reproduction [3]. The exact reason for this is unknown, but assisted hatching and embryo manipulation may play a role [4]. In rare circumstances, monoamniotic twins may also result from the accidental rupture of the intertwin amniotic membrane during amniocentesis [5] or fetoscopic surgery [6, 7] in diamniotic twins. Spontaneous rupture of the amniotic membrane [8] or partial incomplete formation of the intertwin membrane [9] is even rarer.

Conjoined twins are a rare subtype of monoamniotic twins and will be discussed in a separate chapter.

Learning Objectives

- How to diagnose monoamniotic multiple pregnancies
- Recognize risks associated with monoamniotic pregnancies
- Understand the need for close fetal monitoring after viability and be able to describe current monitoring strategies
- Understand reasons for timing and mode of delivery

18.1 Diagnosis of Monoamniotic Twins

Early diagnosis of chorionicity and amnionicity is critical as complication rates are significantly higher in monoamniotic twins than in monochorionic diamniotic or dichorionic twins [10]. Chorionicity is most reliably established by ultrasound early in gestation, but amnionicity can be harder to determine before 10 weeks [11]. The latter is due to the fact that the thin intervening amniotic membrane (◘ Figs. 18.1 and 18.2) may be difficult to appreciate early on, particularly when scanning transabdominally or in challenging imaging conditions. If amnionicity cannot be diagnosed accurately, confirmation of the presence or absence of an intervening membrane should be undertaken after 10 weeks gestation. Other ultrasound factors that may help in determining amnionicity in the first trimester of pregnancy include the presence of cord entanglement [12] (◘ Fig. 18.3), which is virtually omnipresent in monoamniotic twins, and the number of yolk sacs. The latter, however, is not very reliable, as a single yolk sac is only seen in 68% of cases, and up to 32% of monoamniotic twins will present with two yolk sacs [13]. In countries with a well-implemented first trimester screening program, it is very uncommon for the diagnosis not to be made early. If chorionicity and amnionicity cannot be determined by 12 weeks of gestation, referral to an expert center is recommended.

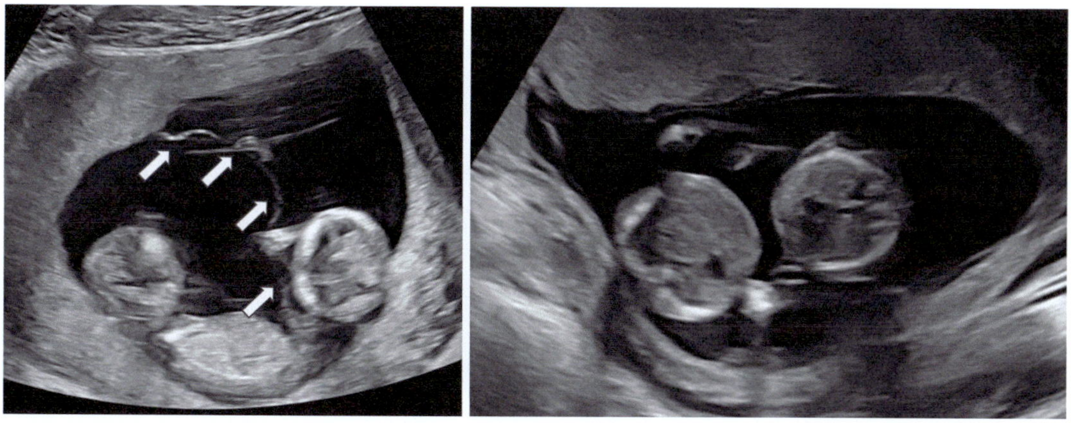

■ **Fig. 18.1** Monochorionic diamniotic **a** and monochorionic monoamniotic **b** twin pregnancies in the first trimester of pregnancy. Note the absence of the intertwin membrane (arrows) in monoamniotic twins

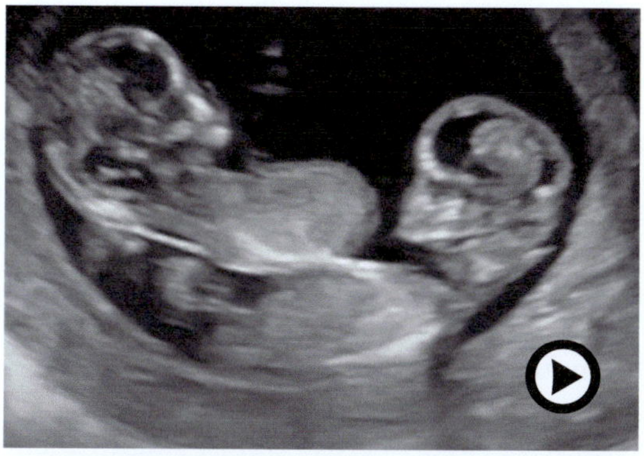

■ **Fig. 18.2** Ultrasound image of a monoamniotic twin pair sharing the same amniotic cavity. (Courtesy from the twin clinic UZ Leuven, Belgium) (https://doi.org/10.1007/000-2tq)

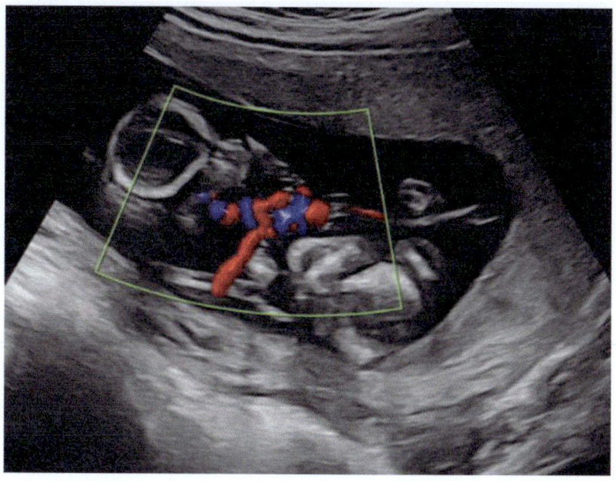

■ **Fig. 18.3** Cord entanglement seen in a set of monoamniotic twins in the first trimester of pregnancy

18.2 Complications of Monoamniotic Twins

18.2.1 Congenital Anomalies

The incidence of congenital anomalies is significantly elevated in monoamniotic twins and studies have described rates between 15% and 25% [14, 15]. In the majority of cases, only one fetus is affected (■ Fig. 18.4), and if both fetuses are affected, anomalies are often discordant. Cardiac anomalies are among the most commonly seen defects and make up about 30% of all defects, but TRAP sequence (described in ► Chap. 18), anencephaly, and other central nervous system anomalies are also common [15].

The high incidence of anomalies has been explained by the delayed cleavage of the embryo as well as imbalances in intertwin blood flow across large artery-to-artery vascular anastomoses at the level of the placenta [16]. This also explains why, in the presence of structural defects, underlying chromosomal anomalies are relatively uncommon (4%) and certainly less frequent than in monochorionic diamniotic twins (15%) or dichorionic twins (25%) [17]. In a very small number of cases, discordant anomalies can be explained by the presence of heterokaryotypic twins [18] or differential gene methylation [19]. Congenital

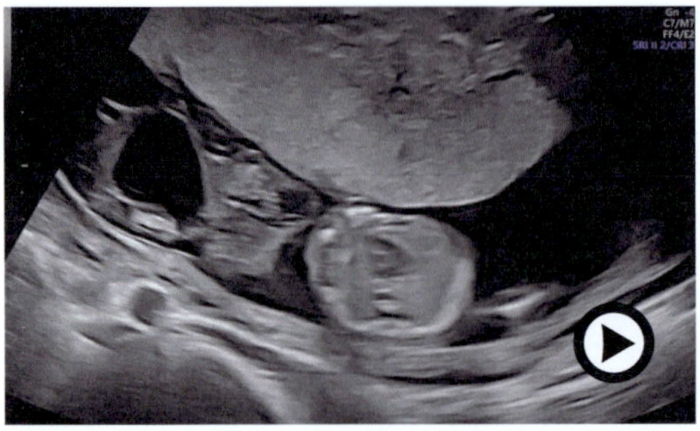

Fig. 18.4 Ultrasound image of a monoamniotic twin pair discordant for body stalk anomaly at 15 weeks. The liver and bowel of one twin protruded in the common extra-amniotic cavity. Since the cord of the affected twin was extra-amniotic, there was no cord entanglement and a selective reduction was performed by intrafetal coagulation. (Courtesy from the twin clinic UZ Leuven, Belgium) (https://doi.org/10.1007/000-2tr)

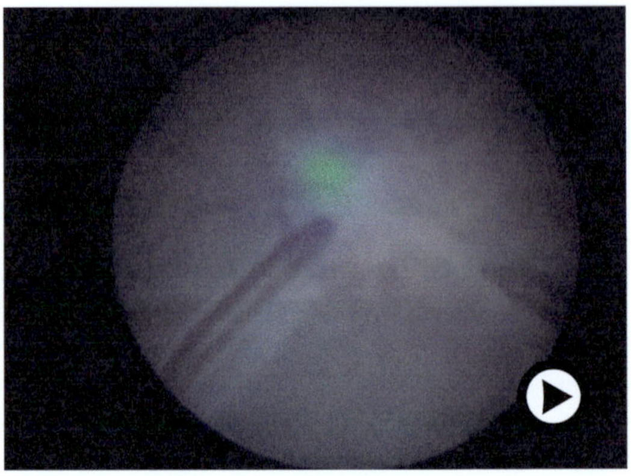

Fig. 18.5 Fetoscopic images of a laser coagulation of the vascular anastomoses for a stage II twin-twin transfusion syndrome at 19.5 weeks. There was polyhydramnios in the shared amniotic sac with one twin without a bladder and the other with a distended bladder. The procedure was hampered by the proximate cord insertions, the large anastomoses, and the entangled cords. The placenta at birth at 33.5 weeks showed no residual anastomoses. (Courtesy from the twin clinic UZ Leuven, Belgium) (https://doi.org/10.1007/000-2ts)

defects, and associated pregnancy termination, play an important role in the high mortality seen in monoamniotic twins [20].

The management of discordant anomalies is highly similar to that in monochorionic diamniotic twins (as reviewed in ▶ Chap. 11) except that, in case of selective reduction, cord transection should be considered to prevent further cord accidents [21], as the umbilical cord of the demised fetus will take the appearance of a "violin string" which is particularly prone to entanglement.

18.2.2 Twin-Twin Transfusion Syndrome

Twin-twin transfusion syndrome (TTTS), which occurs in 10–15% monochorionic diamniotic twins [22], complicates only 2–4% of monoamniotic due to the fact that 98% of all monoamniotic placentas have large balancing bidirectional arterioarterial anastomoses [16]. TTTS is harder to diagnose in monoamniotic twins as the typical combination of oligohydramnios and polyhydramnios is not present. Therefore, TTTS is usually defined as the presence of polyuric polyhydramnios (large bladder in one twin) in combination with an empty bladder in the other twin or Doppler changes characteristic of TTTS.

The outcomes of TTTS treatment in monoamniotic pregnancies were recently reviewed in a meta-analysis by Murgano et al. [23]. They retrieved 17 retrospective cohort studies documenting 890 monoamniotic twin pregnancies, of which 46 were affected by TTTS. In cases not undergoing intervention, miscarriage occurred in 10.7% of fetuses. The incidence of intra-uterine death, neonatal death, and perinatal death was 24.3%, 13.5%, and 32.4%, respectively. Numbers were highly similar in cases undergoing laser therapy (due to the fact that occlusion of the large intertwin anastomoses is often lethal for one or both fetuses) (Fig. 18.5) and outcomes were worse in those undergoing amniodrainage. The number of cases undergoing cord occlusion in this systematic review was too low to draw firm conclusions, but the risk of fetal or perinatal death seemed to be decreased. Importantly, one should consider transection of the cord of the demised fetus after these interventions to prevent further cord accidents [21, 24].

18

18.2.3 (Selective) Intra-Uterine Growth Restriction

The incidence of small-for-gestational-age fetuses and growth restriction is approximately three times higher in monoamniotic twins than in singletons. A birthweight below the 10th centile is seen in 38% of cases [10], and a birth weight below the 3rd centile in 10% [15].

Again however, due to the specific placental configuration of monoamniotic twins, with proximate cord insertions and large anastomoses, the incidence of *selective* fetal growth restriction is lower than in monochorionic diamniotic twins. The average intertwin birth weight discordance in monoamniotic twins is only 8–10% [15, 25] (in comparison with ~15% in diamniotic twins) and a birthweight discordance of more than 25% is only seen in 3% of cases [25]. A significant intertwin weight discordance nevertheless increases the risk of fetal death in monoamniotic twins, but the predictive value of this factor is low, so that it cannot be used as a trigger for intervention [25].

18.2.4 Intrauterine Fetal Death

Although the perinatal mortality of monoamniotic twins has significantly decreased compared to the extremely high rates that were reported previously [26], survival of unselected monoamniotic twin pregnancies is still only 62–70% [2, 10], despite improved surveillance and care. Part of this loss-rate is due to (pregnancy termination for) fetal anomalies. The remainder is largely related to cord-related complications (tight entanglement) and/or acute transfusional processes, resulting in about 15% of deaths after 20 weeks of pregnancy [16, 27]. Attempts at preventing these events by administration of Sulindac, which reduces amniotic fluid volume and hence fetal movements [28], have never found widespread uptake.

18.3 Surveillance of Monoamniotic Twins

Whereas fetal death due to cord complications cannot be prevented prior to fetal viability, preterm delivery becomes an option later in pregnancy and as such, most centers will initiate close surveillance of these pregnancies after viability. Despite the lack of evidence on the best surveillance method, circumstantial evidence suggests that monoamniotic twins which undergo regular surveillance do better than do those which do not have such surveillance, and fetal death rates have decreased over time.

18.3.1 Method of Surveillance

At present, there is not enough evidence to suggest what the best method for monitoring is, and most experts will use a combination of ultrasound surveillance and fetal heart rate monitoring. As discussed above, growth discordance between the fetuses is correlated with increased perinatal risk [25], but has poor predictive value for acute fetal events. On Doppler ultrasound, diastolic notching in the umbilical artery flow pattern [29] or absent or reversed end-diastolic flow [30] is thought to reflect cord compression. However, these flow patterns may persist for long periods of time and are in many cases transient. As a result, they should not be used to justify delivery. Finally, the specificity of fetal heart rate monitoring is questionable, but extended episodes of fetal tachycardia or repeated heart-rate decelerations, for example, will often be considered as triggers for delivery [31]. Given the lack of strong data on optimal triggers for delivery, physician experience plays a critical role in the prevention of unnecessary early delivery or inadequate response to subtle signs of fetal distress. Referral of monoamniotic twins to expert centers for further management and delivery is therefore recommended.

18.3.2 Frequency and Setting of Surveillance

Data are lacking on the optimal frequency of surveillance after viability, but most experts will recommend daily to alternate day fetal heart rate monitoring in combination with ultrasound one to three times per week [15, 27, 32]. Continuous fetal heart rate monitoring is impractical and only feasible in about 50% of cases and therefore not recommended [33].

There has been intense discussion among specialists as to what the best setting for fetal surveillance is: either inpatient or outpatient. Unfortunately, this discussion quickly became clouded and flawed by the fact that in most studies setting of surveillance was strongly linked with method and frequency of surveillance (with less or no surveillance going on in outpatients and surveillance starting later in pregnancy), resulting in higher numbers of fetal deaths in outpatients [31]. Careful analysis of all studies however, shows that, once appropriate surveillance is initiated, the risk of fetal death becomes very low and is likely similar in outpatient and inpatient settings (<5%, ◘ Fig. 18.6) [2, 15, 25, 34].

It is important to note that, in the absence of a clear fetal benefit, hospital admission can be harmful to pregnant women, being associated with an 18-fold increased risk of venous thromboembolism. This risk is even higher in the third trimester and in multiple gestations [35]. Moreover, prolonged hospital admissions incur significant economic and societal costs, and are highly disruptive to family life. In a study of almost 200 women carrying monoamniotic twins, psychiatric symptoms were far more common in the inpatient group compared with the outpatient group (although the difference did not reach statistical significance), with very high rates of hopelessness and despair (42% vs. 24%), thoughts of self-harm or suicide (4% vs. 0%), and postpartum depression (12% vs. 4%) in the inpatients [36].

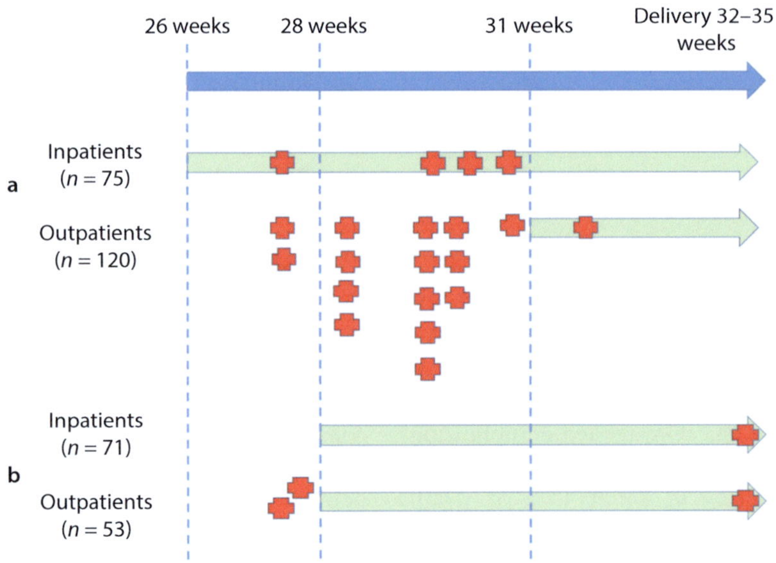

◘ **Fig. 18.6** Diagram illustrating the risk of fetal death with regard to timing of onset of surveillance in the two largest published monoamniotic twin cohorts. Diagram A represents the MonoMono study [32]. Diagram B represents the study by Van Mieghem et al. [15]. The blue arrow on top represents gestational age. The green arrow represents the gestational age during which close surveillance was instituted. The red crosses represent the fetal deaths. Note that the excess fetal deaths in the outpatient cohorts happened before surveillance was initiated

18.4 Timing and Mode of Delivery

Despite close surveillance, a number of acute fetal deaths remain unpredictable, and every unit managing these twins regularly will have knowledge of cases of fetal deaths within hours of a reassuring fetal well-being test. As a result, elective preterm delivery is often recommended when the risk of staying in utero outweighs the risk of delivery. A large multicenter study of nearly 200 monoamniotic twin pairs showed that after 32.6 weeks gestation, the risk of a severe, non-respiratory neonatal complication (death before discharge from the NICU, culture-proven sepsis, necrotizing enterocolitis, retinopathy of prematurity more than grade II, intraventricular hemorrhage more than grade I, or cystic periventricular leukomalacia) is lower than the prospective risk of fetal death (3.1%) [15]. It is nevertheless important to note that, when watched closely, about one third of all monoamniotic twin pregnancies will be delivered prior to their planned delivery date due to abnormal fetal surveillance or other pregnancy complications [37].

In most centers, monoamniotic twins will be delivered by elective cesarean section due to the risk of acute cord entanglement during labor. Additionally, there is a small chance that the umbilical cord of the second twin can be wrapped tightly around the neck of the first twin, mandating cord transection to deliver the first twin – which obviously creates an acute emergency. Nevertheless, some authors continue to advocate vaginal delivery for monoamniotic twins [38].

18.5 Proposed Pregnancy Management Strategy

Based on the available evidence, our current management strategy for monoamniotic twins is as follows:

- Once the diagnosis of monoamnionicity is confirmed in the first trimester of pregnancy, referral to an expert center is recommended.
- At 12–13 weeks gestation, we offer a detailed early anatomy ultrasound [39] and fetal echocardiogram following which patients receive extensive counselling on surveillance and management of monoamniotic twins.
- If the pregnancy is continued, 2-weekly ultrasounds are performed from 14 weeks of gestation onward to assess fetal viability, bladders, amniotic fluid, and fetal Dopplers (umbilical, middle cerebral artery, and ductus venosus) to screen for TTTS and twin anemia-polycythemia sequence.
- Fetal anatomy is reviewed at 20 weeks gestation.
- In otherwise uncomplicated monoamniotic twin pregnancies, patients are offered a counselling session with our neonatologists on the implications of preterm birth around 24 weeks gestation. At this point, the timing of "viability" is determined.
- After "viability," we administer steroids for fetal pulmonary maturation and intensify follow-up, either in an inpatient our outpatient setting, depending on patient preference, geographic location, and patient anxiety. For outpatients, we perform fetal heart rate monitoring and ultrasound three times per week. Inpatients are admitted to our high-risk antenatal ward for daily fetal heart rate monitoring and undergo three ultrasounds per week.
- In the absence of fetal distress or pregnancy complications, elective delivery by cesarean section is done around 33 weeks gestation. If steroids were administered prior to 28 weeks gestation, these may be repeated just prior to delivery.

18.6 Conclusion

Monoamniotic twins are at high risk of adverse pregnancy outcomes, mainly including fetal anomalies and intra-uterine fetal death. Risks can be partially mitigated by close surveillance in expert centers. The optimal surveillance strategy and setting after viability are unclear. Delivery should be undertaken around 33 weeks gestation.

18.6.1 Review Questions

1. How are monoamniotic pregnancies different from diamniotic pregnancies?

2. Explain the etiology of the most common complications in monoamniotic twin pregnancies.

3. Describe the recommended medical management of monoamniotic twin pregnancies.

4. How is the treatment of acardiac twinning in monoamniotic twin pregnancies different from the treatment in dichorionic twins?

18.6.2 Multiple-Choice Questions

1. When does the splitting of a zygote result in a monoamniotic twin pregnancy?
   (a) 1–3 days after fertilization.
   (b) 4–7 days after fertilization.
   (c) 8–14 days after fertilization.
   (d) >14 days after fertilization.

Answer: (c)

2. Amnionicity can accurately be diagnosed by ultrasound based on the
   (a) T sign or lambda sign.
   (b) Confirmation of the presence or absence of an intervening membrane.
   (c) Number of placental masses.
   (d) The number of yolk sacs.

Answer: (b)

3. What is the most common complication of monoamniotic twin pregnancies?
   (a) Fetal congenital anomalies.
   (b) TTTS.
   (c) Fetal death due to cord entanglement.
   (d) Selective growth restriction.

Answer: (a)

4. Which of the following statements about congenital anomalies in monoamniotic twins is true?
   (a) In the majority of cases, both fetuses are affected as they are genetically identical.
   (b) If both fetuses are affected, the anomalies are usually the same.
   (c) Central nerve system anomalies are among the most commonly seen defects and make up about 80% of all defects.
   (d) The high incidence of anomalies has been explained by the delayed cleavage of the embryo.

Answer: (d)

5. Twin-twin transfusion syndrome in monoamniotic twins is characterized by:
   (a) The full Quintero staging system.
   (b) Complicating as much as 25–30% of monoamniotic twins
   (c) Less frequent in monoamniotic twins due to large balancing bidirectional arterioarterial anastomoses.
   (d) The outcomes of TTTS in monoamniotic twins are better than in diamniotic twins.

Answer: (c)

6. Which of the following statement is true regarding antenatal surveillance in monoamniotic twins?
   (a) Continuous fetal heart rate monitoring should be initiated to detect changes in fetal well-being early.

(b) All women should be hospitalized from viability until delivery.
(c) When appropriate surveillance is initiated, the risk of fetal death is likely similar in outpatient and inpatient settings.
(d) There is clear evidence that ultrasound surveillance is more important than fetal heart rate monitoring.

Answer: (c)

Funding:
TVM is supported by a junior faculty award from the Department of Obstetrics and Gynaecology at Mount Sinai Hospital and the University of Toronto.

References

1. Glinianaia SV, Rankin J, Khalil A, Binder J, Waring G, Sturgiss SN, Thilaganathan B, Hannon T. Prevalence, antenatal management and perinatal outcome of monochorionic monoamniotic twin pregnancy: a collaborative multicenter study in England, 2000–2013. Ultrasound Obstet Gynecol. 2019;53:184–92.
2. Madsen C, Søgaard K, Zingenberg H, Jørgensen FS, Rosbach H, Hoseth E, Pedersen LH, Petersen OB. Outcomes of monoamniotic twin pregnancies managed primarily in outpatient care-a Danish multicenter study. Acta Obstet Gynecol Scand. 2019;98(4):479–86.
3. Alikani M, Cekleniak NA, Walters E, Cohen J. Monozygotic twinning following assisted conception: an analysis of 81 consecutive cases. Hum Reprod. 2003;18(9):1937–43.
4. Knopman JM, Krey LC, Oh C, Lee J, McCaffrey C, Noyes N. What makes them split? Identifying risk factors that lead to monozygotic twins after in vitro fertilization. Fertil Steril. 2014;102(1):82.
5. Feldman DM, Odibo A, Campbell WA, Rodis JF. Iatrogenic monoamniotic twins as a complication of therapeutic amniocentesis. Obstet Gynecol. 1998;91(5 Pt 2):815–6.
6. Gordon BJ, Chon AH, Korst LM, Llanes A, Miller DA, Chmait RH. Incidental septostomy after laser surgery for twin-twin transfusion syndrome: perinatal outcomes and antenatal management. Fetal Diagn Ther. 2018;44(4):285–90. https://doi.org/10.1159/000485034.
7. Peeters SH, Stolk TT, Slaghekke F, Middeldorp JM, Klumper FJ, Lopriore E, Oepkes D. Iatrogenic perforation of intertwin membrane after laser surgery for twin-to-twin transfusion syndrome. Ultrasound Obstet Gynecol. 2014;44(5):550–6. https://doi.org/10.1002/uog.13445.
8. Fleming T, Miller T. Spontaneous septostomy in monochorionic diamniotic twins resulting in cord entanglement and fetal demise. Australas J Ultrasound Med. 2012;15(3):103–6.
9. Galjaard S, Moerman P, Corveleyn A, Devlieger R, Lewi L. Partial monochorionic and monoamniotic twin pregnancies: a report of two cases. Ultrasound Obstet Gynecol. 2014;44(6):722–4.
10. Litwinska E, Syngelaki A, Cimpoca B, Frei L, Nicolaides KH. Outcome of twin pregnancies with two live fetuses at 11-13 weeks' gestation. Ultrasound Obstet Gynecol. 2020;55:32–8. https://doi.org/10.1002/uog.21892.
11. Bora SA, Papageorghiou AT, Bottomley C, Kirk E, Bourne T. Reliability of transvaginal ultrasonography at 7-9 weeks' gestation in the determination of chorionicity and amnionicity in twin pregnancies. Ultrasound Obstet Gynecol. 2008;32(5):618–21.
12. Sebire NJ, Souka A, Skentou H, Geerts L, Nicolaides KH. First trimester diagnosis of monoamniotic twin pregnancies. Ultrasound Obstet Gynecol. 2000;16:223–5.
13. Fenton C, Reidy K, Demyanenko M, Palma-Dias R, Cole S, Umstad MP. The significance of yolk sac number in monoamniotic twins. Fetal Diagn Ther. 2019;46(3):193–9.
14. Allen VM, Windrim R, Barrett J, Ohlsson A. Management of monoamniotic twin pregnancies: a case series and systematic review of the literature. BJOG. 2001;108(9):931–6.
15. Van Mieghem T, De Heus R, Lewi L, Klaritsch P, Kollmann M, Baud D, Vial Y, Shah PS, Ranzini AC, Mason L, Raio L, Lachat R, Barrett J, Khorsand V, Windrim R, Ryan G. Prenatal management of monoamniotic twin pregnancies. Obstet Gynecol. 2014;124(3):498–506.
16. Hack KE, van Gemert MJ, Lopriore E, Schaap AH, Eggink AJ, Elias SG, van den Wijngaard JP, Vandenbussche FP, Derks JB, Visser GH, Nikkels PG. Placental characteristics of monoamniotic twin pregnancies in relation to perinatal outcome. Placenta. 2009;30(1):62–5.
17. Li L, He Z, Huang X, Lin S, Wu J, Huang L, Wang Y, Fang Q. Chromosomal abnormalities detected by karyotyping and chromosomal micro-

array analysis in twins with structural anomalies. Ultrasound Obstet Gynecol. 2020;55(4):502–9. https://doi.org/10.1002/uog.20287.
18. Lewi L, Blickstein I, Van Schoubroeck D, Gloning KP, Casteels M, Brandenburg H, Fryns JP, Deprest J. Diagnosis and management of heterokaryotypic monochorionic twins. Am J Med Genet A. 2006;140(3):272–5.
19. Lyu G, Zhang C, Ling T, Liu R, Zong L, Guan Y, Huang X, Sun L, Zhang L, Li C, Nie Y, Tao W. Genome and epigenome analysis of monozygotic twins discordant for congenital heart disease. BMC Genomics. 2018;19(1):428.
20. Prefumo F, Fichera A, Pagani G, Marella D, Valcamonico A, Frusca T. The natural history of monoamniotic twin pregnancies: a case series and systematic review of the literature. Prenat Diagn. 2015;35(3):274–80. https://doi.org/10.1002/pd.4538. Epub 2015 Jan 8.
21. Middeldorp JM, Klumper FJ, Oepkes D, Lopriore E, Kanhai HH, Vandenbussche FP. Selective feticide in monoamniotic twin pregnancies by umbilical cord occlusion and transection. Fetal Diagn Ther. 2008;23(2):121–5.
22. Baxi LV, Walsh CA. Monoamniotic twins in contemporary practice: a single-center study of perinatal outcomes. J Matern Fetal Neonatal Med. 2010;23:506–10.
23. Murgano D, Khalil A, Prefumo F, Van Mieghem T, Rizzo G, Heyborne KD, Melchiorre K, Peeters S, Lewi L, Familiari A, Lopriore E, Oepkes D, Murata M, Anselem O, Buca D, Liberati M, Hack K, Nappi L, Baxi LV, Scambia G, Acharya G, D'Antonio F. Outcome of twin-to-twin transfusion syndrome in monochorionic monoamniotic twin pregnancies: a systematic review and meta-analysis. Ultrasound Obstet Gynecol. 2020;55(3):310–7. https://doi.org/10.1002/uog.21889.
24. Greimel P, Csapo B, Haeusler M, Lang U, Klaritsch P. A modified technique for cord transection in monochorionic monoamniotic twin pregnancies. Fetal Diagn Ther. 2018;44(3):236–40.
25. Saccone G, Khalil A, Thilaganathan B, Glinianaia SV, Berghella V, D'Antonio F, MONOMONO; NorSTAMP; STORK Research Collaboratives. Weight discordance and perinatal mortality in monoamniotic twin pregnancies: analysis of the MONOMONO, NorSTAMP and STORK multiple pregnancy cohorts. Ultrasound Obstet Gynecol. 2020;55(3):332–8.
26. Beasley E, Megerian G, Gerson A, Roberts NS. Monoamniotic twins: case series and proposalfor antenatal management. Obstet Gynecol. 1999;93(1):130–4.
27. Heyborne KD, Porreco RP, Garite TJ, Phair K, Abril D, Obstetrix/Pediatrix Research Study Group. Improved perinatal survival of monoamniotic twins with intensive inpatient monitoring. Am J Obstet Gynecol. 2005;192:96–101.
28. Pasquini L, Wimalasundera RC, Fichera A, Barigye O, Chappell L, Fisk NM. High perinatal survival in monoamniotic twins managed by prophylactic sulindac, intensive ultrasound surveillance, and Cesarean delivery at 32 weeks' gestation. Ultrasound Obstet Gynecol. 2006;28:681–7.
29. Abuhamad AZ, Mari G, Copel JA, Cantwell CJ, Evans AT. Umbilical artery flow velocity waveforms in monoamniotic twins with cord entanglement. Obstet Gynecol. 1995;86:674–7.
30. Rosemond RL, Hinds NE. Persistent abnormal umbilical cord Doppler velocimetry in a monoamniotic twin with cord entanglement. J Ultrasound Med. 1998;17:337–9.
31. Rodis JF, McIlveen PF, Egan JFX, Borgida AF, Turner GW, Campbell WA. Monoamniotic twins: improved perinatal survival with accurate prenatal diagnosis and antenatal fetal surveillance. Am J Obstet Gynecol. 1997;177:1046–9.
32. MONOMONO Working Group. Inpatient vs outpatient management and timing of delivery of uncomplicated monochorionic monoamniotic twin pregnancy: the MONOMONO study. Ultrasound Obstet Gynecol. 2019;53(2):175–83.
33. Quinn KH, Cao CT, Lacoursiere DY, Schrimmer D. Monoamniotic twin pregnancy: continuous inpatient electronic fetal monitoring-an impossible goal? Am J Obstet Gynecol. 2011;204(2):161.e1–6.
34. Van Mieghem T, Shub A. Management of monoamniotic twins: the question is not "where?", but "how?". Ultrasound Obstet Gynecol. 2019;53(2):151–2.
35. Abdul Sultan A, West J, Tata LJ, Fleming KM, Nelson-Piercy C, Grainge MJ. Risk of first venous thromboembolism in pregnant women in hospital: population based cohort study from England. BMJ. 2013;347:f6099.
36. Winkler SS, Mustian MN, Mertz HL. The psychosocial impact of inpatient management of monoamniotic twin gestations. J Matern Fetal Neonatal Med. 2016;29:1877–80.
37. D'Antonio F, Odibo A, Berghella V, Khalil A, Hack K, Saccone G, Prefumo F, Buca D, Liberati M, Pagani G, Acharya G. Perinatal mortality, timing of delivery and prenatal management of monoamniotic twin pregnancy: systematic review and meta-analysis. Ultrasound Obstet Gynecol. 2019;53(2):166–74.
38. Anselem O, Mephon A, Le Ray C, Marcellin L, Cabrol D, Goffinet F. Continued pregnancy

and vaginal delivery after 32 weeks of gestation for monoamniotic twins. Eur J Obstet Gynecol Reprod Biol. 2015;194:194–8.

39. Salomon LJ, Alfirevic Z, Bilardo CM, Chalouhi GE, Ghi T, Kagan KO, Lau TK, Papageorghiou AT, Raine-Fenning NJ, Stirnemann J, Suresh S, Tabor A, Timor-Tritsch IE, Toi A, Yeo G. ISUOG practice guidelines: performance of first-trimester fetal ultrasound scan. Ultrasound Obstet Gynecol. 2013;41(1):102–13. https://doi.org/10.1002/uog.12342.

Key Reading

Glinianaia SV, Rankin J, Khalil A, Binder J, Waring G, Sturgiss SN, Thilaganathan B, Hannon T. Prevalence, antenatal management and perinatal outcome of monochorionic monoamniotic twin pregnancy: a collaborative multicenter study in England, 2000–2013. Ultrasound Obstet Gynecol. 2019;53:184–92.

Hack KE, van Gemert MJ, Lopriore E, Schaap AH, Eggink AJ, Elias SG, van den Wijngaard JP, Vandenbussche FP, Derks JB, Visser GH, Nikkels PG. Placental characteristics of monoamniotic twin pregnancies in relation to perinatal outcome. Placenta. 2009;30(1):62–5.

Litwinska E, Syngelaki A, Cimpoca B, Frei L, Nicolaides KH. Outcome of twin pregnancies with two live fetuses at 11-13 weeks' gestation. Ultrasound Obstet Gynecol. 2020;55:32–8. https://doi.org/10.1002/uog.21892

MONOMONO Working Group. Inpatient vs outpatient management and timing of delivery of uncomplicated monochorionic monoamniotic twin pregnancy: the MONOMONO study. Ultrasound Obstet Gynecol. 2019;53(2):175–83.

Van Mieghem T, De Heus R, Lewi L, Klaritsch P, Kollmann M, Baud D, Vial Y, Shah PS, Ranzini AC, Mason L, Raio L, Lachat R, Barrett J, Khorsand V, Windrim R, Ryan G. Prenatal management of monoamniotic twin pregnancies. Obstet Gynecol. 2014;124:498–506.

Diagnosis and Management of Conjoined Twins

Clifton Brock and Anthony Johnson

Contents

A. Khalil et al. (eds.), *Twin and Higher-order Pregnancies*,
https://doi.org/10.1007/978-3-030-47652-6_19

Trailer

Conjoined twins (CT) are a rare complication of monoamniotic twinning. The true incidence of this complication is difficult to estimate because most women with the diagnosis either choose not to continue the pregnancy or an intrauterine demise ensues. For continuing pregnancies, prognosis is mostly determined by the site fusion and the organs involved. Ultrasound, 3D ultrasound, and magnetic resonance imaging are critical for antenatal diagnosis, careful analysis of the area of fusion, and subsequent prognostication. Only a minority of twins that survive birth will go on to be candidates for surgical separation. Surgical separation should only be attempted at centers with expertise in these procedures, which are complex and frequently associated with residual morbidity. Because the ethical considerations of surgical separation are complex, a palliative care team is critical for understanding patient and her family's goals and preferences.

Definitions

Conjoined twins: A rare complication of monoamniotic twins in which there is fusion between anatomical structures of each twin. Specific organs along the site of fusion may be paired (i.e., one organ for each twin) or singular (i.e., one organ shared between twins).

Thoracopagus twins: The most common type of conjoined twins; they are fused anteriorly from the thorax to the umbilicus typically sharing cardiac structures.

Omphalopagus twins: A type of conjoined twins that are fused anteriorly typically from the sternum to the umbilicus. They are differentiated from thoracopagus twins in that they do not share a heart.

Cephalopagus twins: A type of conjoined twins that are fused primarily at the head and typically share cerebral structures. There are several possible orientations between the twins and fusion may extend rostrally to the level of the umbilicus.

Ischiopagus twins: A type of conjoined twins that are fused at the pelvic outlet. Fusion may extend caudally to the level of the diaphragm. Face-to-face and end-to-end orientations are possible.

Craniopagus twins: A type of conjoined twins that are fused at the head. Usually the cranium and meninges are involved; however, cerebral vasculature may also sometimes be involved. Fusion is not present below the head.

Pygopagus twins: A type of conjoined twins that are fused dorsally at the sacrum.

Parapagus twins: A type of conjoined twins that are fused anterolaterally with side-by-side orientation. The size of the fusion area and organs involved may vary dramatically between pairs of twins of this type.

Rachipagus twins: A type of conjoined twins that are fused posteriorly with the twins oriented facing away from one another. One of the twins is often parasitic.

Learning Objectives

- A general understanding of the history, pathophysiology, embryology, and management of conjoined twins.
- Awareness of the eight types of conjunction and how the site and complexity of fusion dictate the prognosis and availability of postnatal surgical separation.
- An understanding of the roles of antenatal ultrasound, 3D ultrasound, and magnetic resonance imaging for delineation the organs involved in conjunction.
- An overview of postnatal management of conjoined twins that survive birth. This includes non-operative management, emergent surgical separation, and interval elective separation.
- An overview of the ethical issues involved in postnatal management.

19.1 Introduction

Conjoined twins (CT) are a rare complication of monochorionic twining historically viewed as a medical curiosity more than as a manageable condition. This has changed somewhat as successful surgical separation has become possible in selective cases with improved prenatal diagnosis and coordination of care. The true incidence of CT is unknown. Most estimates range between 1:50,000 and 1:250,000 live births; however, several recent reports suggest that the true incidence is more likely to be between 1:20,000 and 1:25,000 [1–7]. In perhaps the largest epidemiological study of CT, Mutchinick et al. calculated an incidence of 1.47:100,000 from a worldwide sample of 26.1 million births [8]. There is regional variation in rates of CT with greater numbers reported in China and Africa (>1:30,000) than in Europe and the United States (<1:50,000) [8]. Female CT are three times more common than male CT.

The first known historical artifact depicting CT is a 17-cm marble statue of parapagus twins, the so-called sisters of Catalhoyuk, dated 6000 BC; it is currently housed in the Anatolian Civilization Museum in Ankara, Turkey [9]. However, a few well-known historical examples of CT dominate the historical landscape. The "Biddenden Maids," were a pair of parapagus sisters born in 1100 in the English agricultural village of Biddenden in the state of Kent. These are the first CT with an extensive historical literature describing their life and times. The twins lived for 34 years fused at the shoulders and hips prior to their demise within 6 hours of one another from an unknown illness [10]. They currently enjoy legendary status in Biddenden. The brothers Chang and Eng Bunker, born in Siam in 1911, are probably the best-known CT. The unfortunate story of their exploitation by PT Barnum at "Freak Shows" across Europe and the United states followed by coinage of the indecorous term "Siamese Twins" has contributed negatively to our cultural understanding and acceptance of CT [11, 12]. The medical circumstances underlying these stories are no less fascinating than the tales themselves.

19.2 Types of Conjoined Twins

The nomenclature of CT, as well as their prenatal and postnatal clinical management and outcomes, are dictated by their shared anatomy. The terminology describing conjunction has evolved, but eventually settled on eight types of twins proposed by Spencer et al., each ending with the suffix "pagus," which means "fixed." The types, in order of estimated incidence, are thoracopagus, omphalopagus, cephalopagus, ischiopagus, pygopagus, craniopagus, parapagus (diprosopus and dicephalus), and rachipagus [13]. Each of these types of CT is illustrated in ◘ Fig. 19.1.

Thoracopagus twins (◘ Fig. 19.1a) are the most common subtype in most large series, accounting for 47–71% of the total [3, 14–21]. These twins usually lie face-to-face, fused from the anterior thorax to the umbilicus; they share a sternum, diaphragm, and upper abdominal wall and the majority share a pericardial sac, heart, and liver [22–24]. For twins with more extensive fusion inferiorly, the term thoraco-omphalopagus is sometimes used. Conjoined hearts, which are common in this group, are nearly always affected by additional major anomalies (◘ Fig. 19.2). In a recent series of 10 thoracopagus twins with conjoined hearts, every twin had additional cardiac anomalies including tricuspid atresia, double outlet right ventricle, transposition of the great arteries, hypoplastic left heart, complete atrioventricular canal defects, and totally anomalous pulmonary venous return among others [23]. This represents the primary source of mortality among these twins. Fusion of the extra-hepatic biliary system has also been described [25, 26].

Omphalopagus twins (◘ Fig. 19.1b) make up about 20% of all CT. They are situated identically to thoracopagus twins (i.e., rostral fusion), but they have a less complex conjunction. Most of these twins share a liver (80%), and about a third share the terminal ileum and colon without rectal involvement [13, 27, 28]. There are always separate hearts (by definition), although the pericardium may be shared. Numerous case reports describe shared biliary anatomy and fusion

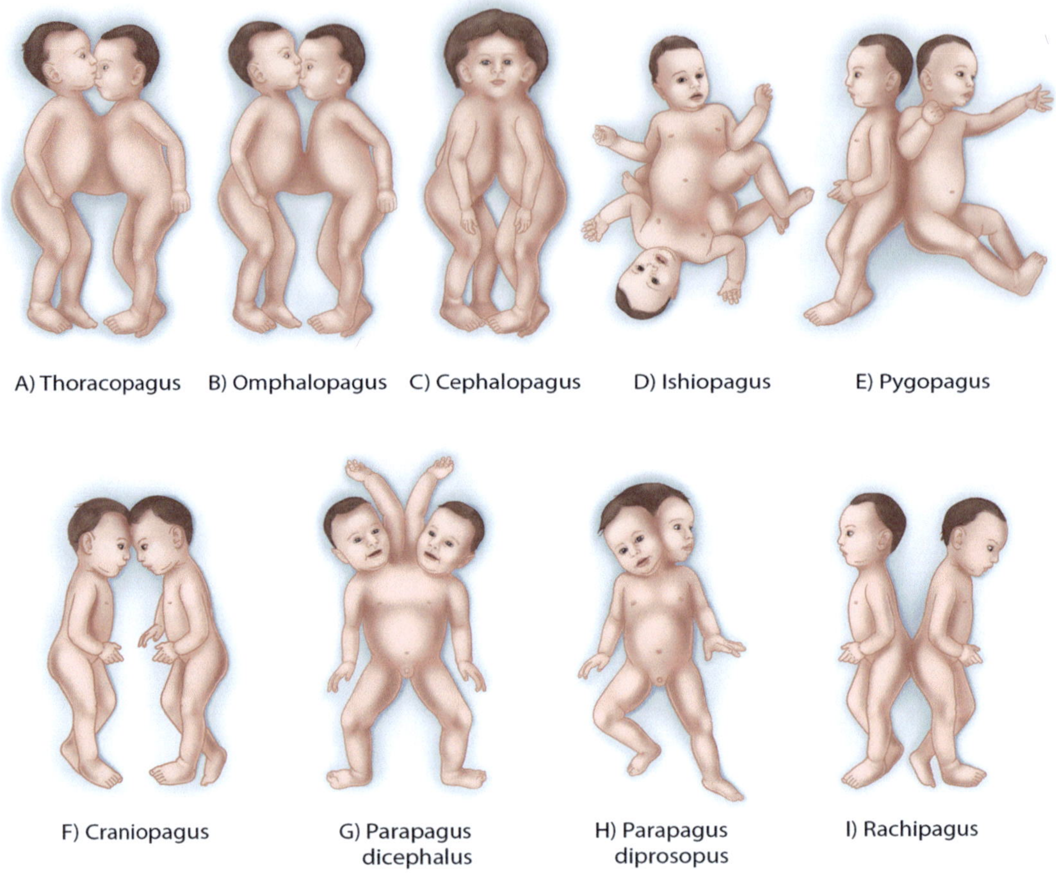

Fig. 19.1 Spencer classification of conjoined twins [13]

extends from the xiphoid to the umbilicus [25]. Because they have the least complex conjunction among CT, they are more likely to survive postnatal surgical separation.

Cephalopagus twins (Fig. 19.1c) are primarily joined at the head. Four varieties of facial presentation may occur including symmetric (two well-formed faces on opposite sides of the head), asymmetric (one well-formed face and one hypotrophic face on opposite sides), deradelphous (one midline face), and deradelphous diprosopous (one midline face with duplication of only some facial features) [29]. There is only one brain; however, some components may be duplicated (i.e., two cerebellums, Fig. 19.3). The fusion may extend rostrally as far as the umbilicus. When the thorax is involved, the twins tend to have separate hearts, lungs, and trachea [30, 31]. When fusion extends lower, the twins usually share the upper gastrointestinal tract with separate ileums, large bowels, and rectums [27, 32]. Cephalopagus twins are inseparable and frequently stillborn. Those that do survive delivery uniformly fail to survive the neonatal period.

Ischiopagus twins (Figs. 19.1d) are joined primarily at the pelvic outlet; however, fusion may present up to the level of the diaphragm and often includes the liver; the twins may be oriented face-to-face or end-to-end (Fig. 19.4). This leads to tremendous variability in the angle between the twins' spines and shared anatomy [28]. They may share portions of the cauda equina, thecal sac, and vertebral bodies [33]. Hemivertebrae and spinal lesions remote from the site of union are also common. There may be two, three, or four lower extremities (dipus, tripus, or tetrapus) and a wide variety of shared and unshared

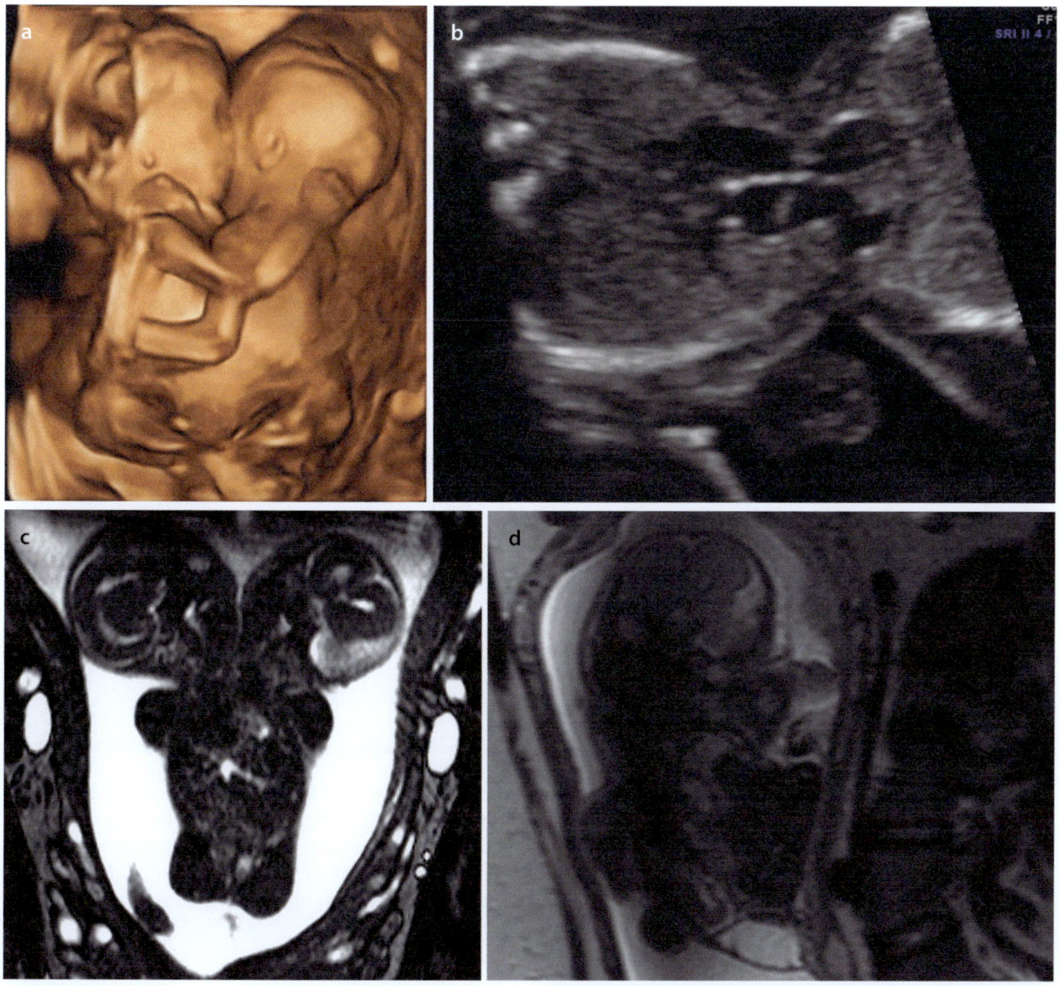

◘ **Fig. 19.2** Two sets of thoracopagus twins **a** 3D ultrasound image of the first pair showing anterior fusion from the sternum to the umbilicus. **b** 2D transverse ultrasound image showing a single shared heart with six chambers centrally located in the fusion between twins. **c** MRI showing the second pair fused more laterally than the first from the lower face to the pelvis. A liver and urinary bladder are shared; however, there are two hearts. **d** MRI showing the fused liver, which is outside of the abdomen

permutations of urinary, genital, and lower gastrointestinal tracts have been reported [33–36]. These include shared urethras and bladders (with varying numbers of ureteral orifices), ureters crossing between twins, cloacas, fused or shared genitals, and anal orifices with or without separate rectums. While the thoraces are separate, cardiac anomalies are present about 10% of the time [28]. These twins are frequently able to be separated when the anatomy if favorable [18].

Pygopagus twins (◘ Fig. 19.1e) are joined dorsally at the sacrum. They have similar urinary, lower gastrointestinal, and neurological malformations to ischiopagus twins without involvement of more superior structures. The twins usually share an anus with or without a common rectum and either one or two urinary bladders [28, 33]. The degree of spinal cord fusion typically determines whether separation is possible. Pygopagus and ischiopagus twins often have long-term urinary and bowel issues in cases of successful separation [33, 36].

Craniopagus twins (◘ Fig. 19.1f), like cephalopagus twins, are joined at the head but fusion typically involves only the skull and meninges while the face and brain are spared. However, cortical fusion and shared cerebral

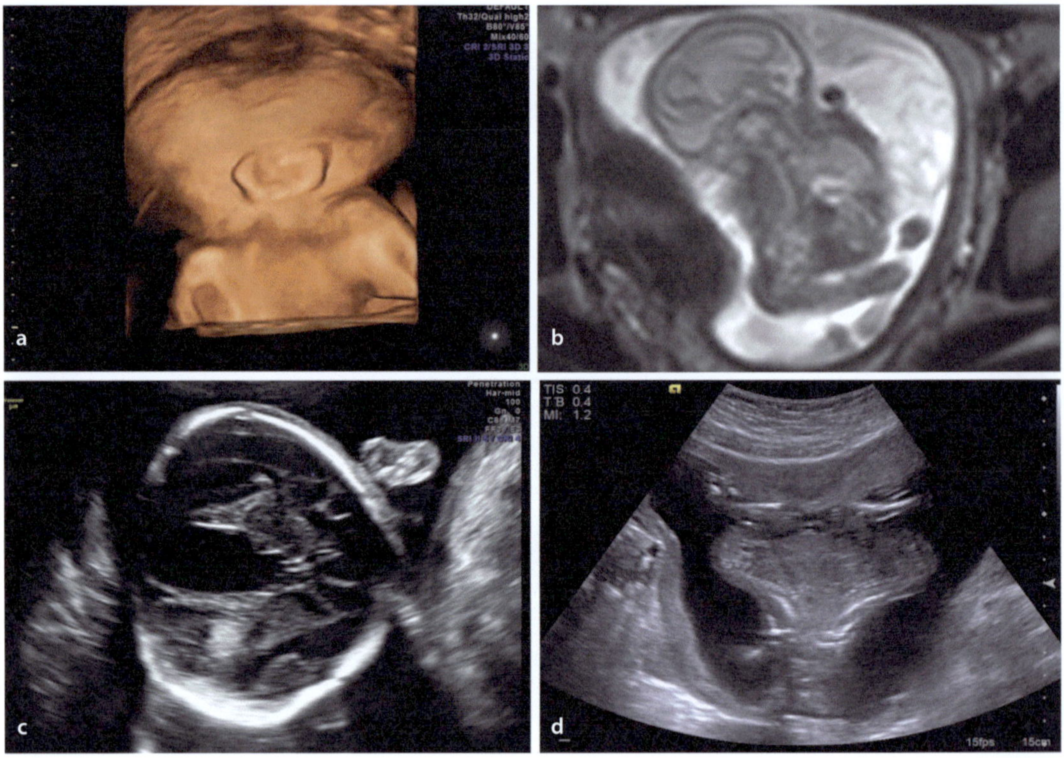

Fig. 19.3 Cephalopagus twins fused from the head to the pelvis. **a** 3D ultrasound image showing anterior fusion of the cranium. There are four ears and one face. **b** MRI showing the twins fused to the umbilicus. There is fused liver and single heart with two spines. **c** Transverse 2D ultrasound image showing a single irregularly shaped cranium. There was a complex brain anomaly with two cerebral hemispheres, a single central ventricle, and two cerebellums. **d** Coronal ultrasound image showing a single liver with bilateral hyperextended spines

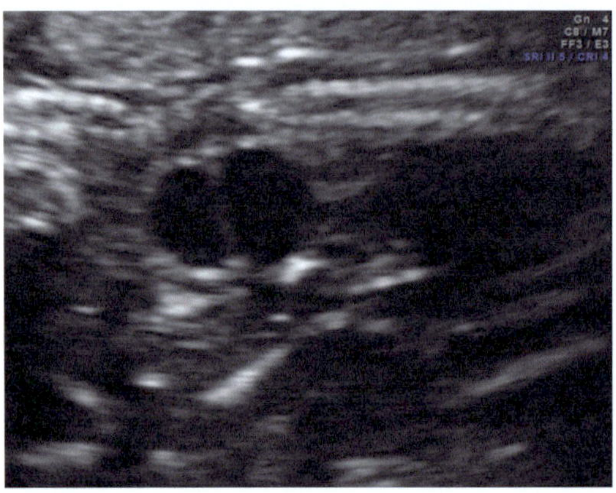

Fig. 19.4 Ischiopagus twins. Sagittal 2D ultrasound image showing tail-to-tail orientation of the sacrums with two separate bladders

vasculature (typically venous) will be seen in upwards of 1/3 of cases. Numerous subclassification systems have been proposed based on the directions the twins are facing, the structures shared, and presence of dural venous communication [37]. While fusion is limited to the head, the majority of these twins have additional issues including cardiac, facial, and gastrointestinal anomalies [37]. Staged separation of these twins with a multidisciplinary team is possible with success often hinging on the degree of dural sinus communication [38–40].

Parapagus twins are fused anterolaterally with extremely variable organ involvement that may include the head, thorax, abdomen, or pelvis; they are positioned side by side [41–44]. The pelvis and abdomen are almost always involved with fusion of the liver and diaphragm; there may be two, three, or four upper limbs. Pelvic involvement may include anal atresia, colovesical fistula, and genitourinary abnormalities [45]. In parapagus disopropus CT, the fusion extends from the pelvis to the cranium, which is typically

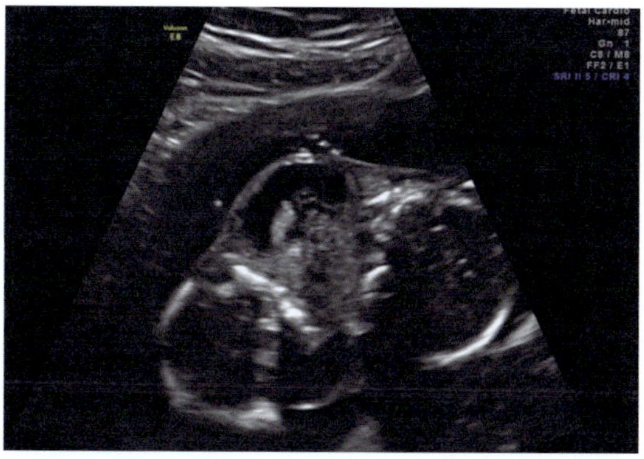

■ **Fig. 19.5** Dicephalic parapagus twins. These twins have anterolateral fusion of the thorax and abdomen. This transverse 2D ultrasound image shows the superior aspect of fusion where bifurcation of two heads can be appreciated. The thorax, shown superiorly, contained pleural and cardiac effusions

lethal (■ Fig. 19.1h). The twins are deemed dithoracic if the pelvis and abdomen are fused with separation above the abdomen. However, when the twins are dicephalic (fused abdomen and thoraces), cardiac anomalies, and often a single heart, are common (■ Figs. 19.1g and 19.5) [14, 46].

Rachipagus twins (■ Fig. 19.1i) are fused posteriorly facing away from one another. The occiput and vertebral bodies are involved to varying degrees, and one of the twins is often parasitic [47–49]. These are the rarest of CT and our understanding of their fusion is limited to case reports [47, 48, 50].

19.3 Pathophysiology/Embryology

The pathophysiology of CT is unknown, and currently available theories do not explain all clinical observations. Nevertheless, the two prevailing theories of CT are fission of a single embryo versus fusion of two early embryos [51, 52]. The fission theory classically accounts for all major types of twins (dichorionic-diamniotic, monochorionic-diamniotic, monochorionic-monoamniotic, and conjoined) and argues that phenotype is determined by the embryological timing of the fission event [52].

According to the fusion theory, conjunction between twins lies along specific anatomic sites where embryological folding or closure occurs and ectoderm is at least transiently absent. Such sites include the diaphragm, oropharyngeal membrane, cloacal membrane, neural tube, and the periumbilical region [51, 53]. The events leading to union occur between 4 and 6 weeks after fertilization when the yolk sac is still prominent. Spencer proposed a "spherical theory" of union in which the two embryos' relative positions on the surface of the yolk sac determine the final configuration [51]. Comparison of the two theories is beyond the scope of this text (reviewed by Spencer); however, some authors believe fusion to be more plausible in light of various clinical observations including cases of diamniotic CT [51, 53, 54]. Regardless of which theory is best describes clinical observations, the practical implication is that the process occurs early and CT are generally detectable at the first obstetric ultrasound.

19.4 Imaging for Detection of Conjoined Twins

CT are readily diagnosed in the first trimester of pregnancy by ultrasound as illustrated in a review of 54 cases diagnosed prior to 15 weeks. Only 18 pairs were suspected before 10 weeks with four of these being false positives [55]. However, diagnosis as early as 7 weeks has been reported [56]. The primary diagnosis in the case of false positives is monochorionic-monoamniotic pregnancy; the distinction between these diagnoses is often made in the late first trimester when fetal movement increases but the fetuses are not found to move independent of one another. The following findings, suspicious for a diagnosis of CT, have been suggested by several authors: two fetuses emerging from a single yolk sac, fetuses lying in the same constant relative position with body parts at the same level, an odd number limbs, shared organs, and single umbilical cords with more than three vessels [45, 57, 58]. Interestingly, increased nuchal translucencies are a common finding in thoracopagus twins thought to be caused by the single hearts' failure to prevent lymphatic stasis in the posterior necks [59]. First trimester detection of CT is paramount to offering early termination, or in cases of triplet pregnancy, selective reduction of the conjoined pair [60–62].

In continuing pregnancies, prenatal imaging is critical for prognostication and planning of surgical separation. A comprehensive anatomy ultrasound at 20 weeks is the first step for estimating the extent of fusion and the organs involved. Fetal echocardiography should be performed in all CT as there is increased risk of heart anomalies even if the chest is not involved in the fusion; severity of cardiac lesions is often underestimated even with detailed prenatal imaging [57, 63]. Three-dimensional ultrasound may be useful in better defining the anatomy of fusion (◘ Figs. 19.2a and 19.3a); however, examples of this is clinically useful are limited to case reports [64–68]. Fetal MRI is increasingly used to provide an enhanced depiction of organ sharing and vascular anatomy. It has become an important tool for prenatal counseling and optimized planning of postnatal surgical management in continuing cases [15, 69–71] (◘ Figs. 19.2c, d and 19.3b).

19.5 Prenatal Issues and Management

Hundreds of documented cases of successfully separated CT and the surgical advancements leading to them have increased optimism for surgical management of CT; however, it is important to emphasize that these represent the minority of cases. In a large series of 36 pairs of CT, 30 (83.3%) were thought to have lethal anomalies [14]. Fourteen pregnancies were terminated after the diagnosis. Among the 16 twins born alive, none survived with seven expiring within 24 hours. In another series of 17 pairs of CT that survived to delivery, five were determined to be inoperable and all expired within 5 days. Seven pairs required emergency separation, of which four of 14 twins survived. The remaining 5 pairs underwent planned separation and experienced more favorable outcomes with eight twins attaining long-term survival [17]. Similarly, a series of 22 pairs of CT by Saguil et al. showed 64% overall mortality for twins born alive [16].

The stillbirth rates for CT are difficult to determine as frequently only live-born twins are reported. Furthermore, most series are from high-volume centers, which lack information regarding fetal demise prior to referral. The high incidence of stillbirth was better emphasized by Martinez-Frias et al., who found rates of stillborn CT to be 99.3 times that of live-born CT in a large database from Spain including 30 years of data [3]. True stillbirth estimates are confounded by the large number of women who terminate CT. In a review of 75 sets of CT detected in the first trimester, Chen et al. reported a termination rate of 80% [72]. This serves as a recapitulation of data from Pajkrt et al. who reported an 82% (41/50) termination rate among CT detected in the first trimester [55].

Termination of pregnancy should clearly be offered to any patient presenting with CT. There are limited data to inform the technical aspects of termination in these cases; however, routine dilation and curettage or evacuation are currently used for this process. After 20 weeks gestational age, transvaginal termination of CT may become technically difficult and hysterotomy may be required [55]. Hence, early detection is critical. While termination by vaginal delivery following induction has been described in the second trimester, this is not ideal [73].

For women who choose to continue the pregnancy, there are similarly scant data to guide antenatal monitoring. Given the high rates of stillbirth, serial ultrasound monitoring should be a cornerstone of any antenatal surveillance plan. As with all monoamniotic twins, delivery by planned Cesarean section likely carries less morbidity than vaginal delivery for these twins [74]. While successful vaginal delivery has been described in the literature, so too have associated birth traumas [75–77]. The optimal timing of delivery is unknown, but planned delivery at 35 weeks gestational age following administration of corticosteroids has been recommended [78].

19.6 Postnatal Management

The management of live-born CT is complex and specific to the site of fusion. Early referral to a tertiary care center with expertise in surgical separation is recommended for twins thought to be potential candidates. Separation requires a well-coordinated multidisciplinary approach with extensive planning and involvement of a variety of pediatric surgical subspecialties. There are three major categories of management for live-born CT:

1. Non-operative management: These cases usually have complex neurological or cardiac fusion such that separation is likely to be lethal or severely disabling. Thoracopagus twins with heart fusion and/or associated complex heart anomalies and craniopagus, cephalopagus, or parapagus disopropus twins with complex cerebral fusion usually fall into this category [23, 79]. These twins are candidates for palliative care, and most survive less than a few days after birth.
2. Emergent surgical separation: Several scenarios may arise where separation must be urgently undertaken. These include cases where one twin has died or has a lethal anomaly, cases with acute injury at the site of fusion, and cases where an omphalocele is present with necrotic tissue. Survival following emergent separation ranges from 8% to 50% [9, 14, 16, 17, 57, 80–82]. The ethical considerations in these cases may be complex. Generally, in cases where both twins may be salvageable, an equal chance should be given to each. In cases where only one twin is salvageable, it is reasonable to make decisions that increase likelihood of survival in one twin with appropriate palliative care provided to other twin [79].
3. Interval elective separation: Carefully selected CT that survive the peripartum period have survival rates between 71% and 100% in experienced hands [9, 14, 16, 17, 57, 80–82]. Such outcomes are more likely for omphalopagus, ischiopagus, craniopagus (without cerebral involvement), and pygopagus twins, although there are examples of successful separation of thoracopagus twins [16]. Separation is usually performed between 6 and 24 months of age. Ethical considerations in this group are also very complex.

CT that survive planned surgical separation frequently have long-term medical complications and varying degrees of disability. Pygopagus and ischiopagus twins, for example, may require extensive post-separation neurologic surgery for a variety of issues including spinal column anomalies, tethered cords, syrinx, and hydrocephalus [33, 83]. To address downstream complications of urinary and lower gastrointestinal tract fusion, they may undergo ileostomy, colostomy, urinary diversion, and bladder augmentation among other procedures [33, 36, 83]. Complications following separation of fused hearts have led some groups towards palliation for thoracopagus twins with complex cardiac lesions [23]. Prediction of long-term sequelae following surgical separation of CT is a difficult task. Data are limited, and each pair of twins will have a unique set of post-operative challenges. This further highlights the importance of early referral to a specialized center with experienced multidisciplinary pediatric subspecialists.

19.6.1 Ethical Considerations

The ethics of managing CT is multifaceted and specific to each set of twins. A practical decision-oriented approach offered by Thomas et al. relies on quantifying the risk of morbidity and mortality of each twin prior to, versus after separation [84]. In cases where both twins are not expected to survive without separation, separation is obligatory as long as at least one survivor without major morbidity is expected. This may involve risk to, or sacrifice of, one of the pair for the other's survival. If major morbidity is expected, separation may not be obligatory, but permissible depending on the values and desires of the patient and her family. If, on the other hand, the twins are expected to survive if they remain conjoined, separation is impermissible if one or both twins are expected to die following the procedure. If both twins are expected to survive, then morbidity and patient preferences become relevant to the permissibility of proceeding with separation. In all cases, involvement of a palliative care team is critical for understanding patient goals and preferences and aiding in communication between the patients (or their family) and the care team.

19.7 Conclusion

CT have captured the imagination of physicians as well as the general public throughout history. This is highlighted by renowned historic examples like the Bunker brothers and the Biddenden Maids. Behind these stories lie an extremely morbid, often lethal and always complex disease. The most common outcome of CT is termination of pregnancy followed by stillbirth and then neonatal demise. The embryology of the disease remains largely speculative, and the epidemiology is difficult to study. Treatment is available in a minority of well-selected cases, and post-separation complications are common.

From a diagnostic standpoint, CT are generally detectable during routine first trimester ultrasound. Prognostication may be improved by more advanced imaging techniques such as 3D ultrasound, fetal echocardiogram, and fetal MRI. Improvements in antenatal care may result from initiatives that promote early establishment of prenatal care and ultrasound. In the same vein, unhindered access to termination of pregnancy is of critical importance. For women who choose to continue their pregnancy, referral to an established and experienced tertiary care center is essential. Finally, advances in surgical techniques may allow more complicated separations to be achieved, but this will affect only a minority of cases.

19.7.1 Review Questions

1. What are the two primary theories describing the embryologic pathophysiology of CT?

2. What are the roles of ultrasound, 3D-ultrasound and fetal MRI in diagnosing and prognosticating cases of CT?

3. What are the most common two outcomes for CT diagnosed in the first trimester?

4. What are the three major categories of postnatal management for CT that survive delivery? What criteria should physicians use to determine the best management strategy?

5. What are the primary ethical considerations in determining whether and when to surgically separate a pair of CT?

19.7.2 Multiple-Choice Questions

1. What is the most likely outcome for the majority of conjoined twins of any type?
   (a) Termination of pregnancy or intrauterine fetal demise.
   (b) Live birth with demise shortly after birth.
   (c) Live birth with emergent separation surgery shortly after birth.
   (d) Live birth with interval elective separation surgery.

Answer: (a)

2. Which of the following is most important to improve the likelihood of neonatal survival in women that choose to continue a pregnancy with a diagnosis of conjoined twins?
   (a) MRI and 3D ultrasound for improved prenatal delineation of the fusion site and organ involvement.
   (b) Early prenatal diagnosis and serial antenatal testing with non-stress tests, biophysical profiles, and Doppler interrogation of fetal vasculature.

(c) Referral to a tertiary care center with expertise in surgical separation of conjoined twins.
(d) A carefully considered plan for mode of delivery at an appropriate gestational age.

Answer: (c)

3. Which of the following is true regarding the ethical considerations of surgical separation of conjoined twins.
(a) Separation is obligatory, even if severe morbidity is expected after the procedure.
(b) Involvement of a palliative team is a reasonable option, but not required, in the setting of planned surgical separation of twins.
(c) Separation is obligatory in cases where both twins are expected to expire in the absence of intervention.
(d) Separation is impermissible if it may involve severe morbidity or sacrifice of one of the twins.

Answer: (c)

References

1. Spitz L. Conjoined twins. Br J Surg. 1996;83(8):1028–30.
2. Edmonds LD, Layde PM. Conjoined twins in the United States, 1970–1977. Teratology. 1982;25(3):301–8.
3. Martinez-Frias ML, Bermejo E, Mendioroz J, et al. Epidemiological and clinical analysis of a consecutive series of conjoined twins in Spain. J Pediatr Surg. 2009;44(4):811–20.
4. Berezowski AT, Duarte G, Rodrigues R, et al. Conjoined twins: an experience of a tertiary hospital in Southeast Brazil. Rev Bras Ginecol Obstet. 2010;32(2):61–5.
5. Tang Y, Zhu J, Zhou GX, Dai L, Wang YP, Liang J. An epidemiological study on conjoined twins in China, from 1996 to 2004. Zhonghua Yu Fang Yi Xue Za Zhi. 2007;41(Suppl):146–9.
6. Liang J, Xu CI, Wang Y. Epidemiological survey of conjoined twins in China. Hua Xi Yi Ke Da Xue Xue Bao. 1999;30(1):56–8.
7. Savona-Ventura C, Grima S, Buttigieg GG. Conjoint twinning in the Maltese Islands. J Obstet Gynaecol. 2009;29(7):599–604.
8. Mutchinick OM, Luna-Munoz L, Amar E, et al. Conjoined twins: a worldwide collaborative epidemiological study of the International Clearinghouse for Birth Defects Surveillance and Research. Am J Med Genet C Semin Med Genet. 2011;157c(4):274–87.
9. Spitz L. Conjoined twins. Prenat Diagn. 2005;25(9):814–9.
10. Bondeson J. The Biddenden maids: a curious chapter in the history of conjoined twins. J R Soc Med. 1992;85(4):217–21.
11. Martin HE. Chang and Eng Bunker, "the original Siamese twins": living, dying, and continuing under the spectator's gaze. J Am Cult (Malden). 2011;34(4):372–90.
12. Bogdan R. Freak show: presenting human oddities for amusement and profit. University of Chicago Press; 1990.
13. Spencer R. Anatomic description of conjoined twins: a plea for standardized terminology. J Pediatr Surg. 1996;31(7):941–4.
14. Brizot ML, Liao AW, Lopes LM, et al. Conjoined twins pregnancies: experience with 36 cases from a single center. Prenat Diagn. 2011;31(12):1120–5.
15. Mackenzie TC, Crombleholme TM, Johnson MP, et al. The natural history of prenatally diagnosed conjoined twins. J Pediatr Surg. 2002;37(3):303–9.
16. Saguil E, Almonte J, Baltazar W, et al. Conjoined twins in the Philippines: experience of a single institution. Pediatr Surg Int. 2009;25(9):775–80.
17. Spitz L, Kiely EM. Experience in the management of conjoined twins. Br J Surg. 2002;89(9):1188–92.
18. Tannuri AC, Batatinha JA, Velhote MC, Tannuri U. Conjoined twins: twenty years' experience at a reference center in Brazil. Clinics (Sao Paulo). 2013;68(3):371–7.
19. el-Gohary MA. Siamese twins in the United Arab Emirates. Pediatr Surg Int. 1998;13(2–3):154–7.
20. Castilla EE, Lopez-Camelo JS, Orioli IM, Sanchez O, Paz JE. The epidemiology of conjoined twins in Latin America. Acta Genet Med Gemellol. 1988;37(2):111–8.
21. Cywes S, Millar AJ, Rode H, Brown RA. Conjoined twins–the Cape Town experience. Pediatr Surg Int. 1997;12(4):234–48.
22. Hoyle RM. Surgical separation of conjoined twins. Surg Gynecol Obstet. 1990;170(6):549–62.
23. Thomas Collins R 2nd, Weinberg PM, Gruber PJ, St John Sutton MG. Conjoined hearts in thoracopagus twins. Pediatr Cardiol. 2012;33(2):252–7.
24. McMahon CJ, Spencer R. Congenital heart defects in conjoined twins: outcome after surgical separation of thoracopagus. Pediatr Cardiol. 2006;27(1):1–12.
25. Meyers RL, Matlak ME. Biliary tract anomalies in thoraco-omphalopagus conjoined twins. J Pediatr Surg. 2002;37(12):1716–9.
26. Saranrittichai S, Niramis R, Siripornadulsilp S, et al. Successful separation of thoracopagus conjoined twins with a single extra-hepatic biliary system. J Med Assoc Thail. 2007;90(5):994–1000.

27. McHugh K, Kiely EM, Spitz L. Imaging of conjoined twins. Pediatr Radiol. 2006;36(9):899–910. quiz 1002–1003
28. Winkler N, Kennedy A, Byrne J, Woodward P. The imaging spectrum of conjoined twins. Ultrasound Q. 2008;24(4):249–55.
29. Grassi R, Esposito V, Scaglione M, et al. Multidetector row CT for depicting anatomic features of cephalothoracopagus varieties: revised approach. Radiographics. 2004;24(5):e21.
30. Kuroda K, Kamei Y, Kozuma S, et al. Cephalopagus conjoined twins. Ultrasound Obstet Gynecol. 2000;16(3):293.
31. Spencer R. Conjoined twins: theoretical embryologic basis. Teratology. 1992;45(6):591–602.
32. Mian A, Gabra NI, Sharma T, et al. Conjoined twins: from conception to separation, a review. Clin Anat. 2017;30(3):385–96.
33. Fieggen AG, Dunn RN, Pitcher RD, Millar AJ, Rode H, Peter JC. Ischiopagus and pygopagus conjoined twins: neurosurgical considerations. Childs Nerv Syst. 2004;20(8–9):640–51.
34. Shapiro E, Fair WR, Ternberg JL, Siegel MJ, Bell MJ, Manley CB. Ischiopagus tetrapus twins: urological aspects of separation and 10-year followup. J Urol. 1991;145(1):120–5.
35. Hoyle RM, Thomas CG Jr. Twenty-three-year follow-up of separated ischiopagus tetrapus conjoined twins. Ann Surg. 1989;210(5):673–9.
36. Lazarus J, Raad J, Rode H, Millar A. Long-term urological outcomes in six sets of conjoined twins. J Pediatr Urol. 2011;7(5):520–5.
37. Harvey DJ, Totonchi A, Gosain AK. Separation of craniopagus twins over the past 20 years: a systematic review of the variables that Lead to successful separation. Plast Reconstr Surg. 2016;138(1):190–200.
38. Dunaway D, Jeelani NU. Staged separation of craniopagus twins. Semin Pediatr Surg. 2015;24(5):241–8.
39. Staffenberg DA, Goodrich JT. Separation of craniopagus conjoined twins with a staged approach. J Craniofac Surg. 2012;23(7 Suppl 1):2004–10.
40. Pai KM, Naidu RC, Raja A, et al. Surgical nuances in the separation of craniopagus twins – our experience and a follow up of 15 years. Neurol India. 2018;66:426–33.
41. Watanabe K, Ono M, Shirahashi M, Ikeda T, Yakubo K. Dicephalus Parapagus conjoined twins diagnosed by first-trimester ultrasound. Case Rep Obstet Gynecol. 2016;2016:8565193.
42. Usang UE, Olasode BJ, Archibong AE, Udo JJ, Eduwem DA. Dicephalus parapagus conjoined twins discordant for anencephaly: a case report. J Med Case Rep. 2010;4:38.
43. Tansel T, Yazicioglu F. Cardiac and other malformations in parapagus twins. Arch Gynecol Obstet. 2004;269(3):211–3.
44. Melo A, Dinis R, Portugal A, Sousa AI, Cerveira I. Early prenatal diagnosis of parapagus conjoined twins. Clin Pract. 2018;8(2):1039.
45. Mathew RP, Francis S, Basti RS, et al. Conjoined twins – role of imaging and recent advances. J Ultrason. 2017;17(71):259–66.
46. Lopes LM, Brizot ML, Schultz R, et al. Twenty-five years of fetal echocardiography in conjoined twins: lessons learned. J Am Soc Echocardiogr. 2013;26(5):530–8.
47. Ratan SK, Rattan KN, Magu S, Rohilla S, Purwar P, Mathur SK. Thoracolumbar rachipagus parasite. Pediatr Surg Int. 2004;20(4):298–300.
48. Rattan KN, Singh J, Dalal P, Sonika P, Rattan A. Sacral Rachipagus parasite: a case report. J Neonatal Surg. 2016;5(2):16.
49. Chadha R, Lal P, Singh D, Sharma A, Choudhury SR. Lumbosacral parasitic rachipagus twin. J Pediatr Surg. 2006;41(1):e45–8.
50. Navaei AA, Habibi Z, Moradi E, Nejat F. Parasitic rachipagus twins; report of two cases. Childs Nerv Syst. 2015;31(6):1001–3.
51. Spencer R. Theoretical and analytical embryology of conjoined twins: part I: embryogenesis. Clin Anat. 2000;13(1):36–53.
52. Kaufman MH. The embryology of conjoined twins. Childs Nerv Syst. 2004;20(8–9):508–25.
53. Spencer R. Theoretical and analytical embryology of conjoined twins: part II: adjustments to union. Clin Anat. 2000;13(2):97–120.
54. Kapur RP, Jack RM, Siebert JR. Diamniotic placentation associated with omphalopagus conjoined twins: implications for a contemporary model of conjoined twinning. Am J Med Genet. 1994;52(2):188–95.
55. Pajkrt E, Jauniaux E. First-trimester diagnosis of conjoined twins. Prenat Diagn. 2005;25(9):820–6.
56. Hill LM. The sonographic detection of early first-trimester conjoined twins. Prenat Diagn. 1997;17(10):961–3.
57. Barth RA, Filly RA, Goldberg JD, Moore P, Silverman NH. Conjoined twins: prenatal diagnosis and assessment of associated malformations. Radiology. 1990;177(1):201–7.
58. Kingston CA, McHugh K, Kumaradevan J, Kiely EM, Spitz L. Imaging in the preoperative assessment of conjoined twins. Radiographics. 2001;21(5):1187–208.
59. Maymon R, Mendelovic S, Schachter M, Ron-El R, Weinraub Z, Herman A. Diagnosis of conjoined twins before 16 weeks' gestation: the 4-year experience of one medical center. Prenat Diagn. 2005;25(9):839–43.
60. Lam YH, Lee CP, Tang MH, Lau E. Thermocoagulation for selective reduction of conjoined twins at 12 weeks of gestation. Ultrasound Obstet Gynecol. 2000;16(3):267–70.
61. Goldberg Y, Ben-Shlomo I, Weiner E, Shalev E. First trimester diagnosis of conjoined twins in a

triplet pregnancy after IVF and ICSI: case report. Hum Reprod. 2000;15(6):1413–5.
62. Sepulveda W, Munoz H, Alcalde JL. Conjoined twins in a triplet pregnancy: early prenatal diagnosis with three-dimensional ultrasound and review of the literature. Ultrasound Obstet Gynecol. 2003;22(2):199–204.
63. Andrews RE, Yates RW, Sullivan ID. The management of conjoined twins: cardiology assessment. Semin Pediatr Surg. 2015;24(5):217–20.
64. Yang PY, Wu CH, Yeh GP, Hsieh CT. Prenatal diagnosis of parapagus diprosopus dibrachius dipus twins with spina bifida in the first trimester using two- and three-dimensional ultrasound. Taiwan J Obstet Gynecol. 2015;54(6):780–3.
65. Ulker K, Akyer SP, Temur I, et al. First trimester diagnosis of parapagus diprosopus dibrachius dipus twins with cranirachischisis totalis by three-dimensional ultrasound. J Obstet Gynaecol Res. 2012;38(2):431–4.
66. Fang KH, Wu JL, Yeh GP, Chou PH, Hsu JC, Hsieh CT. Ischiopagus conjoined twins at 9 weeks of gestation: three-dimensional ultrasound and power Doppler findings. Ultrasound Obstet Gynecol. 2005;25(3):309–10.
67. Bonilla-Musoles F, Raga F, Bonilla F Jr, Blanes J, Osborne NG. Early diagnosis of conjoined twins using two-dimensional color Doppler and three-dimensional ultrasound. J Natl Med Assoc. 1998;90(9):552–6.
68. Biswas A, Chia D, Wong YC. Three-dimensional sonographic diagnosis of cephalothoracopagus janiceps twins at 13 weeks. Ultrasound Obstet Gynecol (England). 2001;18:289–90.
69. Watson SG, McHugh K. Conjoined twins: radiological experience. Semin Pediatr Surg. 2015;24(5):212–6.
70. Unal O, Arslan H, Adali E, Bora A, Yildizhan R, Avcu S. MRI of omphalopagus conjoined twins with a Dandy-Walker malformation: prenatal true FISP and HASTE sequences. Diagn Interv Radiol. 2010;16(1):66–9.
71. Teixeira Castro P, Werner H, Matos AP, Daltro P, Araujo Junior E. Symmetric and ventrally conjoined twins: prenatal evaluation by ultrasound and magnetic resonance imaging and postnatal outcomes. J Matern Fetal Neonatal Med. 2021;34(12):1955–62. https://doi.org/10.1080/14767058.2019.1651282. Epub 2019 Aug 12.
72. Chen CP, Hsu CY, Su JW, et al. Conjoined twins detected in the first trimester: a review. Taiwan J Obstet Gynecol. 2011;50(4):424–31.
73. Mitchell T, Cheng E, Jolley J, Delaney S. Successful induction of labor of late-second-trimester conjoined twins: an alternative to hysterotomy. Obstet Gynecol. 2014;123(2 Pt 2 Suppl 2):469–72.
74. Vaughn TC, Powell LC. The obstetrical management of conjoined twins. Obstet Gynecol. 1979;53(3 Suppl):67s–72s.
75. Harma M, Mil Z, Oksuzler C. Vaginal delivery of dicephalic parapagus conjoined twins: case report and literature review. Tohoku J Exp Med. 2005;205(2):179–85.
76. Tug N, Sahinoglu Z, Cam C, Eren S. Route of delivery of thoracoomphalopagus twins: analysis of three cases. Arch Gynecol Obstet. 2009;280(5):815–8.
77. Sinha M, Gupta R, Gupta P, Tiwari A. Assisted breech vaginal delivery of dicephalus dipus dibrachius conjoined twins: a case report. J Reprod Med. 2015;60(3–4):160–4.
78. O'Brien P, Nugent M, Khalil A. Prenatal diagnosis and obstetric management. Semin Pediatr Surg. 2015;24(5):203–6.
79. Spitz L. Ethics in the management of conjoined twins. Semin Pediatr Surg. 2015;24(5):263–4.
80. O'Neill JA Jr, Holcomb GW 3rd, Schnaufer L, et al. Surgical experience with thirteen conjoined twins. Ann Surg. 1988;208(3):299–312.
81. Rode H, Fieggen AG, Brown RA, et al. Four decades of conjoined twins at Red Cross Children's Hospital–lessons learned. S Afr Med J. 2006;96(9 Pt 2):931–40.
82. Al Rabeeah A. Conjoined twins–past, present, and future. J Pediatr Surg. 2006;41(5):1000–4.
83. Votteler TP, Lipsky K. Long-term results of 10 conjoined twin separations. J Pediatr Surg. 2005;40(4):618–29.
84. Thomas A, Johnson K, Placencia FX. An ethically-justifiable, practical approach to decision-making surrounding conjoined-twin separation. Semin Perinatol. 2018;42(6):381–5.

Key Reading

Brizot ML, Liao AW, Lopes LM, et al. Conjoined twins pregnancies: experience with 36 cases from a single center. Prenat Diagn. 2011;31(12):1120–5.
Martinez-Frias ML, Bermejo E, Mendioroz J, et al. Epidemiological and clinical analysis of a consecutive series of conjoined twins in Spain. J Pediatr Surg. 2009;44(4):811–20.
Mathew RP, Francis S, Basti RS, et al. Conjoined twins – role of imaging and recent advances. J Ultrason. 2017;17(71):259–66.
Votteler TP, Lipsky K. Long-term results of 10 conjoined twin separations. J Pediatr Surg. 2005;40(4):618–29.

Peripartum Care

Contents

Timing of Birth in Uncomplicated Twin Pregnancy

Becky Liu and Asma Khalil

Contents

A. Khalil et al. (eds.), *Twin and Higher-order Pregnancies*,
https://doi.org/10.1007/978-3-030-47652-6_20

Trailer

Twin pregnancies are at higher risk of perinatal morbidity and mortality. Research has shown that the risk of stillbirth significantly increases before 40 weeks in twins, with a degree of variation between different chorionicity and amnionicity. Antenatal complications that are specific or more prevalent in twin pregnancies can occur, contributing to their increased rates of perinatal loss. National recommendations are now in place based on expert opinions and available evidence, in order to mitigate these risks.

Definitions

Stillbirth/intrauterine death: the death of a fetus in utero after 24 weeks' gestation

Neonatal death: the death of an infant from time of birth until 28 days of life

Perinatal loss: the death of a baby in utero after 20 weeks' gestation, or following birth until 28 days of life

Prematurity: the birth of a baby or babies prior to 37 weeks' gestation

Learning Objectives

- To understand the antenatal complications of twin pregnancies
- To understand the gestational age when the risk of stillbirth outweighs the risks of prematurity
- To learn the recommended gestational age for the delivery of different types of twins
- To understand the management of patients who wish to continue their pregnancy beyond the recommended gestation

20.1 Introduction

Twin pregnancies are known to be at an increased risk of perinatal morbidity and mortality compared to singletons. These complications include pre-eclampsia, preterm birth, fetal growth restriction, and stillbirth [1–4]. Efforts must therefore be made to time the delivery of these pregnancies at an appropriate gestation in order to minimize these risks. In this chapter, we focus on the antenatal complications of twin pregnancies, which can contribute to their rates of increased perinatal loss, the gestations where these risks are increased, and the recommended timings of birth in twin pregnancies.

20.2 Antenatal Complications in Twin Pregnancy

20.2.1 Fetal Growth Restriction

In both dichorionic (DC) and monochorionic (MC) twins, the main complications that can affect fetal outcome are fetal growth restriction (FGR) and preterm birth [5]. FGR is associated with an increase in perinatal mortality, which can in turn lead to preterm birth, neurological sequelae, or death in the surviving co-twin [4, 6–8]. DC twins follow a similar growth trajectory as singletons, and slow down after 30 weeks, whereas MC twins have a persistently lower estimated fetal weight (EFW) than singletons throughout the second and third trimesters [9]. This could be contributed to a relative degree of placental insufficiency in twins, or a lack of intrauterine space [5]. An increased growth discordance between the twins is also associated with a significant increase in perinatal death, particularly when the discordance is >25% [10]. An increased rate of pre-eclampsia is seen in FGR in DC twins than those in MC twins, as the aetiology of FGR in DC twins is similar to that of singletons [11].

20.2.2 Preterm Birth

Sixty percent of twin pregnancies can result in spontaneous labour before 37 weeks [12], and 12% before 32 weeks [13]. Preterm birth contributes to the highest proportion of neonatal morbidity and mortality amongst twins [14].

Cervical length measurement at 18–24 weeks is the preferred method of detecting those at risk of preterm birth, where a length of <25 mm is a moderate predictor of preterm birth before 34 weeks [15, 16]. Traditional practice of bed rest, or oral tocolysis, has not shown clear evidence of preventing preterm birth. Recent evidence, however, has suggested that vaginal progesterone may reduce preterm delivery in those women with short cervix, and reduce neonatal mortality and morbidity [17].

20.2.3 Congenital Anomalies

Twins are at a higher risk of congenital anomalies than singletons [18]. Dizygotic twins have a similar per fetus risk of congenital anomalies as singletons, but this risk is 2–3 folds higher in monozygotic twins. Discordant anomalies affect one twin in 1 in 25 DC twins, 1 in 15 monochorionic diamniotic (MCDA) twins, and 1 in 6 monochorionic monoamniotic (MCMA) twins [19, 20]. Congenital heart disease is also six times more prevalent in MC twins than DC twins [21].

20.2.4 Monochorionic-Specific Complications

MC twins are 12 times more likely to be complicated by fetal loss before 26 weeks gestation than DC twins [22], due to the haemodynamic imbalance created by the vascular anastomoses between the two circulations. The main conditions contributing to fetal loss are twin-to-twin transfusion syndrome (TTTS) and early sFGR. After 26 weeks, these twins remain at high risk of stillbirth due to development of other complications such as acute TTTS, twin-anaemia-polycythaemia-sequence (TAPS), and late sFGR [5]. Single twin demise can lead to neurological damage and death in the co-twin, as well as trigger preterm labour.

20.3 Perinatal Mortality with Increasing Gestations

20.3.1 Dichorionic Twins

The risk of stillbirth in twins by 36–37 weeks is similar to those of post mature singletons [23]. The total stillbirth rate after 26 weeks is quoted to be 6.5 in 1000 pregnancies, which remains steady until a significant increase at 38–39 weeks [24]. The main cause has been demonstrated to be secondary to FGR [25]. A large systematic review and meta-analysis on the stillbirth and neonatal complication rates in twins has found that at 36 weeks, the risk of neonatal death was higher than of stillbirth (3.2:1000 vs. 1.5:1000) in DC twins. From 37 weeks however, this relationship was reversed, giving a neonatal death risk of 2.2:1000, and stillbirth risk of 3.4:1000 [26]. This has led to the common practice of delivering uncomplicated DC twins from 37 weeks. ◘ Figure 20.1 highlights the survival rates of both MC and DC twins throughout increasing gestational ages.

20.3.2 Monochorionicity

The rate of stillbirth and neonatal death was significantly higher in MC twins than in DC twins at all gestations, as demonstrated in ◘ Fig. 20.1. The Southwest Thames Obstetric Research Collaboration (STORK) found that the risk for stillbirth after 26 weeks was 19.1:1000 fetuses in MC twins, compared to 6.5:1000 fetuses in DC twins [28]. It has been reported that the stillbirth rates began to increase following 32 weeks, and increased further after 36 weeks in MC twins [25]. The risk of composite neonatal morbidity is reduced after 36 weeks [29]; therefore, the benefit of delivery outweighs the risk of prematurity following this gestation. Given that their risks of complications and perinatal loss are higher than that of DC twins, it was

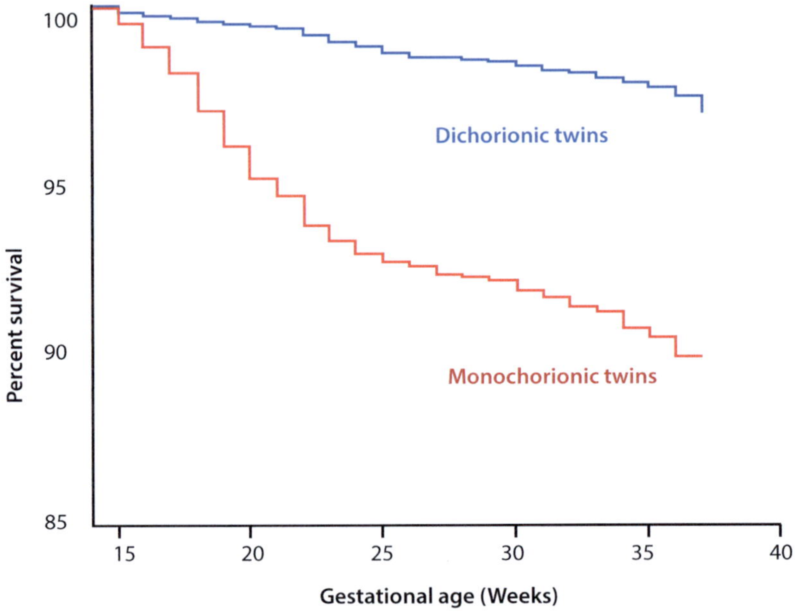

Fig. 20.1 Survival rates of dichorionic and monochorionic twins throughout increasing gestational weeks [27]

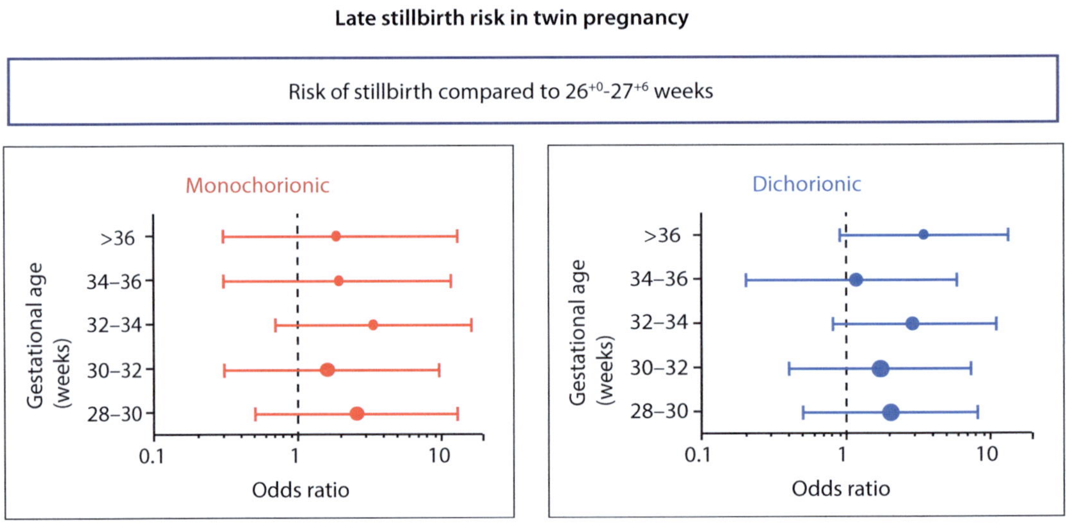

Fig. 20.2 Odds ratios of the risk of stillbirth in monochorionic and dichorionic twin pregnancies compared to 26 + 0–27 + 6 weeks [28]

also suggested by a team of experts that these pregnancies are delivered at an earlier gestation than DC twins [12]. This practice is also supported by the meta-analysis by Cheong-See et al. [26], which found that at 35 weeks, the rate of neonatal death is significantly higher than stillbirth (8.1:1000 vs. 2.8:1000), this difference is less pronounced at 36 weeks (5.4:1000 vs. 4.5:1000), but from 37 weeks, the risk of neonatal death is significantly lower than that of stillbirth (3.6:1000 vs. 9.6:1000) [26]. Figure 20.2 outlines the late stillbirth risk in MC and DC twins compared to 26–27 + 6 weeks.

20.3.3 Monoamnionicity

MCMA twins are at risk of cord entanglement, increased risk of congenital anomalies, as well as the other complications of MC twin pregnancies. Studies have shown that the risk of fetal demise increased from 1.4% at 28 weeks, to 5.1% at 32–34 weeks, and that after 33 weeks' gestation, the risk of fetal demise outweighs the complications of prematurity [30, 31]. Van Mieghem et al. found that the risk of fetal demise from 32 weeks and 4 days exceeded the risk of postnatal non-respiratory neonatal complication [30]. Therefore, it is recommended that these twins are delivered between 32–33 weeks and 6 days, given the higher risk of fetal demise and the earlier increase in this risk compared to DC and MCDA twins [12].

20.4 Triplet Pregnancies

The available data for triplet pregnancies are limited, and often include small cohorts. A recent systematic review has concluded that the risk of perinatal mortality and neurological comorbidity is higher in DC triplets than TC triplets, but the gestational ages at delivery were not significantly different [32]. A national cohort study of multiple pregnancies in Korea found that in triplets, the highest gestation for stillbirth was at 38 weeks, and the lowest at 34 weeks. This risk increased significantly between 34 and 37 weeks (10.8:10,000 to 47.4:10,000), however, given the small number of infant deaths in this study, the risks of expectant management versus delivery were unable to be analysed in this group [33]. MC triplets are exceedingly rare; therefore, no evidence is available to guide the timing of delivery in this cohort. The largest study so far looking into outcomes of these triplets have concluded that the risk of stillbirth in MC triplets is 2.6 fold higher than in TC triplets [34].

20.5 Recommended Practice

The recently updated NICE guideline on twin and triplet pregnancy has made the following recommendations based on expert opinion and available evidence, as outlined in ◘ Table 20.1. Uncomplicated DC twins are recommended to deliver from 37 weeks, MCDA twins from 36 weeks, MCMA twins at 32–33 + 6 weeks, and DC/TC triplets from 35 weeks, with the consideration of a course of antenatal corticosteroids [12]. If any antenatal complications were to arise (TTTS, TAPS, sFGR), the delivery plan should be made on an individualized basis. Any patient who declines elective birth at these gestations should be offered weekly ultrasound to monitor fetal Dopplers and growth 2 weekly, as well as specialist consultant appointments [12].

◘ **Table 20.1** Gestational ages of increased stillbirth risk, and the recommended gestation at delivery, for DC, MCDA, MCMA twins, and TC/DC triplets (NICE guideline) [12]

	Dichorionic (DC)	Monochorionic diamniotic (MCDA)	Monochorionic monoamniotic (MCMA)	Trichorionic/ dichorionic triplets
Increased stillbirth risk	38–39 weeks	36 weeks	32–34 weeks	35 + 6 weeks
Recommended delivery gestation	37 weeks	36 weeks	32–33 + 6 weeks	35 weeks

20.6 Conclusion

Twin pregnancies have an increased risk of antenatal complications and a higher rate of stillbirth. Extensive research has attempted to assess the gestation when this risk is increased, but neonatal morbidity and mortality is not increased due to iatrogenic prematurity. Delivery planning according to chorionicity and antenatal events is crucial in order to mitigate these risks. Patients who are keen to continue their pregnancy must be informed of the risks and monitored closely and counselled sensitively.

20.6.1 Review Questions

1. What are the possible causes of a lower birthweight in multiple pregnancies?

2. What contributory factors cause an increased risk of stillbirth in twins from an earlier gestation?

3. What additional risks are monoamniotic twins exposed to?

4. Why are monochorionic twins advised to deliver earlier than dichorionic twins?

5. What should be considered prior to planning delivery in multiple pregnancies?

20.6.2 Multiple-Choice Questions

1. From what gestation does the risk of stillbirth increase in monochorionic diamniotic twins?
   (a) 34 weeks
   (b) 35 weeks
   (c) 36 weeks
   (d) 37 weeks

Answer: (c)

2. How many times are monochorionic twins are increased risk of fetal loss compared to dichorionic twins prior to 26 weeks?
   (a) 2 times
   (b) 4 times
   (c) 8 times
   (d) 12 times

Answer: (d)

3. How often are monochorionic monoamniotic twins affected by discordant anomalies?
   (a) 1 in 50
   (b) 1 in 25
   (c) 1 in 12
   (d) 1 in 6

Answer: (d)

4. What is the increased risk of stillbirth in monochorionic triplets compared to trichorionic triplets?
   (a) 1.6 fold
   (b) 2.6 fold
   (c) 3.6 fold
   (d) 4.6 fold

Answer: (b)

5. What percentage of intertwin estimated fetal weight discordance is associated with an increased risk of perinatal death?
   (a) >5%
   (b) >10%
   (c) >15%
   (d) >25%

Answer: (d)

References

1. Sairam S, Costeloe K, Thilaganathan B. Prospective risk of stillbirth in multiple-gestation pregnancies: a population-based analysis. Obstet Gynecol. 2002;100:638–41.

2. Ehsanipoor RM, Haydon ML, Lyons Gaffaney C, et al. Gestational age at cervical length measurement and preterm birth in twins. Ultrasound Obstet Gynecol. 2012;40:81–6.
3. Elliott JP, Istwan NB, Collins A, et al. Indicated and nonindicated preterm delivery in twin gestations: impact on neonatal outcome and cost. J Perinatol. 2005;25:4–7.
4. Townsend R, Khalil A. Fetal growth restriction in twins. Best Pract Res Clin Obstet Gynaecol. 2018;49:79–88.
5. Dias T, Akolekar R. Timing of birth in multiple pregnancy. Best Pract Res Clin Obstet Gynaecol. 2014;28(2):319–26.
6. D'Antonio F, Odibo AO, Prefumo F, Khalil A, Buca D, Flacco ME, Liberati M, Manzoli L, Acharya G. Weight discordance and perinatal mortality in twin pregnancy: systematic review and meta-analysis. Ultrasound Obstet Gynecol. 2018;52(1):11–23.
7. Townsend R, Khalil A. Twin pregnancy complicated by selective growth restriction. Curr Opin Obstet Gynecol. 2016;28(6):485–91.
8. Valsky DV, Eixarch E, Martinez JM, Crispi F, Gratacós E. Selective intrauterine growth restriction in monochorionic twins: pathophysiology, diagnostic approach and management dilemmas. Semin Fetal Neonatal Med. 2010;15:342–8.
9. Stirrup OT, Khalil A, D'Antonio F, Thilaganathan B. Fetal growth reference ranges in twin pregnancy: analysis of the Southwest Thames Obstetric Research Collaborative (STORK) multiple pregnancy cohort. Ultrasound Obstet Gynecol. 2015;45(3):301–7.
10. D'Antonio F, Khalil A, Dias T, Southwest Thames Obstetric Research Collaborative (STORK), et al. Early fetal loss in monochorionic and dichorionic twin pregnancies: analysis of the Southwest Thames Obstetric Research Collaborative (STORK) multiple pregnancy cohort. Ultrasound Obstet Gynecol. 2013;41:432–6.
11. Wu D, Huang L, He Z, et al. Pre-eclampsia in twin pregnancies: association with selective intrauterine growth restriction. J Matern Fetal Neonatal Med. 2016;29:1967–71.
12. National Institute for Health and Clinical Excellence. Twin and triplet pregnancy. NICE clinical guideline 137. London: National Institute for Health and Clinical Excellence; 2019.
13. Martin JA, Hamilton BE, Sutton PD, Ventura SJ, Menacker F, Munson ML. Births: final data for 2002. National vital statistics reports, vol. 52, no. 10. Hyattsville: National Center for Health Statistics; 2003.
14. Roberts WE, Morrison JC. Has the use of home monitors, fetal fibronectin, and measurement of cervical length helped predict labor and/or prevent preterm delivery in twins? Clin Obstet Gynecol. 1998;41:95–102.
15. Conde-Agudelo A, Romero R. Prediction of preterm birth in twin gestations using biophysical and biochemical tests. Am J Obstet Gynecol. 2014;211:583–95.
16. Conde-Agudelo A, Romero R, Hassan SS, Yeo L. Transvaginal sonographic cervical length for the prediction of spontaneous preterm birth in twin pregnancies: a systematic review and meta-analysis. Am J Obstet Gynecol. 2010;203:128.e1–12.
17. Romero R, Conde Agudelo A, El-Refaie W, Rode L, Brizot ML, Cetingoz E, Serra V, Da Fonseca E, Abdelhafez MS, Tabor A, Perales A, Hassan SS, Nicolaides KH. Vaginal progesterone decreases preterm birth and neonatal morbidity and mortality in women with a twin gestation and a short cervix: an updated meta-analysis of individual patient data. Ultrasound Obstet Gynecol. 2017;49(3):303–14.
18. Hall JG. Twinning. Lancet. 2003;362:735–43.
19. Lewi L, Jani J, Blickstein I, Huber A, Gucciardo L, Van Mieghem T, Done E, Boes AS, Hecher K, Gratacos E, Lewi P, Deprest J. The outcome of monochorionic diamniotic twin gestations in the era of invasive fetal therapy: a prospective cohort study. Am J Obstet Gynecol. 2008;199:514.e1–8.
20. Baxi LV, Walsh CA. Monoamniotic twins in contemporary practice: a single-center study of perinatal outcomes. J Matern Fetal Neonatal Med. 2010;23:506–10.
21. Pasquini L, Wimalasundera RC, Fisk NM. Management of other complications specific to monochorionic twin pregnancies. Best Pract Res Clin Obstet Gynaecol. 2004;18:577–99.
22. Sebire NJ, Snijders RJ, Hughes K, et al. The hidden mortality of monochorionic twin pregnancies. Br J Obstet Gynaecol. 1997;104:1203–7.
23. Kalyoncu O, Aygun C, Cetinoglu E, et al. Neonatal morbidity and mortality of late-preterm babies. J Matern Fetal Neonatal Med. 2010;23:607–12.
24. Kahn B, Lumey LH, Zybert PA, et al. Prospective risk of fetal death in singleton, twin, and triplet gestations: implications for practice. Obstet Gynecol. 2003;102:685–92.
25. Hack KEA, Derks JB, Elias SG, et al. Increased perinatal mortality and morbidity in monochorionic versus dichorionic twin pregnancies: clinical implications of a large Dutch cohort study. BJOG. 2008;115:58–67.
26. Cheong-See F, Schuit E, Arroyo-Manzano D, Khalil A, Barrett J, Joseph KS, et al. Prospective risk of

stillbirth and neonatal complications in twin pregnancies: systematic review and meta-analysis. BMJ. 2016;354:i4353. https://doi.org/10.1136/bmj.i4353.
27. D'Antonio F, Khalil A, Dias T, Thilaganathan B, Southwest Thames Obstetric Research Collaborative (STORK). Early fetal loss in monochorionic and dichorionic twin pregnancies: analysis of the Southwest Thames Obstetric Research Collaborative (STORK) multiple pregnancy cohort. Ultrasound Obstet Gynecol. 2014;41(6):632–6.
28. Southwest Thames Obstetric Research Collaborative (STORK). Prospective risk of late stillbirth in monochorionic twins: a regional cohort study. Ultrasound Obstet Gynecol. 2012;39(5):500–4.
29. Hack KEA, Derks JB, Elias SG, et al. Perinatal mortality and mode of delivery in monochorionic twin pregnancies ≥32 weeks of gestation: a multicenter retrospective cohort study. BJOG. 2011;118(9):1090–7.
30. Van Mieghem T, De Heus R, Lewi L, et al. Prenatal management of monoamniotic twin pregnancies. Obstet Gynecol. 2014;124:498–506.
31. Ishii K. Prenatal diagnosis and management of monoamniotic twins. Curr Opin Obstet Gynecol. 2015;27(2):159–64.
32. Curado J, D'Antonio F, Papageorghiou AT, Bhide A, Thilaganathan B, Khalil A. Perinatal mortality and morbidity in triplet pregnancy according to chorionicity: systematic review and meta-analysis. Ultrasound Obstet Gynecol. 2019;54(5):589–95.
33. Ko HS, Choi SK, Wie JH, Park IY, Park YG, Shin JC. Optimal timing of delivery based on the risk of stillbirth and infant death associated with each additional week of expectant management in multiple pregnancies: a national cohort study of Koreans. J Korean Med Sci. 2018;33(10):e80.
34. Kawaguchi H, Ishii K, Yamamoto R, Hayashi S, Mitsuda N, Perinatal Research Network Group in Japan. Perinatal death of triplet pregnancies by chorionicity. AJOG. 2013;209:36.e1–7.

Key Reading

Cheong-See F, Schuit E, Arroyo-Manzano D, Khalil A, Barrett J, Joseph KS, et al. Prospective risk of stillbirth and neonatal complications in twin pregnancies: systematic review and meta-analysis. BMJ. 2016;354:i4353. https://doi.org/10.1136/bmj.i4353.

Dias T, Akolekar R. Timing of birth in multiple pregnancy. Best Pract Res Clin Obstet Gynaecol. 2014;28(2):319–26.

Hack KEA, Derks JB, Elias SG, et al. Increased perinatal mortality and morbidity in monochorionic versus dichorionic twin pregnancies: clinical implications of a large Dutch cohort study. BJOG. 2008;115:58–67.

Hack KEA, Derks JB, Elias SG, et al. Perinatal mortality and mode of delivery in monochorionic twin pregnancies ≥32 weeks of gestation: a multicenter retrospective cohort study. BJOG. 2011;118(9):1090–7.

National Institute for Health and Clinical Excellence. Twin and triplet pregnancy. NICE clinical guideline 137. London: National Institute for Health and Clinical Excellence; 2019.

Twin Deliveries – Where Are We Now?

Amir Aviram, Jon F. R. Barrett, Elad Mei-Dan, and Nir Melamed

Contents

A. Khalil et al. (eds.), *Twin and Higher-order Pregnancies*,
https://doi.org/10.1007/978-3-030-47652-6_21

Trailer

The mode of delivery in twin gestation has been a matter of debate for decades. In 2013, the only randomized controlled trial concerning mode of delivery in twin gestations was published, answering some of the most pressing questions in this matter. The Twin Birth Study (TBS) randomized patients carrying dichorionic-diamniotic or monochorionic-diamniotic twins, with the first twin in cephalic presentation, between 32 and 39 weeks of gestation, to planned vaginal versus planned cesarean delivery, and found no significant differences in perinatal or maternal outcomes.

In this chapter, we try to address the known literature before and after the publication of the TBS. We also review the literature with regard to scenarios beyond the scope of the TBS, such as delivery of preterm twins, the impact of chorionicity, combined delivery, and more.

Definitions

CD – Cesarean delivery.

Combined delivery – Vaginal delivery of twin A followed by cesarean delivery of twin B.

DCDA – Dichorionic-diamniotic twins.

External cephalic version – An attempt to turn a non-cephalic fetus to cephalic presentation by an external abdominal manipulation.

Internal podalic version and total breech extraction – An attempt to turn a non-breech fetus to footling presentation by inserting one or both hands into the uterus and grasping one or two feet of the fetus through an intact membrane, and pulling it toward the cervix.

MCDA – Monochorionic-diamniotic twins.

MCMA – Monochorionic-monoamniotic twins.

TOLAC – Trial of labor after previous cesarean delivery.

VBAC – Vaginal birth after previous cesarean delivery.

VD – Vaginal delivery.

Learning Objectives

- The reader will understand the main results and significance of the TBS, and in which situations it is applicable.
- The reader will comprehend the considerations underlying the rationale for the different timing of delivery for DCDA, MCDA, and MCMA twins.
- The reader will know the methods used for delivery of the second twin.
- The reader will be familiar with the literature regarding twin preterm delivery, and twin VBAC.

21.1 Introduction

It is a well-known fact that multiple pregnancies carry higher risk of adverse perinatal outcomes, compared with singleton gestations, mainly attributed to preterm delivery and low birth weight [1–6]. Yet, these are not the only perils awaiting twins. During delivery, apart from the usual indications for cesarean delivery (CD) in singleton pregnancy, delivery of the second twin may be complicated by an unexpected change in fetal lie and presenting part, abruptio placenta following the rapid decompression of the uterus after the delivery of the first twin, prolapsed umbilical cord, changes in cervical dilatation, and more. All of these may lead to a unique mode of delivery – combined delivery, in which twin A is delivered vaginally, and twin B is delivered by a CD.

As such, the conduct of a twin delivery remains one of the most challenging events in the daily practice of obstetricians. The perennial dilemmas that apply to any singleton delivery, such as intra-partum monitoring and operative interventions, are compounded by the presence of the second fetus. In this chapter, we review the evidence concerning the mode of delivery in twin gestations, and address specific clinical scenarios regularly encountered in daily practice.

21.2 Mode of Delivery: Pre-Twin Birth Study Era and Post-Twin Birth Study Era

The literature regarding mode of delivery was limited to observational studies and retrospective cohort studies until the publication of the Twin Birth Study (TBS) in 2013 [7]. Prior to that, only one small-scale RCT was performed, in 1987. In this study, Rabinovici and colleagues aimed to assess the management of a non-vertex twin B [8]. They randomized 60 women carrying twins (in all of which twin B was in breech presentation or transverse lie) to planned vaginal delivery (VD) versus planned CD. All twins A were in cephalic presentation. They did not find any significant differences between the groups in Apgar scores, birth trauma, neonatal morbidity or mortality, but stated that maternal febrile morbidity was significantly higher in the CD group.

As aforementioned, all other studies were mainly observational or retrospective in nature. A systematic review and meta-analysis published in 2011 by Rossi et al. included such manuscripts published in the first decade of the millennium [9]. Their main results showed that while as a general rule the rate of neonatal morbidity of twin A is lower than twin B, it is not associated with mode of delivery, or presentation of twin B. They also reported lower rate of neonatal morbidity of twin A in vaginal delivery (as compared with CD) [9].

In an effort to reconcile different results from different studies, a multi-national, multicenter, randomized, controlled trial was initiated in 2003 [7]. In the TBS, patients were eligible for recruitment between $32^{0/7}$ and $38^{6/7}$ weeks of gestation, if the first twin was in the cephalic presentation, and both fetuses were alive with an estimated weight between 1500 and 4000 g. Exclusion criteria were monoamniotic twins, fetal reduction at 13 or more weeks of gestation, lethal fetal anomaly, contraindication to labor or vaginal delivery (such as fetal compromise, twin B substantially larger than the twin A, previous 2 or more CDs, or vertical uterine incision). Women were randomized to planned VD or planned CD, and delivery was planned between $37^{5/7}$ and $38^{6/7}$ weeks of gestation. Mothers and infants were followed up to 28 days after delivery. The primary outcome was defined as one or more of the following: neonatal mortality, birth trauma, 5-min Apgar score < 4, alteration in consciousness, two or more seizures before 72 h of age, need for assisted ventilation with an endotracheal tube, septicemia or meningitis, necrotizing enterocolitis, bronchopulmonary dysplasia, grade III or IV intraventricular hemorrhage, and cystic periventricular leukomalacia. Additionally, a composite maternal outcome was also defined (one or more of the following): maternal mortality; blood loss ≥1500 ml; need for blood transfusion or need for dilation and curettage after delivery, laparotomy, serious genital tract injury; intraoperative damage to the bladder, ureter, or bowel requiring repair; fistula involving the genital tract; thromboembolism; systemic infection or pneumonia; major medical life-threatening illness; serious wound infection or complication; or other serious maternal complication.

Overall, data were available for a total of 1392 women in each arm, 2783 fetuses/infants in the planned CD arm and 2782 fetuses/infants in the planned VD arm. Approximately 90% of women assigned to the planned CD arm had a CD, 9% had a VD of both twins, and 1% had a combined delivery. In the planned VD arm, 56% patients had a VD, 40% had a CD for both twins, and 4% had a combined delivery. Of this cohort, approximately 75% had DCDA twins (dichorionic-diamniotic), and the rest had MCDA twins (monochorionic-diamniotic).

No differences in the primary composite neonatal outcome or the composite maternal outcome were found between the groups. These results did not change in the pre-specified subgroup analysis according to parity, gestational age at randomization, maternal age, presentation of twin B, chorionicity, or the national perinatal mortality rate of the mother's country of residence. It was found, however, that the second twin was more likely than the first twin to have the primary outcome [7]. The authors of the study concluded that planned CD was not associated with better neonatal or maternal outcomes than planned VD.

While this study was the first (and until today the only) comprehensive, large-scale RCT regarding mode of delivery in twin pregnancies, it still leaves several questions unanswered. First, one of first questions obstetricians face when counselling patients with twin gestation regarding mode of delivery, is the weight difference between the twins. The common notion is that if twin B is substantially larger than twin A, there may be an increased risk for CD or, more even more concerning, entrapment of fetal head when twin B is delivered in breech presentation. One of the TBS exclusion criteria was "second twin substantially larger than the first twin," and fetal weight estimation by ultrasound was not analyzed. As such, the TBS does not answer this question, which is still a matter of debate.

Second, one of the TBS inclusion criteria for institutions was that vaginal delivery of twins will be attended by "a qualified obstetrician who was experienced at vaginal twin delivery, defined a priori as an obstetrician who judged himself or herself to be experienced at vaginal twin delivery and whose department head agreed with this judgment." Naturally, this definition is quite vague. As an attestation, a review of the TBS supplementary material reveals that out of the 59 combined deliveries in the planned VD arm, 35 (~60%) were indicated by fetal malpresentation, and 6 (~10%) by failed attempted version.

Third, the TBS was not designed to answer other pertinent questions regarding multiple deliveries, such as delivery at lower gestational age or lower weight than specified, twin deliveries after previous cesarean section, and – as the TBS implies – higher order multiples. Fourth, the rate of failed attempted vaginal delivery approached 45%. Since the TBS was designed and powered to answer the question of mode of delivery, it was not powered to address the question of risk factors for failed vaginal delivery in twin gestations.

Following the publication of the TBS, several sub-analyses were performed. While not sufficiently powered, they still shed light on several important questions, using the only large-scale, prospective study performed in this area. For example, Mei-Dan et al. sought to explore the differences between planned VD and planned CD for women in the TBS cohort who presented in spontaneous labor. Of the 2804 women included in the original study, 823 in the planned VD group and 612 in the planned CD presented in spontaneous labor. No difference in the rate of primary outcome was found between planned VD and planned CD groups. Similarly, the rates of the individual components of the primary outcome and of maternal adverse outcome were similar between the two groups. The authors concluded that in women with twins who present in spontaneous labor, a policy of planned vaginal delivery compared with CD is not associated with significant differences in neonatal or maternal outcomes [10]. The same group also explored the practice of induction of labor in twin pregnancies. They analyzed the outcomes of 153 women who were induced by prostaglandins, and 215 women who were induced by amniotomy and/or oxytocin alone. No difference in CD rate was found between the groups. In contrast, CD rates were affected by nulliparity, late maternal age, non-cephalic presentation of twin B, and high country's perinatal mortality rate.

There were no differences between induction methods with respect to maternal/neonatal adverse outcomes [11]. The authors concluded that the need for cervical ripening by prostaglandin had no effect on the incidence of CD or adverse outcome in women with twins who require labor induction.

Neonatal outcome at 2 years of age were also assessed in the TBS cohort. Overall, 4603 children from the initial cohort of 5565 infants (83%) were included in the study. The authors found no significant difference in the outcome of death or neurodevelopmental delay (OR 1.04, 95% CI 0.77–1.41), and concluded that a policy of planned CD had no added benefit to children at 2 years of age compared with a policy of planned VD in patients with characteristics similar to the TBS cohort [12].

Hutton and colleagues explored whether maternal outcomes 2 years after delivery, such as urinary stress, fecal or flatus incontinence, were affected by planned mode of delivery in twins. Overall, 2305 women out of the original cohort completed questionnaires at 2 years (82.2% follow-up). The authors found that women in the planned CD group were less likely to experience urinary stress incontinence compared with their CD group counterparts (OR 0.63, 95% CI 0.47–0.83), with no reported difference in the quality of life. No differences were found in fecal or flatus incontinence, or in other maternal outcomes [13].

To conclude, the TBS was an important milestone in twins research, by providing reassurance to obstetricians regarding the feasibility and safety of planned vaginal delivery in twin gestations with matching characteristics to those used in the study.

Several years after the publication of the TBS, these results were further validated by the JUmeaux MODe d'Accouchement (JUMODA) study, a national prospective population-based cohort study in 176 maternity units in France [14]. The inclusion criteria were similar to those of the TBS (twin pregnancies, born at or after 32 weeks of gestation, with a cephalic first twin). More than 5900 women and their neonates were eligible for analysis, of whom roughly 25% had a CD. The authors found that the composite neonatal mortality and morbidity was increased in the planned CD arm (5.2% vs. 2.2%, OR 2.38, 95% CI 1.86–2.05), but this difference was relevant only to those twins delivered prior to 37 weeks of gestation.

21.3 Timing of Delivery

The timing of delivery by either induction of labor or CD is an important consideration in twin delivery. Several reports have attempted to establish the threshold at which the balance between prematurity and excessive maturity tips toward delivery. On the one hand, prematurity is associated with greater morbidity, but on the other hand, prolongation of pregnancy may lead to increased rates of stillbirths [5, 15–24]. Dodd, Crowther, and associates published the results of an RCT on the timing of delivery in uncomplicated twin gestations in 2012 [25]. A total of 235 women (approximately 80% with DCDA twins, and the rest MCDA twins) were randomized to elective delivery at 37 week or from 38 weeks onward. They found that a practice of elective induction of labor or elective CD at 37 weeks of gestation was associated with a significant reduction in the risk of serious adverse outcome for the infant (4.7% vs. 12.2%, $p = 0.005$, RR 0.39, 95% CI 0.20–0.75). They also demonstrated a reduction in the rate of birthweight <3rd percentile (3.0% vs. 10.1%, $p = 0.004$, RR 0.30, 95% CI 0.13–0.67). The authors concluded that elective delivery at 37 weeks should be recommended for women carrying an uncomplicated twin gestation. The results of this study were incorporated into a meta-analysis, which showed similar results. Yet, this meta-analysis consisted of only two studies: one small study of 36 participants and the aforementioned study of 235 participants, thus the results were obviously dominated by the latter [26].

Further support to these findings comes from a retrospective cohort study of 768 twin gestations (601 DCDA and 167 MCDA twins). Burgess et al. found that the nadir of composite neonatal morbidity for MCDA twins occurred at $36^{0/6}$–$36^{6/7}$ weeks' gestation, and for DCDA twins at $37^{0/7}$–$37^{6/7}$ weeks' gestation.

While Dodd and Crowther did include monochorionic twins in their study, they did not stratify the results by chorionicity. Some studies quantified the risk of stillbirth for MCDA twins at 3–4% per week and suggested delivery at 36 weeks [27, 28]. However others suggested that the rate of stillbirth was overestimated in those studies and recommended that, provided that the pregnancy is otherwise uncomplicated, gestation can be advanced until 37 weeks [16, 29].

MCMA (monochorionic-monoamniotic) twins present a different challenge (See ▶ Chap. 17). The cord entanglement that is present in nearly 100% of the cases, along with all other complications of monochorionic gestation, makes their monitoring and the decision-making process regarding timing of delivery challenging. Older reports suggested hospitalization during the third trimester, with early delivery. In 2014, Van Mieghem et al. presented their retrospective data concerning 193 MCMA twin gestations. In their cohort, fetal deaths occurred in 18.1% of fetuses, and neonatal deaths in 5.8%. Overall, the risk of a non-respiratory neonatal complication was lower than the risk of fetal death after $32^{4/7}$ weeks of gestation (95% CI $32^{0/7}$–$33^{4/7}$). They also could not find differences in adverse outcomes between inpatient management and outpatient management, as long as the outpatient management was close and strict [30].

The MONOMONO study was a multinational cohort study of women with MCMA pregnancies, from January 2010 to January 2017. Inclusion criteria were non-anomalous uncomplicated monoamniotic twins, with two live fetuses at $26^{0/7}$ weeks of gestation. The primary outcome was intrauterine fetal death [31]. Out of 195 pregnancies (390 fetuses), the overall perinatal loss rate was 10.8% (peak fetal death rate at 29 weeks of gestation, reaching 4.3%). From $32^{0/7}$ to $36^{6/7}$, no fetal or neonatal deaths were recorded. As with the previous cited study, this study did not find any differences between inpatient management and outpatient strict management of MCMA twins. Combined together, these studies support the elective delivery of MCMA twins at $32^{0/7}$–$34^{0/7}$ weeks of gestation.

21

Of note, as in every case of scheduled delivery prior to 37 completed weeks of gestation, accurate dating of the pregnancy is essential along with parental advice about potential complications, and consideration of administration of antenatal corticosteroids [32].

As for the national guidelines: the American College of Obstetricians and Gynecologists (ACOG) recommends delivery of uncomplicated DCDA, MCDA, and MCMA twins at 38, $34^{0/7}$–$37^{6/7}$, and $32^{0/7}$–$34^{0/7}$ weeks of gestation, respectively [33]. The National Institute for Health and Care Excellence (NICE) guidelines are as follows: 37 weeks for DCDA twins, 36 weeks for MCDA twins, and $32^{0/7}$–$33^{6/7}$ for MCMA twins (after a course of antenatal corticosteroids) [34, 35]. The Royal Australian and New Zealand College of Obstetricians and Gynaecologists (RANZCOG) recommends delivery of the uncomplicated MCDA twin gestation by 37 weeks of gestation [36].

21.4 Delivery of the Second Twin

As aforementioned, in uncomplicated DCDA or MCDA twin pregnancies, after 32 weeks of gestation, if twin A is in cephalic presentation, and regardless of the presentation of twin B, no differences were found in the TBS between planned VD and planned CD. Yet, the delivery of twin B is at times not straightforward, especially in the era of the Term Breech Trial [37], when manual expertise of breech deliveries declined significantly. The main dilemma surrounds the optimal management of the noncephalic twin B – whether an external cephalic version (ECV) should be attempted or whether total breech extraction should be preferred.

Several authors tried to assess the confidence level of trainees in obstetrics in vaginal deliveries of twins. In one of the studies, out of a total of 417 residents only a third felt confident managing the breech second twin, and 28% responded that they would not feel comfortable managing the breech second twin post-residency [38]. The solution to training gaps might be simulations, yet further studies are needed in order to determine the optimal training method for managing the second breech twin [39, 40].

In 1983, Chervenak et al. advocated ECV of the second non-vertex twin after delivery of the first twin in order to achieve delivery of the second in a vertex presentation [41]. ECV was attempted in 25 sets of twins after successful delivery of the first vertex twin. This was successful in 18 of the cases (72%) and was not associated with increased perinatal complications [41]. Subsequent to Chervenak's report, other investigators published similar findings [42, 43]. Others, however, have reported a significantly higher incidence of vaginal delivery with breech extraction compared with ECV for the second non-vertex twin. Because of failed ECV or other complications, CD occurred more frequently if ECV was attempted rather than breech extraction [44–46]. The TBS confirmed this observation with a 95% success rate in patients delivered by breech extraction versus 42% when ECV was attempted, and it therefore now seems conclusive that breech extraction is the optimal procedure for the non-vertex second twin [7]. Interestingly, some have advocated that total breech extraction may even show better results than delivery of the a priori vertex twin B [47].

Breech extraction, with or without internal podalic version, is accomplished in the manner described by Rabinovici et al. [48]: the feet of the second fetus are located through intact membranes and grasped without rupturing the amniotic sac. Gentle and continuous traction is exerted on both feet toward the birth canal. Simultaneously, the operator's other hand is used to dislodge and elevate the fetal head toward the uterine fundus by pressure applied to the abdominal wall. A relaxed uterus is an essential prerequisite for the safe performance of internal version. While epidural provides analgesia it does not provide uterine relaxation as used to be provided by general anesthesia. Tocolysis may be rapidly and safely achieved by the use of 50–100 μg of nitroglycerine given intravenously before the version attempt, membranes are ruptured as late as possible, and only when the fetus is in longitudinal lie.

The unique entity of combined delivery should also be addressed. Several authors along the years have published their findings regarding risk factors for CD of the second twin following VD of the first. According to past reports, the rates of combined delivery are 5–10% [49–52]. Most of these findings come from small-sized, retrospective studies which showed that malpresentation of the second twin is associated with higher rate of combined delivery [53–56]. Combined deliveries were also found to be associated with a higher incidence of maternal and neonatal infectious morbidity [56].

Recently, a sub-analysis of the TBS concerning combined deliveries was published [57]. The rate of non-cephalic presentation of twin B was more than twofold higher in the combined delivery group, and the likelihood of spontaneous version of twin B (a different presentation at delivery compared to the presentation at randomization) was also higher in the combined delivery group. In a multivariable regression model, breech presentation was not significantly associated with combined delivery (aOR 0.99, 95% CI 0.36–2.67), in contrast to transverse/oblique lie (aOR 43.74, 95% CI 15.37–124.49). Combined deliveries were more likely to be associated with fetal/neonatal death or serious neonatal morbidity (13.6% vs. 2.3%, $p < 0.001$), 5-min Apgar score < 7, NICU admissions, abnormal level of consciousness, and prolonged (≥24 h) assisted ventilation.

21.5 Time Interval Between Delivery of Twins

It was previously believed that the time interval between delivery of each twin should be no longer than 30 min, as a prolonged interval placed the second twin at risk of asphyxia from decreased placental circulation [58].

In the TBS, the mean inter-twin delivery interval was 8 min with a range of 1–33 min [7]. Other studies found no correlation between 5-min Apgar scores and inter-twin delivery interval [59, 60]. Rayburn et al. found that perinatal morbidity was lowest with expectant management and subsequent spontaneous delivery regardless of fetal presentation. One small study reported a sixfold increase in the risk of CD for the second twin with a delivery interval greater than 15 min [61].

More recent studies reported different results. For example, Schneuber et al. examined the effect of inter-twin delivery interval on neonatal outcome. In cases where both twins were delivered vaginally ($n = 151$), there was no significant correlation between the inter-twin delivery interval and umbilical cord arterial pH or Apgar scores at 1, 5 and 10 minutes of twin B [62]. Cukierman and associates sought to examine the association between inter-twin delivery interval and short-term perinatal outcomes. They found that adverse neonatal outcome occurred in 201 (58.2%) of the twins (while only 7 had a CD for the second twin), that delivery interval was associated with higher cord lactate, and that low Apgar scores were more frequent with intervals >30 min. The predictors of adverse outcome were gestational age, abnormal fetal heart rate tracing, and breech delivery of the twin B [63].

Most of the studies proved hard to interpret, since most of them do not correlate mode of delivery, set-up (operating room or delivery room) with longer twin-to-twin interval. Naturally, if there is an abnormal fetal heart rate tracing, and an urgent CD is necessary, the inter-twin delivery interval will be longer than an uncomplicated vaginal delivery, if only because the need to transfer to the operating room, administer anesthesia, etc. As such, longer interval is translated to poorer outcomes, but mainly because of the primary indication to intervene, rather than the longer time that intervention caused. It is safe to assume that there is probably some association between the inter-twin delivery interval and deterioration of Apgar scores and umbilical cord pH, yet a clear threshold is hard to establish, and the correlation is probably weak [64–66].

The difficulty arises when fetal heart rate decelerations or bradycardia are detected following delivery of twin A, and delivery of twin B needs to be expedited. In the case of the non-cephalic twin B, an IPV and breech extraction will usually accomplish it quickly. However, great skill and judgment are required in the case of the second twin presenting in a vertex presentation in whom immediate delivery is required. Some will turn to use forceps of vacuum, while others will feel more comfortable with a CD. There are no data available regarding this important clinical dilemma. As long as the delivery is taking place in an operating room, with a patient ready for immediate CD, either method is likely to result in a good fetal outcome, although without the use of the vacuum the CD rate for the second twin will likely be higher.

21.6 Specific Clinical Scenarios

21.6.1 Breech Twin A

The literature regarding the recommended mode of delivery of a non-cephalic twin A is scarce. First, singleton vaginal breech deliveries have been a matter of debate, until the publication of the Term Breech Trial. Another concern with a breech twin A and a cephalic twin B was the potential rare complication of locked twins. This complication is uncommon with an estimated frequency of 1:500–1:800, but the mortality associated with fetal entanglement is extremely high, ranging between 30% and 43% [67–69].

One multicenter retrospective study compared 239 women who had a VD and 374 who had a CD, all of whom had a breech first twin. While lower Apgar scores and higher mortality rates were noted for first twins with birth weight of less than 1500 g, no differences were found between VD and CD for twins with higher birth weight [70]. Another systematic review did not find significant differences between non-cephalic twins A delivered in CD or VD. Nonetheless, the authors only compared the rates of neonatal mortality and 5-min Apgar scores < 7, and for the purpose of non-cephalic twins A included only 8 low-quality observational studies. The authors concluded, "No final conclusion can be drawn due to the small sample sizes and statistical limitations of the included studies" [71].

The Term Breech Trial [37] is one of the pivotal studies in the field of obstetrics. It was published in 2000 and changed obstetrical practices around the world. In this multinational, multi-centered study, 2088 women with singleton gestation in breech presentation were randomized to planned VD versus planned CD. The authors found that perinatal mortality, neonatal mortality, or serious neonatal morbidity were lower in the planned CD group (1.6% vs. 5.0%, $p < 0.001$, RR 0.33, 95% CI 0.19–0.56). While not without controversy, these results were extrapolated to twins as well, and resulted in general agreement that twins in which twin A is in breech presentation should be delivered by CD.

Currently, several national guidelines specifically recommend CD for non-cephalic twin A [34], while others state that the same indications for CD in singleton gestations (such as breech presentation, placenta previa, etc.) should be applied for twins [72]. Other guidelines, such as the ACOG practice bulletin [33], do not address non-cephalic first twin altogether, and one can only assume that it is implied that non-cephalic twin A should be managed the same way as a non-cephalic singleton, i.e., a CD should be offered.

21.6.2 Monochorionic-Monoamniotic Twins

The NICE guidelines, as well as ACOG and Society of Obstetricians and Gynaecologists of Canada (SOGC) guidelines, are unified in their recommendation that CD should be preferred in the case of MCMA twins [33, 34, 72]. The main reason for this recommendation is the concern for cord complications.

21.6.3 Monochorionic-Diamniotic Twins

MCDA twin gestation may be associated with multiple antepartum complications such as twin-to-twin transfusion syndrome, twin anemia-polycythemia sequence, twin reverse arterial perfusion, and selective fetal growth restriction. Even in the absence of recognizable monochorionic-specific complications, monochorionic twins usually experience a higher rate of adverse neonatal outcomes [73–77].

Several studies have attempted to address the issue of mode of delivery of MCDA twins, usually through retrospective analysis [73–80]. Most studies compared delivery outcomes of MCDA twins with those of DCDA twins, and most did not find significant differences between these groups. Nonetheless, these studies were retrospective, with various sample sizes. Most importantly, these studies do not provide practical information and tools that can be used in clinical practice to counsel couples regarding the optimal mode of delivery based on multiple factors, including chorionicity.

In the TBS, 23–25% of women had monochorionic twins, and approximately 2% had unknown chorionicity. While the analysis considered chorionicity as a co-factor for the primary outcome, no direct analysis of the impact of mode of delivery in monochorionic twins was performed [7]. Recently, a subanalysis of the data regarding MCDA twin was completed [81]. The authors found no differences between planned VD and planned CD for MCDA twins.

21.6.4 Preterm Birth and Low Birth Weight

As mentioned, the TBS recruited patients from 32 weeks of gestation and onward. In cases of preterm birth or low birth weight, concerns arise regarding the obstetrical manipulations of a small twin B.

Some studies have shown adverse outcomes associated with VD [82, 83], while other have not [84]. Herbst and Källén compared the outcome of twins B delivered by CD with those delivered by VD. They reported that twins B delivered by CD (due to breech presentation of twin A) prior to 34 weeks of gestation were at lower risk of neonatal death (aOR 0.40, 95% CI 0.17–0.95) [85].

Other reports provided contradictory results. Sentilhes et al. compared neonatal mortality and morbidity in very preterm twins ($26^{0/7}$–$31^{6/7}$) with the first twin in cephalic presentation. Overall, 248 women were included in the planned VD group, of which 86% eventually had a VD, and 63 women in the planned CD group. Planned VD was not found to affect mortality or severe neonatal composite morbidity of either twin [86].

Another population-based study from France explored the impact of planned mode of delivery in preterm twins on outcomes at 2 years of age [87]. Inclusion criteria were women with preterm cephalic first twin who delivered after preterm labor or preterm pre-labor rupture of membranes from $24^{0/7}$ to $34^{6/7}$ weeks of gestation. A total of 276 women were eligible for analysis in the planned VD group, and 107 women in the planned CD group. Overall survival at discharge, survival at discharge without severe morbidity, and survival at 2 years of corrected age without neurosensory impairment were similar between the groups, for both twins.

Dagenais and colleagues performed a systematic review and meta-analysis of the safest mode of delivery for preterm twins, when twin B is in non-cephalic presentation. They found no difference between twins delivered by VD or CD in cephalic/non-cephalic twin pairs at $24^{0/7}$–$27^{6/7}$ weeks. Nonetheless, the confidence intervals were wide, and the I^2 quite large, indicating significant heterogeneity and variety between the studies [88].

Another systematic review and meta-analysis included 15 studies with more than 12,000 infants. CD was associated with a 41% decrease in odds of death between $23^{0/7}$ and $27^{6/7}$ weeks (OR 0.59, 95% CI 0.36–0.95, NNT 8), especially under $24^{6/7}$ weeks of gestation (OR 0.58, 95% CI 0.44–0.75, NNT 7). The odd ratios for $25^{0/7}$ weeks and above were not significant. CD was also protective with regard to severe intraventricular hemorrhage between $23^{0/7}$ and $27^{6/7}$ weeks, yet this effect, as for mortality, was mainly visible in lower gestational ages [89].

The NICE guidelines suggest offering CD for preterm twin deliveries between 26 and 32 weeks when twin A is in non-cephalic presentation. Prior to 26 weeks, their recommendation is that the decision should be individualized [34].

The SOGC guidelines recommend vaginal delivery of both twins as long as their individual weights exceed 1500 g and that twin A is in cephalic presentation. Between 500 and 1500 g, there is no recommendation, as the writers acknowledge the lack of good quality literature [72].

To conclude, neonatal data in twin deliveries are highly variable and depend not only on mode of delivery, but also on neonatal weight, presentations, level of neonatal care, and advances in neonatal resuscitation along the years. With current knowledge, clear gestational age and birthweight thresholds are difficult to determine.

21.6.5 Previous Cesarean Section (Twin VBAC)

While the risks and potential adverse outcomes of trial of labor after a previous CD (TOLAC) were extensively studied for singleton gestations, data for women with twin gestation and a history of CD are less clear.

Cahill and associates compared the rate of successful TOLAC in women with twin (n = 535) or singleton (n = 24,307) pregnancies. They found that while women with twins are less likely to have a TOLAC compared with women with singleton, they had a similar rate of TOLAC failure (aOR 1.1, 95% CI 0.8–1.6), uterine rupture (aOR 1.2, 95% CI 0.3–4.6), or a major maternal morbidity (aOR 1.6, 95% CI 0.7–3.7) [90].

Two meta-analyses addressing twin TOLAC were recently published. In the first one, the authors included 10 studies for a total of 2336 trials of labor and 5736 CD. They reported that the pooled rate for successful TOLAC was 72.2% (95% CI 59.7–83.2%), and the risk for uterine rupture during TOLAC was 0.87% (95% CI 0.51–1.31%). They found that TOLAC was associated with higher risk of neonatal death (RR 3.02, 95% CI 1.07–8.54). The risks of uterine dehiscence, blood transfusions, and hysterectomy were comparable, though the risk of infectious morbidity was higher in the CD group. The authors concluded that twin TOLAC is associated with high success rate and low rate of uterine rupture, and that the finding of higher neonatal mortality rate may be attributed to prematurity [91].

In the second meta-analysis, Kabiri et al. pooled data from 11 cohort studies (8209 twin gestations), of which 2484 were intended for planned VD and 5725 for planned CD [92]. Twin TOLAC was associated with a higher risk of uterine rupture (OR 10.09, 95% CI 4.30–23.69; $I^2 = 68\%$) when compared to twin CD. Nonetheless, when compared with singleton TOLAC, twin TOLAC was not found to differ with regard to the rate of uterine rupture (OR 1.34, 95% CI 0.54–3.31). None of the other adverse outcomes were found to be different between twin TOLAC and CD, and the success rate of twin TOLAC was found to be similar to that of singleton TOLAC (OR 0.85, 95% CI 0.61–1.18).

To conclude, it seems that twin TOLAC is a reasonable and safe option for women carrying twins who had a previous CD, and that the risks and success rates are similar to those reported for TOLAC in singleton pregnancies.

21.7 Higher-Order Multiple Pregnancy

Several authors have attempted to assess the feasibility of vaginal delivery in triplet pregnancies. All these studies are observational and are limited by small sample size.

Alamia et al. [93] recruited 23 sets of triplets. Of the 9 who had a trial of labor, 8 (89%) succeeded; the single intra-partum CD was performed for failure to progress. Additionally, two women with triplets who intended to have a VD had a CD for inadequate fetal monitoring. No differences were found in neonatal mortality, Apgar scores, intracranial hemorrhage, arterial cord blood pH, hospital or neonatal intensive care unit stay, and neonatal weight between the VD and CD groups. Grobman and colleagues reported that 29 out of 33 women (88%) with triplet gestation who had a trial of labor had a vaginal delivery of all three neonates with no differences in neonatal outcomes between the CD and VD groups [94]. In 2004, a group from Paris published their experience with 93 sets of triplets. Out of 78 women who had a trial of labor, 66 delivered all three neonates vaginally (84% success rate), with no significant difference in neonatal outcomes [95].

In 2016, Lappen et al. [96] published their retrospective cohort study of 80 sets of triplets ≥28 weeks of gestation. They compared the results of 24 sets of triplets in the trial of labor group with 56 sets of triplets in the CD group. Interestingly, the rate of successful trial of labor was considerably lower than previously published (4/24, 16.7%). Trial of labor was associated with higher rates of maternal transfusion and neonatal mechanical ventilation.

As for the guidelines, similar to MCMA twins, the NICE, ACOG, and SOGC guidelines are uniform in their recommendation for CD in the case of triplets or higher-order multifetal gestations [33, 34, 72].

21.8 Recommended Conduct of Delivery

- Twin delivery should be undertaken by an experienced practitioner competent in twin deliveries.
- Ultrasonographic examination is a useful adjunct prior to delivery (in order to assess fetal presentations, well-being, and estimated fetal weights) and after delivery of the first twin in order to establish the fetal lie and presentation of the second twin. Depending on the gestational age, up to 20% of second twins will spontaneously change presentation once the first twin is delivered [41].
- Intravenous access should be secured, and blood sent for group and screen in anticipation of postpartum hemorrhage.
- The use of epidural, although not mandatory, is highly recommended. It is the authors' opinion that given the relative high likelihood for obstetrical intervention such as IPV, breech extraction, and/or operative delivery, adequate anesthesia is essential.
- Continuous electronic monitoring is highly recommended. In order to increase maternal comfort by reducing the number of

abdominal straps, and to better differentiate the two twins, the authors prefer a fetal scalp electrode on the leading twin once the membranes are ruptured.
- The use of oxytocin for augmentation may be advantageous, especially after the delivery of the first twin.
- We use double set-up (delivery in the operating room) for all twin gestation. The double set-up arrangement allows for a safe vaginal delivery in the same setting of the delivery room, with extra care taken to provide for spousal chaperoning, skin-to-skin, etc. In addition, if urgent obstetrical intervention is needed, all necessary personnel are in place, and conversion to a cesarean delivery is prompt.
- The third stage of labor should be managed actively to prevent blood loss, using oxytocin, uterine massage, and other uterotonic as needed.

21.8.1 Review Questions

1. What was the main conclusion of the TBS?

2. For which clinical scenarios, the results of the TBS are not applicable?

3. What would be your recommendation regarding timing of delivery for the uncomplicated MCMA twin gestation?

4. What is the recommended mode of delivery for DCDA twins in which twin B is in transverse lie?

5. What would be a proper consultation for a woman with twin gestation and a previous cesarean section, who would like a TOLAC?

21.8.2 Multiple-Choice Questions

1. What was the main conclusion of the TBS?
   (a) Planned VD was associated with higher likelihood of adverse composite neonatal outcomes than planned CD.
   (b) Planned VD was associated with lower likelihood of adverse composite neonatal outcomes than planned CD.
   (c) Planned VD was associated with similar likelihood of adverse composite neonatal outcomes as planned CD.
   (d) Planned VD was associated with higher likelihood of adverse composite maternal outcomes than planned CD.

Answer: (c)

2. For which of the following twin gestations, the results of the TBS are not applicable?
   (a) Twin A cephalic, twin B transverse lie.
   (b) Estimated fetal weight of twin A 1700 g, estimated fetal weight of twin B 1900 g.
   (c) Delivery at 315/7 weeks of gestation.
   (d) Monochorionic-diamniotic twin gestation

Answer: (c)

3. What would be your recommendation regarding timing of delivery for the uncomplicated MCMA twin gestation?
   (a) Elective delivery at 37–38 weeks of gestation.
   (b) Elective delivery at 34–36 weeks of gestation.
   (c) Elective delivery at 32–34 weeks of gestation.
   (d) Elective delivery at 30–32 weeks of gestation.

Answer: (c)

4. Which of the following statements regarding delivery of the second twin is true?
   (a) The preferable method of delivery of a transverse twin B is internal

podalic version and total breech extraction.
(b) The preferable method of delivery of a transverse twin B is external cephalic version and to await vaginal delivery.
(c) The preferable method of delivery of a transverse twin B is cesarean delivery.
(d) The preferable method of delivery of a transverse twin B is watchful waiting for the fetus to assume a longitudinal lie.

Answer: (a)

5. What would be a proper consultation for a woman with twin gestation and a previous cesarean section, who would like a TOLAC?
(a) Twin TOLAC carries higher neonatal and maternal risks than singleton TOLAC.
(b) Twin TOLAC carries similar neonatal and maternal risks as singleton TOLAC.
(c) Twin TOLAC carries lower neonatal and maternal risks than singleton TOLAC.
(d) Previous cesarean section is an absolute contraindication for twin TOLAC.

Answer: (b)

References

1. Sunderam S, Kissin DM, Zhang Y, et al. Assisted reproductive technology surveillance – United States, 2016. MMWR Surveill Summ. 2019;68(4):1–23. https://doi.org/10.15585/mmwr.ss6804a1.
2. Blondel B, Kogan MD, Alexander GR, et al. The impact of the increasing number of multiple births on the rates of preterm birth and low birthweight: an international study. Am J Public Health. 2002;92(8):1323–30. https://doi.org/10.2105/AJPH.92.8.1323.
3. Blondel B, Kaminski M. Trends in the occurrence, determinants, and consequences of multiple births. Semin Perinatol. 2002;26(4):239–49. https://doi.org/10.1053/sper.2002.34775.
4. Blickstein I, Keith LG. Outcome of triplets and high-order multiple pregnancies. Curr Opin Obstet Gynecol. 2003;15(2):113–7. https://doi.org/10.1097/00001703-200304000-00005.
5. Kahn B, Lumey LH, Zybert PA, et al. Prospective risk of fetal death in singleton, twin, and triplet gestations: implications for practice. Obstet Gynecol. 2003;102(4):685–92. https://doi.org/10.1016/S0029-7844(03)00616-1.
6. Cheong-See F, Schuit E, Arroyo-Manzano D, Khalil A, Barrett J, Joseph KS. Prospective risk of stillbirth and neonatal complications in twin pregnancies: systematic review and meta-analysis. BMJ. 2016;354:i4353. https://doi.org/10.1136/bmj.i4353.
7. Barrett JFR, Hannah ME, Hutton EK, et al. A randomized trial of planned cesarean or vaginal delivery for twin pregnancy. N Engl J Med. 2013;369(14):1295–305. https://doi.org/10.1056/NEJMoa1214939.
8. Rabinovici J, Barkai G, Reichman B, Serr DM, Mashiach S. Randomized management of the second nonvertex twin: vaginal delivery or cesarean section. Am J Obstet Gynecol. 1987;156(1):52–6. https://doi.org/10.1016/0002-9378(87)90201-8.
9. Rossi AC, Mullin PM, Chmait RH. Neonatal outcomes of twins according to birth order, presentation and mode of delivery: a systematic review and meta-analysis. BJOG. 2011;118(5):523–32. https://doi.org/10.1111/j.1471-0528.2010.02836.x.
10. Mei-Dan E, Dougan C, Melamed N, et al. Planned cesarean or vaginal delivery for women in spontaneous labor with a twin pregnancy: a secondary analysis of the Twin Birth Study. Birth. 2019;46(1):193–200. https://doi.org/10.1111/birt.12387.
11. Mei-Dan E, Asztalos EV, Willan AR, Barrett JFR. The effect of induction method in twin pregnancies: a secondary analysis for the twin birth study. BMC Pregnancy Childbirth. 2017;17(1):9. https://doi.org/10.1186/s12884-016-1201-8.
12. Asztalos EV, Hannah ME, Hutton EK, et al. Twin Birth Study: 2-year neurodevelopmental follow-up of the randomized trial of planned cesarean or planned vaginal delivery for twin pregnancy. Presented at the annual pregnancy meeting of the Society for Maternal-Fetal Medicine, Atlanta, GA, Feb. 4, 2016. Am J Obstet Gynecol. 2016;214(3):371.e1–19. https://doi.org/10.1016/j.ajog.2015.12.051.
13. Hutton EK, Hannah ME, Willan AR, et al. Urinary stress incontinence and other maternal outcomes 2 years after caesarean or vaginal birth for twin pregnancy: a multicentre randomised trial. BJOG. 2018;125(13):1682–90. https://doi.org/10.1111/1471-0528.15407.
14. Schmitz T, Prunet C, Azria E, et al. Association between planned cesarean delivery and neonatal mortality and morbidity in twin pregnancies. Obstet Gynecol. 2017;129(6):986–95. https://doi.org/10.1097/AOG.0000000000002048.

15. Cheung YB, Yip P, Karlberg J. Mortality of twins and singletons by gestational age: a varying-coefficient approach. Am J Epidemiol. 2000;152(12):1107–16. https://doi.org/10.1093/aje/152.12.1107.
16. Sairam S, Costeloe K, Thilaganathan B. Prospective risk of stillbirth in multiple-gestation pregnancies: a population-based analysis. Obstet Gynecol. 2002;100(4):638–41. https://doi.org/10.1016/S0029-7844(02)02174-9.
17. Imaizumi Y. Perinatal mortality in twins and factors influencing mortality in Japan, 1980-98. Paediatr Perinat Epidemiol. 2001;15(3):298–305. https://doi.org/10.1046/j.1365-3016.2001.00361.x.
18. Puissant F, Leroy F. A reappraisal of perinatal mortality factors in twins. Acta Genet Med Gemellol. 1982;31(3–4):213–9. https://doi.org/10.1017/S000156600000831X.
19. Dodd JM, Crowther CA. Should we deliver twins electively at 37 weeks' gestation? Curr Opin Obstet Gynecol. 2005;17(6):579–83. https://doi.org/10.1097/01.gco.0000188409.62904.a3.
20. Bakr AF, Karkour T. What is the optimal gestational age for twin delivery. BMC Pregnancy Childbirth. 2006;6:3. https://doi.org/10.1186/1471-2393-6-3.
21. Dodd JM, Robinson JS, Crowther CA, Chan A. Stillbirth and neonatal outcomes in South Australia, 1991-2000. Am J Obstet Gynecol. 2003;189(6):1731–6. https://doi.org/10.1016/S0002-9378(03)00854-8.
22. Hartley RS, Emanuel I, Hitti J. Perinatal mortality and neonatal morbidity rates among twin pairs at different gestational ages: optimal delivery timing at 37 to 38 weeks' gestation. Am J Obstet Gynecol. 2001;184(3):451–8. https://doi.org/10.1067/mob.2001.109399.
23. Kato N, Matsuda T. Estimation of optimal birth weights and gestational ages for twin births in Japan. BMC Public Health. 2006;6:45. https://doi.org/10.1186/1471-2458-6-45.
24. Luke B, Minogue JR, Witter F, Keith LG, Johnson TRB. The ideal twin pregnancy: patterns of weight gain, discordancy, and length of gestation. Am J Obstet Gynecol. 1993;169(3):588–97. https://doi.org/10.1016/0002-9378(93)90628-V.
25. Dodd JM, Crowther CA, Haslam RR, Robinson JS. Elective birth at 37 weeks of gestation versus standard care for women with an uncomplicated twin pregnancy at term: the Twins Timing of Birth Randomised Trial. BJOG. 2012;119(8):964–73. https://doi.org/10.1111/j.1471-0528.2012.03356.x.
26. Dodd JM, Deussen AR, Grivell RM, Crowther CA. Elective birth at 37 weeks' gestation for women with an uncomplicated twin pregnancy. Cochrane Database Syst Rev. 2014;2014(2):CD003582. https://doi.org/10.1002/14651858.CD003582.pub2.
27. Barigye O, Pasquini L, Galea P, Chambers H, Chappell L, Fisk NM. High risk of unexpected late fetal death in monochorionic twins despite intensive ultrasound surveillance: a cohort study. PLoS Med. 2005;2(6):0521–7. https://doi.org/10.1371/journal.pmed.0020172.
28. Danon D, Sekar R, Hack KEA, Fisk NM. Increased stillbirth in uncomplicated monochorionic twin pregnancies. Obstet Gynecol. 2013;121(6):1318–26. https://doi.org/10.1097/aog.0b013e318292766b.
29. Breathnach FM, McAuliffe FM, Geary M, et al. Optimum timing for planned delivery of uncomplicated monochorionic and dichorionic twin pregnancies. Obstet Gynecol. 2012;119(1):50–9. https://doi.org/10.1097/AOG.0b013e31823d7b06.
30. Van Mieghem T, De Heus R, Lewi L, et al. Prenatal management of monoamniotic twin pregnancies. Obstet Gynecol. 2014;124(3):498–506. https://doi.org/10.1097/AOG.0000000000000409.
31. Saccone G, Berghella V, Locci M, et al. Inpatient vs outpatient management and timing of delivery of uncomplicated monochorionic monoamniotic twin pregnancy: the MONOMONO study. Ultrasound Obstet Gynecol. 2019;53(2):175–83. https://doi.org/10.1002/uog.19179.
32. Melamed N, Shah J, Yoon EW, et al. The role of antenatal corticosteroids in twin pregnancies complicated by preterm birth. Am J Obstet Gynecol. 2016;215(4):482.e1–9. https://doi.org/10.1016/j.ajog.2016.05.037.
33. Committee on Practice Bulletins—Obstetrics; Society for Maternal–Fetal Medicine. Practice Bulletin No. 169: Multifetal gestations: twin, triplet, and higher-order multifetal pregnancies. Obstet Gynecol. 2016;128(4):e131–46. https://doi.org/10.1097/AOG.0000000000001709.
34. National Institute for Health and Care Excellence. Twin and triplet pregnancy. NICE guideline 137. London: National Institute for Health and Care Excellence; 2019. p. 1–69.
35. Kilby MD, Bricker L. Management of monochorionic twin pregnancy: Green-top Guideline No. 51. BJOG. 2017;124(1):e1–e45. https://doi.org/10.1111/1471-0528.14188.
36. RANZCOG. Management of monochorionic twin pregnancy. BJOG. 2017;124(1):e1–e45. https://doi.org/10.1111/1471-0528.14188.
37. Hannah ME, Hannah WJ, Hewson SA, Hodnett ED, Saigal S, Willan AR. Planned caesarean section versus planned vaginal birth for breech presentation at term: a randomised multicentre trial. Term Breech Trial Collaborative Group. Lancet. 2000;356(9239):1375–83. https://doi.org/10.1016/s0140-6736(00)02840-3.
38. Dotters-Katz SK, Gray B, Heine RP, Propst K. Resident education in complex obstetric procedures: are we adequately preparing tomorrow's obstetricians? Am J Perinatol. 2020;37(11):1155–9. https://doi.org/10.1055/s-0039-1692714.
39. Lepage J, Ceccaldi PF, Remini SA, Plaisance P, Voulgaropoulos A, Luton D. Twin vaginal delivery: to maintain skill – simulation is required. Eur J Obstet Gynecol Reprod Biol. 2019;234:195–9. https://doi.org/10.1016/j.ejogrb.2018.12.038.

40. Easter SR, Gardner R, Barrett J, Robinson JN, Carusi D. Simulation to improve trainee knowledge and comfort about twin vaginal birth. Obstet Gynecol. 2016;128:34s–9s. https://doi.org/10.1097/AOG.0000000000001598.
41. Chervenak FA, Johnson RE, Berkowitz RL, Hobbins JC. Intrapartum external version of the second twin. Obstet Gynecol. 1983;62(2):160–5. http://www.ncbi.nlm.nih.gov/pubmed/6866357. Accessed 18 Nov 2019.
42. Tchabo JG, Tomai T. Selected intrapartum external cephalic version of the second twin. Obstet Gynecol. 1992;79(3):421–3. https://doi.org/10.1097/00006250-199203000-00019.
43. Gocke SE, Nageotte MP, Garite T, Towers CV, Dorcester W. Management of the nonvertex second twin: primary cesarean section, external version, or primary breech extraction. Am J Obstet Gynecol. 1989;161(1):111–4. https://doi.org/10.1016/0002-9378(89)90245-7.
44. Wells SR, Thorp JM, Bowes WA. Management of the nonvertex second twin. Surg Gynecol Obstet. 1991;172(5):383–5. http://www.ncbi.nlm.nih.gov/pubmed/2028373. Accessed 18 Nov 2019.
45. Chauhan SP, Roberts WE, McLaren RA, Roach H, Morrison JC, Martin JN. Delivery of the nonvortex second twin: breech extraction versus external cephalic version. Am J Obstet Gynecol. 1995;173(4):1015–20. https://doi.org/10.1016/0002-9378(95)91319-X.
46. Smith SJ, Zebrowitz J, Latta RA. Method of delivery of the nonvertex second twin: a community hospital experience. J Matern Fetal Med. 1997;6(3):146–50. https://doi.org/10.1002/(SICI)1520-6661(199705/06)6:3<146::AID-MFM5>3.0.CO;2-L.
47. Easter SR, Lieberman E, Carusi D. Fetal presentation and successful twin vaginal delivery. Am J Obstet Gynecol. 2016;214(1):116.e1–116.e10. https://doi.org/10.1016/j.ajog.2015.08.017.
48. Rabinovici J, Barkai G, Reichman B, Serr DM, Mashiach S. Internal podalic version with unruptured membranes for the second twin in transverse lie. Obstet Gynecol. 1988;71(3 Pt 1):428–30. http://www.ncbi.nlm.nih.gov/pubmed/3347429. Accessed 18 Nov 2019.
49. Kurzel RB, Claridad L, Lampley EC. Cesarean section for the second twin. J Reprod Med. 1997;42(12):767–70. http://www.ncbi.nlm.nih.gov/pubmed/9437589. Accessed 1 Feb 2014.
50. Ginsberg NA, Levine EM. Delivery of the second twin. Int J Gynaecol Obstet. 2005;91(3):217–20. https://doi.org/10.1016/j.ijgo.2005.08.017.
51. Bider D, Korach J, Hourvitz A, Dulitzky M, Goldenberg M, Mashiach S. Combined vaginal-abdominal delivery of twins. J Reprod Med. 1995;40(2):131–4. http://www.ncbi.nlm.nih.gov/pubmed/7738923. Accessed 1 Feb 2014.
52. Aviram A, Weiser I, Ashwal E, Bar J, Wiznitzer A, Yogev Y. Combined vaginal-cesarean delivery of twins: risk factors and neonatal outcome-a single center experience. J Matern Fetal Neonatal Med. 2014;28(5):509–14. https://doi.org/10.3109/14767058.2014.927430.
53. Breathnach FM, McAuliffe FM, Geary M, et al. Prediction of safe and successful vaginal twin birth. Am J Obstet Gynecol. 2011;205(3):237.e1–7. https://doi.org/10.1016/j.ajog.2011.05.033.
54. Persad VL, Baskett TF, O'Connell CM, Scott HM. Combined vaginal-cesarean delivery of twin pregnancies. Obstet Gynecol. 2001;98(6):1032–7. http://www.ncbi.nlm.nih.gov/pubmed/11755549.
55. Wen SW, Fung KFK, Oppenheimer L, Demissie K, Yang Q, Walker M. Occurrence and predictors of cesarean delivery for the second twin after vaginal delivery of the first twin. Obstet Gynecol. 2004;103(3):413–9. https://doi.org/10.1097/01.AOG.0000110248.32558.fb.
56. Alexander JM, Leveno KJ, Rouse D, et al. Cesarean delivery for the second twin. Obstet Gynecol. 2008;112(4):748–52. https://doi.org/10.1097/AOG.0b013e318187ccb2.
57. Aviram A, Lipworth H, Asztalos EV, et al. The worst of both worlds – combined deliveries in twin gestations: a subanalysis of the Twin Birth Study, a randomized, controlled, prospective study. Am J Obstet Gynecol. 2019;221(4):353.e1–7. https://doi.org/10.1016/j.ajog.2019.06.047.
58. Rayburn WF, Lavin JP, Miodovnik M, Varner MW. Multiple gestation: time interval between delivery of the first and second twins. Obstet Gynecol. 1984;63(4):502–6.
59. Bartnicki J, Meyenburg M, Saling E. Time interval in twin delivery – the second twin need not always be born shortly after the first. Gynecol Obstet Investig. 1992;33(1):19–20. https://doi.org/10.1159/000294840.
60. Poeschmann PP, van Oppen CAC, Bruinse HW. Delayed interval delivery in multiple pregnancies: report of three cases and review of the literature. Obstet Gynecol Surv. 1992;47(3):139–47. https://doi.org/10.1097/00006254-199203000-00001.
61. Smith GCS, Shah I, White IR, Pell JP, Dobbie R. Mode of delivery and the risk of delivery-related perinatal death among twins at term: a retrospective cohort study of 8073 births. BJOG. 2005;112(8):1139–44. https://doi.org/10.1111/j.1471-0528.2005.00631.x.
62. Schneuber S, Magnet E, Haas J, et al. Twin-to-twin delivery time: neonatal outcome of the second twin. Twin Res Hum Genet. 2011;14(6):573–9. https://doi.org/10.1375/twin.14.6.573.
63. Cukierman R, Heland S, Palmer K, Neil P, da Silva Costa F, Rolnik DL. Inter-twin delivery interval, short-term perinatal outcomes and risk of caesarean for the second twin. Aust N Z J Obstet Gynaecol. 2019;59(3):375–9. https://doi.org/10.1111/ajo.12867.
64. Benito M, De Bonrostro C, Agustín A, Roca M, Campillos JM, Castán S. Impact of intertwin interval on short-term neonatal outcomes of the second twin in dichorionic pregnancies with vaginal

delivery. Int J Gynecol Obstet. 2019;145(2):193–8. https://doi.org/10.1002/ijgo.12790.
65. Leung TY, Lok IH, Tam WH, Leung TN, Lau TK. Deterioration in cord blood gas status during the second stage of labour is more rapid in the second twin than in the first twin. BJOG. 2004;111(6):546–9. https://doi.org/10.1111/j.1471--0528.2004.00133.x.
66. Tal A, Peretz H, Garmi G, Zafran N, Romano S, Salim R. Effect of inter-twin delivery interval on umbilical artery pH and Apgar score in the second twin. Birth. 2018;45(1):37–42. https://doi.org/10.1111/birt.12317.
67. Nissen ED. Twins: collision, impaction, compaction, and interlocking. Obstet Gynecol. 1958;11(5):514–26. http://www.ncbi.nlm.nih.gov/pubmed/13553155. Accessed 16 Nov 2019.
68. Rydhström H, Cullberg G. Pregnancies with growth-retarded twins in breech-vertex presentation at increased risk for entanglement during delivery. J Perinat Med. 1990;18(1):45–50. https://doi.org/10.1515/jpme.1990.18.1.45.
69. Khunda S. Locked twins. Obstet Gynecol. 1972;39(3):453–9. http://www.ncbi.nlm.nih.gov/pubmed/5019321. Accessed 16 Nov 2019.
70. Blickstein I, Goldman RD, Kupferminc M. Delivery of breech first twins: a multicenter retrospective study. Obstet Gynecol. 2000;95(1):37–42. https://doi.org/10.1016/S0029-7844(99)00474-3.
71. Bisschop CNS, Vogelvang TE, May AM, Schuitemaker NWE. Mode of delivery in noncephalic presenting twins: a systematic review. Arch Gynecol Obstet. 2012;286(1):237–47. https://doi.org/10.1007/s00404-012-2294-6.
72. Barrett J, Blocking A. Management of twin pregnancies (part I). J SOGC. 2000;22(7):519–29. https://doi.org/10.1016/s0849-5831(16)30135-5.
73. Sung J-H, Kim SH, Kim Y-M, et al. Neonatal outcomes of twin pregnancies delivered at late-preterm versus term gestation based on chorionicity and indication for delivery. J Perinat Med. 2016;44(8):903–11. https://doi.org/10.1515/jpm-2015-0401.
74. Hack KEA, Derks JB, Elias SG, et al. Increased perinatal mortality and morbidity in monochorionic versus dichorionic twin pregnancies: clinical implications of a large Dutch cohort study. BJOG. 2008;115(1):58–67. https://doi.org/10.1111/j.1471--0528.2007.01556.x.
75. Hjortø S, Nickelsen C, Petersen J, Secher NJ. The effect of chorionicity and twin-to-twin delivery time interval on short-term outcome of the second twin. J Matern Fetal Neonatal Med. 2014;27(1):42–7. https://doi.org/10.3109/14767058.2013.799657.
76. Armson BA, O'Connell C, Persad V, Joseph KS, Young DC, Baskett TF. Determinants of perinatal mortality and serious neonatal morbidity in the second twin. Obstet Gynecol. 2006;108(3 Pt 1):556–64. https://doi.org/10.1097/01.AOG.0000227747.37184.0a.
77. Garabedian C, Poulain C, Duhamel A, Subtil D, Houfflin-Debarge V, Deruelle P. Intrapartum management of twin pregnancies: are uncomplicated monochorionic pregnancies more at risk of complications than dichorionic pregnancies? Acta Obstet Gynecol Scand. 2015;94(3):301–7. https://doi.org/10.1111/aogs.12558.
78. Yamashita A, Ishii K, Taguchi T, et al. Adverse perinatal outcomes related to the delivery mode in women with monochorionic diamniotic twin pregnancies. J Perinat Med. 2014;42(6):769–75. https://doi.org/10.1515/jpm-2014-0072.
79. Oldenburg A, Rode L, Bødker B, et al. Influence of chorionicity on perinatal outcome in a large cohort of Danish twin pregnancies. Ultrasound Obstet Gynecol. 2012;39(1):69–74. https://doi.org/10.1002/uog.10057.
80. Sau A, Chalmers S, Shennan A, Fox G, Maxwell D. Short communication: vaginal delivery can be considered in monochorionic diamniotic twins. BJOG. 2006;113(5):602–4. https://doi.org/10.1111/j.1471-0528.2006.00887.x.
81. Aviram A, Lipworth H, Asztalos EV, et al. Delivery of monochorionic twins – lessons learned from the twin birth study, a randomized, controlled, prospective study (unpublished data). Toronto; 2019.
82. Bergenhenegouwen LA, Meertens LJE, Schaaf J, et al. Vaginal delivery versus caesarean section in preterm breech delivery: a systematic review. Eur J Obstet Gynecol Reprod Biol. 2014;172(1):1–6. https://doi.org/10.1016/j.ejogrb.2013.10.017.
83. Tucker Edmonds B, McKenzie F, Macheras M, Srinivas SK, Lorch SA. Morbidity and mortality associated with mode of delivery for breech periviable deliveries. Am J Obstet Gynecol. 2015;213:70.e1–12. https://doi.org/10.1016/j.ajog.2015.03.002.
84. Kayem G, Combaud V, Lorthe E, et al. Mortality and morbidity in early preterm breech singletons: impact of a policy of planned vaginal delivery. Eur J Obstet Gynecol Reprod Biol. 2015;192:61–5. https://doi.org/10.1016/j.ejogrb.2015.06.019.
85. Herbst A, Källén K. Influence of mode of delivery on neonatal mortality in the second twin, at and before term. BJOG. 2008;115(12):1512–7. https://doi.org/10.1111/j.1471-0528.2008.01899.x.
86. Sentilhes L, Oppenheimer A, Bouhours AC, et al. Neonatal outcome of very preterm twins: policy of planned vaginal or cesarean delivery. Am J Obstet Gynecol. 2015;213(1):73.e1–7. https://doi.org/10.1016/j.ajog.2015.02.020.
87. Sentilhes L, Lorthe E, Marchand-Martin L, et al. Planned mode of delivery of preterm twins and neonatal and 2-year outcomes. Obstet Gynecol. 2019;133(1):71–80. https://doi.org/10.1097/AOG.0000000000003004.
88. Dagenais C, Lewis-Mikhael AM, Grabovac M, Mukerji A, McDonald SD. What is the safest mode of delivery for extremely preterm cephalic/non-cephalic twin pairs? A systematic review and meta-analyses. BMC Pregnancy Childbirth.

2017;17(1):397. https://doi.org/10.1186/s12884-017-1554-7.
89. Grabovac M, Karim JN, Isayama T, Liyanage SK, McDonald SD. What is the safest mode of birth for extremely preterm breech singleton infants who are actively resuscitated? A systematic review and meta-analyses. BJOG. 2018;125(6):652–63. https://doi.org/10.1111/1471-0528.14938.
90. Cahill A, Stamilio DM, Paré E, et al. Vaginal birth after cesarean (VBAC) attempt in twin pregnancies: is it safe? Am J Obstet Gynecol. 2005;193:1050–5. https://doi.org/10.1016/j.ajog.2005.06.038.
91. Shinar S, Agrawal S, Hasan H, Berger H. Trial of labor versus elective repeat cesarean delivery in twin pregnancies after a previous cesarean delivery – a systematic review and meta-analysis. Birth. 2019;46(4):550–9. https://doi.org/10.1111/birt.12434.
92. Kabiri D, Masarwy R, Schachter-Safrai N, et al. Trial of labor after cesarean delivery in twin gestations: systematic review and meta-analysis. Am J Obstet Gynecol. 2019;220(4):336–47. https://doi.org/10.1016/j.ajog.2018.11.125.
93. Alamia VJ, Royek AB, Jaekle RK, Meyer BA. Preliminary experience with a prospective protocol for planned vaginal delivery of triplet gestations. Am J Obstet Gynecol. 1998;179. Mosby Inc.:1133–5. https://doi.org/10.1016/s0002-9378(98)70119-x.
94. Grobman WA, Peaceman AM, Haney EI, Silver RK, MacGregor SN. Neonatal outcomes in triplet gestations after a trial of labor. Am J Obstet Gynecol. 1998;179(4):942–5. https://doi.org/10.1016/s0002-9378(98)70193-0.
95. Alran S, Sibony O, Luton D, et al. Maternal and neonatal outcome of 93 consecutive triplet pregnancies with 71% vaginal delivery. Acta Obstet Gynecol Scand. 2004;83(6):554–9. https://doi.org/10.1111/j.0001-6349.2004.00516.x.
96. Lappen JR, Hackney DN, Bailit JL. Maternal and neonatal outcomes of attempted vaginal compared with planned cesarean delivery in triplet gestations. Am J Obstet Gynecol. 2016;215. Mosby Inc.:493.e1–6. https://doi.org/10.1016/j.ajog.2016.04.054.

Key Reading

Aviram A, Lipworth H, Asztalos EV, et al. The worst of both worlds – combined deliveries in twin gestations: a subanalysis of the Twin Birth Study, a randomized, controlled, prospective study. Am J Obstet Gynecol. 2019;221(4):353.e1–7.

Barrett JFR, Hannah ME, Hutton EK, et al. A randomized trial of planned cesarean or vaginal delivery for twin pregnancy. N Engl J Med. 2013;369(14):1295–305.

Breathnach FM, McAuliffe FM, Geary M, et al. Optimum timing for planned delivery of uncomplicated monochorionic and dichorionic twin pregnancies. Obstet Gynecol. 2012;119(1):50–9. https://doi.org/10.1097/AOG.0b013e31823d7b06.

Chauhan SP, Roberts WE, McLaren RA, Roach H, Morrison JC, Martin JN. Delivery of the nonvortex second twin: breech extraction versus external cephalic version. Am J Obstet Gynecol. 1995;173(4):1015–20.

Dodd JM, Deussen AR, Grivell RM, Crowther CA. Elective birth at 37 weeks' gestation for women with an uncomplicated twin pregnancy. Cochrane Database Syst Rev. 2014;2014(2):CD003582.

Hack KEA, Derks JB, Elias SG, et al. Increased perinatal mortality and morbidity in monochorionic versus dichorionic twin pregnancies: clinical implications of a large Dutch cohort study. BJOG. 2008;115(1):58–67.

Kabiri D, Masarwy R, Schachter-Safrai N, et al. Trial of labor after cesarean delivery in twin gestations: systematic review and meta-analysis. Am J Obstet Gynecol. 2019;220(4):336–47.

Rossi AC, Mullin PM, Chmait RH. Neonatal outcomes of twins according to birth order, presentation and mode of delivery: a systematic review and meta-analysis. BJOG. 2011;118(5):523–32.

Sentilhes L, Oppenheimer A, Bouhours AC, et al. Neonatal outcome of very preterm twins: policy of planned vaginal or cesarean delivery. Am J Obstet Gynecol. 2015;213(1):73.e1–7.

Van Mieghem T, De Heus R, Lewi L, et al. Prenatal management of monoamniotic twin pregnancies. Obstet Gynecol. 2014;124(3):498–506.

Analgesia and Anaesthetic Considerations for Twins and Higher-Order Pregnancies

M. A. Clayton, R. L. May, and D. N. Lucas

Contents

A. Khalil et al. (eds.), *Twin and Higher-order Pregnancies*,
https://doi.org/10.1007/978-3-030-47652-6_22

Trailer

Women presenting with twins and higher-order pregnancy are a high-risk group for peripartum complications, including the need for operative delivery. Anaesthetic support is likely to be required to provide analgesia and anaesthesia to these women. The anaesthetic team should be involved in the multidisciplinary team caring for these patients during the antenatal, peripartum, and postpartum periods. The physiological changes of pregnancy are exaggerated in multiple pregnancy. This chapter describes the implications this has for the safe and effective provision of anaesthesia and anaesthetic strategies for the delivery of twins and higher-order pregnancy.

Definitions

Obstetric team – comprises the obstetrician, anaesthetist, and the midwife.

Neuraxial anaesthesia – spinal/epidural/combined-spinal-epidural anaesthesia.

Learning Objectives

- Understand the implications of the physiological changes associated with multiple pregnancy for the provision of anaesthesia and analgesia for these patients
- Understand that multiple pregnancy is a high-risk condition, and is best managed with early multidisciplinary team input

22.1 Introduction

Since 1980 and the start of assisted reproductive technologies, the birth rate for twins and higher-order multiples have risen significantly in high-income countries. The world's first set of twins conceived using in vitro fertilisation were born in Australia in 1981. In the United States, the birth rate for twins has risen from 18.9 per 1000 live births in 1980 to 32.6 per 1000 live births in 2018 [1]. In the United Kingdom, about 1 in every 65 births today are twins, triplets or more, representing a significant increase from 1984 when 1 in every 100 births was multiple births [2].

Twins and higher-order pregnancy are at high risk of caesarean section and pre-term delivery and also maternal complications such as post-partum haemorrhage and pre-eclampsia. Compared to a singleton pregnancy, there is an increased likelihood of obstetric intervention and anaesthesia being required.

The principle anaesthetic considerations for twins and multiple births are as follows:

- Management of the exaggerated physiological adaptation to pregnancy.
- The increased likelihood of the development of obstetric complications.
- The increased likelihood of obstetric intervention being required at delivery.

22.2 Physiological Adaptation to Pregnancy with Twins and Higher-Order Pregnancy

During pregnancy, anatomical and physiological changes occur to meet the metabolic demands of the mother and fetus. Oxygen consumption increases during pregnancy as a result of increased demands of the fetus, placenta, and uterine muscle (two-thirds of total consumption) and also due to the increased oxygen requirements of the maternal myocardium, kidneys, and respiratory muscles (one-third of total consumption) [3]. Oxygen requirements and concomitant carbon dioxide production can rise by as much as 60% [4]. The increased maternal and fetal demands for oxygen are higher in twin pregnancies. Oxygen consumption is greater in women with twins and higher-order pregnancy compared with singleton gestations [5]. During a singleton pregnancy, there is a decrease in the functional residual capacity (FRC) as a result of the expansion of the gravid uterus and movement of the diaphragm in a cephalad direction [6]. There can be as much as a 20% decrease in the FRC in the upright position and up to 30% decrease in the supine position. There is also a fall in the expiratory reserve volume with a corresponding rise in inspiratory volume. Pregnancy is also associated with an increase in minute ventilation; this occurs predominantly due to an increased tidal volume as there is a minimal change in respiratory rate. The arterial partial pressure of carbon dioxide falls, with an average PaCO2 of 4 kPa at term.

It might be assumed that the increased size of the uterus in twin and higher-order pregnancies would lead to even greater diaphragmatic displacement and thoracic wall changes than singleton pregnancy with an even more significant impact on static lung volumes and other respiratory parameters. However, there is limited evidence to support this assumption. A cross-sectional study of respiratory function looked at a range of respiratory indices, including FRC and expiratory reserve volume (ERV), in women with twin and singleton pregnancies and compared the results with non-pregnant women [7]. There were differences observed between pregnant women (twin and singleton pregnancies) and non-pregnant women in the mean FRC and ERV of women measured in the third trimester. There were also differences observed between pregnant (singleton and twin pregnancies) and non-pregnant women in minute ventilation measures in all three trimesters. However, there were no significant differences demonstrated in respiratory function between healthy women with twin compared to singleton pregnancies.

Nevertheless, the combined effects of an increase in oxygen consumption and decreased FRC would suggest that a woman pregnant with twins/higher-order multiples would be particularly vulnerable to developing hypoxaemia during episodes of apnoea, even with careful pre-oxygenation. Increased minute ventilation and a reduced FRC facilitate gas exchange at the alveoli leading to an increased rate of uptake of volatile anaesthetic agents and more rapid changes in depth of anaesthesia. When a pregnant woman requires mechanical ventilation, it is important to be aware that excessive hyperventilation can lead to severe alkalosis and a left shift of the oxygen dissociation curve resulting in reduced oxygen transfer to the fetus.

Other anatomical changes in the respiratory system that can have an impact on anaesthesia include the effect of capillary engorgement on the nasopharyngeal and oropharyngeal tissue – leading to swelling and increased friability of the tissues. The glottic opening can be reduced in size, and it is recommended that size 7.0 and smaller endotracheal tubes are used for intubation in any pregnant woman [8].

The cardiovascular system undergoes significant adaptation during a healthy singleton pregnancy. Stroke volume increases secondary to an increase in both end-diastolic volume and ventricular muscle wall mass, and this combined with an increased heart rate, leads to an increase in cardiac output. Cardiac output can increase by as much as 50% with most of this increase occurring by 24 weeks gestation [3]. In twins and higher multiple gestations, as a result of the increased fetal mass and maternal weight gain, maternal cardiac function undergoes even more dramatic changes. Cardiac output in a twin pregnancy is 15% higher than that of a singleton pregnancy; a larger increase in left atrial diameter is seen, consistent with volume overload [9]. Cross-sectional and longitudinal studies utilising echocardiography in women with twin pregnancies have identified evidence of increased cardiovascular parameters, including left ventricular end-diastolic and end-systolic dimensions, left ventricular mass, and ejection fraction [10].

Women with twin pregnancies are more vulnerable to aortocaval compression (or supine hypotensive syndrome). This typically occurs after 20 weeks gestation, although it can be earlier in twin pregnancy when a woman is lying supine [11]. The gravid uterus can cause compression of the inferior vena cava and, to a lesser extent, the aorta, with reduced blood flow back to the maternal heart. The resultant drop in venous return decreases cardiac output leading to maternal hypotension. Symptoms such as pallor, sweating, nausea, and vomiting can occur, and in severe cases, profound maternal hypotension, loss of consciousness, cardiovascular collapse, and fetal depression [12]. Due to the increased morbidity and mortality to mother and baby, the obstetric team must be aware and recognize this as a potential cause of hypotension in the pregnant patient. If it is suspected, manoeuvres to correct it must be immediately undertaken, including moving the woman to the full left lateral position.

In a woman with a singleton pregnancy, plasma volume can increase by as much as 45%, while the increase in red blood cell mass is only 20% resulting in a dilutional physiological anaemia of pregnancy [13]. In twin and higher-order pregnancy, there is an even greater increase in plasma volume. Alongside this, women with twin pregnancies are at high risk of iron deficiency because of maternal, fetal, and placental demands. Therefore, women with twin pregnancy have an even greater vulnerability to developing anaemia. One study identified a prevalence of anaemia in 45% of women with twins or higher-order pregnancies during the third trimester. This was four times higher than the expected national prevalence reported for women who were carrying singletons [14].

22.3 Obstetric Complications and Implications for Anaesthesia

Obstetric complications (maternal and fetal) of twins are discussed and are summarised in ▶ Box 22.1.

Twin pregnancies are at higher risk of pre-term delivery; 50% of twin pregnancies deliver before 37 weeks, and 10% deliver before 32 weeks of gestation [15]. Surgical intervention such as cervical cerclage can reduce preterm birth rates in singleton pregnancy but have shown mixed results in twins; a systematic review and meta-analysis of cerclage placement was beneficial for the reduction of preterm birth and the prolongation of pregnancy in twin pregnancies with a cervical length of <15 mm or dilated cervix of >10 mm, but the benefit of cerclage based on history alone was less certain in twin pregnancies with normal cervical length [16]. Anaesthesia may be required to support surgical interventions such as cerclage during twin pregnancy. There are no prospective or large retrospective studies comparing regional or general anaesthesia for cervical cerclage, and both techniques have been used safely [17].

If preterm labour occurs, tocolytic therapy may be initiated or magnesium sulphate for neuroprotection. These pharmacologic agents can interact with anaesthesia and can increase the risk of post-partum haemorrhage.

Twin to twin transfusion syndrome is a complication of multiple gestations in which arteriovenous vascular communications occur in a monochorionic placenta. This leads to an imbalance of blood flow between the developing fetuses, where one fetus becomes the 'donor', and the other becomes the 'recipient'. The recipient fetus can develop polycythaemia, polyhydramnios, and hydrops fetalis, while the donor can develop oligohydramnios and anaemia. Twin to twin transfusion syndrome is associated with high fetal mortality if it develops before 26 weeks of gestation. Mortality can be reduced with selective laser photocoagulation of communicating vessels to the vascular anastomoses between the twins. Regional or local anaesthesia is preferred, but the use of general anaesthesia has also been described [18].

There is an increased incidence of maternal morbidity and mortality in multiple gestation pregnancies. A population-based cohort study from The Netherlands calculated the rate of severe acute maternal morbidity in multiple pregnancies and examined a range of possible risk indicators. The overall incidence of severe acute maternal morbidity was 7.0 per 1000 deliveries and 6.5 and 28.0 per 1000 for singletons and multiple pregnancies, respectively [19]. Risk indicators for developing severe acute maternal morbidity in women with multiple pregnancies were age greater than 40 years, nulliparity, and use of assisted reproductive techniques. These findings have been confirmed by another large population-based study. Compared to women with singleton pregnancies, women with twin pregnancies had a fourfold increased risk for severe maternal complications, both before and after delivery [20]. The authors estimated that 20% of the association between twin pregnancy and intrapartum or post-partum severe acute maternal morbidity was mediated by caesarean delivery. Triplet and quadruplet pregnancies have significantly higher risks than twin pregnancies for most maternal and neonatal complications [21].

Box 22.1 Complications of Twin or Higher-Order Pregnancy

Maternal	Fetal
Preterm labour/delivery Preeclampsia Gestational diabetes Placental abruption Instrumental delivery/caesarean section Post-partum haemorrhage	Placental abruption Fetal demise/loss Low birth weight Intrauterine growth restriction Congenital anomalies Cord entanglement Twin to twin transfusion syndrome Malpresentation

Twin pregnancy is a risk factor of post-partum haemorrhage (PPH), primarily as a result of uterine overdistension leading to uterine atony. Significant maternal and peripartum factors for PPH and transfusion in twin pregnancy include nulliparity, pregestational or gestational diabetes, intrapartum magnesium sulphate, a haematocrit <30%, admission platelets <100,000/μL and administration of general anaesthesia, higher gestational age at ≥41 weeks, and hypertensive disorders of pregnancy [22]. Women with twin pregnancies are at increased risk of pre-eclampsia compared to singleton pregnancies [23]. A population-based study estimated that the risk of pre-eclampsia in twin pregnancies was three- to fourfold that of singleton pregnancies, regardless of maternal age, parity, smoking, maternal comorbidity, or in vitro fertilisation. This study found that the risk of gestational hypertension was not increased in women with twin pregnancies after adjustment for the main risk factors [24].

22.4 Anaesthesia for Twin Deliveries

The mode of delivery is discussed.

22.4.1 Labour Analgesia

Epidural analgesia (whether initiated with a combined spinal epidural or epidural alone) offers clear advantages to a labouring woman: it causes minimal depression to the fetus in the event of preterm labour, it can facilitate intrapartum monitoring of the fetus, and it can be rapidly extended to provide anaesthesia in the event of operative delivery being required or when internal podalic version is required for a second twin. The National Institute for Health and Care Excellence (NICE) [25] and the American College of Obstetricians and Gynaecologists (ACOG) [26] both recommend that it should be offered to women planning vaginal delivery. One consideration in the provision of neuraxial analgesia in twin or higher-order pregnancy is the risk of thrombocytopenia. Thrombocytopenia occurs more commonly in twin and higher-order pregnancies. A retrospective analysis of platelet counts in over 7000 women who delivered at a large US medical centre was compared with platelet counts of non-pregnant women, singleton and multiple pregnancies were included [27]. Women with twin pregnancy had lower platelet counts in all three trimesters and at the time of delivery than the women who had uncomplicated singleton pregnancies, but the difference at the time of delivery was not significant. There are limited data about triplet pregnancies; one study that analysed platelet counts in twin and triplet pregnancies found that 43% of women with triplet pregnancy had a platelet count of less than 100 × 10/9/L compared to 4.3% of women with twin pregnancy [28]. In the absence of documented thrombocytopenia and an otherwise healthy twin pregnancy, it is not mandatory to check either the platelet count or clotting profile before siting neuraxial anaesthesia. For triplets and higher-order pregnancy, it would seem be prudent to check the platelet count before undertaking neuraxial anaesthesia, although in the emergency setting, the balance of risks versus benefits would likely support the provision of neuraxial anaesthesia.

Low-dose solutions of local anaesthetic combined with an opioid are preferred for maintenance of labour epidural analgesia. Particular care must be taken when establishing labour epidural analgesia to avoid aortocaval compression. Labour epidurals must be actively reviewed to ensure that they are effective and therefore more likely to be successfully converted to provide anaesthesia in the event of operative delivery being required for one or both twins. A well-established risk factor for failure to convert labour epidural analgesia to anaesthesia is an increased number of bolus 'top-ups' administered during labour [29]. Where any concern exists about the quality of labour analgesia, there should be early consideration of re-siting the epidural.

22.4.2 Anaesthesia for Caesarean Section

Spinal anaesthesia (alone as 'single-shot' or as part of a combined spinal-epidural) is the preferred anaesthetic technique for caesarean section. Spinal anaesthesia-induced maternal hypotension can occur in up to three-quarters of women in the absence of prophylactic measures, causing maternal nausea and vomiting and impaired uteroplacental perfusion leading to fetal acidaemia. Although women with twins or higher-order pregnancies may be particularly vulnerable to aortocaval compression which can excavate spinal hypotension, it has been demonstrated that patients with twin pregnancy do not exhibit greater haemodynamic instability during spinal anaesthesia for caesarean section compared to those with a singleton pregnancy [30]. There are very little data to guide anaesthetic management for caesarean section in triplet pregnancy. A retrospective case series evaluated the effects of regional anaesthetic techniques for caesarean section in triplet pregnancies on maternal and neonatal outcome [31]. Ninety-six women with triplet pregnancies were delivered by caesarean section, of which 91 received regional anaesthesia. The authors found a statistically significant decrease in systolic blood pressure was demonstrated immediately after the induction of spinal as compared to epidural anaesthesia. The total volume of crystalloid solution and the cumulative dose of ephedrine were significantly larger in the spinal group than the epidural group. The authors commented that the decrease in systolic blood pressure remained within the physiological range and did not seem to be clinically significant. It is important to highlight that this series was undertaken before the era of the ubiquitous use of alpha-agonist drugs in the management of spinal hypotension. Careful attention to uterine displacement with left lateral tilt and the use of prophylactic vasopressors can obviate the risk of hypotension. Alpha-agonist drugs are the most appropriate agents to treat or prevent hypotension following spinal anaesthesia. An international consensus statement on the management of hypotension during caesarean section under spinal anaesthesia was published in 2017 and recommended phenylephrine given via infusion [32]. Fluid co-loading should be used in addition to vasopressors [33].

Multiple pregnancy can result in decreased lumbosacral cerebrospinal fluid volume. This is thought to be due to venous engorgement secondary to vena cava compression, shrinking the subarachnoid space. It has been suggested that dose reduction of local anaesthetic for spinal anaesthesia in women with twins or higher-order pregnancy would be appropriate, to minimise the risk of high neuraxial block. Jawan et al. demonstrated that women with multiple pregnancy had a more rapid onset and a greater cephalospread of local anaesthetic than women with singleton pregnancy [34]. However, Ngan Kee did not reach the same conclusion, finding similar vasopressor requirements and haemodynamic and neonatal outcomes between twin and singleton caesarean section [30]. Additionally, Behfouraz et al. also found similar local anaesthetic requirements for epidural anaesthesia for elective caesarean section in higher-order (triplets and quadruplets) pregnancies compared to singleton pregnancies [35]. Any difference with height of neuraxial block in women with twins or higher-order pregnancies is unlikely to be of clinical significance. The decision to reduce the dose of local anaesthetic has to be carefully balanced against the risk of inadequate block necessitating a second neuraxial technique or even general anaesthesia, both of which arguably carry increased risk. Where genuine concerns exist, a combined spinal-epidural technique that enables a smaller spinal dose to be used with an epidural top-up if required may be appropriate; however, most authorities would advocate standard spinal dosing.

The provision of general anaesthesia to a woman with a twin or higher-order pregnancy follows the same principles as for any pregnant woman. The principle concerns are around the management of the obstetric airway: minimising both the risk of aspiration of gastric contents and the development of hypoxaemia, and the potential for difficult or failed tracheal intubation. The Obstetric Anaesthetists' Association and Difficult Airway Society guidelines (OAA/DAS) for the management of difficult and failed tracheal intubation in obstetrics provide three algorithms to support safe airway management. The first algorithm details how to provide safe general anaesthesia, emphasising preparation and team planning. The second algorithm describes management once a failed intubation has been declared. The third algorithm deals with the management of a 'can't intubate can't oxygenate' situation. This algorithm emphasises that oxygenation rather than intubation is now the priority.

An significant recent advance in airway management in anaesthesia has been the advent of videolaryngoscopy [36]. The role of videolaryngoscopy in obstetric general anaesthesia has been subject to less scrutiny than in other areas of anaesthesia, likely because of the difficulties of research in this group of patients; smaller overall numbers of general anaesthetics are given, and most occur in the extreme urgency of the Category 1 caesarean section. There are a small but growing number of studies and case reports that do support the use of videolaryngoscopy in obstetrics. These, and extrapolation from the non-obstetric population suggest that videolaryngoscopy is becoming an essential tool for obstetric anaesthetists [37].

The OAA/DAS guidelines for the management of difficult and failed tracheal intubation in obstetrics recommend that videolaryngoscopy should be immediately available for all general obstetric anaesthetics.

It is standard practice for the anaesthetist to administer a uterotonic after delivery at caesarean section. Care should be taken to ensure that this is not given before BOTH babies are delivered. Uterotonic agents given accidentally before delivery can have catastrophic consequences for the neonate. A UK survey of drug errors in obstetric anaesthesia reported cases where oxytocin had inadvertently been administered before delivery [38].

22.5 Anaesthetic Planning for Twin and Higher-Order Pregnancy

In the UK, NICE recommends that birth plans and wishes should be discussed with the mother from 24 weeks onwards in multiple pregnancy, given the increased likelihood of premature delivery [25]. Similarly, analgesia during labour or caesarean section should be addressed by 28 weeks at the latest. The anaesthetic team should be aware at an early stage of any woman with a multiple pregnancy presenting to labour ward, with early discussions between the mother, the anaesthetist, and the obstetrician regarding labour analgesia and delivery options.

There is no consensus over where vaginal delivery should occur – in the labour room or the operating theatre. Neither NICE nor ACOG make specific recommendations. FIGO recommends that delivery should occur in a setting where there is immediate recourse to operative delivery if necessary [39]. The question of whether the anaesthetist should attend all vaginal twin deliveries remains [40]. A survey of practice in California highlighted the lack of consensus regarding the appropriate location for vaginal twin deliveries and the role of the anaesthetist [41]. Two-thirds of responders reported that vaginal twin deliveries were performed in the operating theatre and 55% that an anaesthetist was present. Practice should be dictated by local guidelines and individualised risk assessment, considering the potential for complications arising with delivery of the babies and the risk of immediate complications such as postpartum haemorrhage.

22.5.1 Review Questions

1. What are the main physiological changes in twin and higher-order pregnancies of direct relevance to anaesthesia?

2. Describe a strategy for neuraxial anaesthesia for caesarean section in twin and higher-order pregnancies.

3. Describe the principles of safe general anaesthesia for caesarean section in a twin or higher-order pregnancy.

22.5.2 Multiple-Choice Questions

1. Anatomical and physiological changes in higher-order pregnancies include:
   (a) An increased functional residual capacity and a decreased expiratory reserve volume
   (b) Increased minute ventilation mostly explained by increased tidal volume
   (c) An increase in cardiac output 15% higher than with a singleton pregnancy
   (d) An increase in lumbosacral CSF volume
   (e) Dilutional anaemia more pronounced than in singleton pregnancies

FTTFT

2. In multiple pregnancy:
   (a) Supine hypotensive syndrome can present from 24 weeks gestation
   (b) Tocolytic therapy reduces the risk of post-partum haemorrhage
   (c) General anaesthesia is the preferred anaesthetic technique when laser photocoagulation therapy for twin to twin transfusion syndrome is required
   (d) The risk of serious complications in pregnancy and labour is at least twice that of singleton pregnancies
   (e) There is a lower risk of preeclampsia compared to singleton pregnancies

FFFTF

3. Risk factors for postpartum haemorrhage include:
   (a) Multiparity
   (b) Intrapartum magnesium
   (c) Regional anaesthesia
   (d) Haematocrit <30%
   (e) Preeclampsia

TTFTT

4. When providing anaesthesia for operative delivery in multiple order pregnancies:
   (a) Spinal dose should always be reduced because of the risk of a high spinal
   (b) Co-loading with fluids is only required if the mother is hypotensive before administration of anaesthesia
   (c) Phenylephrine is the recommended first-line vasopressor and should be used prophylactically with spinal anaesthesia
   (d) Uterotonics should be administered after delivery of the first twin
   (e) Clotting profile and platelet count should always be checked before administration of neuraxial anaesthesia

FFTFF

5. When providing general anaesthesia for caesarean section for multiple pregnancy
   (a) Rapid changes in depth of anaesthesia occur in a spontaneously ventilating parturient due to a reduced FRC and increased minute ventilation
   (b) Hypoventilation can cause alkalosis, a left shift of the oxygen dissociation curve, and impaired oxygen delivery to the fetus
   (c) Pre-oxygenation is more effective with high flow nasal oxygen than with a standard facemask
   (d) Multiple pregnancy is an independent risk factor for difficult intubation

(e) Videolaryngoscopy should be considered as an aid to facilitate intubation

TFFFT

6. When providing anaesthesia for preterm delivery in twin pregnancies
   (a) Spinal dose should be reduced proportional to the gestation of the fetuses
   (b) Epidural anaesthesia is contraindicated below 28 weeks gestation
   (c) Pre-oxygenation for general anaesthesia is not required below 28 weeks gestation
   (d) Magnesium sulphate may be considered for fetal neuroprotection
   (e) Nausea and vomiting is a late sign of aortocaval compression

FFFTF

7. Regarding twin pregnancy
   (a) Incidence has been rising rapidly in low-income countries whilst remaining relatively stable in high-income countries
   (b) A large diameter endotracheal tube (size 7.0 or above) should be used if intubation is required as the increased diaphragmatic splinting requires higher airway pressures
   (c) Left atrial dilation consistent with volume overload is typical
   (d) Supine parturients are at risk of aortocaval compression from 20 weeks gestation onwards
   (e) General anaesthesia is contraindicated for cervical cerclage

FFTFF

8. Risk factors for severe maternal morbidity in multiple pregnancy include:
   (a) Multiparity
   (b) Age greater than 30 years
   (c) Use of assisted reproductive technologies
   (d) Caesarean section
   (e) Diabetes

FFTTT

Patient Testimonials

When the doctors told me I would have to have a caesarean section at 32 weeks I was very upset and worried about my twins. It was very reassuring to have a spinal anaesthetic and be able to see my babies being born and cared for immediately by the neonatal doctors. I was able to see them before they went to neonatal unit which I wouldn't have been able to do if I had a general anaesthetic.

I didn't have an epidural with my first baby and didn't intend to with my next baby. I had to see the anaesthetist when I was 30 weeks pregnant. She explained why an epidural was a good idea as I was having twins. I'm glad I saw her early on, as it gave me time to think about it and speak to my partner. I did have an epidural when I was in labour (which was great), and my twins were both born normally.

References

1. Birth rate for twins in the United States from 1980 to 2018 (per 1,000 live birth). https://www.statista.com/statistics/276017/us-twin-birth-rate/.
2. https://www.nhs.uk/conditions/pregnancy-and-baby/what-causes-twins/
3. Sanghavi M, Rutherford JD. Cardiovascular physiology of pregnancy. Circulation. 2014;130(12):1003–8.
4. Head B, Ferguson J III, Ferguson J II. Cardiorespiratory physiology of pregnancy. Glob Libr Women's Med. 2008; https://doi.org/10.3843/GLOWM.10159.
5. Suzuki S, Shinagawa S, Chihara H, et al. Resting oxygen consumption in patients with twin pregnancy. Arch Gynecol Obstet. 2005;271(2):152–3.
6. Hegewald MJ, Crapo RO. Respiratory physiology in pregnancy. Clin Chest Med. 2011;32(1):1–13.

7. McAuliffe F, Kametas N, Costello J, Rafferty GF, Greenough A, Nicolaides K. Respiratory function in singleton and twin pregnancy. BJOG. 2002;109(7):765–9.
8. Knight M, Nair M, Tuffnell D, Shakespeare J, Kenyon S, Kurinczuk JJ, MBRRACE-UK, editors. Saving lives, improving mothers' care – lessons learned to inform maternity care from the UK and Ireland confidential enquiries into maternal deaths and morbidity 2013–15. Oxford: National Perinatal Epidemiology Unit, University of Oxford; 2017.
9. Hunter S, Robson SC. Adaptation of the maternal heart in pregnancy. Br Heart J. 1992;68:540–3.
10. Estensen ME, Beitnes JO, Grindheim G, et al. Altered maternal left ventricular contractility and function during normal pregnancy. Ultrasound Obstet Gynecol. 2013;41(6):659–66.
11. Kerr MG, Scott DB, Samuel E. Studies of the inferior vena cava in late pregnancy. Br Med J. 1964;1(5382):532–3.
12. Murphy CJ, McCaul CL, Thornton PC. Maternal collapse secondary to aortocaval compression. Int J Obstet Anesth. 2015;24(4):393–4.
13. de Haas S, Ghossein-Doha C, van Kuijk SM, van Drongelen J, Spaanderman ME. Physiological adaptation of maternal plasma volume during pregnancy: a systematic review and meta-analysis. Ultrasound Obstet Gynecol. 2017;49(2):177–87.
14. Ru Y, Pressman EK, Cooper EM, et al. Iron deficiency and anemia are prevalent in women with multiple gestations. Am J Clin Nutr. 2016;104(4):1052–60.
15. Murray SR, Stock SJ, Cowan S, Cooper ES, Norman JE. Spontaneous preterm birth prevention in multiple pregnancy. Obstet Gynaecol. 2018;20(1):57–63.
16. Li C, Shen J, Hua K. Cerclage for women with twin pregnancies: a systematic review and metaanalysis. Am J Obstet Gynecol. 2019;220(6):543–557.e1.
17. Ioscovich A, Popov A, Gimelfarb Y, et al. Anesthetic management of prophylactic cervical cerclage: a retrospective multicenter cohort study. Arch Gynecol Obstet. 2015;291(3):509–12.
18. Rossi AC, Kaufman MA, Bornick PW, Quintero RA. General vs local anesthesia for the percutaneous laser treatment of twin-twin transfusion syndrome. Am J Obstet Gynecol. 2008;199(2):137.e1–7.
19. Witteveen T, Van Den Akker T, Zwart JJ, Bloemenkamp KW, Van Roosmalen J. Severe acute maternal morbidity in multiple pregnancies: a nationwide cohort study. Am J Obstet Gynecol. 2016;214(5):641.e1–10.
20. Madar H, Goffinet F, Seco A, Rozenberg P, Dupont C, Deneux-Tharaux C. Severe acute maternal morbidity in twin compared with singleton pregnancies. Obstet Gynecol. 2019;133(6):1141–50.
21. Luke B, Brown MB. Maternal morbidity and infant death in twin vs triplet and quadruplet pregnancies. Am J Obstet Gynecol. 2008;198(4):401.e1–10.
22. Blitz MJ, Yukhayev A, Pachtman SL, Reisner J, Moses D, Sison CP, Greenberg M, Rochelson B. Twin pregnancy and risk of postpartum hemorrhage. J Matern Fetal Neonatal Med. 2020;33(22):3740–5.
23. Bartnik P, Kosinska-Kaczynska K, Kacperczyk J, et al. Twin chorionicity and the risk of hypertensive disorders: gestational hypertension and pre-eclampsia. Twin Res Hum Genet. 2016;19(4):377–82.
24. Laine K, Murzakanova G, Sole KB, et al. Prevalence and risk of pre-eclampsia and gestational hypertension in twin pregnancies: a population-based register study. BMJ Open. 2019;9:e029908.
25. National Institute for Health and Care Excellence. Twin and triplet pregnancy. London: NICE; 2019. Available from: https://www.nice.org.uk/guidance/ng137
26. Committee on Practice Bulletins—Obstetrics; Society for Maternal–Fetal Medicine. Practice Bulletin No. 169: Multifetal gestations: twin, triplet, and higher-order multifetal pregnancies. Obstet Gynecol. 2016;128(4):e131–46.
27. Reese JA, Peck JD, Deschamps DR, et al. Platelet counts during pregnancy. N Engl J Med. 2018;379(1):32–43.
28. Morikawa M, Yamada T, Kataoka S, et al. Changes in antithrombin activity and platelet counts in the late stage of twin and triplet pregnancies. Semin Thromb Hemost. 2005;31(3):290–6.
29. Bauer ME, Kountanis JA, Tsen LC, Greenfield ML, Mhyre JM. Risk factors for failed conversion of labor epidural analgesia to cesarean delivery anesthesia: a systematic review and meta-analysis of observational trials. Int J Obstet Anesth. 2012;21(4):294–309.
30. Ngan Kee WD, Khaw KS, Ng FF, Karmakar MK, Critchley LA, Gin T. A prospective comparison of vasopressor requirement and hemodynamic changes during spinal anesthesia for cesarean delivery in patients with multiple gestation versus singleton pregnancy. Anesth Analg. 2007;104(2):407–11.
31. Marino T, Goudas LC, Steinbok V, Craigo SD, Yarnell RW. The anesthetic management of triplet cesarean delivery: a retrospective case series of maternal outcomes. Anesth Analg. 2001;93(4):991–5.
32. Kinsella SM, Carvalho B, Dyer RA, et al. International consensus statement on the management of hypotension with vasopressors during caesarean section under spinal anaesthesia. Anaesthesia. 2018;73(1):71–92.
33. Fitzgerald JP, Fedoruk KA, Jadin SM, Carvalho B, Halpern SH. Prevention of hypotension after spinal anaesthesia for caesarean section: a systematic review and network meta-analysis of ran-

domised controlled trials. Anaesthesia. 2020;75(1): 109–21.
34. Jawan B, Lee JH, Chong ZK, Chang CS. Spread of spinal anaesthesia for caesarean section in singleton and twin pregnancies. Br J Anaesth. 1993;70(6):639–41.
35. Behforouz N, Dounas M, Benhamou D. Epidural anaesthesia for caesarean delivery in triple and quadruple pregnancies. Acta Anaesthesiol Scand. 1998;42:1088–91.
36. Scott-Brown S, Russell R. Video laryngoscopes and the obstetric airway. Int J Obstet Anesth. 2015;24(2):137–46.
37. Lucas DN, Vaughan DJA. Videolaryngoscopy and obstetric anaesthesia. Br J Anaesth. 2017;119(3):549.
38. Yentis SM, Randall K. Drug errors in obstetric anaesthesia: a national survey. Int J Obstet Anesth. 2003;12:246–9.
39. FIGO Working Group on Good Clinical Practice in Maternal-Fetal Medicine. Good clinical practice advice: management of twin pregnancy. Int J Gynaecol Obstet. 2019;144(3):330–7.
40. Tsen LC. The more the merrier: should anesthesiologists be present for multiple births? Int J Obstet Anesth. 2008;17(3):205–7.
41. Carvalho B, Saxena A, Butwick A, Macario A. Vaginal twin delivery: a survey and review of location, anesthesia coverage and interventions. Int J Obstet Anesth. 2008;17(3):212–6.

Key Reading

Bauer ME, Kountanis JA, Tsen LC, Greenfield ML, Mhyre JM. Risk factors for failed conversion of labor epidural analgesia to cesarean delivery anesthesia: a systematic review and meta-analysis of observational trials. Int J Obstet Anesth. 2012;21(4):294–309.

Kinsella SM, Carvalho B, Dyer RA, et al. International consensus statement on the management of hypotension with vasopressors during caesarean section under spinal anaesthesia. Anaesthesia. 2018;73(1):71–92.

National Institute for Health and Care Excellence. Twin and triplet pregnancy. London: NICE; 2019. Available from: https://www.nice.org.uk/guidance/ng137.

Maternal Complications in Multifetal Pregnancy

Paul Ian Ramler and Thomas van den Akker

Contents

A. Khalil et al. (eds.), *Twin and Higher-order Pregnancies*,
https://doi.org/10.1007/978-3-030-47652-6_23

Trailer

Although attention for fetal complications of multifetal pregnancies prevails in modern obstetric teaching and literature, it is a moral and medical imperative to also consider the health of the woman herself in clinical decision-making. Multifetal pregnancy poses her at increased risk of antepartum and peripartum complications compared to singleton pregnancies. It is important to be aware of such risks, and to, as much as possible, avoid iatrogenic multifetal pregnancies as well as medical procedures without medical indication, both of which may be harmful to the woman.

Definitions

Maternal mortality: Death of a woman while pregnant or within 42 days of termination of pregnancy, irrespective of the duration and site of the pregnancy, from any cause related to or aggravated by the pregnancy or its management but not from accidental or incidental causes [1].

Maternal near miss: Women who nearly died but survived a complication during pregnancy, childbirth, or within 42 days of termination of pregnancy [2].

Pregnancy-induced hypertension: Hypertension (systolic blood pressure ≥140 mmHg and/or diastolic blood pressure ≥90 mmHg) arising de novo after 20 weeks' gestation in absence of proteinuria and without biochemical or hematological abnormalities [3].

Preeclampsia: Presence of de novo hypertension after 20 weeks of gestation with proteinuria and/or acute kidney injury, liver dysfunction, neurological features, hemolysis or thrombocytopenia, and/or fetal growth restriction [3].

Eclampsia: Onset of convulsions in women with preeclampsia [3].

Postpartum hemorrhage: The World Health Organization defines postpartum hemorrhage as blood loss of 500 mL or more within 24 hours after birth [4]. However, many countries use their own definition. In the Netherlands, postpartum hemorrhage is defined as blood loss of at least 1000 mL within 24 hours after birth [5], while in the United Kingdom postpartum hemorrhages are divided into minor (500–1000 mL) and major (1000 mL or more) bleeds [6]. Major bleeds are subdivided into moderate (1001–2000 mL) and severe (more than 2000 mL) [6].

Peripartum (pregnancy-related) hysterectomy: Surgical removal of the uterus during pregnancy up to 42 days postpartum [7].

Learning Objectives

- Increase awareness of possible adverse maternal outcomes in multifetal pregnancy.
- Distinguish commoner milder complaints from more severe pathological conditions.

23.1 Background

In present-day obstetrics, much of the clinicians' time and attention are devoted to the wellbeing of the fetus, and perhaps even more so in multifetal pregnancies, where multiple fetuses are at risk of complications. It remains nonetheless a moral and medical imperative to also consider the impact of the multifetal pregnancy on the health of the woman herself. Pregnancy-related physiological changes and altered anatomical relationships involving almost every organ system of the body occur in women with multifetal pregnancies to an even larger extent. Multifetal pregnancy generally places the woman at a significantly increased risk of antepartum and peripartum complications.

Considering possible negative impact on the health of the woman with a multifetal pregnancy should also inform fertility treatment, during which iatrogenic multifetal pregnancies should be avoided as much as possible. The health of the woman with a multifetal pregnancy must also be addressed early during antenatal care, and appropriate follow-up of possible maternal complications organized with the same attentiveness as that of fetal complications. Peripartum care including decisions related to mode of birth should strive to achieve optimal birth outcomes for the woman as much as her children. The third stage of labor requires particular attention in women with a multifetal pregnancy.

Better understanding of possible antepartum, intrapartum, and postpartum complications could help the managing clinician or midwife anticipate and mitigate the effects of multifetal pregnancies on maternal health. Engaging into a conversation with the pregnant woman and her partner about the importance of considering her own health throughout the pregnancy will help ensure that their perspectives are included in clinical decision-making and will contribute to the best possible pregnancy outcome.

23.2 Physiological Alterations and Maternal Complaints

Towards the end of the first trimester, when maternal serum concentrations of β-hCG peak highest, women with multifetal pregnancies may experience extreme nausea, vomiting, and dehydration requiring hospital admission more frequently compared to woman with a singleton pregnancy [8, 9].

Maternal blood volume increases even higher in twin compared to singleton pregnancies: 50 to 60 percent versus 40–50 percent [10]. While the increase in red blood cell volume is around 30 percent in both singleton and multifetal pregnancies, the expansion of plasma volume is significantly higher in women carrying twins compared to singleton pregnancies [10]. This plasma augmentation, combined with greater iron needs, predisposes to a higher incidence of anemia in multifetal pregnancies [11].

Furthermore, an increase in maternal blood volume modified by a decrease in vascular resistance due to elevated prostaglandin levels results in a 20-percent additional increase in maternal cardiac output in women carrying twins compared to singleton pregnancies [12, 13]. In addition, diastolic blood pressure at term increases more rapidly in women with a multifetal pregnancy [14, 15].

Accelerated uterine growth in a multifetal pregnancy, often resulting in a total uterine volume double that of a singleton pregnancy, may lead to the uterus compressing abdominal viscera and lungs, and to increased maternal discomfort and complaints of dyspnea [16].

23.3 Generally Milder Antepartum Maternal Morbidity with Possible Adverse Impact on the Fetus

Although not all studies confirm this finding, it appears that gestational diabetes is more common in multifetal pregnancies [17–24]. Diagnosis and management of gestational diabetes are similar to that in a singleton pregnancy. Gestational diabetes is associated with an increased risk of preeclampsia [25]. At the same time, it may be argued that women with gestational diabetes are sometimes unjustifiably labelled as “high risk,” which may lead to medical interventions, including cesarean section, being performed in these women without evidence-based indication [26]. The most important risks associated with gestational diabetes are fetal rather than maternal, and generally related to a higher incidence of macrosomia. The latter may result in adverse pregnancy outcome, including shoulder dystocia [27].

A similar risk pattern exists for intrahepatic cholestasis of pregnancy (ICP), a liver disease characterized by pruritus (often including the palms and soles) and increasing bile acids due to impaired release of bile from liver cells [28]. The prevalence of ICP is increased in twin pregnancies compared to singleton pregnancies [29–33] and appears to be even higher in higher-order gestations [34]. ICP occurs in the late second and/or third trimester and is associated with increased risk of stillbirth in singleton pregnancies with serum total bile acids above 100 μmol/L according to a meta-analysis [35]. Of note, the same study found no association between stillbirth and peak total bile acids in women with multifetal pregnancies, but conclusions are limited by small numbers [35].

Pruritus associated with ICP needs to be distinguished from pruritic urticarial papules and plaques of pregnancy (PUPPP), the commonest dermatosis in pregnancy [36]. PUPPP is of unknown etiology and not associated with fetal or maternal morbidity or mortality [36]. Two studies reported higher incidences of PUPPP in multifetal pregnancies [37, 38].

23.4 Potentially Severe Peripartum Maternal Morbidity

Women with multifetal pregnancies are at increased risk of most obstetric complications, and for a number of conditions the risk increase is very considerable. It is important that obstetric clinicians and midwives are aware of these increased risks and remain vigilant throughout the pregnancy. Although installing unnecessary fear of complications in pregnant women carrying a multifetal gestation should be avoided, it is important that women themselves are made aware of signs and symptoms related to these complications, so that they may seek timely medical advice.

23.4.1 Hypertensive Disorders of Pregnancy

Hypertensive disorders are associated with perinatal and maternal morbidity and mortality [39–42]. Both pregnancy-induced hypertension and preeclampsia are more likely to develop in women with a multifetal pregnancy [43, 44]. Twin pregnancies are associated with a twofold increased risk of developing pregnancy-induced hypertension compared with singleton pregnancies, and there is an even larger risk increase in triplet pregnancies [45]. Prevalence of pregnancy-induced hypertension from a gestational age of 28 weeks increases with the number of fetuses a woman carry: one in fifteen women with a singleton pregnancy, one in eight with twins, and one in five with triplets [46].

Preeclampsia in multifetal pregnancy is more commonly of early onset, and there is a threefold risk of developing preeclampsia in multifetal compared to singleton pregnancies [41, 47, 48]. Antenatal use of low-dose aspirin leads to a reduction of preeclampsia in women at risk [49]. The World Health Organization and American College of Obstetricians and Gynecologists consider women with multifetal pregnancies at high risk of preeclampsia and recommend aspirin from as early as 12 weeks' gestation until birth [50, 51]. The Royal College of Obstetricians and Gynaecologists of the United Kingdom considers women with multifetal pregnancies at moderate risk of developing preeclampsia and advises aspirin to pregnant women with more than one moderate risk factor [52]. Nevertheless, quality of the evidence supporting use of aspirin for prevention of preeclampsia in multifetal pregnancies is relatively low [53].

Incidence of pregnancy-related hypertensive disorders is not associated with zygosity or chorionicity [54, 55], but women with a multifetal pregnancy following any reproductive-assisted technology are at increased risk of developing pregnancy-induced hypertension [56]. Following in vitro fertilization and gamete intrafallopian transfer, the risk of preeclampsia is doubled compared to women who conceived spontaneously [57].

Pre-pregnancy obesity (BMI $\geq$30 kg/m^2) is associated with increased risk of developing pregnancy-induced hypertension and preeclampsia in twin pregnancies [58–60]. For twin pregnancies, the Institute of Medicine recommends a gestational weight gain of 16.8–24.5 kg for women with a normal body mass index (BMI 18.5–24.9 kg/m^2), 14.1–22.7 kg for overweight women (BMI 25.0–29.9 kg/m^2), and 11.3–19.1 kg for obese women (BMI $\geq$30 kg/m^2) [61]. It remains unclear whether excessive weight gain in twin pregnancy is associated with pregnancy-induced hypertension and preeclampsia [62, 63]. Gestational weight gain in multifetal pregnancy and its relation to maternal outcome is a neglected area of research, but intensified surveillance of hypertensive disorders in obese women appears justified [64].

23.4.2 Venous Thromboembolism

Risk of venous thromboembolism during pregnancy and postpartum period is increased in multifetal pregnancies [47, 65–68]. This risk is partly related to a higher proportion of cesarean sections in multifetal pregnancies, as well as increased risks of preeclampsia and postpartum hemorrhage. All of these are known risk factors for venous thromboembolism [65, 66, 68–72] and must be considered in decisions related to starting postpartum thromboprophylaxis, particularly in women who had a multifetal pregnancy.

The Royal College of Obstetricians and Gynaecologists of the United Kingdom acknowledges multifetal pregnancy as a risk factor for venous thromboembolism in the postpartum period, but recommends postpartum thromboprophylaxis only in case of one or more additional risk factors (such as a BMI $\geq$30 kg/m^2, immobility, preeclampsia, or postpartum hemorrhage above 1000 mL) [73]. The Dutch Society of Internal Medicine recommends postpartum thromboprophylaxis in multifetal pregnancies after every in-labor cesarean section or after elective cesarean section with one additional risk factor (such as smoking, preeclampsia, or fetal growth restriction) [74].

23.4.3 Postpartum Hemorrhage

Women who give birth to multiple babies have a twofold increased risk of postpartum hemorrhage [43, 47]. This increased risk is thought to be the result of uterine distention in multifetal pregnancy leading to uterine atony [75]. Among women with multifetal pregnancies who give birth vaginally, the risk of postpartum hemorrhage is even three-and-a-half fold increased in labors beyond a gestational age of 39 weeks and two-and-a-half fold in case of a combined birth weight over 5500 grams, induction of labor, oxytocin augmentation, and/or duration of labor beyond 24 hours [76].

Postpartum hemorrhage requiring packed red blood cells is significantly more common in multifetal pregnancies [77, 78]. Women with multifetal pregnancies who gave birth by cesarean section are even 10 times more likely to receive packed red blood cells compared to women who gave birth vaginally [79]. Considering that cesarean section itself is a risk factor for postpartum hemorrhage [80–82], mode of birth in multifetal pregnancy should be carefully scrutinized and cesarean sections should be performed on appropriate indications.

Compared to women with singleton pregnancies, women with multifetal pregnancies have a four-times elevated risk of receiving eight or more units of packed red bloods cells due to postpartum hemorrhage [83] and a five-times elevated risk of major obstetric hemorrhage (defined as having been transfused at least four units of packed cells, or having had peripartum hysterectomy or uterine artery embolization) [84]. The other way around, among women with major obstetric hemorrhage, multifetal pregnancy was found to be a risk factor for peripartum hysterectomy and uterine artery embolization [85, 86]. One study found a nearly 24-fold increased risk of peripartum hysterectomy for women with higher-order pregnancies compared to women with singletons [87].

A multifetal pregnancy after any assisted reproductive technology is associated with higher risks of preeclampsia, placenta previa, and placental abruption [56, 88], which in turn are significant risk factors for postpartum hemorrhage [89–91]. The risk of peripartum hysterectomy due to obstetric hemorrhage is also increased in women who conceived through assisted reproductive technology [86]. This should only strengthen the motivation to prevent iatrogenic multifetal pregnancies as much as possible.

Nevertheless, every birth attendant should be vigilant for postpartum hemorrhage during childbirth in multifetal pregnancies. An active management of the third stage of labor with administration of oxytocin to women giving birth to multiple babies is advised [4]. No evidence was found to suggest that any other uterotonic agent is more effective than oxytocin in preventing postpartum hemorrhage in multifetal pregnancy [92]. As with any birth, the first step in managing postpartum hemorrhage includes uterine massage, administration of uterotonic agents, and fluid resuscitation. In case of refractory hemorrhage, surgical interventions should be resorted to in time, along with measures to correct coagulopathy. Surgical approaches consist of intrauterine balloon tamponade, uterine compression sutures, uterine artery ligation or embolization, and peripartum hysterectomy. Following cesarean section in multifetal pregnancy, one study group found a high success rate for uterine compression sutures in case of bleeding due to uterine atony refractory to uterine massage and uterotonics [93].

23.4.4 Other Rare Conditions

Acute fatty liver of pregnancy (AFLP, 5.0 per 100.000 maternities) and amniotic fluid embolism (AFE, 0.8–1.8 per 100.000 maternities) are serious and life-threatening obstetric emergencies [94, 95]. AFLP is characterized by maternal liver dysfunction and aberrant fatty acid metabolism and may lead to maternal and fetal complications, including death. A prospective national study of AFLP in the United Kingdom showed that 10 out of 52 women (18%) with AFLP had a twin pregnancy [94]. AFE is a condition that occurs when amniotic fluid or fetal cells enter the maternal circulation and trigger a severe “anaphylaxis-like” reaction, starting with cardiorespiratory arrest, which, if survived, is followed by an excessive clotting disorder and severe postpartum hemorrhage. Risk of AFE is considerably increased in women with a multifetal pregnancy [95].

23.5 Severe Acute Maternal Morbidity and Maternal Mortality

A multi-country study conducted by the World Health Organization found an increased risk for most severe maternal outcomes in twin pregnancies compared to singleton pregnancies [96]. Another study found that the composite outcome of severe acute maternal morbidity (defined as major obstetric hemorrhage, (pre-)eclampsia, pulmonary embolism, stroke, psychiatric disorder, organ dysfunction, intensive care admission, and laparotomy following vaginal birth) was four times higher in women with twins compared to singletons [97]. The commonest underlying causal conditions of severe acute maternal morbidity were major obstetric hemorrhage and hypertensive disorders [97].

A nationwide study in the Netherlands found a similar fourfold elevated risk of severe acute maternal morbidity (composite outcome of intensive care unit admission, uterine rupture, eclampsia, and major obstetric hemorrhage) in multifetal pregnancies [84]. This study found no significant difference between mono- and dichorionic twins, but the risk of severe acute maternal morbidity was doubled in women having conceived through in vitro fertilization or intracytoplasmic sperm injection [84]. Overall, the risk of severe maternal morbidity was found to be higher in pregnancies after in vitro fertilization, but path analysis estimates that more than 20 percent of this risk is mediated by multifetal pregnancies [98].

The risk of maternal mortality in women with a multifetal pregnancy is more than four times elevated compared to women with singleton pregnancies [84, 96, 99]. Embolism, hemorrhage, hypertensive disorders, and infection are the most frequent causes for women with multifetal and singleton pregnancies alike [99]. However, women with a multifetal pregnancy were 3–4 times more likely to die from these causes irrespective of age, race, marital status, and level of education [99].

23.6 Summary

In conclusion, the risk of maternal morbidity and mortality is significantly increased in women with a multifetal pregnancy [96], with particular increases in women with pre-pregnancy obesity [58], higher-order gestations [100], and those who conceived through assisted reproductive technology [98]. Considering that use of fertility treatments in many high-income countries has been associated with a substantial rise in the rate of multifetal pregnancies [101, 102], we may improve maternal health by preventing iatrogenic multifetal pregnancies as much as possible. It is imperative to retain awareness of possible maternal complications associated with multifetal pregnancies and encourage clinicians to closely monitor women with a multifetal pregnancy antenatally and intrapartum. Birth of a multifetal gestation should always take place in a maternity ward with access to blood products, intensive care, and surgical expertise.

23.6.1 Review Questions

1. Of which conditions are women with multifetal pregnancies at increased risk?

2. Which groups of women with a multifetal pregnancy are at particular risk of maternal morbidity?

3. Which clinical considerations must be taken into account when caring for women with a multifetal pregnancy antenatally? And during the peripartum period?

23.6.2 Multiple-Choice Questions

1. The maternal blood volume increases even higher in twin pregnancies compared to singleton pregnancies, mainly due to a disproportionally large increase of:
   (a) Red blood cell volume
   (b) Blood plasma volume

2. Which of the following is not associated with an increased risk of pregnancy-induced hypertension in multifetal pregnancy:
   (a) Chorionicity
   (b) Pre-pregnancy obesity
   (c) Higher-order gestation
   (d) In vitro fertilization

3. Women with multifetal pregnancies following assisted reproductive technology are at increased risk of:
   (a) Preeclampsia
   (b) Pregnancy-induced hypertension
   (c) Massive obstetric hemorrhage
   (d) All of the above

4. Among women with a multifetal pregnancy who give birth vaginally, the risk of postpartum hemorrhage is especially increased in:
   (a) Gestational age beyond 38 weeks
   (b) Duration of labor less than 24 hours
   (c) Combined birth weight >5500 grams
   (d) Spontaneous onset of labor

5. The risk of maternal mortality in women with a multifetal pregnancy compared to women with a singleton pregnancy is:
   (a) Not increased
   (b) Doubled
   (c) Increased threefold
   (d) Increased fourfold

Patient Testimonials

A woman carrying twins was seen for a regular checkup at the antenatal clinic at 32 weeks' gestation. Although the woman complained about a mild headache, her blood pressure was not recorded. One week later, she presented with increased headache, visual scotoma, and general malaise. Her blood pressure was 190/135 mmHg and she had mild proteinuria. She was transferred to the antenatal ward and treated with oral nifedipine only. Magnesium sulfate was not started. One-on-one care was not provided and her blood pressure was not recorded until 2 hours later by which time her situation had deteriorated. She died from intracranial hemorrhage.

References

1. World Health Organization. The WHO application of ICD-10 to deaths during pregnancy, childbirth and puerperium: ICD MM. Publication date: 2012. ISBN: 978 92 4 154845 8. Accessible on: https://apps.who.int/iris/bitstream/handle/10665/70929/9789241548458_eng.pdf;jsessionid=A660C360F3FD05CF80085A0EA22059B1?sequence=1
2. Say L, Souza JP, Pattinson RC, WHO working group on Maternal Mortality and Morbidity classifications. Maternal near miss–towards a standard tool for monitoring quality of maternal health care. Best Pract Res Clin Obstet Gynaecol. 2009;23(3):287–96.
3. Brown MA, Magee LA, Kenny LC, et al. Hypertensive disorders of pregnancy: ISSHP classification, diagnosis, and management recommendations for international practice. Hypertension. 2018;72(1):24–43.
4. World Health Organization. WHO recommendations for the prevention and treatment of postpartum haemorrhage. Publication date: 2012. ISBN: 978 92 4 154850 2. Accesible on: https://apps.who.int/iris/bitstream/handle/10665/75411/9789241548502_eng.pdf?sequence=1
5. Nederlandse Vereniging voor Obstetrie en Gynaecologie. NVOG-richtlijn Hemorrhagia Postpartum (HPP). Arnhem: NVOG; 2013. Accessible on: https://www.nvog.nl/wp-content/uploads/2018/02/Hemorrhagia-postpartum-HPP-3.0-14-11-2013.pdf
6. Mavrides E, Allard S, Chandraharan E, Collins P, Green L, Hunt BJ, Riris S, Thomson AJ, on behalf of the Royal College of Obstetricians and Gynaecologists. Prevention and Management of Postpartum Haemorrhage. BJOG. 2017;124(5):e106–e49.
7. Schaap T, Bloemenkamp K, Deneux-Tharaux C, et al. Defining definitions: a Delphi study to develop a core outcome set for conditions of severe maternal morbidity. BJOG. 2019;126(3):394–401.
8. Louik C, Hernandez-Diaz S, Werler MM, Mitchell AA. Nausea and vomiting in pregnancy: maternal characteristics and risk factors. Paediatr Perinat Epidemiol. 2006;20(4):270–8.
9. Fiaschi L, Nelson-Piercy C, Deb S, King R, Tata LJ. Clinical management of nausea and vomiting in pregnancy and hyperemesis gravidarum across primary and secondary care: a population-based study. BJOG. 2019;126(10):1201–11.
10. Pritchard JA. Changes in the blood volume during pregnancy and delivery. Anesthesiology. 1965;26:393–9.
11. Ru Y, Pressman EK, Cooper EM, et al. Iron deficiency and anemia are prevalent in women with multiple gestations. Am J Clin Nutr. 2016;104(4):1052–60.
12. Kametas NA, McAuliffe F, Krampl E, Chambers J, Nicolaides KH. Maternal cardiac function in twin pregnancy. Obstet Gynecol. 2003;102(4):806–15.
13. Kuleva M, Youssef A, Maroni E, et al. Maternal cardiac function in normal twin pregnancy: a longitudinal study. Ultrasound Obstet Gynecol. 2011;38(5):575–80.
14. Macdonald-Wallis C, Lawlor DA, Fraser A, May M, Nelson SM, Tilling K. Blood pressure change in normotensive, gestational hypertensive, pre-eclamptic, and essential hypertensive pregnancies. Hypertension. 2012;59(6):1241–8.
15. Campbell DM. Maternal adaptation in twin pregnancy. Semin Perinatol. 1986;10(1):14–8.
16. Redford DH. Uterine growth in twin pregnancy by measurement of total intrauterine volume. Acta Genet Med Gemellol. 1982;31(3–4):145–8.
17. Schwartz DB, Daoud Y, Zazula P, et al. Gestational diabetes mellitus: metabolic and blood glucose parameters in singleton versus twin pregnancies. Am J Obstet Gynecol. 1999;181(4):912–4.
18. Sivan E, Maman E, Homko CJ, Lipitz S, Cohen S, Schiff E. Impact of fetal reduction on the incidence of gestational diabetes. Obstet Gynecol. 2002;99(1):91–4.
19. Roach VJ, Lau TK, Wilson D, Rogers MS. The incidence of gestational diabetes in multiple pregnancy. Aust N Z J Obstet Gynaecol. 1998;38(1):56–7.
20. Rauh-Hain JA, Rana S, Tamez H, Wang A, Cohen B, Cohen A, et al. Risk for developing gestational diabetes in women with twin pregnancies. J Matern Fetal Neonatal Med. 2009;22(4):293–9.
21. Weissman A, Drugan A. Glucose tolerance in singleton, twin and triplet pregnancies. J Perinat Med. 2016;44(8):893–7.
22. Buhling KJ, Henrich W, Starr E, et al. Risk for gestational diabetes and hypertension for women with twin pregnancy compared to singleton pregnancy. Arch Gynecol Obstet. 2003;269(1):33–6.
23. Henderson CE, Scarpelli S, LaRosa D, Divon MY. Assessing the risk of gestational diabetes in twin gestation. J Natl Med Assoc. 1995;87(10):757–8.
24. Naidoo L, Jailal I, Moodley J, Desai R. Intravenous glucose tolerance tests in women with twin pregnancy. Obstet Gynecol. 1985;66(4):500–2.
25. Weissgerber TL, Mudd LM. Preeclampsia and diabetes. Curr Diab Rep. 2015;15(3):9.
26. Naylor CD, Sermer M, Chen E, Sykora K. Cesarean delivery in relation to birth weight and gestational glucose tolerance: pathophysiology or practice style? Toronto Trihospital Gestational Diabetes Investigators. JAMA. 1996;275(15):1165–70.
27. Hartling L, Dryden DM, Guthrie A, Muise M, Vandermeer B, Donovan L. Benefits and harms of treating gestational diabetes mellitus: a systematic review and meta-analysis for the U.S. Preventive Services Task Force and the National Institutes

of Health Office of Medical Applications of Research. Ann Intern Med. 2013;159(2):123–9.
28. Kremer AE, Oude Elferink RP, Beuers U. Pathophysiology and current management of pruritus in liver disease. Clin Res Hepatol Gastroenterol. 2011;35(2):89–97.
29. Gonzalez MC, Reyes H, Arrese M, et al. Intrahepatic cholestasis of pregnancy in twin pregnancies. J Hepatol. 1989;9(1):84–90.
30. Glantz A, Marschall HU, Mattsson LA. Intrahepatic cholestasis of pregnancy: relationships between bile acid levels and fetal complication rates. Hepatology. 2004;40(2):467–74.
31. Cui Y, Xu B, Zhang X, He Y, Shao Y, Ding M. Diagnostic and therapeutic profiles of serum bile acids in women with intrahepatic cholestasis of pregnancy-a pseudo-targeted metabolomics study. Clin Chim Acta. 2018;483:135–41.
32. Grymowicz M, Czajkowski K, Smolarczyk R. Pregnancy course in patients with intrahepatic cholestasis of pregnancy treated with very low doses of ursodeoxycholic acid. Scand J Gastroenterol. 2016;51(1):78–85.
33. Garcia-Flores J, Canamares M, Cruceyra M, et al. Clinical value of maternal bile acid quantification in intrahepatic cholestasis of pregnancy as an adverse perinatal outcome predictor. Gynecol Obstet Investig. 2015;79(4):222–8.
34. Savander M, Ropponen A, Avela K, et al. Genetic evidence of heterogeneity in intrahepatic cholestasis of pregnancy. Gut. 2003;52(7):1025–9.
35. Ovadia C, Seed PT, Sklavounos A, et al. Association of adverse perinatal outcomes of intrahepatic cholestasis of pregnancy with biochemical markers: results of aggregate and individual patient data meta-analyses. Lancet. 2019;393(10174):899–909.
36. Matz H, Orion E, Wolf R. Pruritic urticarial papules and plaques of pregnancy: polymorphic eruption of pregnancy (PUPPP). Clin Dermatol. 2006;24(2):105–8.
37. Cohen LM, Capeless EL, Krusinski PA, Maloney ME. Pruritic urticarial papules and plaques of pregnancy and its relationship to maternal-fetal weight gain and twin pregnancy. Arch Dermatol. 1989;125(11):1534–6.
38. Elling SV, McKenna P, Powell FC. Pruritic urticarial papules and plaques of pregnancy in twin and triplet pregnancies. J Eur Acad Dermatol Venereol. 2000;14(5):378–81.
39. Hauth JC, Ewell MG, Levine RJ, et al. Pregnancy outcomes in healthy nulliparas who developed hypertension. Calcium for Preeclampsia Prevention Study Group. Obstet Gynecol. 2000;95(1):24–8.
40. Buchbinder A, Sibai BM, Caritis S, et al. Adverse perinatal outcomes are significantly higher in severe gestational hypertension than in mild preeclampsia. Am J Obstet Gynecol. 2002;186(1):66–71.
41. Steegers EA, von Dadelszen P, Duvekot JJ, Pijnenborg R. Pre-eclampsia. Lancet. 2010;376(9741):631–44.
42. Say L, Chou D, Gemmill A, et al. Global causes of maternal death: a WHO systematic analysis. Lancet Glob Health. 2014;2(6):e323–33.
43. Conde-Agudelo A, Belizan JM, Lindmark G. Maternal morbidity and mortality associated with multiple gestations. Obstet Gynecol. 2000 Jun;95(6 Pt 1):899–904.
44. Sibai BM, Hauth J, Caritis S, et al. Hypertensive disorders in twin versus singleton gestations. National Institute of Child Health and Human Development Network of Maternal-Fetal Medicine Units. Am J Obstet Gynecol. 2000;182(4):938–42.
45. Luke B, Brown MB. Contemporary risks of maternal morbidity and adverse outcomes with increasing maternal age and plurality. Fertil Steril. 2007;88(2):283–93.
46. Day MC, Barton JR, O'Brien JM, Istwan NB, Sibai BM. The effect of fetal number on the development of hypertensive conditions of pregnancy. Obstet Gynecol. 2005;106(5 Pt 1):927–31.
47. Walker MC, Murphy KE, Pan S, Yang Q, Wen SW. Adverse maternal outcomes in multifetal pregnancies. BJOG. 2004;111(11):1294–6.
48. Long PA, Oats JN. Preeclampsia in twin pregnancy–severity and pathogenesis. Aust N Z J Obstet Gynaecol. 1987;27(1):1–5.
49. Duley L, Meher S, Hunter KE, Seidler AL, Askie LM. Antiplatelet agents for preventing preeclampsia and its complications. Cochrane Database Syst Rev. 2019;2019(10):CD004659.
50. The American College of Obstetricians and Gynecologists. ACOG Practice Bulletin No. 202: gestational hypertension and preeclampsia. Obstet Gynecol. 2019;133(1):e1–e25.
51. World Health Organization. WHO recommendations for prevention and treatment of pre-eclampsia and eclampsia. Publication date: 2011. ISBN: 978 92 4 154833 5 Accessible on: https://apps.who.int/iris/bitstream/handle/10665/44703/9789241548335_eng.pdf?sequence=1
52. National Institute for Health and Care Excellence. Hypertension in pregnancy: diagnosis and management. Clinical guideline [NG133]. Publication date: 2019. Accessible on: https://www.nice.org.uk/guidance/ng133
53. Bergeron TS, Roberge S, Carpentier C, Sibai B, McCaw-Binns A, Bujold E. Prevention of preeclampsia with aspirin in multiple gestations: a systematic review and meta-analysis. Am J Perinatol. 2016;33(6):605–10.
54. Feng B, Zhai J, Cai Y. Effect of twin pregnancy chorionic properties on maternal and fetal outcomes. Taiwan J Obstet Gynecol. 2018;57(3):351–4.
55. Lucovnik M, Blickstein I, Lasic M, et al. Hypertensive disorders during monozygotic and dizy-

gotic twin gestations: a population-based study. Hypertens Pregnancy. 2016;35(4):542–7.
56. Qin J, Wang H, Sheng X, Liang D, Tan H, Xia J. Pregnancy-related complications and adverse pregnancy outcomes in multiple pregnancies resulting from assisted reproductive technology: a meta-analysis of cohort studies. Fertil Steril. 2015;103(6):1492–508, e1–7.
57. Lynch A, McDuffie R Jr, Murphy J, Faber K, Orleans M. Preeclampsia in multiple gestation: the role of assisted reproductive technologies. Obstet Gynecol. 2002;99(3):445–51.
58. Fox NS, Roman AS, Saltzman DH, Klauser CK, Rebarber A. Obesity and adverse pregnancy outcomes in twin pregnancies. J Matern Fetal Neonatal Med. 2014;27(4):355–9.
59. Lucovnik M, Blickstein I, Verdenik I, Trojner-Bregar A, Tul N. Maternal obesity in singleton versus twin gestations: a population-based matched case-control study. J Matern Fetal Neonatal Med. 2015;28(6):623–5.
60. Al-Obaidly S, Parrish J, Murphy KE, Maxwell C. Maternal pre-gravid body mass index and obstetric outcomes in twin gestations. J Perinatol. 2014;34(6):425–8.
61. The American College of Obstetricians and Gynecologists. ACOG Committee opinion no. 548: weight gain during pregnancy. Obstet Gynecol. 2013;121(1):210–2.
62. Pettit KE, Lacoursiere DY, Schrimmer DB, Alblewi H, Moore TR, Ramos GA. Maternal and neonatal outcomes in women with twin pregnancies with excessive gestational weight gain. J Matern Fetal Neonatal Med. 2016;29(13):2182–5.
63. Fox NS, Saltzman DH, Kurtz H, Rebarber A. Excessive weight gain in term twin pregnancies: examining the 2009 Institute of Medicine definitions. Obstet Gynecol. 2011;118(5):1000–4.
64. Bodnar LM, Pugh SJ, Abrams B, Himes KP, Hutcheon JA. Gestational weight gain in twin pregnancies and maternal and child health: a systematic review. J Perinatol. 2014;34(4):252–63.
65. Virkus RA, Lokkegaard E, Lidegaard O, et al. Risk factors for venous thromboembolism in 1.3 million pregnancies: a nationwide prospective cohort. PLoS One. 2014;9(5):e96495.
66. Jacobsen AF, Skjeldestad FE, Sandset PM. Incidence and risk patterns of venous thromboembolism in pregnancy and puerperium–a register-based case-control study. Am J Obstet Gynecol. 2008;198(2):233, e1–7
67. Henriksson P, Westerlund E, Wallen H, Brandt L, Hovatta O, Ekbom A. Incidence of pulmonary and venous thromboembolism in pregnancies after in vitro fertilisation: cross sectional study. BMJ. 2013;346:e8632.
68. James AH, Jamison MG, Brancazio LR, Myers ER. Venous thromboembolism during pregnancy and the postpartum period: incidence, risk factors, and mortality. Am J Obstet Gynecol. 2006;194(5):1311–5.
69. Jacobsen AF, Skjeldestad FE, Sandset PM. Ante- and postnatal risk factors of venous thrombosis: a hospital-based case-control study. J Thromb Haemost. 2008;6(6):905–12.
70. Lindqvist P, Dahlback B, Marsal K. Thrombotic risk during pregnancy: a population study. Obstet Gynecol. 1999;94(4):595–9.
71. Sultan AA, Tata LJ, West J, et al. Risk factors for first venous thromboembolism around pregnancy: a population-based cohort study from the United Kingdom. Blood. 2013;121(19):3953–61.
72. Liu S, Liston RM, Joseph KS, et al. Maternal mortality and severe morbidity associated with low-risk planned cesarean delivery versus planned vaginal delivery at term. CMAJ. 2007;176(4): 455–60.
73. The Royal College of Obstetricians and Gynaecologists. Reducing the Risk of Venous Thromboembolism during Pregnancy and the Puerperiom. Green-top Guideline No 37a. 2015.
74. Nederlandse Internisten Vereniging. Tromboseprofylaxe bij vrouwen na een sectio caesarea. Publication date: 2016. Accessible on: https://richtlijnendatabase.nl/richtlijn/antitrombotisch_beleid/preventie_vte_in_de_verloskunde/trombo-embolie_na_een_sectio_caesarea.html
75. Gill P PA, Van Hook MD JW. Uterine Atony. [Updated 2019 May 2019]. In: StatPearls [Internet] Treasure Island (FL): StatPearls Publishing. 2020 Jan. Accessible on: https://www.ncbi.nlm.nih.gov/books/NBK493238/#_NBK493238_pubdet_
76. Suzuki S, Kikuchi F, Ouchi N, et al. Risk factors for postpartum hemorrhage after vaginal delivery of twins. J Nippon Med Sch. 2007;74(6): 414–7.
77. Marocchini M, Lauferon J, Quantin C, Sagot P. Postpartum hemorrhage with transfusion: trends, near misses, risk factors and management at the scale of a perinatal network. J Gynecol Obstet Hum Reprod. 2017;46(5):455–60.
78. Kramer MS, Berg C, Abenhaim H, et al. Incidence, risk factors, and temporal trends in severe postpartum hemorrhage. Am J Obstet Gynecol. 2013;209(5):449, e1–7
79. Blitz MJ, Yukhayev A, Pachtman SL, et al. Twin pregnancy and risk of postpartum hemorrhage. J Matern Fetal Neonatal Med. 2019;5:1–6.
80. Nyflot LT, Sandven I, Stray-Pedersen B, et al. Risk factors for severe postpartum hemorrhage: a case-control study. BMC Pregnancy Childbirth. 2017;17(1):17.
81. Davey MA, Flood M, Pollock W, Cullinane F, McDonald S. Risk factors for severe postpartum haemorrhage: a population-based retrospective cohort study. Aust N Z J Obstet Gynaecol. 2019;60(4):522–32.
82. Butwick AJ, Ramachandran B, Hegde P, Riley ET, El-Sayed YY, Nelson LM. Risk factors for severe postpartum hemorrhage after cesarean delivery: case-control studies. Anesth Analg. 2017;125(2):523–32.

83. Ramler PI, van den Akker T, Henriquez D, et al. Women receiving massive transfusion due to postpartum hemorrhage: a comparison over time between two nationwide cohort studies. Acta Obstet Gynecol Scand. 2019;98(6):795–804.
84. Witteveen T, Van Den Akker T, Zwart JJ, Bloemenkamp KW, Van Roosmalen J. Severe acute maternal morbidity in multiple pregnancies: a nationwide cohort study. Am J Obstet Gynecol. 2016;214(5):641, e1-e10.
85. Zwart JJ, Dijk PD, van Roosmalen J. Peripartum hysterectomy and arterial embolization for major obstetric hemorrhage: a 2-year nationwide cohort study in the Netherlands. Am J Obstet Gynecol. 2010;202(2):150, e1–7
86. Maraschini A, Lega I, D'Aloja P, et al. Women undergoing peripartum hysterectomy due to obstetric hemorrhage: a prospective population-based study. Acta Obstet Gynecol Scand. 2019;99(2):274–82.
87. Francois K, Ortiz J, Harris C, Foley MR, Elliott JP. Is peripartum hysterectomy more common in multiple gestations? Obstet Gynecol. 2005;105(6):1369–72.
88. Karami M, Jenabi E, Fereidooni B. The association of placenta previa and assisted reproductive techniques: a meta-analysis. J Matern Fetal Neonatal Med. 2018;31(14):1940–7.
89. auf Altenstadt JFS, Hukkelhoven CW, van Roosmalen J, Bloemenkamp KW. Pre-eclampsia increases the risk of postpartum haemorrhage: a nationwide cohort study in the Netherlands. PLoS One. 2013;8(12):e81959.
90. Fan D, Xia Q, Liu L, et al. The incidence of postpartum hemorrhage in pregnant women with placenta previa: a systematic review and meta-analysis. PLoS One. 2017;12(1):e0170194.
91. Kainer F, Hasbargen U. Emergencies associated with pregnancy and delivery: peripartum hemorrhage. Dtsch Arztebl Int. 2008;105(37):629–38.
92. National Institute for Health and Care Excellence. Twin and triplet pregnancy – evidence reviews for interventions to prevent postpartum haemorrhage in the third stage of labour. Clinical guideline [NG137]. Publication date: 2019. Accessible on: https://www.nice.org.uk/guidance/ng137/evidence/i-interventions-to-prevent-postpartum-haemorrhage-in-the-third-stage-of-labour-pdf-6898605381
93. Kim ML, Hur YM, Ryu H, Lee MJ, Seong SJ, Shin JS. Clinical outcomes of prophylactic compression sutures for treatment of uterine atony during the cesarean delivery of twins. BMC Pregnancy Childbirth. 2020;20(1):40.
94. Knight M, Nelson-Piercy C, Kurinczuk JJ, Spark P, Brocklehurst P, System UKOS. A prospective national study of acute fatty liver of pregnancy in the UK. Gut. 2008;57(7):951–6.
95. Fitzpatrick KE, van den Akker T, Bloemenkamp KWM, et al. Risk factors, management, and outcomes of amniotic fluid embolism: a multicountry, population-based cohort and nested case-control study. PLoS Med. 2019;16(11):e1002962.
96. Santana DS, Cecatti JG, Surita FG, et al. Twin pregnancy and severe maternal outcomes: the World Health Organization multicountry survey on maternal and newborn health. Obstet Gynecol. 2016;127(4):631–41.
97. Madar H, Goffinet F, Seco A, Rozenberg P, Dupont C, Deneux-Tharaux C. Severe acute maternal morbidity in twin compared with singleton pregnancies. Obstet Gynecol. 2019;133(6):1141–50.
98. Le Ray C, Pelage L, Seco A, Bouvier-Colle MH, Chantry AA, Deneux-Tharaux C, et al. Risk of severe maternal morbidity associated with in vitro fertilisation: a population-based study. BJOG. 2019;126(8):1033–41.
99. MacKay AP, Berg CJ, King JC, Duran C, Chang J. Pregnancy-related mortality among women with multifetal pregnancies. Obstet Gynecol. 2006;107(3):563–8.
100. Luke B, Brown MB. Maternal morbidity and infant death in twin vs triplet and quadruplet pregnancies. Am J Obstet Gynecol. 2008;198(4):401, e1–10
101. El-Toukhy T, Bhattacharya S, Akanda VA, on behalf of the Royal College of Obstetricians and Gynaecologists. Multiple pregnancies following assisted conception: scientific impact paper no. 22. BJOG. 2018;125(5):e12–e8.
102. Kulkarni AD, Jamieson DJ, Jones HW, et al. Fertility treatments and multiple births in the United States. N Engl J Med. 2013;369(23):2218–25.

Key Reading

Madar H, Goffinet F, Seco A, Rozenberg P, Dupont C, Deneux-Tharaux C. Severe acute maternal morbidity in twin compared with singleton pregnancies. Obstet Gynecol. 2019;133(6):1141–50.

Santana DS, Cecatti JG, Surita FG, et al. Twin pregnancy and severe maternal outcomes: the world health organization multicountry survey on maternal and newborn health. Obstet Gynecol. 2016;127(4):631–41.

Witteveen T, Van Den Akker T, Zwart JJ, Bloemenkamp KW, Van Roosmalen J. Severe acute maternal morbidity in multiple pregnancies: a nationwide cohort study. Am J Obstet Gynecol. 2016;214(5):641, e1–e10.

Postnatal Care

Contents

Breastfeeding Twins and Multiples

Sophie Russell and Neal Russell

Contents

A. Khalil et al. (eds.), *Twin and Higher-order Pregnancies*,
https://doi.org/10.1007/978-3-030-47652-6_24

Trailer

The benefits of breastfeeding for both mother and child have been widely documented. Women who are expecting twins or higher order multiples face additional challenges with breastfeeding when compared to feeding a singleton, such as higher rates of obstetric complications, prematurity and neonatal unit admission. Strategies for improving breastfeeding in singletons are well documented and supported by evidence, but there is a need for a greater focus on strategies to improve breastfeeding in twins.

Learning Objectives

After studying this chapter, you will be better able to:

- Understand the basic physiology of breastfeeding multiples
- Appreciate the importance of antenatal support and preparation to facilitate breastfeeding in multiples.
- Describe the common problems with breastfeeding multiples
- Explain methods to overcome them

24.1 Benefits of Breastfeeding

Breastfeeding is associated with significant benefits to both mothers and babies, and evidence suggests that scaling up breastfeeding to optimum levels globally could prevent more than 800,000 child deaths [1].

For the child, breastfeeding reduces the risk of infections such as pneumonia and diarrhoea, may also reduce the risk of obesity and diabetes, and is associated with increased intelligence. For the mother, breastfeeding reduces the risk of breast cancer, contributes to birth spacing by delaying menstruation in exclusively breastfeeding mothers, and is associated with reductions in ovarian cancer and type 2 diabetes. Indeed it is estimated that 20,000 breast cancer-related deaths could be prevented by scaling up breastfeeding [1].

Beyond health benefits, it is well recognised that the bond between mothers and their infants is enhanced by breastfeeding, with positive psychological effects.

24.2 Challenges

Despite the clear health and psychological benefits, rates of breastfeeding are highly variable globally, with particularly low rates in some high-income countries such as the United Kingdom. For multiple births, breastfeeding may present additional challenges beyond the obvious challenge of caring for additional infants, and breastfeeding rates in multiple births are usually lower than for singletons [2]. As an example, in the United Kingdom breastfeeding rates are approximately 25% for multiples at 3 months versus 40% for singletons.

Multiple pregnancy is associated with a greater risk of preterm birth, operative delivery, and obstetric and perinatal complications in general, leading to a greater likelihood of admission to neonatal units, with a consequent challenges for initiating the maternal-newborn dyad and decrease in breastfeeding rates. The increasing association of multiple births with in vitro fertilisation (IVF) may also be associated with increased complications and lead to similar risk factors.

The increased rate of complications in twin pregnancies may also contribute to increased anxiety in mothers in general, in addition to specific concerns around feeding. Mothers of twins and multiples are less likely to intend to initiate breastfeeding [3] as well as to maintain it, and are more likely to be concerned about feeding and milk supply.

Indeed, early initiation of breastfeeding is likely to be more challenging especially after operative delivery or neonatal unit admission, but is also compromised by practical difficulties initiating important practices such as skin-to-skin care.

24.2.1 Preterm Multiples

Lower gestational age is strongly associated with multiple pregnancy and has an important influence on the ability of infants and mothers to breastfeed. The effect is seen even comparing early term and late term infants, with lower rates of breastfeeding at 37 compared to 40 weeks [4], but preterm infants (<37 weeks) face the greatest challenges. Aside from interference with the maternal-newborn dyad associated with neonatal admission and need for invasive procedures such as ventilation support in the first few days, preterm newborns may have less ability to initiate sucking and breastfeeding, depending on their gestational age. First, due to an increased rate of complications at lower gestational ages, twins may be too unwell to breastfeed, due to respiratory distress, or sepsis for example. Even without being unwell, the sucking reflex, and coordination with swallowing and breathing may be reduced in preterm infants due to neurological immaturity, particularly before 32 weeks gestation, when nasogastric feeding is normally required. Furthermore, mothers' milk supply is also often less after preterm delivery, which may be exacerbated with delayed onset of feeding and reliance on expression of breastmilk rather than direct sucking. This may exacerbate concerns about insufficient milk, which together with the focus on promoting growth in preterm infants and high milk requirements may lead to a need (real or perceived) for additional preterm formula milk.

Nevertheless, receiving breast milk is particularly important for preterm newborns, not only due to the aforementioned benefits, but especially due to the benefit of breast milk for preventing necrotising enterocolitis. Women with preterm twins therefore require extra support to initiate and maintain breast milk supply for their preterm infants and establish breastfeeding, with use where possible of breast milk fortification (supplemented with nutrients, particularly protein, calcium and phosphate) for growth concerns rather than preterm formula where possible. When there are concerns over quantity of breastmilk, donor milk is preferable (after screening) particularly in preterm infants.

24.3 Chronicity

There are limited data on the breastfeeding rates of twins according to their chronicity. It is believed that the breastfeeding rates of MC twins are lower than DC twins and that this is primarily related to the higher rate of complications including complication that do not occur within the DC group (TTTS) and number of premature deliveries within the MC cohort.

Mothers should be advised that breastfeeding all chronicity's of twins is possible, but it can be more difficult in extremes of prematurity and when complications arise. In these situations, it may be possible for mothers to express breast milk prior to establishing breastfeeding.

24.4 International Recommendations on Breastfeeding

The World Health Organisation (WHO) recommends early initiation of, and exclusive breastfeeding up to 6 months of age, followed by introduction of complimentary foods and continued breastfeeding up to 2 years of age or beyond.

Given that most twins are born in hospital, the 10 steps of the UNICEF/WHO Baby Friendly Hospital Initiative are as relevant for multiple births as for singletons.

Baby Friendly Hospital Initiative: 10 steps	
Critical management procedures	
1a	Comply fully with the International Code of Marketing of Breast-milk Substitutes and relevant World Health Assembly resolutions.
1b	Have a written infant feeding policy that is routinely communicated to staff and parents.
1c	Establish ongoing monitoring and data-management systems.
2	Ensure that staff have sufficient knowledge, competence and skills to support breastfeeding.
Key clinical practices	

Baby Friendly Hospital Initiative: 10 steps	
3	Discuss the importance and management of breastfeeding with pregnant women and their families.
4	Facilitate immediate and uninterrupted skin-to-skin contact and support mothers to initiate breastfeeding as soon as possible after birth.
5	Support mothers to initiate and maintain breastfeeding and manage common difficulties.
6	Do not provide breastfed newborns any food or fluids other than breast milk, unless medically indicated.
7	Enable mothers and their infants to remain together and to practise rooming-in 24 hours a day.
8	Support mothers to recognize and respond to their infants' cues for feeding.
9	Counsel mothers on the use and risks of feeding bottles, teats and pacifiers.
10	Coordinate discharge so that parents and their infants have timely access to ongoing support and care.

Source: WHO/UNICEF 2018: Ten steps to successful breastfeeding (revised 2018). Available at ► https://www.who.int/nutrition/bfhi/ten-steps/en/ [Accessed on 14.12.2019]

Implementation of the 10 steps has been shown to be associated with increasing rates of breastfeeding, with an increasing effect the more steps are implemented [5]. In particular, interventions such as kangaroo mother care, skin-to-skin contact, peer support, breast milk expression, staff training and formal accreditation as a Baby Friendly Hospital are also associated with greater breastfeeding rates [6].

24.5 Improving Breastfeeding Rates in Multiple Births

A common misconception is that mothers of twins and higher order multiples will not be able to produce enough breast milk to feed their babies. Mothers should be made aware that they are able to provide enough milk to breastfeed multiple infants, and that mothers of multiples on average produce more milk [7]. Research shows breastfeeding mums of triplets can produce three litres a day, whilst the average male singleton baby drinks 831 ml a day [8]. However, despite the overall evidence for support of breastfeeding, the overall evidence for twin and multiple births is far more limited. A recent systematic review concluded that the evidence on support for breastfeeding strategies in randomised controlled trials in twins is inconclusive and of limited quality [9]. Given the challenges, there is a need for a greater focus on evidence-based strategies for improving breastfeeding rates in twins. Nevertheless, there are several recommended approaches, which are likely to improve breastfeeding rates in twins and should be encouraged. Importantly, each infant should be treated as an individual and feeding and growth expectations should be adapted to their specific needs, which may be different to their sibling(s).

24.5.1 Antenatal Period

Given that multiple pregnancies are usually detected during pregnancy in settings with ultrasonography available, interventions to support breastfeeding can and should ideally begin during the antenatal period. This is particularly important given the decreased intention of mothers of multiples to breastfeed. Education, counselling and support during the antenatal period are likely to be important for improving breastfeeding rates in twins and higher order multiples and should be encouraged. Specialist services with advice tailored to multiple pregnancies may also improve confidence in mothers intending to breastfeed.

Antenatal expression of breast milk is an area of recent interest and may theoretically also be a potential strategy, but it has limited scientific evidence [10]. Although concerns about the potential for causing preterm delivery were not supported by a recent study of expression in diabetic mothers if they started expressing after 36 weeks gestation [11], more evidence would be required to recommend this practice routinely in twins.

24.5.2 Immediate Postpartum Period

Mothers may require additional support in the immediate postpartum period to initiate skin-to-skin care of multiples due to the practical challenges, and they will require support for early expression of breastmilk for newborns who are unable to breastfeed.

24.5.3 Admission to a Neonatal Unit

In neonatal units, mothers require a dedicated space for expression of milk, as well as opportunities for skin-to-skin and kangaroo mother care, and minimal disruption to the maternal-newborn dyad. Family-centred care is also increasingly promoted in neonatal units [9] and may also help promote bonding and breastfeeding.

24.5.4 Postnatal Wards and Early Discharge

Term multiples, as well as moderately preterm babies between 34 and 37 weeks of age, are often discharged early, and may receive limited support for breastfeeding on general postnatal wards. Breastfeeding therefore requires more targeted support for these infants both on postnatal wards and in the community [12].

24.6 Techniques for Breastfeeding

Each infant is different, and mothers should be made aware that one rule may not always apply, and patterns may change over time. Although it may be convenient to feed infants together, some infants may have different feeding patterns, particularly when they are of different weights, which may need to be adapted to, and it may be easier to feed one infant at a time. As such, many mothers use a combination of separate and simultaneous feeding. The mother should be supported to find the method and pattern that works for her, which may take some time. It is preferable to alternate breasts for each baby however, particularly as each breast may produce different amounts of milk.

The mother may require extra support for positioning and attachment, particularly in the first few days and when performing simultaneous feeding. Below are examples of different positioning methods that may be considered.

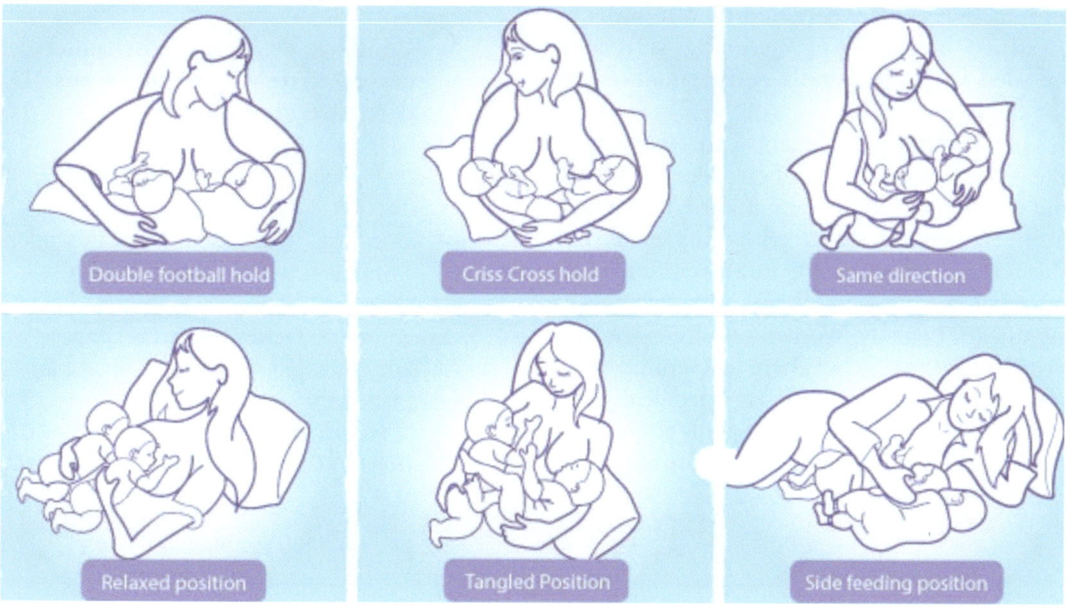
Double football hold
Criss Cross hold
Same direction
Relaxed position
Tangled Position
Side feeding position

Image credit Lansinoh.co.uk

Expression of milk may also be an important strategy for relieving pressure on the mother by allowing others to assist with feeding, to feed babies who are sick, to relieve breastfeeding difficulties such as sore nipples, or as a long-term strategy for feeding. Mothers should be supported to express milk where necessary, but should also be aware that if babies can breastfeed then expressing milk is not necessary per se.

Both hand expression and pumps (manual or electric) are possible, with some limited evidence that the latter may produce slightly more milk. Feeding or expression should start early, ideally within 6 hours of life, and should be regular, approximately 8 times a day. Adding an extra expression at night when milk production is high, or a double pump may help to increase supply. Special attention should be paid to sterilising equipment and adequate storage of breast milk to avoid contamination, and volumes should follow the normal recommendation by weight for singletons.

Mothers of multiples may require greater support at home after discharge, with more frequent visits, support groups, and ultimately greater social support and maternity leave. This support must be practical, but women may also need additional emotional support given the increased risk of postnatal depression in twins. After a period of 6 months of exclusive breastfeeding, weaning is recommended with the same recommendations as for singletons.

In summary, women can exclusively breastfeed twins and higher order multiples, but numerous challenges makes this much more challenging than feeding singletons. For this reason, breastfeeding rates are often lower in twins, meaning they may miss out on the significant benefits. Women require extra support to feed twins, but there are limited studies on methods of support specifically for twins, and therefore most evidence comes from singletons. There is a need for more evidence on how best to support breastfeeding of twins, at the same time as supporting women to make an informed choice about how to feed their babies.

24.7 Higher Order Multiples

There is little high quality research on breastfeeding higher orders multiples. However, there is some evidence that suggests mothers can produce enough milk to exclusively breastfeed triplets [8] as the mechanism behind breastfeeding is based on supply and demand. Mothers should be informed and reassured that it is physically possible to breastfeed higher order multiples with an emphasis on the mother creating a social support network to support her with the demands of feeding more than one infant. This can be difficult if the mother has little support or when the mother has to coordinate having different babies admitted to NICU. In these situations, expression of milk or donor milk can be considered. Depending on availability and the wishes of the mother, different methods of supplementary feeding may also be considered.

24.7.1 Review Questions

1. List >2 benefits of breastfeeding for the baby
   - Bonding, decreased gastroenteritis, decreased respiratory infections, IQ, decreased mortality

2. List >2 benefits of breastfeeding for the mother
   - Bonding, decreased breast cancer, decreased type 2 diabetes

3. What are 3 factors affecting breastfeeding rates in twins and multiple pregnancies
   - *Answer: Preterm, higher complications, NICU admission*

24.7.2 Multiple-Choice Questions (Choose 1 Answer)

1. Expression of antenatal breast milk is one strategy in improving breastfeeding rates in twins. It is advisable to start expression after
   - (a) The mother has given birth
   - (b) After 24 weeks of pregnancy
   - (c) After 36 weeks of pregnancy
   - (d) After 30 weeks of pregnancy
   - (e) After 35 weeks

2. Research shows the average male singleton baby drinks 831 mls a day whilst the average triplet mum produces
   - (a) 3 litres of milk a day
   - (b) 2 litres of milk a day
   - (c) 1.5 litres of milk a day
   - (d) 1 litre of milk a day
   - (e) 900 mls of milk a day

3. In premature twins, the sucking reflex and coordination of swallowing and breathing is hinder prior to
   - (a) 30 weeks gestation
   - (b) 28 weeks gestation
   - (c) 35 weeks gestation
   - (d) 36 weeks gestation
   - (e) 32 weeks gestation

Patient Testimonials

"I found breastfeeding my twins a lovely way to bond with them, this was important to me as they spent 2 weeks in NICU. I found breastfeeding quite time consuming until my midwife showed me how to breastfeed them both at the same time."

"I didn't get much support from the hospital with breastfeeding my twins, I had two other children and was keen to get home but in hindsight I wished I had stayed in the hospital a bit longer to learn how to feed both of the twins at the same time."

"I went to a breastfeeding twins group and I am so pleased I did, the other mums were so helpful with passing on tips, they have been an excellent on-going support group. I would definitely recommend that mums of twins link up with other multiple parents."

"I had a very difficult delivery with my twins and I felt exhausted afterwards, I had little support and would not have managed without formula."

References

1. Victora CG, Bahl R, Barros AJD, França GVA, Horton S, Krasevec J, et al. Breastfeeding in the 21st century: epidemiology, mechanisms, and lifelong effect. Lancet. 2016;387(10017):475–90. https://doi.org/10.1016/S0140-6736(15)01024-7.
2. Porta R, Capdevila E, Botet F, Ginovart G, Moliner E, Nicolàs M, et al. Breastfeeding disparities between multiples and singletons by NICU discharge. Nutrients. 2019;11(9):2191.
3. Lutsiv O, Pullenayegum E, Foster G, Vera C, Giglia L, Chapman B, et al. Women's intentions to breastfeed: a population-based cohort study. BJOG. 2013;120(12):1490–8. Available from: http://www.ncbi.nlm.nih.gov/pubmed/23859024
4. Lutsiv O, Giglia L, Pullenayegum E, Foster G, Vera C, Chapman B, et al. A population-based cohort study of breastfeeding according to gestational age at term delivery. J Pediatr. 2013;163(5):1283–8.
5. Pérez-Escamilla R, Martinez JL, Segura-Pérez S. Impact of the Baby-friendly Hospital Initiative on breastfeeding and child health outcomes: a systematic review. Vol. 12, Maternal and Child Nutrition. Blackwell Publishing Ltd; 2016. p. 402 17.
6. Renfrew MJ, Craig D, Dyson L, McCormick F, Rice S, King SE, et al. Breastfeeding promotion for infants in neonatal units: a systematic review and economic analysis. Health Technol Assess. 2009;13(40):1–146, iii–iv. Available from: http://www.ncbi.nlm.nih.gov/pubmed/19728934
7. Flidel-Rimon O, Shinwell ES. Breast feeding twins and high multiples. Arch Dis Child Fetal Neonatal Edn. 2006;91(5):F377–80.
8. Kent JC, et al. Volume and frequency of breastfeedings and fat content of breast milk throughout the day. Pediatrics. 2006;117(3):e387–95.
9. Chapman T, Pincombe J, Harris M. Antenatal breast expression: a critical review of the literature. Midwifery. 2013;29(3):203–10.
10. Forster DA, Moorhead AM, Jacobs SE, Davis PG, Walker SP, McEgan KM, et al. Advising women

with diabetes in pregnancy to express breast-milk in late pregnancy (Diabetes and Antenatal Milk Expressing [DAME]): a multicentre, unblinded, randomised controlled trial. Lancet. 2017;389(10085):2204–13.
11. Roué J-M, Kuhn P, Maestro ML, Maastrup RA, Mitanchez D, Westrup B, et al. Eight principles for patient-centred and family-centred care for newborns in the neonatal intensive care unit. Arch Dis Child. 2017;102(4):F364–8. Available from: http://www.ncbi.nlm.nih.gov/pubmed/28420745
12. Whitford HM, Wallis SK, Dowswell T, West HM, Renfrew MJ. Breastfeeding education and support for women with twins or higher order multiples. Cochrane Database Syst Rev. 2017;28(2):CD012003.

Key Reading

Guidance for health professionals on feeding twins, triplets and higher order multiples. Royal College of Midwives, Royal College of Paediatrics and Child Health, and Royal College of Nursing. Available at http://www.multiplebirths.org.uk/MBF_Professionals_Final.pdf

Lancet series breastfeeding.

Successful Breastfeeding, Royal College of Midwives London 2002, 3rd ed., Churchill Livingstone.

UNICEF – Baby friendly hospital initiative.

WHO Breastfeeding guidance.

Perinatal Depression and Psychiatric Considerations

Femke Vanwetswinkel and Titia Hompes

Contents

A. Khalil et al. (eds.), *Twin and Higher-order Pregnancies*,
https://doi.org/10.1007/978-3-030-47652-6_25

25

Trailer

Perinatal depression (PND) is one of the most common complications of pregnancy. Estimates of prevalence range from 10% to 20%. The perinatal period is associated with complex and unique biological, socio-environmental, and psychological changes for each woman. PND is a burdensome disorder with a profound intrusive impact on the (expectant) mother (to be), her (unborn) child, but also the supporting system. PND is heterogeneous in presentation with likely multifactorial etiologies for each woman. Apart from psychosocial factors, researchers investigated potential underlying endocrinological, immunological, and (epi)genetic factors associated with PND. The Edinburgh Postnatal Depression Scale (EPDS) is the gold standard for detection. The main goals of treating PND are to reduce maternal psychiatric symptoms and to support maternal–child attachment. A stepped-care approach is advocated, in which mild to moderate symptoms should be treated with psychotherapeutic interventions, whereas women with severe symptoms or women who do not respond to nonpharmacological treatment, pharmacological treatment can be suggested. A weighted decision should be made.

Definitions

Perinatal period = period starting from conception to 12 months after birth

PND = perinatal depression

EPDS = Edinburgh Postnatal Depression Scale

DSM-5 definition of a MDD with postpartum onset = major depressive episode (MDD) with symptoms start during pregnancy or in the 4 weeks following delivery

Suicidality = broad concept that can range from suicidal thoughts to suicidal attempts as well as completed suicides themselves

Learning Objectives

After reading this chapter, the readers should be able to define PND and recognize the associated symptoms. The risk factors and underlying pathophysiology of a PND must be understood. The reader must gain insight into the treatment options, both therapeutic and medicinal.

25.1 Introduction

The perinatal period (pregnancy and the first postnatal year) is a period of important changes and great adjustment. It is a period of emotional ambivalence, where high intense positive affect go hand in hand with difficult negative emotions and, consequently, vulnerability to emotional problems such as depression [1].

"Life" is programmed in the early beginning. The first 1000 days (from conception until age two) can be considered as the most intense period of life, in which every human being is formed. In no other period of life, so many biological and as socio-emotional developmental milestones have to be reached. Therefore, the environment in which these developments take place is crucial, since organ structures and functions are formed under the influence of the environment and need to last a lifetime. Spending these 1000 days (even partially) in circumstances of parental depression places a burden on the child's development [2, 3]. Perinatal depression (PND) can have a significant adverse impact on the mother, her child, and the supporting environment (e.g., partner and family). PND is heterogeneous in presentation and most likely has multifactorial etiologies for each woman. Hence, the precise mechanisms that guide these intergenerational transmissions are largely unknown.

Since the use of assisted reproduction techniques, the rates of twins and triplets have significantly increased. After a debilitating period of subfertility, couples may idealize a twin pregnancy. On the other hand, the news of a twin pregnancy may also cause anxiety because of the increased perinatal risks. Multiple pregnancy often causes more discomfort and requires greater psychosocial adaptation from parents than a singleton pregnancy. Furthermore, the physical changes that accompany pregnancy can strongly influence body image and self-confidence, which are important risk factors for PND. Obviously, sleep deprivation and increased workload are associated with the postpartum and these are even more common in twin or triplet pregnancies [4, 5]

25.2 Prevalence

Perinatal depression – comprising minor and major depressive episodes – is one of the most common complications of pregnancy [6, 7]. The estimated point prevalence of major depressive disorder is estimated in the 3·1–4·9% range during pregnancy and around 5% the first 3 months postpartum. Similarly, estimated point prevalence for minor depression is around 11% in pregnancy and 13% in the first 3 months postpartum. In addition, the period prevalence of depression during pregnancy and the first 3 months after delivery are estimated at 18.4% (12.7% having major depression) and 19.2% (7.1% having major depression), respectively [8–10]. According to a systematic review by Woody et al. (2017) [11], the overall pooled prevalence for PND is 11.9%. There were insufficient data to calculate the pooled incidence. There was a clear discrepancy between the low- and medium-income countries and the high-income countries on the other hand. It is suggested that 33% of postnatal depression has its onset during pregnancy and 27% already pre-pregnancy [12]. Moreover, PND is a burdensome disorder with a profound intrusive impact on the expectant mother, her (unborn) child, but also the supporting system [13].

The question arises whether the prevalence of PND is higher in twin and higher-order pregnancies. Most studies focus on the postpartum period, and only limited data are available on the prenatal period. Furthermore, most studies did not control for the baseline presence of depression before conception.

In a systematic review, the overall prevalence of PND in twin and higher-order pregnancies was estimated between 12.2% and 19% [14]. Ross et al. (2011) concluded that there is an association between multiple births and postpartum depression during the first postpartum year. Some smaller studies have demonstrated an increased prevalence of depression as well as anxiety in multiple pregnancies [4]. If further studies would confirm these data, this may warrant targeted interventions for this population.

Ross et al. (2011) indicated little or no increased risk for postpartum depression among women who use assisted reproductive technology (ART) to conceive versus women with naturally conceived multiple pregnancies. They pointed out that the women using ART differ from other childbearing women, because their pregnancy is planned, they are more likely to have a stable relationship and have a higher economic status [14]. Additionally, the meta-analysis by Van den akker et al. (2016) concluded that mothers of ART multiple births were significantly more likely to have depression and stress than mothers of ART singletons, but were no different from mothers of naturally conceived multiples [15].

Determining the prevalence of PND is associated with several methodological issues. First of all, the screening tools to assess depression as well as the time point of assessment within the studies vary greatly. Furthermore, different definitions of PND are applied. As a consequence, it is often not possible to differentiate between transient maternal distress and clinically significant postpartum depression. Third, the sample sizes of the study populations are often small and appropriate comparison groups lack. Additionally, most studies lack control of maternal psychiatric history and other important sociodemographic predictors of depression. The latter is of course a serious limitation. On the other hand, some studies specifically exclude women with a known psychiatric history. Finally, most of the studies do not control for the use of ART, whereas this is crucial information, since ART and the occurrence of multiple births are correlated and subfertility as well as the associated reproductive treatments can cause stress, anxiety, and depression [14].

25.3 Diagnosis and Presentation

Currently DSM and International Classification of Diseases (ICD) do not categorize PND as a separate diagnosis. DSM-IV defined PND as an episode of major depressive disorder with onset within 4 weeks of delivery [16]. According to DSM-5 a specifier "with peripartum onset" can be added to a major depressive episode (MDD) if the symptoms start during pregnancy or in the 4 weeks following delivery [17]. The ICD, 11th Edition (ICD-11), uses a time frame of 6 weeks postpartum to identify "mental and behavioral disorders associated with the puerperium," without psychotic symptoms. A distinction can be made between mild and severe depression [18].

One of the main issues is the short timeframe used in these definitions. It is debated to further extend this timeframe to 6 months unto 1 year postpartum given the numerous, unique biological, psychological, and social traits and factors that extend beyond 4 weeks after delivery [19, 20].

The presentation of PND largely resembles the presentation of MDD outside the perinatal period. Depressed mood and/or loss of interest or pleasure must be present, together with five or more additional symptoms: changes in weight or appetite, psychomotor retardation or agitation, fatigue or loss of energy, concentration difficulties, sleep disturbances (insomnia or hypersomnia), feelings of worthlessness or excessive or inappropriate guilt, and recurrent thoughts of death and/or suicidal ideation. The symptoms must have been present for 2 weeks and must cause significant distress or functional impairment. When at least two but less than five symptoms are present in the depressive episode, this is defined as minor depression. On the other hand, the presentation and content of PND might differ from MDD outside the perinatal period. PND might be accompanied by a reduction in mother–child bonding, as well as important feelings of guilt and insufficiency towards/concerning motherhood. Furthermore, isolation on an emotional and social level might occur more often, since women are ashamed of having these negative feelings and thoughts during a period, which is supposed to be a joyful period according to societal perception.

Diagnosing PND is challenging. Often PND is under-recognized because some symptoms (fatigue, sleep disturbance, changes in weight or appetite) are perceived to be normal during the perinatal period [17].

When the depression is severe, suicidality may be present. This is a broad concept that can range from suicidal thoughts to suicidal attempts as well as completed suicides themselves. Suicide is one of the leading causes of maternal and perinatal mortality. Therefore, early detection and intervention may prevent self and infant harm [9]. The exact incidence is difficult to determine, because of the stigma associated with suicidality during the perinatal period [21]. Roughly one in 50 suicides in women aged 16–50 years and one in 25 suicides in women aged 20–35 years take place in the perinatal period [22].

PND is the largest risk factor for maternal suicide and infanticide [23]. Furthermore, a prospective longitudinal research by Martini et al. (2019) revealed that a history of suicide attempt is associated with suicidality and therefore an additional important risk factor. On the other hand, living with a partner and social support significantly reduced the odds. Other risk and protective factors associated with PND are discussed below [21]. Khalifeh et al. showed that suicide during the perinatal period is often violent and more likely to occur in women with a depression diagnosis and recent illness onset, whereas this depression was less likely to be actively treated, particularly with medication [22].

A large retrospective trial by Gressier et al. (2017) studied women admitted with their child to a mother-baby unit (MBU) during the first year after birth. They concluded that more than 11% attempted suicide during the perinatal period, with two thirds of these attempts taking place in the postpartum period. Women attempting to commit suicide during pregnancy have different psychopathological and environmental profiles compared to those, attempting suicide during the postnatal period. Pregnancy suicide attempts are mostly linked to addictive behaviors and a history of miscarriage, which suggests pregnancy-related stress and/or difficulties which interfere with the pregnancy, whereas post-partum suicide attempts are more associated with mood regulation and younger age [24].

25.4 Subtypes and Course of Perinatal Depression

Recently, there has been increasing evidence that depressed mothers cannot be considered a homogeneous group [25–27]. Different subtypes of PND have been defined. Three different dimensions measured by the Edinburgh Postnatal Depression Scale (see below) were taken into account: depressed mood, anxiety, and anhedonia. On the basis of these dimensions, five distinct subtypes of PND were identified: severe anxious depression, moderate anxious depression, anxious anhedonia, pure anhedonia, and resolved depression. There are clear differences between these subtypes in terms of time of onset and symptom characteristics. Women with the subtype anxious anhedonia for example were more likely to have onset of symptoms in the postpartum period, and this subtype was associated with more severe depression [26]. On the other hand, the most depressed group in the study of the international postpartum depression: action towards causes and treatment (PACT) consortium was characterized by an onset of symptoms during pregnancy and more obstetric complications [25]. Furthermore, poor partner involvement is shown to be associated with increasing depressive symptoms during pregnancy [28].

With regard to the course of PND, further differences are observed. Although the majority of women recover from a PND, the depression can become chronic in a relatively large subgroup [27, 29]. Approximately 30% of postpartum-depressed mothers from community samples, and 50% of mothers with PND from clinical samples remained depressed beyond the first postnatal year [27]. These women also have an increased risk of approximately 40% for subsequent postnatal and non-postnatal relapse [10, 30, 31]. These findings are supported by the data from Torres et al. (2019). In their prospective study, only 66.3% of the mothers with a PND achieved full remission at 12 months postpartum, and for 9.7% of women, depressive symptoms persisted after 2 years of follow-up [29]. A perceived lower quality of partner relationship, a history of depression, sexual abuse, lower-quality maternal care, higher parental stress, contextual risk factors, and personality-related vulnerability have been consistently found to predict a chronic course of postpartum depression [27].

Furthermore, there is evidence for an increase of depressive symptomatology during pregnancy over the past decades, despite improvement of protective factors. Potential explanations may be greater awareness, high social expectations, and the influence of social media [32].

25.5 Postpartum Blues

Up to 80% of the women experience postpartum or baby blues. The onset is typically day two or three after delivery and last less than 10 days. The symptoms peak between 3 and 5 days after birth. It is important to mention that the postpartum blues is not considered to be pathological, but part of normal hormonal changes during the postpartum period. The syndrome is characterized by emotional liability (euphoria versus misery), anxiety, irritability, restlessness, insomnia, poor concentration, tearfulness, and hypersensitivity. The relationship between postpartum blues and postpartum depression remains unclear. There is limited evidence that the intensity of the blues may predict the later development of depression, but no systematic research has confirmed this. Also, the impact of multiple births on the incidence of postpartum blues remains unknown. But it is highly probable that caring for more than one baby would cause more psychological stress for a mother [5, 33].

25.6 Risk Factors

In their recent review, Kimmel et al. (2019) state that the perinatal period is associated with complex and unique biological, socio-environmental, and psychological changes for each woman. Whether or not a PND is present depends on a complex combination of risk and protective factors. As a consequence, every woman has a unique mix of factors that are dysregulated or imbalanced [9, 19, 34, 35].

The most important risk factors are a personal history of depression, anxiety or trauma, as well as a family history of (perinatal) depression. Furthermore, the lack of social support is a common risk factor. Pregnant women and women in postpartum need both emotional and practical support. Support from their partner is essential, but a wider network they can rely on is needed. If this is missing, feelings of loneliness and hopelessness may arise. With regard to personality characteristics, it is known that neuroticism, low self-esteem, and perfectionism are more frequently associated with PND. Other risk factors that may play a role are ambivalence toward pregnancy, obstetrical stressors, and socio-economic status [5, 9, 36, 37].

The abovementioned risk factors apply to singleton as well as multiple pregnancies. Twin and higher-order pregnancies entail more specific risk factors such as prematurity, obstetric complications, use of ART, and operative delivery. These risk factors are more common among multiple birth mothers [38].

After birth, the prevalence of PND is also associated with child factors. The risk of prematurity is greater with twin and higher-order pregnancies and requires a larger adjustment of the parents, both practically and emotionally. Premature newborns may be more difficult to feed and need more vigilant care. Difficult temperament, low adaptability, and unsettled behavior can further implicate care. Separation of mother and infants is common with prematurity and can be a contributing factor to PND.

Taking care of two or more infants at the same time is exhausting, especially when it is impossible to meet the needs of the infants at the same time. This can lead to a sense of guilt and hopelessness [5].

25.7 Screening

Even though PND is highly prevalent (10–20%), it is estimated that only around 40% of the cases are detected, around 20% receive any form of treatment, and 3–5% achieve remission (Milgrom & Gemill 2015; Cox, Sowa, Meltzer-Brody, & Gaynes, 2016; Flynn, Davis, Marcus, Cunningham, & Blow, 2004; Kimmel et al. 2019). Factors that might influence under-identification and treatment seem to be the heterogeneity of PND clinical presentation, stigma associated with PND, lack of transportation, difficulty obtaining child care to attend appointments, complex decision-making around whether to take medication during the perinatal period, and lack of adequate availability of perinatal mental health care providers (Goodman, 2009; Hansotte, Payne, & Babich, 2017; Kimmel et al. 2019).

A positive screening indicates that the likelihood of a possible depression is increased. Therefore, it is very important that a proper diagnosis is made, based on clinical judgment. Furthermore, a thorough psychiatric history, medication history, as well as the impact on functioning must be assessed. Ideally, this should take place during preconception counseling [39].

The purpose of screening tools in PND is its rapid detection and treatment in order to reduce the associated morbidity and mortality. During the prenatal and postnatal period, there is an increased contact with care providers, but nevertheless, still too little attention is paid to potential PND. Over the past years, there has been an ongoing debate about the benefits of depression screening during the perinatal period as a routine component of adequate maternity care. Screening programs seem to have positive results. However, there is an important need for appropriate, longitudinal, "real world" evaluations of the effectiveness of PND screening and broader psychosocial assessment programs (Reilly et al. 2019). It is important to also offer a follow-up procedure and treatment if indicated [11, 37, 40].

Currently, The Edinburgh Postnatal Depression Scale (EPDS) is the gold standard to detect PND [41]. This scale was initially developed for the postpartum period, but it has also been validated for assessment during pregnancy [42]. It contains a 10-item list regarding depression, including the presence of suicidal thoughts, and anxiety symptoms during the past 7 days. Every item has four possible answers, scored zero to three. The total score ranges from 0 to 30. Different threshold values have been suggested, with a value of 10 or more suggesting possible depression and a value of 13 or more indicating probable depression. In the systematic review by Woody et al. the EPDS cut-off for PND used in the included studies ranged from 10 to 15 [9, 11].

25.8 Pathophysiology

Until present, the pathophysiological mechanisms of PND remain unrevealed. Apart from psychosocial factors, researchers investigated potential underlying endocrinological, immunological, and (epi)genetic factors associated with PND [9, 43, 44].

A possible hypothesis regarding the pathophysiology of PND is based on the extensive fluctuations of reproductive hormones during the perinatal period. The postpartum is characterized by a rapid decline in estrogen, progesterone, and allopregnanolone levels, which may affect neurotransmission and neuroplasticity in the central nervous system. Brain-derived neurotrophic factor (BDNF) is probably associated with this process [43, 45]. Oxytocin has also been studied in connection to PND [43]. Furthermore, endocrinological changes seem to be associated with PND, such as hypothalamic–pituitary–adrenal (HPA) axis dysfunction and thyroid hormone alterations [43, 45]. Neuroimmune pathways might also be connected to PND, for example decreased levels of ω3-polyunsaturated fatty acids (PUFAs), IL-6, and leptin [43, 45].

Furthermore, the systematic review by Figueiredo et al. explored the potential influence of genetic factors on the symptoms of PND [44]. They account for potential genetic–environmental interactions. Specifically, during late pregnancy and the early postpartum period women appear to be more susceptible to genetic factors or epigenetic modifications. Since this period is characterized by strong changes in estrogen levels, there is speculation about a possible role of estrogen as a neuromodulator with possible effects on neuroplasticity [44].

However, certain forms of PND likely have stronger biologic underpinnings, whereas other forms may be more strongly influenced by the contribution of psychosocial factors [9, 43]. Further research is needed.

25.9 Perinatal Bereavement

Twin and higher-order pregnancies are associated with increased risk of complications, including prematurity, congenital fetal anomalies, and perinatal mortality. Depending on the chorionicity, these complications may either affect one twin with a healthy co-twin or have consequences for both. Prematurity and congenital abnormalities require major adjustments from (future) parents and may entail heartbreaking ethical dilemmas. These may involve grief for the loss of an imagined child and the gradual adjustment to the reality of the actual infant. Loss of an infant during pregnancy, stillbirth, or neonatal death may encompass a complex psychological paradox with mourning and detachment on the one hand and attachment on the other hand [5, 46].

25.10 Treatment

25.10.1 General Recommendations

Efficient treatment of PND is imperative [9]. The main goals of treating PND are to reduce maternal psychiatric symptoms and to support maternal–child bonding [43]. Untreated PND is associated with increased risk for negative outcomes in mother and child during the perinatal period [47–49].

Women with PND are more likely to misuse alcohol, nicotine, and other substances during pregnancy, which could negatively impact pregnancy outcomes. Untreated PND may be associated with low birthweight, increased risk of preterm delivery, gestational hypertension, and perinatal death [39, 50].

Antenatal maternal depression and anxiety have been associated with a range of adverse outcomes for the child such as preterm birth, impaired mother–infant bonding, and impaired cognitive and socio-emotional development of the child (emotional problems, symptoms of ADHD, conduct disorders, impaired cognitive function, schizophrenia, and possibly autism) [39].

All women should receive information about PND and the potential treatment options, including the potential benefits and harms of each treatment. The psychiatric symptoms, severity of the depression, psychiatric history, and preferences of the woman must be taken into account. Social support and adequate sleep should be optimized [43].

A stepped-care approach is advocated, in which the intensity of the intervention matches the severity and acuity of the clinical presentation. Mild to moderate symptoms should be treated with psychotherapeutic interventions, whereas pharmacological treatment should be suggested for women with severe symptoms or women who do not respond to nonpharmacological treatment [43].

Obviously, not only the treatment, but also the prevention of PND is mandatory. In a large review by O'Connor et al., there was evidence for the effectiveness of counseling-based interventions like depression-focused cognitive behavior therapy (CBT) and interpersonal psychotherapy (IPT) in the prevention of PND [51].

25.10.2 Nonpharmacological Therapy

A recent review, on the effect of PND treatment for mothers on parenting and child development, found promising findings exist for IPT, CBT, maternal–child interaction guidance, and other interventions including massage and psychotherapeutic group support; it is difficult to draw any definitive conclusions regarding any one treatment that shows the most potential to influence maternal and infant outcomes. Letourneau et al. (2017) concluded that there is insufficient evidence available to make policy or practice recommendations. Further research in this area is recommended [52].

25.10.2.1 Interpersonal Therapy (IPT)

IPT is a validated form of psychotherapy with a focus on the interpersonal context and the changes and stressors that can lead to depressive symptoms. It is not surprising that this form of psychotherapy is helpful for PND, since the theme of role change during pregnancy and postpartum plays an important role. This form of therapy can also be useful if there are problems in the interpersonal context, such as relationship problems or little social support, because these are known risk factors for PND [53, 54].

A systematic review by Sockol et al. (2018) and a meta-analysis by van Ravensteyn et al. (2017) assessed the efficacy of IPT during pregnancy. In prevention studies, IPT was effective for reducing depressive symptoms and the prevalence of depressive episodes. In treatment studies, IPT reduced symptoms of depression and anxiety and improved relationship quality, social adjustment, and social support [53, 54].

25.10.2.2 Cognitive Behavioral Therapy (CBT)

The principle idea of CBT is the assumption that thoughts (dysfunctional patterns of cognition) have an influence on our behavior and on how we feel, and vice versa. The techniques used in CBT focus on changing the content of these irrational cognitions [54, 55].

Results of the meta-analysis by Sockol et al. (2015) and van Ravensteyn et al. (2017) provide evidence of CBT being effective in the treatment and prevention of PND, with small to moderate effects as a result [54, 55].

25.10.2.3 Mindfulness-Based Interventions (MBI)

Mindfulness can be defined as a mental state that is characterized by focusing on the present moment and awareness of present feelings, thoughts, and bodily sensations. MBI are relatively new and are effective in the prevention and treatment of depression and anxiety, especially by reducing the levels of rumination. Despite promising results in the general population, between-group analyses failed to find any significant post-intervention benefits of MBI for depression, anxiety, or stress in comparison to control conditions in a recent meta-analysis by Taylor et al. [56]

25.10.3 Pharmacologic Treatment

25.10.3.1 General Recommendations

As previously reported, the current guidelines agree on psychotherapy (especially cognitive behavioral therapy) as initial treatment for mild to moderate new depressive episodes versus antidepressants for severe depression.

The start or modification of antidepressant therapy during pregnancy or postpartum should be based on an individual assessment of the risks and benefits in each particular case. This must be properly discussed with the future parents and all care providers involved. Clear information about the risks of the medication, as well as the risks of untreated disease must be discussed extensively. It is advised to avoid switching medication during pregnancy unless the benefits outweigh the risks. Equally, suddenly stopping medication should be avoided to prevent withdrawal symptoms. Monotherapy is preferred, with the lowest effective dose. In women with severe PND, it is recommended that delivery should take place in hospital [39]. For ongoing depression, there is an ongoing debate on whether or not antidepressants can and should be discontinued [50].

In the past, much of the data regarding the risks of medication in the perinatal period have been retrospective. Fortunately, during recent years, there have been larger prospective cohort studies. Molenaar et al. (2018) reviewed 16 Clinical Practice Guidelines (CPG), half of which were exclusively on perinatal management, the other half were general guidelines with a section on perinatal recommendations. Most of the guidelines recommend sertraline and citalopram during pregnancy. Breastfeeding is encouraged with sertraline as preferred medication. Most of the guidelines agree on avoiding paroxetine during pregnancy, because of increased risk of congenital cardiovascular malformations in the newborn. Therefore, paroxetine is not the preferred treatment for new episodes, but on the other hand switching antidepressants for ongoing treatment is discouraged [50]. Fluoxetine was marked "unfavorable" by five guidelines due to its long half-life and its presence in breast milk.

A recent study analyzed prescribing patterns during pregnancy for antipsychotics (APs), antidepressants (ADs), and mood-stabilizing antiepileptics (AEDs) in Denmark from 2000 to 2016. A marked increase in the prevalence of the use of ADs during pregnancy was seen from 2000 to 2011 (from 6 to 41 per 1000 pregnancies ending in a delivery), but currently they appear slightly in decline. Age, smoking, obesity, and social status were generally associated with increased use of psychotropic drugs [57].

25.10.3.2 Congenital Malformation

Serotonin is essential for healthy fetal development during embryogenesis. SSRIs cross the placental barrier and block serotonin reuptake transporter (SERT) sites, disturbing the free movement of serotonin during this critical phase of development, which can impact morphogenesis and organogenesis [58, 59].

Despite the available research, there is no general consensus regarding the risk of in utero antidepressant exposure and congenital malformations. The association between antidepressant use during pregnancy and congenital malformations could be explained by the underlying maternal depression, unaccounted potential confounders, lack of statistical power, etc. The available literature is limited on singleton pregnancies and multiple pregnancies are mostly excluded, due to the known increased risk of adverse pregnancy outcomes. Furthermore, miscarriage is usually excluded, although this can be an indicator of severe malformations [59].

According to the 2018 NICE guideline, there was some evidence for a statistically significant association between all SSRIs and congenital malformations (p = 0.04) with an absolute risk difference of 9 more per 1000 [60]. Regarding the risk of cardiac malformations, the cohort-study by Huybrechts et al. (2014) suggested no increase in the risk of cardiac malformations attributable to antidepressant use during the first trimester [61]. A Nordic population-based study by Furu et al. (2015) confirms these findings. Although the prevalence of septal defects and right ventricular outflow tract defects was higher in exposed infants, the lack of an association in the sibling-controlled analyses points against a teratogenic effect of these drugs [62].

Regarding the specific SSRIs, paroxetine was statistically associated with congenital (p = 0.05), major congenital (p = 0.04), and cardiac (p = 0.006) malformations, and fluoxetine with major congenital (p = 0.008) and cardiac (p = 0.02) malformations with absolute risk differences ranging from 3 to 8 more per 1000. There was some evidence for a statistically significant association between citalopram and escitalopram and ventricular septal defects with absolute risk difference of 4 and 9 more per 1000, respectively [60].

25.10.3.3 Pregnancy Outcome

The effect of antidepressant use and pregnancy outcome was extensively studied by Ross et al. (2014) in their systematic review and meta-analysis. They concluded that there was no significant association between antidepressant medication exposure and miscarriage. Gestational age and preterm delivery were statistically significantly associated with antidepressant exposure (mean difference [MD] [weeks], 0.45; 95% CI, 0.64–0.25; P < 0.001; and OR, 1.55; 95% CI, 1.38–1.74; P < 0.001, respectively). Also, antidepressant exposure during pregnancy was significantly associated with lower birth weight (MD [grams], −74; 95% CI, 117–31; P = 0.001). When this comparison group was limited to depressed mothers without antidepressant exposure, there no longer was a significant association. Antidepressant exposure was significantly associated with lower Apgar scores at 1 and 5 minutes (Ross 2014). SSRIs are also known for their increased risk of bleeding [14].

25.10.3.4 Poor Neonatal Adaptation Syndrome (PNAS) and Persistent Pulmonary Hypertension of the Newborn (PPHN)

Multiple studies support the existence of a poor neonatal adaptation syndrome (PNAS) after in utero exposure to SSRIs. The most common symptoms are irritability, constant crying, sleep disturbances, respiratory problems, tremors, hypotonia, vomiting, and feeding difficulties. Most symptoms develop within 2 days after birth, are usually mild, and disappear spontaneously.

Due to the absence of validated questionnaires for neonatal withdrawal based on SSRI use of the mother, the Finnegan questionnaire is frequently used. The Finnegan score assesses withdrawal symptoms based on addiction of the mother, but this has not been validated for withdrawal based on SSRI use in the mother [39, 63, 64]. Klinger et al. (2011) showed that infants who developed PNAS had normal cognitive ability, but were at an increased risk for social–behavioral abnormalities. Therefore, they concluded that follow-up evaluation of symptomatic neonates should be considered [63].

Another risk associated with SSRI use during pregnancy is persistent pulmonary hypertension of the newborn (PPHN). Serotonin has a role in the development and modulation of the lungs, and this could be a factor in the development of PPHN [10]. The findings of a large network meta-analysis by Masarwa et al. (2019) suggest that exposure to SSRIs during pregnancy is associated with a twofold increased risk for PPHN. Sertraline is most likely to have the lowest risk for PPHN compared to other SSRIs [65].

25.10.4 Review Questions

1. Define a PND.

2. Which symptoms are associated with a PND?

3. How to screen for a PND?

4. Which factors play a role in the pathophysiology of PND

5. What are the treatment options of PND?

25.10.5 Multiple-Choice Questions

1. What is the prevalence of major and minor PND?
   (a) 10–20%
   (b) <5%
   (c) 5–10%
   (d) >20%

Answer: (a)

2. Which of the following symptoms are not mentioned in the definition of a MDD according to the DSM 5?
   (a) Suicidality
   (b) Sleep disturbances
   (c) Loss of interest
   (d) Panic attacks

Answer: (d)

3. What is the percentage of women who suffer from postpartum blues?
   (a) 50%
   (b) 80%
   (c) 20%
   (d) 40%

Answer: (b)

4. Which SSRI should be avoided during pregnancy because of increased risk of congenital cardiovascular malformations in the newborn?
   (a) Sertraline
   (b) Escitalopram
   (c) Paroxetine
   (d) Fluoxetine

Answer: (c)

5. Which questionnaire is currently considered the gold standard for PND screening?
   (a) EPDS
   (b) STAI
   (c) HAMD
   (d) MINI

Answer: (a)

References

1. Zeanah C. Handbook of infant mental health. 4th ed. New York & London: The Guilford Press; 2019.
2. Roseboom T. De eerste 1000 dagen – Het fundamentele belang van een goed begin vanuit biologisch, medisch en maatschappelijk perspectief. Utrecht: de Tijdstroom; 2018.
3. Van den Bergh BRH, van den Heuvel MI, Lahti M, Braeken M, de Rooij SR, Entringer S, et al. Prenatal developmental origins of behavior and mental health: the influence of maternal stress in pregnancy. Neurosci Biobehav Rev. 2017;S0149-7634(16):30734–5.
4. Benute GR, Nozzella DC, Prohaska C, Liao A, de Lucia MC, Zugaib M. Twin pregnancies: evaluation of major depression, stress, and social support. Twin Res Hum Genet. 2013;16(2):629–33.
5. Fisher J, Stocky A. Maternal perinatal mental health and multiple births: implications for practice. Twin Res. 2003;6(6):506–13.
6. Kendig S, Keats JP, Hoffman MC, Kay LB, Miller ES, Simas TAM, et al. Consensus bundle on maternal mental health: perinatal depression and anxiety. J Midwifery Womens Health. 2017;62(2):232–9.
7. Wisner KL, Sit DK, McShea MC, Rizzo DM, Zoretich RA, Hughes CL, et al. Onset timing, thoughts of self-harm, and diagnoses in postpartum women with screen-positive depression findings. JAMA Psychiat. 2013;70(5):490–8.
8. Gavin NI, Gaynes BN, Lohr KN, Meltzer-Brody S, Gartlehner G, Swinson T. Perinatal depression: a systematic review of prevalence and incidence. Obstet Gynecol. 2005;106(5 Pt 1):1071–83.
9. Kimmel MC, Bauer A, Meltzer-Brody S. Toward a framework for best practices and research guidelines for perinatal depression research. J Neurosci Res. 2019;98(7):1255–67.
10. Howard LM, Molyneaux E, Dennis CL, Rochat T, Stein A, Milgrom J. Non-psychotic mental disorders in the perinatal period. Lancet. 2014;384(9956):1775–88.
11. Woody CA, Ferrari AJ, Siskind DJ, Whiteford HA, Harris MG. A systematic review and meta-regression of the prevalence and incidence of perinatal depression. J Affect Disord. 2017;219:86–92.
12. Heron J, O'Connor TG, Evans J, Golding J, Glover V, Team AS. The course of anxiety and depression through pregnancy and the postpartum in a community sample. J Affect Disord. 2004;80(1):65–73.
13. Atif N, Lovell K, Rahman A. Maternal mental health: the missing "m" in the global maternal and child health agenda. Semin Perinatol. 2015;39(5):345–52.
14. Ross LE, McQueen K, Vigod S, Dennis CL. Risk for postpartum depression associated with assisted reproductive technologies and multiple births: a systematic review. Hum Reprod Update. 2011;17(1):96–106.
15. van den Akker O, Postavaru GI, Purewal S. Maternal psychosocial consequences of twins and multiple births following assisted and natural conception: a meta-analysis. Reprod Biomed Online. 2016;33(1):1–14.
16. American Psychiatric Publishing. Diagnostic and statistical manual of mental disorders. 4th ed. Arlington: American Psychiatric Publishing; 2000.
17. American Psychiatric Publishing. Diagnostic and statistical manual of mental disorders. 5th ed. Arlington: American Psychiatric Publishing; 2013.
18. Prevention CfDCa. International classification of diseases, 11th revision, clinical modification (ICD-11-CM). Geneva: WHO; 2019.
19. O'Hara MW, Wisner KL. Perinatal mental illness: definition, description and aetiology. Best Pract Res Clin Obstet Gynaecol. 2014;28(1):3–12.
20. Sharma V, Mazmanian D. The DSM-5 peripartum specifier: prospects and pitfalls. Arch Womens Ment Health. 2014;17(2):171–3.
21. Martini J, Bauer M, Lewitzka U, Voss C, Pfennig A, Ritter D, et al. Predictors and outcomes of suicidal ideation during peripartum period. J Affect Disord. 2019;257:518–26.
22. Khalifeh H, Hunt IM, Appleby L, Howard LM. Suicide in perinatal and non-perinatal women in contact with psychiatric services: 15 year findings from a UK national inquiry. Lancet Psychiatry. 2016;3(3):233–42.
23. Lindahl V, Pearson JL, Colpe L. Prevalence of suicidality during pregnancy and the postpartum. Arch Womens Ment Health. 2005;8(2):77–87.
24. Gressier F, Guillard V, Cazas O, Falissard B, et al. Risk factors for suicide attempt in pregnancy and the post-partum period in women with serious mental illnesses. J Psychiatr Res. 2017;84:284–91.
25. Consortium PDATCaTP. Heterogeneity of postpartum depression: a latent class analysis. Lancet Psychiatry. 2015;2(1):59–67.
26. Putnam KT, Wilcox M, Robertson-Blackmore E, Sharkey K, Bergink V, Munk-Olsen T, et al. Clinical phenotypes of perinatal depression and time of symptom onset: analysis of data from an international consortium. Lancet Psychiatry. 2017;4(6):477–85.
27. Vliegen N, Casalin S, Luyten P. The course of postpartum depression: a review of longitudinal studies. Harv Rev Psychiatry. 2014;22(1):1–22.
28. Boekhorst MGBM, Beerthuizen A, Van Son M, Bergink V, Pop VJM. Psychometric aspects of the Tilburg pregnancy distress scale: data from the HAPPY study. Arch Womens Ment Health. 2019;23(2):215–9.
29. Torres A, Gelabert E, Roca A, Navarro P, Plaza A, Subirà S, et al. Course of a major postpartum depressive episode: a prospective 2 years naturalistic follow-up study. J Affect Disord. 2019;245:965–70.
30. Cooper PJ, Murray L. Course and recurrence of postnatal depression. Evidence for the specificity

of the diagnostic concept. Br J Psychiatry. 1995;166(2):191–5.
31. Wisner KL, Perel JM, Peindl KS, Hanusa BH. Timing of depression recurrence in the first year after birth. J Affect Disord. 2004;78(3):249–52.
32. Pop V, van Son M, Wijnen H, Spek V, Denollet J, Bergink V. Increase of depressive symptomatology during pregnancy over 25 years' time in four population based cohorts. J Affect Disord. 2019;259:175–9.
33. Marcus SM, Heringhausen JE. Depression in childbearing women: when depression complicates pregnancy. Prim Care. 2009;36(1):151–65, ix.
34. Vigod SN, Wilson CA, Howard LM. Depression in pregnancy. BMJ. 2016;352:i1547.
35. Howard LM, Piot P, Stein A. No health without perinatal mental health. Lancet. 2014;384(9956):1723–4.
36. Lancaster CA, Gold KJ, Flynn HA, Yoo H, Marcus SM, Davis MM. Risk factors for depressive symptoms during pregnancy: a systematic review. Am J Obstet Gynecol. 2010;202(1):5–14.
37. O'Hara MW, McCabe JE. Postpartum depression: current status and future directions. Annu Rev Clin Psychol. 2013;9:379–407.
38. Choi Y, Bishai D, Minkovitz CS. Multiple births are a risk factor for postpartum maternal depressive symptoms. Pediatrics. 2009;123(4):1147–54.
39. McAllister-Williams RH, Baldwin DS, Cantwell R, Easter A, Gilvarry E, Glover V, et al. British Association for Psychopharmacology consensus guidance on the use of psychotropic medication preconception, in pregnancy and postpartum 2017. J Psychopharmacol. 2017;31(5):519–52.
40. Milgrom J, Gemmill A, editors. Identifying perinatal depression and anxiety: evidence-based practice in screening, psychosocial assessment and management. Chichester: Wiley; 2015.
41. Cox JL, Holden JM, Sagovsky R. Detection of postnatal depression. Development of the 10-item Edinburgh Postnatal Depression Scale. Br J Psychiatry. 1987;150:782–6.
42. Bergink V, Kooistra L, et al. Validation of the Edinburgh Depression Scale during pregnancy. J Psychosom Res. 2011;70(4):385–9.
43. Meltzer-Brody S, Howard LM, Bergink V, Vigod S, Jones I, Munk-Olsen T, et al. Postpartum psychiatric disorders. Nat Rev Dis Primers. 2018;4:18022.
44. Figueiredo FP, Parada AP, de Araujo LF, Silva WA, Del-Ben CM. The influence of genetic factors on peripartum depression: a systematic review. J Affect Disord. 2015;172:265–73.
45. Serati M, Redaelli M, Buoli M, Altamura AC. Perinatal major depression biomarkers: a systematic review. J Affect Disord. 2016;193:391–404.
46. Meaney S, Corcoran P, O'Donoghue K. Death of one twin during the perinatal period: an interpretative phenomenological analysis. J Palliat Med. 2017;20(3):290–3.
47. Muzik M, Bocknek EL, Broderick A, Richardson P, Rosenblum KL, Thelen K, et al. Mother-infant bonding impairment across the first 6 months postpartum: the primacy of psychopathology in women with childhood abuse and neglect histories. Arch Womens Ment Health. 2013;16(1):29–38.
48. Shonkoff J, Philips D. From neurons to neighborhoods: the science of early childhood development. Washington, DC: National Academies Press; 2000.
49. Kimmel M, Clive M, Gispen F, Guintivano J, Brown T, Cox O, et al. Oxytocin receptor DNA methylation in postpartum depression. Psychoneuroendocrinology. 2016;69:150–60.
50. Molenaar NM, Kamperman AM, Boyce P, Bergink V. Guidelines on treatment of perinatal depression with antidepressants: an international review. Aust N Z J Psychiatry. 2018;52(4):320–7.
51. O'Connor E, Senger CA, Henninger ML, Coppola E, Gaynes BN. Interventions to prevent perinatal depression: evidence report and systematic review for the US preventive services task force. JAMA. 2019;321(6):588–601.
52. Letourneau NL, Dennis CL, Cosic N, Linder J. The effect of perinatal depression treatment for mothers on parenting and child development: a systematic review. Depress Anxiety. 2017;34(10):928–66.
53. Sockol LE. A systematic review and meta-analysis of interpersonal psychotherapy for perinatal women. J Affect Disord. 2018;232:316–28.
54. van Ravesteyn LM, Lambregtse-van den Berg MP, Hoogendijk WJ, Kamperman AM. Interventions to treat mental disorders during pregnancy: a systematic review and multiple treatment meta-analysis. PLoS One. 2017;12(3):e0173397.
55. Sockol LE. A systematic review of the efficacy of cognitive behavioral therapy for treating and preventing perinatal depression. J Affect Disord. 2015;177:7–21.
56. Lever Taylor B, Cavanagh K, Strauss C. The effectiveness of mindfulness-based interventions in the perinatal period: a systematic review and meta-analysis. PLoS One. 2016;11(5):e0155720.
57. Damkier P, Christensen LS, Broe A. Patterns and predictors for prescription of psychotropics and mood-stabilizing antiepileptics during pregnancy in Denmark 2000-2016. Br J Clin Pharmacol. 2018;84(11):2651–62.
58. Sadler TW. Selective serotonin reuptake inhibitors (SSRIs) and heart defects: potential mechanisms for the observed associations. Reprod Toxicol. 2011;32(4):484–9.
59. Bérard A, Zhao JP, Sheehy O. Antidepressant use during pregnancy and the risk of major congenital malformations in a cohort of depressed pregnant women: an updated analysis of the Quebec Pregnancy Cohort. BMJ Open. 2017;7(1):e013372.
60. NICE. Antenatal and postnatal Mental Health. The NICE guideline on clinical management and service guidance – Updated edition: The Royal

Psychological Society and the Royal College of Psychiatrists (National Institute for Health and Care Excellence – National Collaborating Centre for Mental Health); 2018.
61. Huybrechts KF, Palmsten K, Avorn J, Cohen LS, Holmes LB, Franklin JM, et al. Antidepressant use in pregnancy and the risk of cardiac defects. N Engl J Med. 2014;370(25):2397–407.
62. Furu K, Kieler H, Haglund B, Engeland A, Selmer R, Stephansson O, et al. Selective serotonin reuptake inhibitors and venlafaxine in early pregnancy and risk of birth defects: population based cohort study and sibling design. BMJ. 2015;350:h1798.
63. Klinger G, Frankenthal D, Merlob P, Diamond G, Sirota L, Levinson-Castiel R, et al. Long-term outcome following selective serotonin reuptake inhibitor induced neonatal abstinence syndrome. J Perinatol. 2011;31(9):615–20.
64. Levinson-Castiel R, Merlob P, Linder N, Sirota L, Klinger G. Neonatal abstinence syndrome after in utero exposure to selective serotonin reuptake inhibitors in term infants. Arch Pediatr Adolesc Med. 2006;160(2):173–6.
65. Masarwa R, Bar-Oz B, Gorelik E, Reif S, Perlman A, Matok I. Prenatal exposure to selective serotonin reuptake inhibitors and serotonin norepinephrine reuptake inhibitors and risk for persistent pulmonary hypertension of the newborn: a systematic review, meta-analysis, and network meta-analysis. Am J Obstet Gynecol. 2019;220(1):57, e1–e13.

Key Reading

Gavin NI, Gaynes BN, Lohr KN, Meltzer-Brody S, Gartlehner G, Swinson T. Perinatal depression: a systematic review of prevalence and incidence. Obstet Gynecol. 2005;106(5 Pt 1):1071–83.

Kimmel MC, Bauer A, Meltzer-Brody S. Toward a framework for best practices and research guidelines for perinatal depression research. J Neurosci Res. 2019;98(7):1255–67.

McAllister-Williams RH, Baldwin DS, Cantwell R, Easter A, Gilvarry E, Glover V, Green L, et al. British Association for Psychopharmacology consensus guidance on the use of psychotropic medication preconception, in pregnancy and postpartum 2017. J Psychopharmacol. 2017;31(5):519–52.

Meltzer-Brody S, Howard LM, Bergink V, Vigod S, Jones I, Munk-Olsen T, Honikman S, Milgrom J. Postpartum psychiatric disorders. Nat Rev Dis Primers. 2018;4:18022.

Ross LE, McQueen K, Vigod S, Dennis CL. Risk for postpartum depression associated with assisted reproductive technologies and multiple births: a systematic review. Hum Reprod Update. 2011;17(1):96–106.

Van den Akker O, Postavaru GI, Purewal S. Maternal psychosocial consequences of twins and multiple births following assisted and natural conception: a meta-analysis. Reprod Biomed Online. 2016;33(1):1–14.

Postnatal Neonatal Assessment in Monochorionic Twins

Enrico Lopriore

Contents

A. Khalil et al. (eds.), *Twin and Higher-order Pregnancies*,
https://doi.org/10.1007/978-3-030-47652-6_26

Trailer

Monochorionic twins are not only at increased risk of severe complications during pregnancy, but also after birth. Antenatal disorders such as twin-twin transfusion syndrome (TTTS) and twin anaemia-polycythaemia sequence (TAPS) may leave temporary or permanent marks in survivors and require specific management during the neonatal period. As most TTTS and TAPS survivors are born prematurely, these neonates are primarily at risk for morbidity associated with prematurity. Additionally, specific complications related to TTTS and TAPS may occur in neonatal survivors including cardiovascular morbidity (right ventricular outflow tract obstruction and persistent pulmonary hypertension of the newborn, renal failure and haematological disorders. The most important and dreaded complication in survivors is cerebral injury, as it may have profound and lifelong impact on these infants. In this chapter, we summarize the different risks of neonatal morbidity and discuss postnatal assessment and management in the various subgroups of complicated monochorionic twins.

Learning Objectives

After reading this chapter, readers should be able to recognize the differences between twin-twin transfusion syndrome, twin anaemia-polycythaemia sequence and acute peripartum twin-twin transfusion syndrome. The reader should gain insight into the management options and diagnostic work-up in complicated monochorionic twins.

26.1 Introduction

Twins, either dichorionic or monochorionic, have higher neonatal morbidity and mortality rates compared to singletons, mainly due to the higher rate of prematurity and low birth weight [1–3]. Monochorionic twins carry a higher risk compared to dichorionic twins due to their unique placenta architecture with vascular anastomoses which can lead to inter-twin blood transfusion. When the inter-twin transfusion is unbalanced, severe disorders such as twin-twin transfusion syndrome (TTTS) and twin anaemia-polycythaemia sequence (TAPS) may occur.

As the majority of TTTS and TAPS survivors are born prematurely, these neonates are at risk for morbidity associated with prematurity, including respiratory disease, necrotizing enterocolitis, retinopathy of prematurity and cerebral injury [4, 5]. Additionally, specific complications related to the complicated monochorionic pregnancy may occur in neonatal survivors including cardiovascular morbidity, renal failure, haematological disorders, ischaemic limb injury and pseudo-amniotic bands syndrome [5–8]. The most important and dreaded complication in survivors is cerebral injury, as it may have profound and lifelong impact on these infants. In this chapter, we summarize the risks of neonatal morbidity and discuss postnatal assessment in the various subgroups of complicated monochorionic twins.

26.2 Cerebral Injury and Neurologic Assessment

Cerebral injury is the most feared complication in survivors of complicated monochorionic pregnancies. The risk for cerebral injury is highest for single survivors after intrauterine demise of their co-twin, caused by severe hypovolaemia and anaemia following acute exsanguination and blood loss from the surviving fetus into their dying or dead sibling through patent vascular connections [9–11]. Up to one third of co-twins may suffer from severe brain injury and, as a consequence, up to one fourth may develop severe long-term neurodevelopmental impairment. Importantly, fetoscopic laser surgery protects against cerebral injury after single fetal demise, provided that the surgery is complete and no anastomoses are missed.

In TTTS, the incidence of cerebral injury has dropped considerably since the introduction of laser therapy and reported ranges are now between 2% and 18% [12–19]. In our own centre, the incidence has decreased since the start of our laser surgery program in 2000 from 14% in the first 5 years, to 6% in the most recently studied cohort treated between 2011 and 2014 [20, 21]. Various reasons have been suggested to explain the decrease in brain injury, including improvement in laser technique, learning curve effect, both associated with a decrease in post-operative complications such as post-laser TAPS or recurrent TTTS. In a large cohort of 1023 TTTS pregnancies, post-operative TAPS and recurrence of TTTS after laser, both known to be caused by residual anastomoses, were associated with increased risk of cerebral injury [22, 23].

Several types of cerebral injury have been described in the literature, including (cystic) periventricular leukomalacia (PVL), cerebral white-matter cysts, intraventricular haemorrhage (IVH), ventricular dilatation, cerebral atrophy and arterial ischaemic stroke. Fetal and neonatal MRI studies have shed more light on brain abnormalities detected in TTTS in the last decade. Several studies have reported additional findings of MRI compared to ultrasound alone, including polymicrogyria and other migrational disorders, sinus thrombosis, and more subtle signs of ischaemia such as loss of white matter volume [17, 23–27]. Donors and recipients are equally affected by cerebral injury, although the occurrence of middle cerebral artery stroke seems to be a specific risk for recipients [15, 23, 28]. The range of cerebral injury reported by different groups is quite wide, which is due to varying definitions of cerebral injury, differences in the timing and frequency of imaging, and the fact that some centres do not routinely perform cranial imaging in all TTTS survivors.

Prematurity is still more the rule than the exception in TTTS and TAPS pregnancies, making survivors prone to postnatally acquired cerebral damage related to (extreme) prematurity, especially IVH and PVL. Prematurity and low birth weight (with birth weight being strongly correlated with gestational age) have in fact been proven to be the most important risk factors for severe cerebral injuries in survivors of TTTS [15, 19]. Reduction of severe prematurity in complicated monochorionic pregnancies could hypothetically be achieved by reduction of the risk of PPROM and intrauterine infection through further technical improvements in fetoscopic surgery (e.g. by developing smaller fetoscopic instruments). Besides postnatal brain injury caused by prematurity, antenatally acquired cerebral lesions are more common in the context of complicated monochorionic pregnancies compared to dichorionic twins, presumably because of the severe nature of TTTS and TAPS during pregnancy [15]. When antenatal in origin, cerebral injury in donors is thought to be mainly caused by impaired cerebral perfusion as the result of haemodynamic imbalance and inter-twin shifts of blood, leading to hypoxic-ischaemic insults. Polycythaemia and hyperviscosity with subsequent vascular sludging are the presumed mechanisms for cerebral injury in recipients.

Given the remaining risk of cerebral injury for TTTS and TAPS survivors, routine standardized antenatal and postnatal cerebral imaging protocols are strongly recommended to accurately evaluate origin, timing and type of damage. MRI may play a larger role in determining cerebral injury in the future. Increased awareness of the increased risk by neonatologists and paediatricians may improve neonatal and paediatric care for these children. The clinical relevance of neuroimaging findings should be determined using long-term neurodevelopmental outcome data until at least school age in all survivors of complicated monochorionic twin pregnancies. An overview of the suggested diagnostic evaluations in complicated monochorionic twins at birth is summarized in ◘ Table 26.1.

26.3 Cardiac Morbidity and Cardiovascular Assessment

Monochorionic twins are at an increased risk of developing congenital heart defects (CHDs) compared to singletons and dichorionic twins) [8]. The development of acquired CHDs in this specific group of twins is associated with TTTS. In a recent systematic review and meta-analysis, we estimated the preva-

Table 26.1 Recommended or suggested postnatal evaluations in complicated monochorionic twins

	Recommended	Suggested	Comments
Haemoglobin levels at birth	YES	–	Determine intertwin haemoglobin difference
Reticulocyte count at birth	YES	–	Measure count in ‰, and calculate reticulocyte ratio
Cerebral ultrasound	YES	–	Preferably on day 1 (to rule out antenatal injury)
Echocardiography	–	YES	In recipient twins with TTS (to rule out RVOTO or PPHN)
Renal function	–	YES	In donor twins with TTS treated with amnioreduction or not successfully treated with laser
Albumin, total protein	–	YES	In donor twins with TAPS
Hearing test	YES	–	In donor twins with TAPS (see ▶ Chap. 17)
Placental dye injection	YES	–	See ▶ Chap. 3

lence of CHD in monochorionic twins to be 59 per 1000 live births, which is more than 6 times higher compared to singleton live births [29]. In TTTS survivors, the risk appears to be even higher, with a 12-fold increased risk compared to singletons. The estimated prevalence in these neonates is 111.3 per 1000 live births. The increased incidence of CHDs can mainly be attributed to the risk of right ventricular outflow tract obstruction (RVOTO) (35/1000 TTTS twin live births vs. 0.5/1000 singleton live births), primarily in the recipient twin [8]. The exact pathophysiologic mechanisms leading to RVOTO in recipient twins in TTTS is not entirely known. Hypothetically, chronic cardiac overload and hypervolaemia in these recipients may result in shear stress and ventricular hypertrophy, which can cause abnormal development of the cardiac valves through a cascade of events. Shear stress causes endothelial changes, and right ventricular hypertrophy and severe tricuspid valve regurgitation lead to diminished flow across the right ventricular outflow tract, which may impair growth and development of the right ventricular outflow tract.

In addition, recipient twins with TTTS are also at increased risk of persistent pulmonary hypertension of the newborn (PPHN) [8]. PPHN is probably the result of both increased pulmonary vascular resistance (PVR) from vasoactive substances and chronic volume overload [30, 31]. This chronic volume loading might cause remodelling of the pulmonary vasculature, which could result in neonatal PPHN. In a recent case-control study, we reported that the prevalence of PPHN requiring inhaled nitric oxide (iNO) in TTTS twins was 40 per 1000 live births (24/598, 95% confidence interval [CI] 2.7–5.9%) compared to 4 per 1000 live births (2/493, 95% CI 0.1–1.5%) in uncomplicated monochorionic twins (odds ratio [OR] 10.3, 95% CI 2.4–43.9; $p = 0.002$) [32]. Several risk factors were independently associated with PPHN including severe prematurity (OR 3.3, 95% CI 1.0–11.4), recipient status (OR 3.9, 95% CI 1.4–11.0) and the presence of anaemia at birth (OR 7.2, 95% CI 1.8–29.6) [32]. Based on these findings, clinicians caring for neonates with TTTS should be aware of the 10-fold increased risk of PPHN compared to uncomplicated monochorionic twins. Importantly, as the development of severe PPHN is difficult to predict, we advise that all TTTS twins should be delivered in a tertiary care centre with iNO treatment options.

In view of the severe clinical course and need for adequate and prompt treatment with iNO in case of PPHN and surgical intervention with balloon valvuloplasty in case of RVOTO, perinatologists should be aware of the increased risk of these severe cardiovascular complications in TTTS. In addition, given the higher risk of CHD, we recommend an expert fetal echocardiogram in all MC twins and follow-up scans in the event of TTTS. We also suggest that postnatal cardiac evaluation should be performed in all TTTS survivors.

26.4 Haematological Disorders and Blood Counts Assessment

In TTTS, haemoglobin differences are already present antenatally, but may also be encountered at birth [33, 34]. The presence of haemoglobin differences after delivery depends on the type of antenatal treatment. In TTTS twins treated with fetoscopic laser coagulation, no significant differences in haemoglobin levels between donor twins and recipient twins are found. On the other hand, in TTTS twins treated conservatively, donor twins have lower haemoglobin levels at birth compared to recipients. Donors may be severely anaemic, whereas recipients may suffer from severe hyperviscosity-polycythaemia.

In TAPS, large inter-twin haemoglobin differences at birth (>8 g/dL) are typically found. TAPS is based on chronic unbalanced inter-twin transfusion. Donor twins have therefore chronic anaemia and often require a blood transfusion at birth but are usually haemodynamically stable. On the other hand, recipient twins may be severely polycythaemic and require a partial exchange transfusion [35, 36]. Due to hyperviscosity, recipients may suffer from vascular limb necrosis or severe cerebral injury [37, 38]. Donor twins with TAPS always have a highly increased reticulocyte count and the ratio of reticulocyte counts between donor and recipient is >1.7. Reticulocyte count should always be measured to distinguish between TAPS (high reticulocyte count ratio >1.7) and acute peripartum TTTS (low reticulocyte count ratio <1.7). Examination of the placenta is also crucial to discriminate between the two disorders. One of the diagnostic criteria for TAPS is based on the detection of small anastomoses after careful placenta injection. However, placenta injection is not always easy and is only performed in a few specialized centres. Alternatively, examination of the maternal side of the placenta can help perinatologists, since in TAPS the placenta share of the recipient is much darker compared to the pale placenta share of the donor. In acute peripartum TTTS, no colour difference is detected between the two placenta shares.

In acute peripartum TTTS, large inter-twin haemoglobin differences are also always present at birth due to acute transfusion through large superficial anastomoses [39]. The diagnostic criteria for acute peripartum TTTS are based on a large difference in haemoglobin levels of >8 g/dL at birth in the absence of chronic TTTS or TAPS. Presence of oligo-polyhydramnios antenatally (criterion for chronic TTTS) or large reticulocyte count ratio and minuscule anastomoses (criterion for TAPS) should therefore be ruled out before reaching the diagnosis of acute peripartum TTTS. However, in most case reports reticulocyte count or placenta injection studies were not performed and TAPS could not be ruled out. We suspect that the majority of these reported cases were wrongly diagnosed and were probably TAPS cases. In our experience, TAPS occurs more frequently than acute peripartum TTTS. The donor in case of acute peripartum TTTS suffers from acute blood loss which may lead to hypovolaemic shock requiring an acute blood transfusion or an acute 0.9% NaCl bolus to increase the blood volume and blood pressure. Recipient twins on the other hand may need partial exchange transfusion in case of severe polycythaemia-hyperviscosity. Importantly, haemoglobin levels are often measured directly after birth, but in case of acute blood loss or transfusion, equilibration of haemoglobin levels occurs only several hours after the event. In case of suspected acute peripartum TTTS, haemoglobin level measurements should therefore be repeated approximately 4–6 hours after birth to determine the true haemoglobin levels. Clinical and haematological differences between TAPS and acute peripartum TTTS are summarized in ◘ Table 26.2.

Interestingly, haemoglobin differences also occur in uncomplicated monochorionic

Table 26.2 Differences between TAPS and acute peripartum TTTS

	Twin anaemia-polycythaemia sequence (TAPS)	Acute peripartum TTTS
Haemoglobin difference at birth	>8 g/dL	>8 g/dL
Reticulocyte count in donor (‰)	High	Normal
Reticulocyte count ratio	>1.7	<1.7
Placenta anastomoses	Only few minuscule	Large superficial (AA or VV)
Maternal side of placenta	Clear colour difference	No colour difference
Clinical signs donor at birth	No/minimal signs of hemodynamic imbalance	Hypovolaemic shock

twins and dichorionic twins [40]. These differences are often found when delivered vaginally, but not after caesarean delivery. Second-born twins delivered vaginally have higher haemoglobin levels compared to first-born twins [40]. Since dichorionic twins have their own separate placenta without vascular anastomoses, haemoglobin differences in dichorionic twins cannot only be explained by inter-twin transfusion. We hypothesized that the haemoglobin differences are related to the timing of cord clamping. Delayed cord clamping is associated with higher haemoglobin levels at birth due to increased placento-fetal transfusion. We suspect that the umbilical cord of first-born twins is clamped relatively earlier than the cord of second-born twins, and that this could lead to the difference in haemoglobin levels. An alternative explanation for haemoglobin differences in uncomplicated monochorionic twins is unbalanced intra-partum transfusion. Due to differences in pressure gradients and uterine contractions, relatively more blood might flow from twin 1 to twin 2 resulting in a higher haemoglobin level in twin 2. Another hypothesis is that after birth of twin 1, twin 2 might receive blood from both placenta shares through the anastomoses (so-called acute placento-fetal transfusion), resulting in a higher haemoglobin level.

Not much is known on the occurrence of other haematological complications such as thrombocytopenia or leukopenia in TTTS and TAPS survivors. Thrombocytopenia is known to occur more often in case of polycythaemia. Therefore, polycythaemic recipient twins with TTTS may be at risk for thrombocytopenia at birth. In a small study in TAPS survivors, we indeed found that thrombocytopenia occurred quite often (in 45% of cases), in particular in recipient twins (63%) and less frequently in donor twins (26%) [36]. In another recent study in TTTS and TAPS survivors, we found that leukocyte counts at birth in twins with TTTS or TAPS were similar between donors and recipients, but TAPS donors were at an increased risk of leukopenia [41]. Overall, TTTS and TAPS donors seem to be at an increased risk of early-onset neonatal sepsis compared to recipient twins.

In conclusion, since haematological disorders (anaemia, polycythaemia, thrombocytopenia and leukocytopenia) often occur, we recommend routine measurement at birth of full blood counts (including reticulocyte count) in all (complicated monochorionic twins.

26.5 Renal Disorders and Biochemical Assessment

In both TTTS and TAPS, knowledge on biochemical abnormalities is scarce. We previously hypothesized that inter-twin blood transfusion through the vascular anastomoses allows not only inter-twin flow of red blood cells, but also inter-twin flow of nutrients and proteins and can lead to biochemical disorders. In addition, inter-twin circulatory and haemodynamic imbalance can lead to renal hypo-or hyperperfusion and eventually to renal dysfunction.

In a recent study, we found that TTTS donors (not treated with laser surgery) and TAPS donors had significantly lower albumin levels compared to recipient twins [42, 43]. In TTTS twins treated with fetoscopic laser surgery, no inter-twin differences in albumin were detected. Our findings suggest that vascular anastomoses not only allow significant loss of haemoglobin, but also loss of albumin. Hypothetically, hypoalbuminemia in donor twins may also result from a decreased production in the liver due to a subordinate physical condition of these donor twins. However, we did not analyse other proteins or other parameters for the function of the liver such as the coagulation. Furthermore, since renal dysfunction occurs more often in donor twins treated conservatively, hypoalbuminemia in donor twins might also result from proteinuria and renal loss. Irrespective of the aetiologic mechanisms, given the higher risk of severe hypoalbuminemia, we suggest that serum albumin be measured in all donors with TAPS or with TTTS treated conservatively [42, 43].

Importantly, donor twins with TTTS suffer during pregnancy from severe renal hypoperfusion resulting in hypovolaemia, oliguria and oligohydramnios. Several studies in TTTS twins treated *conservatively* reported various renal complications in TTTS twins after birth [44–49]. Renal function in TTTS twins treated *with laser surgery* is less investigated. Beck et al. found in a small group of 18 children (TTTS twins treated with laser surgery) at median age 3 year no renal dysfunction [50]. However, accurate renal follow-up should take much longer. We recently evaluated creatinine levels in the first week after birth and urine output in TTTS twins treated with laser surgery compared to TTTS twins treated conservatively and found that renal dysfunction (defined as creatinine level >100 μmol/L) occurs less often in twins treated with laser surgery compared to twins treated conservatively (7.1% vs. 37.9%) [51]. In TTTS twins treated conservatively, we found a high risk of oliguria in donors (>90%) and lower blood pressure at birth [51]. Higher creatinine levels may reflect a state of chronic hypovolaemia due to chronic blood loss (pre-renal hypothesis). Circulatory imbalance could reduce renal perfusion and glomerular perfusion pressure. This theory is supported by the lower blood pressure and lower urine output in conservatively treated TTTS donors. An alternative hypothesis may be that elevated creatinine levels could result from chronic hypoxia and anaemia (renal hypothesis). Alternatively, hormonal dysfunction may also affect TTTS twins. Besides the concept of unbalanced inter-twin blood transfusion, there is also evidence for an adaptive response of the renal, endocrine and cardiovascular system to alter blood volume and causing twin oligo-polyhydramnios sequence (TOPS). Several studies have reported on highly abnormal values of hormones. In donor fetuses, plasma and amniotic vasopressin levels are higher compared to recipients. Oligohydramnios and higher creatinine levels in donors may therefore occur as a consequence of vasopressin-mediated reduction in fetal urine output [52]. In autopsy studies in TTTS twins, overexpression of the renin protein and transcript with evidence of renin synthesis was observed in donor kidneys. In recipients, renin expression was virtually absent and probably down-regulated [53–55]. Fetal atrial natriuretic peptide (ANP), brain natriuretic peptide (BNP) and endothelin levels are higher in recipient twins compared to donor twins [56, 57]. Hypervolaemia causes stretch of the cardiac atria and release of ANP and BNP which have natriuretic and vasodilatory properties resulting in polyuria and polyhydramnios. Although these hormonal reactions seem to be sufficient, increased release of renin and vasopressin in hypotensive- hypovolaemic donors and increased release of ANP and BNP in hypertensive-hypervolaemic recipients, the placental anastomoses facilitate exchange of these hormones and cause paradoxic effects [55].

In TAPS, donor twins do not have oligohydramnios reflecting a different antenatal situation compared to TTTS twins. However, we found that donor twins with TAPS have higher creatinine levels compared to recipients, and renal dysfunction occurred more often in donor twins compared to recipients twins (26.0% vs. 6.3%) [58]. Besides, donors had a lower blood pressure at birth and lower urine production. Our data suggest that chronic blood loss in donor twins may not only lead to anaemia and hypoalbuminemia, but may also affect the short-term renal function [58]. Our hypothesis is that chronic anaemia in donor twins causes hypoxia and results in an increased risk for renal dysfunction. We also evaluated renal function in uncomplicated monochorionic twins and compared larger twins to smaller twins. No differences between these twins were found. The overall incidence of short-term renal dysfunction in uncomplicated monochorionic twins was 7.7% (8/104). The assessment of short-term renal function in our studies was only based on routine measurements at our neonatal nursery including urine production, creatinine and urea levels during the first week. Whether renal dysfunction may also have long-term consequences such as impaired renal function in adult age requires further investigation. Due to the large reserve capacity of the kidney, serum creatinine could be normal for a long time. When children grow older and particularly during the growth spurt, renal insufficiency might become evident. Renal injury which may occur in donor twins may have permanent effects up to adult age, warranting further long-term investigations. This is in analogy with the 'Brenner hypothesis' which states that retardation of renal development may give rise to increased postnatal risk for systemic hypertension as well as enhanced risk of expression of renal disease [59].

26.6 Conclusion

Complicated monochorionic twins are at increased risk for cerebral, cardiovascular, haematological and biochemical disorders in the neonatal period. We therefore recommend routine evaluation in survivors using cranial ultrasound examination, echocardiography and laboratory investigations. However most studies focused on TTTS and TAPS survivors, whereas other complicated monochorionic twins such as monoamniotic twins, selective fetal growth restriction and twin reversed arterial perfusion sequence (TRAP) are probably also at risk for postnatal complications in the neonatal period, warranting further investigations. Given the rarity of these diseases, close collaboration between obstetricians and neonatologists and multicentre participation is of paramount importance to improve our understanding of neonatal morbidity in complicated monochorionic twins.

26.6.1 Review Questions

1. Should we perform a cranial ultrasound in all complicated monochorionic twins at birth to rule out cerebral injury?

2. Which cardiovascular complications can occur in recipient twins with TTS?

3. What are the differences between TAPS and acute peripartum TTS?

26.6.2 Multiple-Choice Questions

1. What is the prevalence of cerebral injury in TTTS treated with laser?
   (a) <5%
   (b) 5–10%
   (c) 10–20%
   (d) >20%

Answer: (b)

2. What is the risk for cerebral injury for single survivors after intrauterine demise of their co-twin (in case of patent anastomoses)?
   (a) 10–20%
   (b) 20–30%
   (c) 30–40%
   (d) >40%

Answer: (c)

? 3. What is the increased risk of congenital heart disease (CHD) in TTTS compared to singletons?
   (a) 3-fold increased risk of CHD
   (b) 6-fold increased risk of CHD
   (c) 9-fold increased risk of CHD
   (d) 12-fold increased risk of CHD

Answer: (d)

? 4. What is the increased risk of persistent pulmonary hypertension of the neonate (PPHN) in TTTS compared to singletons?
   (a) 2-fold increased risk of PPHN
   (b) 5-fold increased risk of PPHN
   (c) 10-fold increased risk of PPHN
   (d) 15-fold increased risk of PPHN

Answer: (c)

? 5. What is the best way of differentiating between acute peripartum TTS and TAPS in neonates at birth?
   (a) Assess the intertwin skin colour difference
   (b) Determine the reticulocyte count ratio
   (c) Determine the haemoglobin difference
   (d) Assess the hemodynamic condition of the twins

Answer: (b)

References

1. Kiely JL. The epidemiology of perinatal mortality in multiple births. Bull N Y Acad Med. 1990;66:618–37.
2. McCarthy BJ, Sachs BP, Layde PM, Burton A, Terry JS, Rochat R. The epidemiology of neonatal death in twins. Am J Obstet Gynecol. 1981;141:252–6.
3. Grothe W, Ruttgers H. Twin pregnancies: an 11-year review. Acta Genet Med Gemellol. 1985;34:49–58.
4. Halvorsen CP, Sverker E, Dellgren A, Grunnewald C, Kublickas M, Westgren M, Norman M. Survival and neonatal outcome after fetoscopic guided laser occlusion (FLOC) of twin-to-twin transfusion syndrome (TTTS) in Sweden. J Perinat Med. 2012;40(5):533–8.
5. Lopriore E, Oepkes D, Walther FJ. Neonatal morbidity in twin-twin transfusion syndrome. Early Hum Dev. 2011;87(9):595–9.
6. Verbeek L, Slaghekke F, Sueters M, Middeldorp JM, Klumper FJ, Haak MC, Oepkes D, Lopriore E. Hematological disorders at birth in complicated monochorionic twins. Expert Rev Hematol. 2017;10(6):525–32.
7. Wohlmuth C, Boudreaux D, Moise KJ, Johnson A, Papanna R, Bebbington M, Gardiner HM. Cardiac pathophysiology in twin-twin transfusion syndrome: new insights into its evolution. Ultrasound Obstet Gynecol. 2018;51(3):341–8.
8. Manning N, Archer N. Cardiac manifestations of twin-to-twin transfusion syndrome. Twin Res Hum Genet. 2016;19(3):246–54.
9. Hillman SC, Morris SK, Kilby MD. Co-twin prognosis after single fetal death: a systematic review and meta-analysis. Obstet Gynecol. 2011;118(4):928–40.
10. van Klink JM, van Steenis A, Steggerda SJ, Genova L, Sueters M, Oepkes D, Lopriore E. Single fetal demise in monochorionic pregnancies: incidence and patterns of cerebral injury. Ultrasound Obstet Gynecol. 2015;45(3):294–300.
11. Adegbite AL, Castille S, Ward S, Bajoria R. Prevalence of cranial scan abnormalities in preterm twins in relation to chorionicity and discordant birth weight. Eur J Obstet Gynecol Reprod Biol. 2005;119(1):47–55.
12. van Klink JM, Koopman HM, van Zwet EW, Oepkes D, Walther FJ, Lopriore E. Cerebral injury and neurodevelopmental impairment after amnioreduction versus laser surgery in twin-twin transfusion syndrome: a systematic review and meta-analysis. Fetal Diagn Ther. 2013;33(2):81–9.
13. Lenclen R, Ciarlo G, Paupe A, Bussieres L, Ville Y. Neurodevelopmental outcome at 2 years in children born preterm treated by amnioreduction or fetoscopic laser surgery for twin-to-twin transfusion syndrome: comparison with dichorionic twins. Am J Obstet Gynecol. 2009;201(3):291, e1–5.
14. Senat MV, Deprest J, Boulvain M, Paupe A, Winer N, Ville Y. Endoscopic laser surgery versus serial amnioreduction for severe twin-to-twin transfusion syndrome. N Engl J Med. 2004;351(2):136–44.
15. Spruijt MS, Steggerda SJ, Rath ME, Zwet E, Oepkes D, Walther FJ, Lopriore E. Cerebral injury in twin-twin transfusion syndrome treated with fetoscopic laser surgery. Obstet Gynecol. 2012;120(1):15–20.
16. Chmait RH, Chon AH, Schrager HM, Llanes A, Hamilton AH, Vanderbilt DL. Neonatal cerebral lesions predict 2-year neurodevelopmental impairment in children treated with laser surgery for twin-twin transfusion syndrome. J Matern Fetal Neonatal Med. 2019;32(1):80–4.

17. Quarello E, Molho M, Ville Y. Incidence, mechanisms, and patterns of fetal cerebral lesions in twin-to-twin transfusion syndrome. J Matern Fetal Neonatal Med. 2007;20(8):589–97.
18. Korsakissoka M, Groussolles M, Dicky O, Alberge C, Casper C, Azogui-Assouline C. Mortality, morbidity and 2-years neurodevelopmental prognosis of twin to twin transfusion syndrome after fetoscopic laser therapy: a prospective, 58 patients cohort study. J Gynecol Obstet Hum Reprod. 2018;47(10):555–60.
19. Vanderbilt DL, Schrager SM, Llanes A, Chmait RH. Prevalence and risk factors of cerebral lesions in neonates after laser surgery for twin-twin transfusion syndrome. Am J Obstet Gynecol. 2012;207(4):320, e1–6.
20. Spruijt MS, Lopriore E, Tan RN, Slaghekke F, Klumper FJ, Middeldorp JM, Haak MC, Oepkes D, Rijken M, less v KJM. Long-term neurodevelopmental outcome in twin-to-twin transfusion syndrome: is there still room for improvement? J Clin Med. 2019;8(8):1226.
21. Lopriore E, van Wezel-Meijler G, Middeldorp JM, Sueters M, Vandenbussche F, Walther FJ. Incidence, origin, and character of cerebral injury in twin-to-twin transfusion syndrome treated with fetoscopic laser surgery. Am J Obstet Gynecol. 2006;194(5):1215–20.
22. Lewi L, Deprest J, Hecher K. The vascular anastomoses in monochorionic twin pregnancies and their clinical consequences. Am J Obstet Gynecol. 2013;208(1):19–30.
23. Stirnemann J, Chalouhi GE, Essaoui M, Bahi-Buisson N, Sonigo P, Millischer A, Lapillonne A, Guigue V, Salomon LJ, Ville Y. Fetal brain imaging following laser surgery in twin-to-twin surgery. BJOG. 2018;125(9):1186–91.
24. Ascher R, Sorge I, Thome U, Hirsch FW, Bläser A, Kiess W, Merkenschlager A. Severe gyration and migration disorder in fetofetal transfusion syndrome: two case reports and a review of the literature on the neurological outcome of children with lesions on neuroimaging. Childs Nerv Syst. 2018;34(1):155–63.
25. Merhar SL, Kline-Fath BM, Meinzen-Derr J, Schibler KR, Leach JL. Fetal and postnatal brain MRI in premature infants with twin-twin transfusion syndrome. J Perinatol. 2013;33(2):112–8.
26. Griffiths PD, Sharrack S, Chan KL, Bamfo J, Williams F, Kilby MD. Fetal brain injury in survivors of twin pregnancies complicated by demise of one twin as assessed by in utero MR imaging. Prenat Diagn. 2015;35(6):583–91.
27. Robinson AJ, Teoh M, Edwards A, Fahey MC, Goergen S. Fetal brain injury in complicated monochorionic pregnancies: diagnostic yield of prenatal MRI following surveillance ultrasound and influence on prognostic counselling. Prenat Diagn. 2017;37(6):611–27.
28. Rossi AC, D'Addario V. Comparison of donor and recipient outcomes following laser therapy performed for twin-twin transfusion syndrome: a meta-analysis and review of literature. Am J Perinatol. 2009;26(1):27–32.
29. Gijtenbeek M, Shirzada MR, Ten Harkel ADJ, Oepkes D, Haak C, Congenital Heart M. Defects in monochorionic twins: a systematic review and meta-analysis. J Clin Med. 2019;24(8):6.
30. Habli M, Michelfelder E, Livingston J, Harmon J, Lim FY, Polzin W, Crombleholme T. Acute effects of selective fetoscopic laser photocoagulation on recipient cardiac function in twin-twin transfusion syndrome. Am J Obstet Gynecol. 2008;199:412, e1–6.
31. Wohlmuth C, Gardiner HM, Diehl W, Hecher K. Fetal cardiovascular hemodynamics in twin-twin transfusion syndrome. Acta Obstet Gynecol Scand. 2016;95:664–71.
32. Gijtenbeek M, Haak MC, Ten Harkel DJ, Te Pas AB, Middeldorp JM, Klumper FJCM, van Geloven N, Oepkes D, Lopriore E. Persistent pulmonary hypertension of the newborn in twin-twin transfusion syndrome: a case-control study. Neonatology. 2017;112(4):402–8.
33. Berry SM, Puder KS, Bottoms SF, Uckele JE, Romero R, Cotton DB. Comparison of intrauterine hematologic and biochemical values between twin pairs with and without stuck twin syndrome. Am J Obstet Gynecol. 1995;172:1403–10.
34. Denbow M, Fogliani R, Kyle P, Letsky E, Nicolini U, Fisk N. Haematological indices at fetal blood sampling in monochorionic pregnancies complicated by feto-fetal transfusion syndrome. Prenat Diagn. 1998;18:941–6.
35. Ashwal E, Yinon Y, Fishel-Bartal M, Tsur A, Chayen B, Weisz B, Lipitz S. Twin anemia-polycythemia sequence: perinatal management and outcome. Fetal Diagn Ther. 2016;40:28–34.
36. Lopriore E, Slaghekke F, Oepkes D, Middeldorp JM, Vandenbussche FP, Walther FJ. Hematological characteristics in neonates with twin anemia-polycythemia sequence (TAPS). Prenat Diagn. 2010;30:251–5.
37. Stranak Z, Korcek P, Hympanova L, Kyncl M, Krofta L. Prenatally acquired multiple limb ischemia in a very low birth weight monochorionic twin. Fetal Diagn Ther. 2017;41(3):237–8.
38. Robyr R, Lewi L, Salomon LJ, Yamamoto M, Bernard JP, Deprest J, Ville Y. Prevalence and management of late fetal complications following successful selective laser coagulation of chorionic plate anastomoses in twin-to-twin transfusion syndrome. Am J Obstet Gynecol. 2006;194:796–803.
39. Lopriore E, Holtkamp N, Sueters M, Middeldorp JM, Walther FJ, Oepkes D. Acute peripartum twin-twin transfusion syndrome: incidence, risk factors, placental characteristics and neonatal outcome. J Obstet Gynaecol Res. 2014;40(1):18–24.
40. Verbeek L, Zhao DP, Middeldorp JM, Oepkes D, Hooper SB, Te Pas AB, Lopriore E. Haemoglobin discordances in twins: due to differences in timing of cord clamping? Arch Dis Child Fetal Neonatal Ed. 2017;102(4):F324–8.

41. Visser GL, Tollenaar LSA, Bekker V, Te Pas AB, Lankester AC, Oepkes D, Lopriore E, Verbeek L. Leukocyte counts and other hematological values in twin-twin transfusion syndrome and twin anemia-polycythemia sequence. Fetal Diagn Ther. 2019;1:1–6.
42. Verbeek L, Middeldorp JM, Hulzebos CV, Oepkes D, Walther FJ, Lopriore E. Hypoalbuminemia in donors with twin-twin transfusion syndrome. Fetal Diagn Ther. 2013;33(2):98–102.
43. Verbeek L, Slaghekke F, Hulzebos CV, Oepkes D, Walther FJ, Lopriore E. Hypoalbuminemia in donors with twin anemia-polycythemia sequence: a matched case-control study. Fetal Diagn Ther. 2013;33(4):241–5.
44. Oberg KC, Pestaner JP, Bielamowicz L, Hawkins EP. Renal tubular dysgenesis in twin-twin transfusion syndrome. Pediatr Dev Pathol. 1999;2:25–32.
45. Barr M Jr, Sedman AB, Heidelberger KP. Renal tubular dysgenesis in twins. Pediatr Nephrol. 1998;12:408–13.
46. Chiang MC, Lien R, Chao AS, Chou YH, En Chen YJ. Clinical consequences of twin-to-twin transfusion. Eur J Pediatr. 2003;162:68–71.
47. De Paepe ME, Stopa E, Huang C, Hansen K, Luks FI. Renal tubular apoptosis in twin-to-twin transfusion syndrome. Pediatr Dev Pathol. 2003;6:215–25.
48. Cincotta RB, Gray PH, Phythian G, Rogers YM, Chan FY. Long term outcome of twin-twin transfusion syndrome. Arch Dis Child Fetal Neonatal Ed. 2000;83:F171–6.
49. Lopriore E, Nagel HT, Vandenbussche FP, Walther FJ. Long-term neurodevelopmental outcome in twin-to-twin transfusion syndrome. Am J Obstet Gynecol. 2003;189:1314–9.
50. Beck M, Graf C, Ellenrieder B, Bokenkamp A, Huber A, Hecher K, Bartmann P. Long-term outcome of kidney function after twin-twin transfusion syndrome treated by intrauterine laser coagulation. Pediatr Nephrol. 2005;20:1657–9.
51. Verbeek L, Joemmanbaks FA, Quak JME, Sukhai RN, Middeldorp JM, Oepkes D, Lopriore E. Renal function in neonates with twin-twin transfusion syndrome treated with or without fetoscopic laser surgery. Eur J Pediatr. 2017;176(9):1209–15.
52. Bajoria R, Ward S, Sooranna SR. Influence of vasopressin in the pathogenesis of oligohydramnios-polyhydramnios in monochorionic twins. Eur J Obstet Gynecol Reprod Biol. 2004;113:49–55.
53. Mahieu-Caputo D, Dommergues M, Delezoide AL, Lacoste M, Cai Y, Narcy F, Jolly D, Gonzales M, Dumez Y, Gubler MC. Twin-to-twin transfusion syndrome. Role of the fetal renin-angiotensin system. Am J Pathol. 2000;156:629–36.
54. Kilby MD, Platt C, Whittle MJ, Oxley J, Lindop GB. Renin gene expression in fetal kidneys of pregnancies complicated by twin-twin transfusion syndrome. Pediatr Dev Pathol. 2001;4:175–9.
55. Mahieu-Caputo D, Meulemans A, Martinovic J, Gubler MC, Delezoide AL, Muller F, Madelenat P, Fisk NM, Dommergues M. Paradoxic activation of the renin-angiotensin system in twin-twin transfusion syndrome: an explanation for cardiovascular disturbances in the recipient. Pediatr Res. 2005;58:685–8.
56. Bajoria R, Ward S, Chatterjee R. Natriuretic peptides in the pathogenesis of cardiac dysfunction in the recipient fetus of twin-twin transfusion syndrome. Am J Obstet Gynecol. 2002;186:121–7.
57. Bajoria R, Sullivan M, Fisk NM. Endothelin concentrations in monochorionic twins with severe twin-twin transfusion syndrome. Hum Reprod. 1999;14:1614–1618.66.
58. Verbeek L, Slaghekke F, Favre R, Vieujoz M, Cavigioli F, Lista G, Oepkes D, Lopriore E. Short-term postnatal renal function in twin anemia-polycythemia sequence. Fetal Diagn Ther. 2016;39(3):192–7.
59. Brenner BM. The etiology of adult hypertension and progressive renal injury: an hypothesis. Bull Mem Acad R Med Belg. 1994;149:121–5.

Key Readings

Lopriore E, Oepkes D, Walther FJ. Neonatal morbidity in twin-twin transfusion syndrome. Early Hum Dev. 2011;87(9):595–9.

Spruijt MS, Lopriore E, Tan RN, Slaghekke F, Klumper FJ, Middeldorp JM, Haak MC, Oepkes D, Rijken M, van Klink JM. Less long-term neurodevelopmental outcome in twin-to-twin transfusion syndrome: is there still room for improvement? J Clin Med. 2019;8(8):1226.

Childhood Development

Content

Cerebral Palsy and Long-Term Neurodevelopmental Impairment in Complicated Monochorionic Twin Pregnancy

J. M. M. van Klink, M. S. Spruijt, and Enrico Lopriore

Contents

A. Khalil et al. (eds.), *Twin and Higher-order Pregnancies*,
https://doi.org/10.1007/978-3-030-47652-6_27

Trailer

This chapter gives an update on the current level of knowledge of the neurological and long-term neurodevelopmental outcome in complicated monochorionic twin pregnancy, including twin-twin transfusion syndrome, twin anemia-polycythemia sequence, selective fetal growth restriction, twin reversed arterial perfusion, severe discordant anomalies, and single fetal demise. Risk factors for adverse long-term outcome are highlighted and future research- and care suggestions are provided.

Learning Objectives

After reading the chapter, the reader is able to

- Understand and explain the importance of long-term neurodevelopmental assessment of MC twins.
- Define long-term neurodevelopmental impairment (NDI).
- Describe the long-term outcome for the different MC twin pregnancy complications.
- Summarize risk factors for adverse outcome.
- Enumerate the requirements for a structured long-term follow-up program for MC twins.
- Elaborate on future care and research suggestions.

27.1 Introduction

Due to major improvements in prenatal ultrasound examinations, an increasing number of monochorionic (MC) twin pregnancy complications are being detected prior to birth [1]. Early detection and interventions for the management of MC twin complications have been proven successful to prevent permanent organ damage including severe damage to the developing fetal brain. To evaluate these interventions and optimize care for complicated MC twin pregnancies, long-term follow-up of surviving twins is essential. The aim of this chapter is threefold: to summarize current knowledge on the neurological and neurodevelopmental outcome in complicated MC twin pregnancies, to identify risk factors for adverse long-term outcome, and to provide future research- and care suggestions.

27.2 Long-Term Neurodevelopmental Outcome in Twin-Twin Transfusion Syndrome

Twin-twin transfusion syndrome (TTTS) is one of the most lethal conditions in perinatal medicine. Management options include serial amnioreduction and fetoscopic laser coagulation of placental vascular anastomoses. Amnioreduction aims to reduce pressure on the chorionic plate and cervix improving placental blood flow and increasing pregnancy duration [2]. However, amnioreduction is a symptomatic therapy; hence, both fetuses remain exposed to TTTS and are often born very premature. Fetoscopic laser coagulation of the placental vascular anastomoses addresses the underlying cause of TTTS and has proven to be superior to serial amnioreduction with higher (dual) survival rates, prolonged pregnancy (32 vs. 29 weeks gestational age, respectively), and a significant reduction of the risk of cerebral injury [3, 4]. Since the introduction of fetoscopic laser coagulation in the early 1990s, survival rate has improved from 55 to 74% at present [5, 6]. The most important outcome measure for the evaluation of new interventions is however long-term neurodevelopment of survivors. Now, a growing number of studies are gradually shedding more light on the wide range of long-term morbidity associated with TTTS.

The following sections focus on the neurological and long-term neurodevelopmental outcome in TTTS survivors treated with either serial amnioreduction or fetoscopic laser surgery.

27.2.1 CP and Long-Term Neurodevelopmental Impairment in TTTS Survivors

Advancing techniques, increasing survival rates, and improving short-term outcome necessitate a greater knowledge on the impact of TTTS and its management on long-term neurodevelopment of survivors. A better understanding of the impact on child development over time will allow more accurate counseling of parents and targeted interventions to optimize child development when needed. This requires international collaboration, to obtain large enough sample size and statistical power, using a standardized follow-up regimen including uniform and clearly defined criteria for long-term neurodevelopmental impairment (NDI). NDI is a standard composite outcome defined as at least one of the following: cerebral palsy (CP), severe motor and/or cognitive developmental delay, bilateral blindness, or deafness requiring amplification with hearing aids. Determining NDI involves a follow-up regimen that includes a physical and neurological examination and an assessment of cognitive and motor development using standardized developmental tests such as the Bayley Scales of Infant and Toddler Development performed by certified examiners.

The incidence and type of long-term NDI in TTTS survivors treated with either amnioreduction or laser surgery is outlined in the following two sections.

27.2.1.1 Long-Term Neurodevelopmental Outcome in TTTS Treated with Amnioreduction

Following amnioreduction, CP occurs in 5% to 23% (overall 14%) and NDI in 14% to 26% (overall 20%) of TTTS survivors [7]. The long-term follow-up studies are summarized in ◘ Table 27.1. The large discrepancy in outcome is due to considerable differences in methodology between studies and heterogeneity within the case series. A clear definition of NDI was often not reported in the amnioreduction studies, and detailed information on individual observations of impairment was generally lacking. In addition, not all follow-up studies included standardized developmental tests. All studies included a small number of children (20 to 52 children) and, as a consequence, the investigators were unable to assess whether NDI was due to confounders such as prematurity or growth restriction [5].

In the 2004 Eurofetus trial, neurological outcome at 6 months of age of TTTS survivors treated with amnioreduction was less favorable compared to TTTS survivors treated with laser surgery, 52% vs. 31% survivors with severe neurological sequelae, respectively ($P = 0.003$) [5]. However, the long-term neurodevelopmental outcome was similar between the two treatment groups [16]. Unfortunately, the long-term evaluation did not take into account that in a relatively large percentage (22%; 20/93) of live-born neonates in the amnioreduction group, intensive care treatment was withdrawn due to severe cerebral injury. Had these children survived, the differences in long-term neurodevelopmental outcome between both groups could have been much more evident. Disease-free survival or NDI rate could not be calculated from the results since individual cases of impairment were not reported.

27.2.1.2 Long-Term Neurodevelopmental Outcome in TTTS Treated with Laser Surgery

The reported incidence of CP and NDI following laser surgery ranges from 2% to 18% (overall 6%) and from 4% to 18% (overall 10%), respectively [7, 18–24]. ◘ Table 27.2 summarizes the neurodevelopmental follow-up studies after laser surgery. Again, it is difficult to compare the results of these studies and to combine these data to provide an accurate rate of long-term impairment. The methods vary widely with regard to the timing of assessments, inclusion criteria, the definition of NDI, and the use of appropriate outcome measures and controls.

The number of twins included for follow-up ranges from 13 to 278 children and the age

Table 27.1 Long-term neurodevelopmental outcome in twin-twin transfusion syndrome treated with amnioreduction

Author, Year	Outcome measure	CP % (n/N)	NDI % (n/N)	Comments
1. Reisner, 1993 [8]	Neurologic exam at 5 to 53 months	19 (5/27)	NA	100% inclusion, no developmental test, 70% <18 months at FUP, no controls
2. Mari, 2000 [9]	Clinical records, discussion parent/pediatrician, speech or physical therapy at >24 months	5 (2/42)	NA	*N* = 1 lost to FUP, 16% NND, no developmental test, no controls
3. Cincotta, 2000 [10]	Neurologic exam, physiotherapy assessment, Griffiths scale at 2 to 4.5 years	13 (3/23)	22 (5/23)	100% inclusion, 18% NND, gestation matched twin controls
4. Haverkamp, 2001 [11]	Neurologic exam, Denver screening test, Griffiths scale at mean age 24 months	23 (9/40)	23 (9/40)	18% lost to FUP, no controls
5. Frusca, 2003 [12]	Neurologic exam, Griffiths scale at mean age 24 months	16 (5/31)	26 (8/31)	100% inclusion, 35% <24 months at FUP, no controls
6. Lopriore, 2003 [13]	Neurologic exam, school functioning at mean age 6.2 years	21 (6/29)	NA	100% inclusion, no developmental test, 17% (5/29) special needs education, no controls
7. Dickinson, 2005 [14]	Neurologic exam, general health questionnaire, VABS, CBCL, Bayley scales, Stanford-Binet Intelligence Scale	6 (3/52)	14 (7/52)	94% inclusion, majority born <30 weeks, contemporaneous regional control cohort
8. Lenclen, 2009 [15]	Neurologic exam, ASQ at 24 months	19 (4/21)	NA	*N* = 1 lost to FUP, GA at birth 24–34 weeks, NDI not reported, gestation-matched DC controls
9. Salomon, 2010 [16]	Neurologic exam, ASQ, Wechsler scales up to 6 years	13 (6/47)	NA	25% lost to FUP at 6 years, 36% NND, NDI not reported, no controls
10. Li, 2011 [17]	Neurologic exam, Enjoji development scale, Wechsler scales at mean age 6.3 (3 to 12) years	15 (3/20)	20 (4/20)	8% lost to FUP, small study size, 10% mild NDI, majority mild TTTS cases
Total **Range**		**14% (46/332)** **5–23%**	**20% (33/166)** **14–26%**	

CP cerebral palsy, *NDI* neurodevelopmental impairment defined as CP, severe cognitive/motor delay (<-2SD), blindness/deafness, *NA* not assessed, *FUP* follow-up, *TTTS* twin-twin transfusion syndrome, *NND* neonatal death, *VABS* Vineland Adaptive Behavior Scales, *CBCL* Child behavior checklist, *GA* gestational age, *ASQ* Ages and Stages Questionnaire, *DC* dichorionic

at follow-up assessment from 1 month to 6 years. The majority of studies performed their assessments at an adjusted age of 2 years. At this young age, it is possible to discover major developmental abnormalities that require and benefit from early intervention. However, developmental outcomes assessed during early childhood are only moderate pre-

27

Table 27.2 Long-term neurodevelopmental outcome in twin-twin transfusion syndrome treated with laser surgery

Author, year	Outcome measure	CP % (n/N)	NDI % (n/N)	Comments
1. De Lia, 1999 [25]	Neurologic exam at 14 ± 10 months	4 (3/93)	NA	100% inclusion, no developmental test, no controls
2. Sutcliffe, 2001 [26]	Neurologic exam, Griffiths scale at mean age 24 (17–32) months	9 (6/66)	9 (6/66)	19% lost to FUP, 47% information GP, 54% incomplete test, no controls
3. Banek, 2003 [27]	Neurologic exam, Griffiths scale, Snijders-Oomen intelligence test at median age 22 months	11 (10/89)	11 (10/89)	100% inclusion, severe developmental delay not included as criterion for NDI, 11% minor neurologic deficiencies, rate, no controls
4. Graef, 2006 [28]	Neurologic exam, Griffiths scale, Snijders-Oomen intelligence test at median age 3 years 2 months	6 (10/167)	8 (13/167)	98% inclusion, sub-optimal/ incomplete developmental tests, 7% minor neurologic deficiencies, no controls
5. Lenclen, 2009 [15]	Neurologic exam, ASQ at 2 years	10 (9/88)	NA	98% inclusion, no developmental test, gestation-matched DC controls
6. Lopriore, 2009 [29]	Neurologic exam, Bayley scales at 2 years	6 (17/278)	18 (50/278)	94% inclusion, 2 TTTS-pregnancies treated >26 weeks' gestation, no controls
7. Salomon, 2010 [16]	Neurologic exam, ASQ, Wechsler scales up to 6 years	12 (9/73)	NA	25% lost to FUP at 6 years, 36% NND, NDI not reported, no controls
8. Gray, 2011 [30]	Neurologic exam, Griffiths and Bayley scales at 2.1 (1.8–3.8) years	4 (5/113)	12 (14/113)	97% inclusion, mixed developmental tests, for example, second and third version Bayley scales, 3 pregnancies treated >26 weeks' gestation, no controls
9. Chang, 2012 [31]	Neurologic exam, Bayley scales at corrected age 1 year	5 (3/59)	7 (4/59)	97% inclusion, small study size, follow-up at young age, no controls
10. Graeve, 2012 [32]	Neurologic exam, Kaufman assessment battery, national screening, questionnaires at 6 years	NA	9 (17/151)	25% lost to FUP, CP not reported, 47% (89/190) neurologic exam, 43% (82/190) intelligence test
11. McIntosh, 2014 [33]	General health questionnaire and Wechsler scales at 3 to 5 years	2 (1/50)	4 (2/50)	16% lost to FUP, no neurologic exam, small sample size, no controls
12. Vanderbilt, 2014 [34]	Amiel Tieson exam, Battelle developmental inventory at 2 years	3 (3/100)	4 (4/100)	50% lost to FUP with majority Quintero stage IV, no controls

Table 27.2 (continued)

Author, year	Outcome measure	CP % (n/N)	NDI % (n/N)	Comments
13. Tosello, 2014 [18]	ASQ at up to 5 years	6 (2/35)	NA	20% lost to FUP, small sample size, 31% (11/35) at least one ASQ score <-2SD
14. van Klink, 2015 [35]	Neurologic exam, Bayley scales at 2 years	3 (6/216)	10 (22/216)	94% inclusion, FUP in 2 of the 5 participating trial centers
15. Müllers, 2015 [19]	Individual correspondence and pediatric evaluation at median age 4 years (6 months-7 years)	4 (4/106)	NA	90% inclusion, no developmental test, 14% (15/106) "neurodevelopmental concerns": speech-language (*n* = 7), behavior (*n* = 2), motor delay (*n* = 2), CP (*n* = 4), no controls
16. Campos, 2016 [20]	Clinical exam, Bayley screening test at 5.5 (± 1.4) and 9.8 (± 1.9) months	18 (6/33)	NA	100% inclusion, small sample size, inadequate test score: 18% cognitive domain, 9% receptive- and 21% expressive communication, 24% fine- and 24% gross motor, 22 term singleton controls
17. Sananès, 2016 [36]	ASQ at 2 to 5 years	NA	NA	44% lost to FUP with majority Quintero I, no neurological exam, 14% (17/126) at least one ASQ score <-2SD: 4% communication, 4% fine- and 6% gross motor, 6% problem solving, 3% social skills, no controls
18. Korsakissok, 2018 [21]	ASQ at mean 59.3 months (24–96), non-standardized questionnaire parents, information attending physician	5 (3/58)	12 (7/58)	45% lost to FUP, 30% moderate neurological abnormalities, parent-rated learning disabilities, attending physician-rated rehabilitation needs and last objective neurological exam
19. Sommer, 2018 [22]	Evaluation CP using GMFCS, hearing and vision at 18 months corrected GA	15 (2/13)	NA	No developmental test, small sample size, preterm (<29 weeks GA) TTTS survivors vs. preterm DC twins without TTTS
20. Schou, 2019 [23]	ASQ at 25 months ±11, telephone interview parents	6 (5/86)	11 (9/86)	Mixed follow-up methods, TTTS survivors higher risk NDI compared to uncomplicated MC twins
21. Spruijt, 2019 [24]	Bayley scales at 2 years	2 (4/258)	4 (10/241)	15% lost-to follow-up, follow-up at 2 years
Total **Range**		**6% (108/1981)** **2–18%**	**10% (168/1674)** **4–18%**	

CP cerebral palsy, *NDI* neurodevelopmental impairment, *NA* not assessed, *TTTS* twin-twin transfusion syndrome, *NND* neonatal death, *FUP* follow-up, *ASQ* Ages and Stages Questionnaire, *GP* general practitioner, *GA* gestational age, *DC* is dichorionic, *SD* standard deviation

Of note: Two studies [13, 37] are not included in this table because the included children are more fully described in the multi-center follow-up of these studies [29, 35]

dictors of long-term neurodevelopment, particularly for scores on cognitive tests and academic performance. Although some studies followed their cohort until 6 years of age, some developmental problems including learning difficulties or autism spectrum disorder cannot be detected until later on, once the children start becoming more socially and academically challenged at school age. Longer-term follow-up is required to understand the clinical relevance (of milder forms) of impairments diagnosed in early childhood.

Several risk factors for long-term NDI have been identified, including advanced gestational age at laser surgery and high TTTS Quintero stage, low gestational age at birth, low birth weight, and severe neonatal morbidity including severe cerebral injury [7, 29]. The association between advanced gestational age at laser and Quintero stage with long-term impairment suggests that increasing disease severity may not only lead to increased perinatal mortality but also to increased long-term morbidity. The prognostic value of severe ante- or postnatal cerebral injury for long-term impairment is subject of debate. Large prospective multicenter studies with stringent neuroimaging- and long-term follow-up protocols could provide more clarity around the association between these important outcomes. Low gestational age at birth and low birth weight are well-recognized risk factors for long-term impairment: severe NDI in children born preterm is very frequent and is inversely related with diminishing gestational age and birth weight.

Nevertheless, long-term outcome in TTTS survivors seems to improve with time, especially with regard to CP and severe NDI. Several factors may explain this improvement in disease-free survival such as improvements in fetal and neonatal care strategies (monitoring and management options), increased awareness and knowledge of (potential) treatable complications in TTTS, and learning curve effect associated with a highly technical procedure such as laser surgery. Now, a shift towards an increase in mild to moderate impairments can be expected. Using Ages and Stages Questionnaire (ASQ) up to 5 years of age, Tosello et al. (2014) considered 31% of questionnaires as abnormal that is, at least one developmental domain below the cut-off [18]. Müllers et al. (2015) reported "ongoing neurodevelopmental concerns" in 14% (4/106) of survivors at a median age of 4 years including speech and language concerns, behavioral concerns, for example, autism, mild motor delay, and CP grade I [19]. In addition, Campos et al. (2016) reported the frequency of an inappropriate Bayley screening test performance for their TTTS group: 18% for the cognitive domain, 9% for receptive communication, 21% for expressive communication, 24% for fine motor, and 24% for gross motor skills [20]. Spruijt et al. (2019) reported Bayley-III scores below 85 (−1 SD) in 21% (50/232) of TTTS survivors [24]. These results imply that, even in children without obvious NDI, subtle problems may occur including mild CP and neurocognitive impairments. These "subtle" problems can have a significant impact on the care and educational requirements of children throughout life.

27.3 Long-Term Neurodevelopmental Outcome in Twin Anemia-Polycythemia Sequence

TAPS may occur spontaneously in up to 5% of MC pregnancies or after TTTS treated with laser surgery (post-laser TAPS) in up to 16% [38]. Data on the neurological and neurodevelopmental outcome in TTTS survivors who developed TAPS after laser surgery are confined to three small case series. In a case series of three post-laser TAPS twin pairs, one TAPS donor and one TAPS recipient had NDI; bilateral deafness at 9.5 years old and spastic paralysis at 2 years old, respectively [39]. Slaghekke and van Klink detected severe cerebral injury in 4%, NDI in 9%, and cognitive delay (<-1 SD) in 17% of post-laser TAPS survivors [38]. Risk factors for decreased cognitive scores were low gestational age at birth and low birth weight as well as intrauterine transfusion. The NDI rate in post-laser TAPS seems to be comparable to the rate of impairment in twins with TTTS treated with laser surgery (~10%).

Ashwal and colleagues (2015) compared perinatal outcome of 8 spontaneous- and 2 post-laser TAPS cases to gestational age-matched uncomplicated MC twins [40]. The rate of severe cerebral injury on postnatal ultrasound was similar in the TAPS- and control group (5% vs. 2.5%, $P = 0.61$). In addition, severe neonatal morbidity was comparable between groups. These conclusions are however limited due to the small sample size and the "mild" TAPS stages (stage 1 to 2) of the 10 cases [41]. In a recent long-term follow-up study by Tollenaar et al. (2019), NDI was detected in 9% of spontaneous TAPS survivors, and was higher in donors (18%) than in recipients (3%) [42]. Overall, donors showed higher rates of mild (−1 SD) cognitive impairment (35% vs. 18%), and lower rates of disease-free survival (45% vs. 80%) than recipients. Additionally, a high rate of bilateral deafness was observed in TAPS donors, 15% versus 0% in recipients. In all donors, deafness was based on auditory neuropathy spectrum disorder. The exact cause for the high rate of deafness in donor twins is unclear. Importantly, this finding is not observed in TTTS donors or children that suffered from chronic fetal anemia based on erythrocyte alloimmunization [43]. Furthermore, the prevalence of deafness in TAPS donors is higher compared to the prevalence of deafness in NICU infants (1–3%) [44]. Aside from severe anemia, NDI was strongly depending on gestational age at birth, once again illustrating the profound impact of prematurity on lifelong outcome.

27.4 Long-Term Neurodevelopmental Outcome in Selective Fetal Growth Restriction

Selective fetal growth restriction (sFGR) occurs in up to 25% of MC twin pregnancies and is related to unequal placental sharing in which the growth-restricted fetus has a small placental share and a velamentous cord insertion [45]. The optimal management in MC twins with sFGR is not clear, and international consensus on the best treatment strategy is lacking. Whether fetal surgery (fetoscopic laser coagulation of vascular anastomoses, selective reduction) or obstetric interventions (elective preterm birth) may improve the (long-term) outcome remains to be determined. How to balance the benefit from prolonging pregnancy in preventing prematurity-related injury against the risk of single fetal demise and concomitant damage to the co-twin is a clinical challenge and warrants further study. On the other hand, the invasiveness of fetal therapy is associated with complications such as preterm premature rupture of membranes (PPROM) and preterm delivery.

Systematic review shows that the incidence of severe cerebral injury in MC twins with sFGR varies greatly from 0% to 33%, with an estimated average of 8% [46]. The highest incidence of cerebral injury is reported in the pregnancies complicated by single fetal demise of a co-twin, in pregnancies with abnormal umbilical artery Doppler findings and in cohorts with a lower gestational age at birth. The results of these observational and case controlled studies should be interpreted with care due to different inclusion criteria, various definitions of sFGR, and different outcome measures.

◘ Table 27.3 summarizes the long-term neurodevelopmental follow-up studies performed in MC twins with sFGR. Most remarkable is the between-study variation in the definition of sFGR which obviously hampers the ability to compare and combine the results. The most commonly used definition is a birth weight discrepancy of 20% or more. Swamy and colleagues report on the developmental outcome at school age of 51 pairs of MC twins with a growth discrepancy ranging from 20% to 56% [53]. The more severely growth restricted co-twin had a three point average lower cognitive score compared to their co-twin, with the largest within-pair difference on mathematics and memory skills. The authors showed a significant positive association of within-pair birth weight differences and cogni-

Table 27.3 Long-term neurodevelopmental outcome in monochorionic twins complicated by selective fetal growth restriction

Author, year	Definition sFGR	Outcome measure	CP % (n/N)	NDI % (n/N)	Comments
1. Adegbite, 2004 [47]	Birthweight discordance ≥20% and abdominal circumference ≤5th	Griffiths scale at 24 months	19 (5/26)	42 (11/26)	GA: 24–34 weeks, GA-matched DC twins, no difference test score small vs large twin
2. Hack, 2009 [48]	Birthweight discordance ≥20%	Griffiths scale at 22 months	0 (0/14)	1 (1/14)	Small twin lower test scores (trend)
3. Edmonds, 2010 [49]	Birthweight discordance as a continuous variable	Wechsler scales at 7–17 years	Excluded	NA	*N* = 71 >32 weeks GA, small twin lower Wechsler verbal IQ
5. Halling, 2016 [50]	Birthweight discordance ≥20%	Bayley scales at 24–42 months	NA	NA	*N* = 24: No analysis small vs. large MC twin, sFGR MC twins lower Bayley scores vs. sFGR DC twins
4. Vedel, 2017 [51]	Birthweight discordance >75th	ASQ up to 48–60 months	NA	NA	*N* = 119: No difference ASQ small vs large twin
6. Rustico, 2017 [52]	Estimated fetal weight <10th small twin or estimated fetal weight difference ≥20%	No developmental test, evaluation at 8 years	5 (4/80) small 5 (5/111) large	6 (5/80) small 5 (6/111) large	No developmental test, more mild NDI in small vs large twin
7. Swamy, 2018 [53]	Birthweight discordance ≥20%	British Ability Scales, Strength Difficulties Questionnaire at mean age 6.3 years	2 (3/58) 1 small 2 large	Excluded	12% (6/51) complicated by TTTS, twins with CP/NDI excluded from analysis cognitive scores
Total Range			**6% (17/289) 5–19%**	**9% (23/254) 1–42%**	

sFGR selective fetal growth restriction, *FUP* follow-up, *CP* Cerebral palsy, *NDI* neurodevelopmental impairment, *GA* is gestational age, *DC* dichorionic, *ASQ* Ages and Stages Questionnaire.

tive scores at school age. Consistent findings were published by Edmonds and colleagues in 71 MC twin pairs between the ages of 7 and 18 years [49]. The authors found a relationship between the severity of the growth discrepancy and lower verbal intelligence scores in the smaller twin. This suggests a continued effect of fetal growth restriction.

FGR not only has an immediate impact on health but also has an adverse impact on health throughout life, most notably on the risk of insulin resistance, cardiovascular disease, and neurodevelopmental disorders [54, 55]. A mechanistic explanation for these long-term effects likely involves epigenetic changes that persistently alter the regulation of genes controlling growth and metabolism [56]. The study of MC twins discordant for fetal growth represents a powerful approach to discover the epigenetic mechanisms that are disturbed in FGR and contribute to adverse effects on health throughout the life course [57]. MC twins discordant for fetal growth share their genome, gender, maternal factors and, apart from the factors that led to divergent growth, experienced the same in utero conditions and gestational age at birth.

The discovery of an epigenetic signature that defines twins who are at increased neurodevelopmental risk already at birth will not only shed light on the processes that are disturbed in the twins but will help to identify those children who need extra surveillance and support. Also, the signature may be applied as a surrogate marker to evaluate the long-term effects of prenatal interventions including fetal therapy and, for example, novel therapies focusing on promoting placental function in sFGR. Insight into long-term outcomes will lead to improved prognostics, which are essential in parent counseling and crucial in the process of forming a management protocol specifically for twins with sFGR to optimally monitor and support their development [58].

27.5 Long-Term Neurodevelopmental Outcome in Twin Reversed Arterial Perfusion and Severe Discordant Anomalies

In specific complicated MC pregnancies, selective reduction can be offered as an alternative management option with the aim to optimize the chances of healthy survival of the co-twin. Indications include, among others, twin reversed arterial perfusion (TRAP), and severe discordant congenital anomalies. Available techniques include bipolar cord coagulation, radiofrequency ablation, cord occlusion by ligation, or photocoagulation of umbilical vessels and laser coagulation of placental anastomoses. Survival rates of the co-twin of 65 to 92% have been reported depending on indication and technique [59]. A large consecutive cohort of 131 MC pregnancies reported an overall perinatal survival rate of 67% after selective reduction, with higher survival (86%) when intervention was performed after 18 weeks' gestation compared to interventions before 18 weeks (47%) [60]. Neonatal morbidity, mainly due to severe cerebral injury or secondary to prematurity, affects ~7% of survivors [59].

Long-term neurodevelopmental follow-up of the surviving twin is limited to small case series ranging from 6 to 84 survivors [61–66]. The reported incidences of CP and NDI after selective reduction range from 0% to 8% and from 0 to 12%, respectively. ◘ Table 27.4 summarizes the long-term neurodevelopmental follow-up studies after selective reduction for various MC twin complications. Delabaere and colleagues (2013) reviewed all consecutive cases of umbilical cord occlusion performed for complicated MC twin pregnancies over a 16-year period [64]. Pediatric follow-up at 5 years (range: 6 months to 15 years) was based on medical records and updated by phone calls to the parents. CP was diagnosed in 8% (2/26) and NDI in 12% (3/26) of survivors. Important risk factors for adverse outcome include PPROM, low gestational age at birth, low birth weight, and severe neonatal morbidity including severe cerebral injury [65]. Multi-center efforts are of paramount importance to entangle those factors leading to adverse perinatal and long-term outcome including the indication for selective reduction as well as technique. In addition, *routine cerebral imaging should be performed in all survivors to rule out severe cerebral injury and determine etiology and timing of possible injury.* In case of cerebral injury, MRI may play an important role in investigating the correlation between antenatal and postnatal imaging findings. Increased awareness may improve neonatal and pediatric care for these

Table 27.4 Long-term neurodevelopmental outcome in monochorionic twins treated with selective reduction for various complications

Author, year	Indication and technique	CP % (n/N)	NDI % (n/N)	Comments
1. Robyr, 2005 [61]	TRAP *n* = 12, TTTS *n* = 19, discordant anomaly *n* = 5 Bipolar cord coagulation	0 (0/36)	3 (1/36)	100% inclusion, no developmental test: pediatric follow-up at 1 month to 5 years (range)
2. Lewi, 2006 [62]	TRAP *n* = 14, TTTS *n* = 18, discordant anomaly *n* = 24, sFGR *n* = 5 Laser and/or bipolar cord coagulation	0 (0/67)	2 (1/67)	MC twins and triplets, no formal criteria NDI, 55/67 (82%) children assessed with standardized developmental test: Bayley scales or Snijders-Oomen intelligence test at median age 1.3 years (12 months to 6 years), 12/67 (18%) information GP
3. Moise, 2008 [63]	TTTS *n* = 3, discordant anomaly *n* = 3 Radiofrequency ablation	0 (0/6)	NA	Small study (*n* = 6), no developmental test: phone call to parents at mean age 4 months (2.3 to 6.6 months)
4. Lanna, 2012 [67]	TTTS *n* = 30, TRAP *n* = 2, discordant anomaly *n* = 26, sFGR *n* = 26 Bipolar cord coagulation	1 (1/84)	NA	Standardized developmental test: Griffiths scale and neurological exam, no developmental test (questionnaire) for children born at other hospital at 1 to 9 years (range), normal neurological development in 98% (82/84): TOP *n* = 1 and NND *n* = 4 due to severe cerebral injury
4. Delabaere, 2013 [64]	TTTS *n* = 10, TRAP *n* = 9, discordant anomaly *n* = 4, sFGR *n* = 3 Bipolar cord coagulation, ligation	8% (2/26)	12% (3/26)	No developmental test: medical records or phone call to parents at mean age 5 years (6 months to 15 years)
5. van Klink, 2015 [65]	TTTS *n* = 25, TRAP *n* = 19, discordant anomaly *n* = 21, sFGR *n* = 8, other *n* = 1 Bipolar-, interstitial-, fetoscopic laser cord coagulation, radiofrequency ablation	3% (2/74)	7% (5/74)	16% lost to follow-up, standardized developmental tests: Bayley or Wechsler scales at median age 55 months (25 months to 12 years)
6. Wang, 2017 [66]	TTTS *n* = 5, TRAP *n* = 1, discordant anomaly *n* = 8, sFGR *n* = 3 Radiofrequency ablation	0% (0/17)	0% (0/17)	No developmental test: follow-up interview at 6 months to 3 years
Total **Range**		**2% (5/310)** **0–8%**	**5% (10/220)** **0–12%**	

CP cerebral palsy, *NDI* neurodevelopmental impairment, *sFGR* selective fetal growth restriction, *GP* general practitioner, *TOP* termination of pregnancy

children. However, following *selective reduction, the majority of MC pregnancies are discharged from specialized care in tertiary fetal medicine centers to the referring hospital. Information at discharge regarding the management of these pregnancies should therefore include ante- and postnatal cerebral imaging in the surviving co-twin.*

27.6 Neurodevelopmental Outcome After Single Fetal Demise in Monochorionic Twin Pregnancies

Single fetal demise in MC twin pregnancies with patent vascular anastomoses poses a high risk for severe cerebral injury in the surviving co-twin. Using meta-analysis, Hillman and colleagues reported severe cerebral injury in 34% and long-term NDI in 26% of survivors after fetal demise of the co-twin [68].

Cerebral injury following single fetal demise is mostly of hypoxic-ischemic origin and spares the brainstem and cerebellum [69, 70]. Focal brain lesions are more frequent in MC pregnancies complicated by TTTS or in those where an intervention has been performed. An important risk factor for severe cerebral injury is single fetal demise later in pregnancy [69, 71, 72]. The placental anastomoses grow larger with increasing gestational age and therefore the impact of acute exsanguination is thought to be greater.

A (inter)national database should be developed to register all cases with single fetal demise in order to study the natural history and possible risk factors for adverse long-term outcome. Stringent neuroimaging protocols to accurately evaluate the incidence and nature of antenatal cerebral injury and to investigate the correlation between antenatal and postnatal imaging findings are strongly recommended. The clinical relevance of these findings should then be determined using long-term neurodevelopmental outcome data of all MC pregnancies with single fetal demise until at least childhood.

27.7 Conclusion

Although an increasing number of twins are being born alive after severe MC pregnancy complications, knowledge on long-term development is still limited, especially on potential risk factors for adverse outcome and mild to moderate impairments. The majority of follow-up studies available are observational, cross-sectional in design, and do not allow for examination of child development over time. The studies are generally limited by small sample size and power and do not include matched controls. In addition, standardized neurodevelopmental testing and clearly specified criteria for impairment are lacking. Core outcome sets for the evaluation of care of MC twin pregnancy are essential and could help standardize outcome collection and reporting in follow-up studies [73].

The results of long-term follow-up studies are further hampered by relative high lost-to-follow-up rates. High lost-to-follow-up rates can lead to biased reports of impairment, likely resulting in underestimation, since parents with low educational levels and those with children with severe developmental delay are most likely to drop out of follow-up programs [74, 75]. In addition, in countries where families have to travel long distances to the follow-up clinic, parents are more likely to refrain from participating. Assessments using e-consults or (web-based) questionnaires such as the ASQ could be more feasible to avoid large loss to follow-up rates.

The importance of long-term follow-up studies lies in both the necessity of evaluating fetal therapy and care of complicated MC twin pregnancies as well as in evidence-based counseling of future parents. In addition, when a center decides to treat fetuses in utero, with the knowledge that a significant proportion will develop long-term morbidity, this center also has the responsibility to ensure that survivors will eventually receive the care they need. Long-term follow-up should be an integrated component in the care of complicated MC twin pregnancies. Unfortunately,

Table 27.5 Proposition follow-up assessments according to age in years

Fetus	Neonate	2 years	5 years	8 years	12 years	16 years
Brain development: Cerebral imaging (cranial ultrasound, MRI)						
	Senses: Hearing screening and test, (sensorineural) deafness or hearing loss, ROP screening, vision test, (bilateral) blindness or vision loss					
	Physical: General health, growth, neurological exam, cerebral palsy (GMFCS), gross motor development, DCD					
	Cognitive development: Bayley scales/Ages and Stages Questionnaire, Wechsler scales (IQ)					
	Academic: Pre-academic skills, special needs education, number of grades below age-appropriate level					
	Neuropsychological: Learning problems (dyslexia, dyscalculia), language (expressive and receptive), executive functioning, attention, visual spatial abilities, memory, fine motor development					
	Psychosocial and behavior: Behavioral assessment, internalizing and externalizing behavior (Achenbach system), social skills, quality of life, sleep, daily functioning (Vineland Adaptive Behavioral Scales)					
	Developmental disorders: Attention deficit, hyperactivity, autism spectrum, mood and anxiety					

MRI magnetic resonance imaging, *ROP* retinopathy of prematurity, *GMFCS* gross motor functioning classification system, *DCD* developmental coordination disorder, *IQ* intelligence quotient

long-term neurodevelopmental studies are costly and difficult to perform and, consequently, hard to realize. Challenges include, among others, tracking families, motivating families to participate, organizing follow-up assessments with trained pediatricians and child psychologists, as well as complete data acquisition and analysis. Structured long-term follow-up programs of MC twins require a dedicated follow-up team including fetal medicine specialists, neonatologists, physiotherapists, child psychologists, and research nurses.

It is crucial to continuously assess child development including formal psychological testing and standardized measures of well-documented psychometric quality, with increasing reliability of results with increasing age of surviving MC twins. A proposition for long-term assessment according to age in years is presented in Table 27.5.

Multicenter efforts are of utmost importance to study the natural history in complicated MC pregnancies and the effect of interventions to determine optimal management (timing and type of intervention). The ideal study design to evaluate new interventions in the management of complicated MC twin pregnancies is an adequately powered randomized controlled trial with "survival without NDI" as primary outcome. An international registry to record and evaluate the outcome in large groups of MC twins is of paramount importance to increase current knowledge in specific subgroups.

27.7.1 Multiple-Choice Questions

1. Neurodevelopmental impairment (NDI):
   - (a) Is a direct consequence of extreme prematurity
   - (b) Represents a standard composite outcome including cerebral palsy, severe cognitive and/or motor delay (-2SD), bilateral blindness, and/or deafness requiring hearing aids
   - (c) Can be diagnosed using information from parents and/or the attending pediatrician
   - (d) Is more frequent in TTTS donor twins compared to TTTS recipient twins

Answer: (b)

2. The optimal evaluation of the management of complicated MC twin pregnancy concerns:
   (a) The technical success of fetal treatment
   (b) The rate of cerebral palsy
   (c) Dual survival
   (d) Survival without neurodevelopmental impairment

Answer: (d)

3. Which of the following is true
   I. All TTTS survivors born premature will develop long-term impairment.
   II. Structured long-term follow-up programs of MC twins require a dedicated follow-up team including fetal medicine specialists, neonatologists, physiotherapists, child psychologists, and research nurses.
   III. Cerebral injury at birth equals long-term impairment.
   IV. TAPS donors are at increased risk of neurodevelopmental impairment compared to TAPS recipient twins.
   (a) Only IV is true.
   (b) I and II are true.
   (c) II and IV are true.
   (d) All are false.

Answer: (c)

27.7.2 Essay Questions

Question 1: How would you set up your own structured follow-up program for MC twins? Describe how you would face the different challenges of follow-up including tracking families, motivating families to participate, organizing follow-up assessments, data acquisition, and analysis. Which healthcare professional should do which task? And, which developmental domains do you want to assess at what age and why?

References

1. Deprest J, et al. Fetoscopic surgery: encouraged by clinical experience and boosted by instrument innovation. Semin Fetal Neonatal Med. 2006;11:398–412.
2. Hecher K, et al. Long-term outcomes for monochorionic twins after laser therapy in twin-to-twin transfusion syndrome. Lancet Child Adolesc Health. 2018;2(7):525–35.
3. Rossi AC, D'Addario V. Laser therapy and serial amnioreduction as treatment for twin-twin transfusion syndrome: a metaanalysis and review of literature. Am J Obstet Gynecol. 2008;198(2):147–52.
4. van Klink JMM, et al. Cerebral injury and neurodevelopmental impairment after amnioreduction versus laser surgery in twin-twin transfusion syndrome: a systematic review and meta-analysis. Fetal Diagn Ther. 2013;33:81–9.
5. Senat MV, et al. Endoscopic laser surgery versus serial amnioreduction for severe twin-to-twin transfusion syndrome. N Engl J Med. 2004;351:136–44.
6. Slaghekke F, et al. Fetoscopic laser coagulation of the vascular equator versus selective coagulation for twin-to-twin transfusion syndrome: an open-label randomised controlled trial. Lancet. 2014;383(9935):2144–51.
7. van Klink JM, et al. Long-term neurodevelopmental outcome in survivors of twin-to-twin transfusion syndrome. Twin Res Hum Genet. 2016;19(3):255–61.
8. Reisner DP, et al. Stuck twin syndrome: outcome in thirty-seven consecutive cases. Am J Obstet Gynecol. 1993;169(4):991–5.
9. Mari G, et al. Long-term outcome in twin-twin transfusion syndrome treated with serial aggressive amnioreduction. Am J Obstet Gynecol. 2000;183(1):211–7.
10. Cincotta RB, et al. Long term outcome of twin-twin transfusion syndrome. Arch Dis Child Fetal Neonatal Ed. 2000;83:F171–6.
11. Haverkamp F, et al. Neurodevelopmental risks in twin-to-twin transfusion syndrome: preliminary findings. Eur J Paediatr Neurol. 2001;5:21–7.
12. Frusca T, et al. Pregnancies complicated by twin-twin transfusion syndrome: outcome and long-term neurological follow-up. Eur J Obstet Gynecol Reprod Biol. 2003;107(2):145–50.
13. Lopriore E, et al. Long-term neurodevelopmental outcome in twin-to-twin transfusion syndrome treated with fetoscopic laser surgery. Am J Obstet Gynecol. 2007;196(3):231–4.
14. Dickinson JE, et al. The long term neurologic outcome of children from pregnancies complicated by twin-to-twin transfusion syndrome. BJOG. 2005;112(1):63–8.

15. Lenclen R, et al. Neurodevelopmental outcome at 2 years in children born preterm treated by amnioreduction or fetoscopic laser surgery for twin-to-twin transfusion syndrome: comparison with dichorionic twins. Am J Obstet Gynecol. 2009;201(3):291–5.
16. Salomon LJ, et al. Long-term developmental follow-up of infants who participated in a randomized clinical trial of amniocentesis vs laser photocoagulation for the treatment of twin-to-twin transfusion syndrome. Am J Obstet Gynecol. 2010;203(5):444–7.
17. Li X, et al. Prognosis and long-term neurodevelopmental outcome in conservatively treated twin-to-twin transfusion syndrome. BMC Pregnancy Childbirth. 2011;11(1):32.
18. Tosello B, et al. Short and medium-term outcomes of live-born twins after fetoscopic laser therapy for twin-twin transfusion syndrome. J Perinat Med. 2014;42(1):99–105.
19. Mullers SM, et al. Outcome following selective fetoscopic laser ablation for twin to twin transfusion syndrome: an 8 year national collaborative experience. Eur J Obstet Gynecol Reprod Biol. 2015;191:125–9.
20. Campos D, et al. Twin-twin transfusion syndrome: neurodevelopment of infants treated with laser surgery. Arq Neuropsiquiatr. 2016;74(4):307–13.
21. Korsakissok M, et al. Mortality, morbidity and 2-years neurodevelopmental prognosis of twin to twin transfusion syndrome after fetoscopic laser therapy: a prospective, 58 patients cohort study. J Gynecol Obstet Hum Reprod. 2018;47(10):555–60.
22. Sommer J, et al. Outcomes of extremely premature infants with twin-twin transfusion syndrome treated by laser therapy. J Perinatol. 2018;38(11):1548–55.
23. Schou KV, et al. Long-term neurodevelopmental outcome of Monochorionic twins after laser therapy or umbilical cord occlusion for twin-twin transfusion syndrome. Fetal Diagn Ther. 2019;46(1):20–7.
24. Spruijt MS, et al. Long-term neurodevelopmental outcome in twin-to-twin transfusion syndrome: is there still room for improvement? J Clin Med. 2019;8(8):1226.
25. De Lia JE, Kuhlmann RS, Lopez KP. Treating previable twin-twin transfusion syndrome with fetoscopic laser surgery: outcomes following the learning curve. J Perinat Med. 1999;27(1):61–7.
26. Sutcliffe AG, et al. Outcome for children born after in utero laser ablation therapy for severe twin-to-twin transfusion syndrome. BJOG. 2001;108(12):1246–50.
27. Banek CS, et al. Long-term neurodevelopmental outcome after intrauterine laser treatment for severe twin-twin transfusion syndrome. Am J Obstet Gynecol. 2003;188(4):876–80.
28. Graef C, et al. Long-term neurodevelopmental outcome of 167 children after intrauterine laser treatment for severe twin-twin transfusion syndrome. Am J Obstet Gynecol. 2006;194(2):303–8.
29. Lopriore E, et al. Risk factors for neurodevelopment impairment in twin-twin transfusion syndrome treated with Fetoscopic laser surgery. Obstet Gynecol. 2009;113(2, Part 1):361–6.
30. Gray PH, et al. Neurodevelopmental outcome and risk factors for disability for twin-twin transfusion syndrome treated with laser surgery. Obstet Gynecol Surv. 2011;66(6):344–5.
31. Chang YL, et al. The neurological outcomes of surviving twins in severe twin-twin transfusion syndrome treated by fetoscopic laser photocoagulation at a newly established center. Prenat Diagn. 2012;32:893–6.
32. Graeve P, et al. Neurodevelopmental outcome at 6 years of age after intrauterine laser therapy for twin-twin transfusion syndrome. Acta Paediatr. 2012;101:1200–5.
33. McIntosh J, et al. Long term developmental outcomes of pre-school age children following laser surgery for twin-to-twin transfusion syndrome. Early Hum Dev. 2014;90(12):837–42.
34. Vanderbilt DL, et al. Predictors of 2-year cognitive performance after laser surgery for twin-twin transfusion syndrome. Am J Obstet Gynecol. 2014;211(4):388.e1–7.
35. van Klink JM, et al. Neurodevelopmental outcome at 2 years in twin-twin transfusion syndrome survivors randomized for the Solomon trial. Am J Obstet Gynecol. 2015;214(1):113.e1–7.
36. Sananes N, et al. Evaluation of long-term neurodevelopment in twin-twin transfusion syndrome after laser therapy. Prenat Diagn. 2016;36(12):1139–45.
37. van Klink JM, et al. Improvement in neurodevelopmental outcome in survivors of twin-twin transfusion syndrome treated with laser surgery. Am J Obstet Gynecol. 2014;210(6):540.e1–7.
38. Slaghekke F, et al. Neurodevelopmental outcome in twin anemia-polycythemia sequence after laser surgery for twin-twin transfusion syndrome. Ultrasound Obstet Gynecol. 2014;44(3):316–21.
39. Taniguchi K, et al. Twin anemia-polycythemia sequence after laser surgery for twin-twin transfusion syndrome and maternal morbidity. Fetal Diagn Ther. 2015;37(2):148–53.
40. Ashwal E, et al. Twin Anemia-polycythemia sequence: perinatal management and outcome. Fetal Diagn Ther. 2016;40(1):28–34.
41. Tollenaar LS, et al. Twin Anemia polycythemia sequence: current views on pathogenesis, diagnostic criteria, perinatal management, and outcome. Twin Res Hum Genet. 2016;19(3):222–33.
42. Tollenaar LSA, Lopriore E, Slaghekke F, Oepkes D, Middeldorp JM, Haak MC, Klumper FJCM, Tan RNGB, Rijken M, Van Klink JMM. High risk of long-term neurodevelopmental impairment in donor twins with spontaneous twin anemia-polycythemia sequence. Ultrasound Obstet Gynecol. 2020;55(1):39–46. https://doi.org/10.1002/uog.20846.

43. Lindenburg IT, Smits-Wintjens VE, van Klink JM, Verduin E, van Kamp IL, Walther FJ, Schonewille H, Doxiadis II, Kanhai HH, van Lith JM, van Zwet EW, Oepkes D, Brand A, Lopriore E, LOTUS Study Group. Long-term neurodevelopmental outcome after intrauterine transfusion for hemolytic disease of the fetus/newborn: the LOTUS study. Am J Obstet Gynecol. 2012;206(2):141.e1–8.
44. Jayagobi PA, Yeoh A, Hee KYM, Sok Bee Lim L, Choo KP, Kun Kiaang HT, Lazaroo D, Daniel LM. Hearing screening outcome in neonatal intensive care unit graduates from a tertiary care Centre in Singapore. Child Care Health Dev. 2020;46(1):104–10.
45. Lopriore E, et al. Neonatal morbidity in growth-discordant monochorionic twins: comparison between the larger and the smaller twin. Twin Res Hum Genet. 2012;15(4):541–6.
46. Inklaar MJ, et al. Cerebral injury in monochorionic twins with selective intrauterine growth restriction: a systematic review. Prenat Diagn. 2014;34(3):205–13.
47. Adegbite AL, et al. Neuromorbidity in preterm twins in relation to chorionicity and discordant birth weight. Am J Obstet Gynecol. 2004;190(1):156–63.
48. Hack KE, et al. Long-term neurodevelopmental outcome of monochorionic and matched dichorionic twins. PLoS One. 2009;4(8):e6815.
49. Edmonds CJ, et al. The effect of intrauterine growth on verbal IQ scores in childhood: a study of monozygotic twins. Pediatrics. 2010;126(5):e1095–101.
50. Halling C, et al. Neuro-developmental outcome of a large cohort of growth discordant twins. Eur J Pediatr. 2016;175(3):381–9.
51. Vedel C, et al. Short- and long-term perinatal outcome in twin pregnancies affected by weight discordance. Acta Obstet Gynecol Scand. 2017;96(2):233–42.
52. Rustico MA, et al. Selective intrauterine growth restriction in monochorionic twins: changing patterns in umbilical artery Doppler flow and outcomes. Ultrasound Obstet Gynecol. 2017;49(3):387–93.
53. Swamy RS, et al. Cognitive outcome in childhood of birth weight discordant monochorionic twins: the long-term effects of fetal growth restriction. Arch Dis Child Fetal Neonatal Ed. 2018;103(6):F512–6.
54. Barker DJ. Adult consequences of fetal growth restriction. Clin Obstet Gynecol. 2006;49(2):270–83.
55. Gluckman PD, et al. Effect of in utero and early-life conditions on adult health and disease. N Engl J Med. 2008;359(1):61–73.
56. Heijmans BT, et al. Persistent epigenetic differences associated with prenatal exposure to famine in humans. Proc Natl Acad Sci U S A. 2008;105(44):17046–9.
57. Groene SG, et al. TwinLIFE: the twin longitudinal investigation of FEtal discordance. Twin Res Hum Genet. 2019;22(6):617–22.
58. Groene SG, et al. The impact of selective fetal growth restriction or birth weight discordance on long-term neurodevelopment in Monochorionic twins: a systematic literature review. J Clin Med. 2019;8(7):944.
59. Rossi AC, D'Addario V. Umbilical cord occlusion for selective feticide in complicated monochorionic twins:a systematic review of the literature. Am J Obstet Gynecol. 2009;200:123–9.
60. van den Bos EM, et al. Perinatal outcome after selective feticide in monochorionic twin pregnancies. Ultrasound Obstet Gynecol. 2013;41(6):653–8.
61. Robyr R, Yamamoto M, Ville Y. Selective feticide in complicated monochorionic twin pregnancies using ultrasound-guided bipolar cord coagulation. BJOG. 2005;112:1344–8.
62. Lewi L, et al. Pregnancy and infant outcome of 80 consecutive cord coagulations in complicated monochorionic multiple pregnancies. Am J Obstet Gynecol. 2006;194(3):782–9.
63. Moise KJ Jr, et al. Radiofrequency ablation for selective reduction in the complicated monochorionic gestation. Am J Obstet Gynecol. 2008;198(2):198.e1–5.
64. Delabaere A, et al. Pediatric outcome after selective feticide for 30 complicated monochorionic twin pregnancies. Gynecol Obstet Fertil. 2013;41(2):85–9.
65. van Klink JM, et al. Long-term neurodevelopmental outcome after selective feticide in monochorionic pregnancies. Br J Obstet Gynaecol. 2015;122(11):1517–24.
66. Wang HM, et al. Radiofrequency ablation for selective reduction in complex monochorionic multiple pregnancies: a case series. Taiwan J Obstet Gynecol. 2017;56(6):740–4.
67. Lanna MM, et al. Bipolar cord coagulation for selective feticide in complicated monochorionic twin pregnancies: 118 consecutive cases at a single center. Ultrasound Obstet Gynecol. 2012;39:407–13.
68. Hillman SC, Morris RK, Kilby MD. Co-twin prognosis after single fetal death. A systematic review and meta-analysis. Obstet Gynecol. 2011;118(4):928–40.
69. Klink JM, et al. Single fetal demise in monochorionic pregnancies: incidence and patterns of cerebral injury. Ultrasound Obstet Gynecol. 2015;45(3):294–300.
70. Conte G, et al. Brain-injured survivors of Monochorionic twin pregnancies complicated by single intrauterine death: MR findings in a multicenter study. Radiology. 2018;288(2):582–90.
71. O'Donoghue K, et al. Interstitial laser therapy for fetal reduction in monochorionic multiple preg-

nancy: loss rate and association with aplasia cutis congenita. Prenat Diagn. 2008;28:535–43.
72. Mackie FL, Morris RK, Kilby MD. Fetal brain injury in survivors of twin pregnancies complicated by demise of one twin: a review. Twin Res Hum Genet. 2016;19(3):262–7.
73. Perry H, et al. A core outcome set for the evaluation of treatments for twin-twin transfusion syndrome. Ultrasound Obstet Gynecol. 2018;54(2):255–61.
74. Aylward GP, et al. Who goes and who stays: subject loss in a multicenter, longitudinal follow-up study. J Dev Behav Pediatr. 1985;6:3–8.
75. Wolke D, et al. Follow-up of preterm children: important to document dropouts. Lancet. 1995;345(8947):447.

Key Reading

Hecher K, et al. Long-term outcomes for monochorionic twins after laser therapy in twin-to-twin transfusion syndrome. Lancet Child Adolesc Health. 2018;2(7):525–35.

Rossi AC, D'Addario V. Laser therapy and serial amnioreduction as treatment for twin-twin transfusion syndrome: a metaanalysis and review of literature. Am J Obstet Gynecol. 2008;198(2):147–52.

van Klink JMM, et al. Cerebral injury and neurodevelopmental impairment after amnioreduction versus laser surgery in twin-twin transfusion syndrome: a systematic review and meta-analysis. Fetal Diagn Ther. 2013;33:81–9.

Research, Registries and Parent Views

Contents

Research Studies in Twins and Multiple Pregnancy

Janine R. Lam, Becky Liu, Kate Murphy, and Asma Khalil

Contents

A. Khalil et al. (eds.), *Twin and Higher-order Pregnancies*,
https://doi.org/10.1007/978-3-030-47652-6_28

Trailer

This chapter outlines the key research priorities for the health of twins and multiples from the Global Twins and Multiples Priority Setting Partnership. These priorities are considered significant by families of twins and multiples and clinicians and researchers who work with twins and multiples. The top ten and 89 priorities from five key areas are discussed: antenatal care, intrapartum and postpartum care, neonatal and paediatric health, child psychiatry and development, and parental and family health. Existing findings and future directions for research are outlined.

Definitions

Perinatal morbidity: Complications in the fetus occurring during pregnancy from 20 weeks' gestation, during delivery, or up to 28 days post birth.

Perinatal mortality: Fetal deaths with a gestational age of 20 weeks or more, or infant deaths that occur at less than 28 days of age.

Growth restriction: A pathological restriction of the fetus in reaching its full genetic growth potential.

Neonatal unit admission: An infant that requires extra support or treatment (ventilation, antibiotics, inotropes, etc.) in an intensive neonatal ward.

Postpartum or postnatal depression: Depression or anxiety experienced by a parent that may occur between 1 and 3 weeks or up to 1 year following childbirth [1].

Learning Objectives

For the areas of antenatal care, postpartum care, neonatal and paediatric health, child psychiatry and development, and parental and family health:

1. To understand key research priorities for families of twins and multiples, clinicians who work with twins and multiples, and researchers who study the health of twins and multiples
2. To gain an overview of existing findings for the above key research priorities
3. To understand where future research in these areas should focus

28.1 Introduction

This chapter highlights the research priorities considered most significant for the future health of twins and multiples and their families. The Global Twins and Multiples Priority Setting Partnership [2] brought together families of twins and multiples and clinicians and researchers who work with twins and multiples to determine these priorities; see Fig. 28.1. The top ten and 89 priorities from five key areas will be discussed: antenatal care, intrapartum and postpartum care, neonatal and paediatric health, child psychiatry and development, and parental and family health.

The top ten priorities are as follows:

Antenatal Care

- How can we prevent maternal complications in multiple pregnancies?
- Would staff with specialist training in multiple pregnancies improve outcomes in these pregnancies?
- How are higher-order multiple pregnancies best managed?

Intrapartum and Postpartum Care

- What are the short- and long-term maternal health risks following a multiple pregnancy?
- What prenatal factors (including changes to lifestyle, health history, per-

28

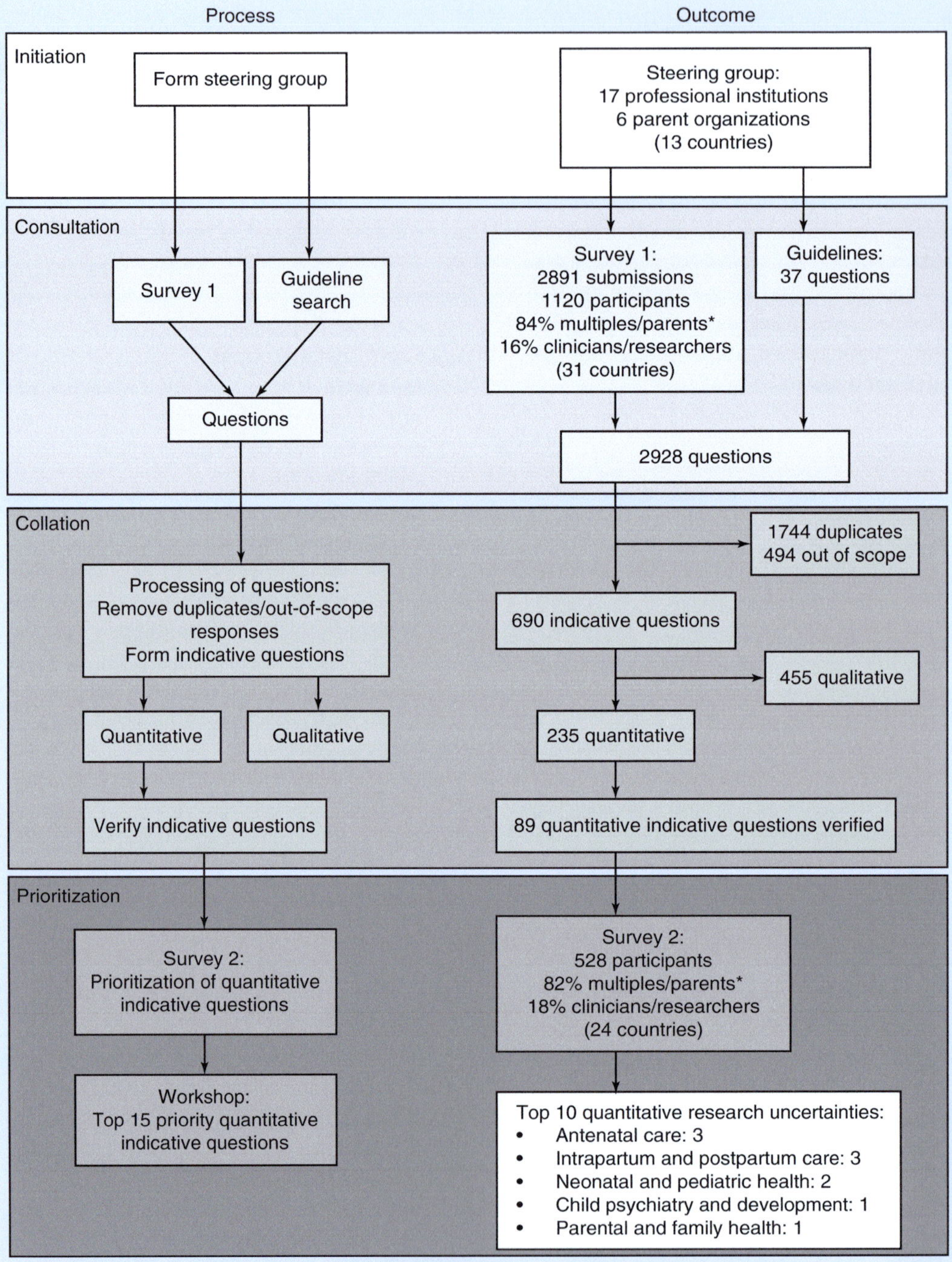

Fig. 28.1 Flowchart of priority-setting process for global research on health of multiples and their families. *Includes multiples, parents of multiples, carers of multiples, and representatives from parent and multiples groups

sonality characteristics) and supports for parents of multiples have the most benefit on birth and ongoing health outcomes for both parents and their children?

Neonatal and Paediatric Health

- What are the expected growth patterns of small-for-gestational-age multiples? How can we assess the growth of infant multiples and ensure that they follow a satisfactory growth trajectory?
- How can we reduce multiples' admission to the neonatal unit? If admitted, how can we reduce multiples' length of stay in the neonatal unit?
- What are the short- and long-term outcomes in multiple pregnancies? How are these outcomes affected by antenatal events and medical interventions?

Child Psychiatry and Development

- What parental interventions can improve the developmental outcomes (i.e. speech, language, education) of multiples?

Parental and Family Health

- What interventions prevent and support postnatal mental-health problems in parents of multiples?

The objectives of this chapter are to discuss a few of the key research priorities for the health of twins and multiples; provide an overview of existing findings for the above key research priorities; and to explain where future research in these areas should focus.

28.2 Antenatal Care

28.2.1 Background

Twin and multiple pregnancies are exceptional experiences for both families and clinicians; however, they carry an increased risk of complications. Mothers are predisposed to increased risks of pre-eclampsia, preterm delivery, and postpartum haemorrhage (PPH). Twins and multiples have an increased incidence of fetal growth restriction (FGR), stillbirth, fetal anomalies, as well as monochorionic-specific complications such as twin-twin transfusion syndrome (TTTS), and twin anaemia polycythaemia sequence (TAPS) [3–8].

An analysis by the World Health Organization Multicountry Survey on Maternal and Newborn Health (WHOMCS 2010–2011) found that the rate of maternal death was four times higher in twin pregnancies than singletons, and maternal near miss was three times higher [9]. Dichorionic twins have a five-fold increased risk of stillbirth compared to singletons, and this is increased 13-fold in monochorionic twins [10, 11]. It is recommended by the National Institute for Health and Care Excellence (NICE) guidelines that women with multiple pregnancies should receive care by a specialist team of midwives, Obstetricians, and sonographers with the relevant expertise in the management of multiple pregnancies to allow early recognition of antenatal complications and reduce poor outcomes [12].

Higher-order multiple pregnancies are associated with even higher rates of miscarriage and preterm birth than twins [13]. Previously, no clear consensus was in place regarding the antenatal care, monitoring, or timing of delivery of these pregnancies. Recently, the NICE guideline was updated to include the care and surveillance of triplets, specifically, to provide guidance to clinicians on the most optimal pathway of care [12].

28.2.2 What Previous Research Has Told Us

Traditionally, multiple pregnancies have often been excluded from trials. However, in recent years, both researchers and clinicians have recognised the need to focus on the requirements of multiple pregnancies. This is reflected in the increasing numbers of studies in this area. And in the last few years, national and international guidelines have been developed to guide clinicians on the management and surveillance of these pregnancies, as well as the recognition of multiple specific complications.

Closer surveillance of monochorionic pregnancies is now recommended, together with the identification of monochorionic-specific complications, as well as the indications for referral to a fetal medicine centre [12]. A Delphi consensus was reached to unify the diagnosis of selective fetal growth restriction [14], and twin-specific growth charts have been designed and incorporated into practice to minimise overdiagnosis and unnecessary intervention [15]. Furthermore, low-dose Aspirin is now routinely recommended in multiple pregnancies with an aim to prevent preterm pre-eclampsia, although the evidence for this is still unclear, and optimisation of haemoglobin levels through regular monitoring antenatally. An enhanced care team should also be available for referrals (including physiotherapists, dieticians, and mental health professionals), with specialist experience in multiple pregnancies [12].

Research has identified that miscarriage and very preterm delivery rates can be reduced through selective fetal reduction of higher-order multiples [16, 17]. This option is now routinely offered to all couples with these pregnancies [18]. Their antenatal surveillance pathway and timing of delivery depend on chorionicity, as dichorionic triplets are at higher risk of adverse outcome than trichorionic triplets [19]; however, very few cases of the outcomes of monochorionic triplets have been described due to the rarity of the condition.

28.2.3 Future Research

Despite recent recommendations for specialist care for multiples, further research is required to assess the difference in outcomes in centres prior to, and after this change. The benefits of Aspirin in pre-eclampsia prevention in multiples is still unclear, as is the prediction and prevention of preterm deliveries. Recent research has also aimed to assess perinatal outcomes in triplet pregnancies, and further research is underway to study outcomes in monochorionic triplets to provide more information for their optimal care.

28.3 Intrapartum and Postpartum Care

28.3.1 Background

As discussed, women with twin and multiple pregnancies are at an increased risk of perinatal morbidity and mortality [9]. The current recommendation is that both vaginal and Caesarean delivery are safe in twins, provided they are over 32 weeks gestation, the presenting twin in cephalic, there are no Obstetric contraindications, or significant size discrepancies. Monoamniotic twins and higher-order multiples are recommended to have a Caesarean section [12]. Women with multiple pregnancies are at an increased risk of pre-eclampsia and PPH and are therefore offered an active third stage in labour, a group and save taken at the onset of labour, and are given additional uterotonics if there are more risk factors for bleeding [12].

The recovery of the mother following birth is felt to be a particular concern amongst parents and clinicians. The emotional and physical well-being of the mother can impact on her ability to care for her infants, and if unrecognised, suboptimal maternal health can lead to long-term impacts on herself, the children, and the rest of the family [20]. One question prioritised by the Global Twins and Multiples

Priority Setting Partnership was "What are the short- and long-term maternal health risks following a multiple pregnancy?"

28.3.2 What Previous Research Has Told Us

Data looking into maternal health postnatally are scarce. One large Cochrane review investigated the difference in outcomes between vaginal and Caesarean delivery in twin pregnancies [21]. No differences were found between the mode of delivery and maternal mortality or short-term morbidity. Furthermore, there were no differences in the ability to breastfeed, or the rate of postnatal depression.

The Twin Birth Study was an international randomised controlled trial that compared outcomes of the neonates following vaginal or Caesarean delivery. Hutton et al. performed the first twin postnatal maternal analysis on the women from this trial, which provided insight into the quality of life of mothers 3 months after birth [22]. Of the sample, 86% of women in all groups stated they were happy in their relationship with their partner; 11–15% reported urinary incontinence; 3.8% faecal incontinence, and 23% scored >10 points on the Edinburgh Postnatal Depression scale (total 30). In the study, 84–86% of these women continued to breastfeed after 3 months. There were no significant differences between women who had a planned vaginal delivery compared with those who had a planned Caesarean delivery [20].

28.3.3 Future Research

The study above analyses maternal health 3 months postnatally, but long-term follow-up may be useful to identify the development of physical and mental health issues in the future. A comparison to singleton mothers postnatally may also be useful to compare the prevalence of medical comorbidities and limitations to quality of life.

28.4 Neonatal and Paediatric Health

28.4.1 Background

Twins and higher-order multiples have a lower birth weight than singletons [23, 24]. From 30 weeks gestation, the growth of dichorionic twins fall behind that of singletons, and monochorionic twins tend to have a persistently slower growth throughout the gestations [15]. Triplets begin to fall behind the growth of singletons after 30 weeks, and behind twins after 34 weeks [24]. By 40 weeks, the birthweight difference between twins and singletons are as large as 640 g for male babies and 480 g for female babies [25]. Given that twins are at a higher risk of preterm delivery, they are highly likely to be of lower weight at birth. One research priority proposed by the Global Twin and Multiples Priority Setting Partnership was "What are the expected growth patterns of small-for-gestational-age multiples? How can we assess the growth of infant multiples and ensure that they follow a satisfactory growth trajectory?"

As previously discussed, these babies are at higher risk of adverse perinatal outcomes, thereby increasing their likelihood of neonatal unit admissions. These admissions are largely due to prematurity, fetal growth restriction, and monochorionic-specific complications [25]. This can affect early parent-child relationship bonding and have an emotional and financial impact on the families [26]. In addition, these admissions increase the costs of healthcare. (The Global Twins and Multiples Priority Setting Partnership also recognised methods to reduce the rate and duration of neonatal unit admissions needed to be investigated [2].)

28

28.4.2 What Previous Research Has Told Us

Existing research has resulted in the development of growth charts specifically for twins and multiples. Stirrup et al. have analysed the antenatal growth charts of a large cohort of twin pregnancies, and based on these patterns, they derived growth charts specific to twin pregnancies [15]. Twin birthweight centiles according to sex and gestational age have also been proposed by Li et al. [25]. Further, triplet antenatal growth ranges have been published [24, 27], although triplet-specific growth charts are not yet used in practice. However to date, there is little information on normal twin infant growth trajectories based on birthweight and gestational age at birth.

It is well established that there are clear patterns between gestational age at birth and twin and multiple outcomes. A systematic review analysed the prospective risks of neonatal morbidity and mortality in twin pregnancies, and found that the most prevalent neonatal morbidity after 34 weeks was admission to the neonatal unit [28]. All neonatal morbidities (respiratory distress syndrome, septicaemia, and admission to neonatal unit) were reduced in twins with increasing gestational age at delivery. After 37 weeks in dichorionic twins, and after 36 weeks in monochorionic twins, the risk of stillbirth outweighed the risk of neonatal death [28]. Luke et al. found that the increased cost of neonatal unit admissions was more highly contributed to prematurity rather than plurality [29]; therefore, further research into the reduction of preterm deliveries may also aid the reduction of neonatal unit admissions.

28.4.3 Future Research

Infant growth charts specific to twins according to gestational age of delivery, as well as birthweight, may allow us to assess normal growth trajectory after birth. Further research is required to find ways to reduce neonatal unit admissions – this may include identification and prevention of preterm deliveries, early diagnosis and treatment of monochorionic specific complications, and avoiding unnecessary preterm deliveries.

28.5 Child Psychiatry and Development

28.5.1 Background

Twins and multiples born premature are also at increased risk of developmental delay, in part due to low birthweight [30, 31]. One significant area of delayed development in twins is speech and language [32, 33]. Although researchers agree speech and language delay in twins is usually mild, it is prevalent [34, 35]. One audit found delays in speech and language to be the most prevalent ongoing neurodevelopmental concern in twins who had been treated with selective fetoscopic laser ablation for TTTS [35]. Further, both families of multiples and clinicians feel the trajectories of speech and language development in twins warrant further investigation [2]. The specific question prioritised by the Global Twins and Multiples Priority Setting Partnership was "What are the speech and language developmental trajectories of twins?"

28.5.2 What Previous Research Has Told Us

Previous research on the speech and language development in twins has established several patterns of note in early childhood. Rutter et al. found the language ability of twins to be behind that of single birth children by 1.7 months at the age of 20 months and 3.1 months at the age of 3 years [36]; Mittler et al.'s study found twins experienced a delay in language by 6 months at the age of 4 years. (Studies have found language delay in twins to range depending on study methodology [34, 36–38]).

Further, delay in language ability has been found to be a particular problem for male twins [36, 37] with studies finding a 6–8 month lag in twin males compared with twin females

[37–39]. At 30 months of age, Hay et al. found twin boys to be 8 months behind twin girls in expressive language and 6 months behind on verbal comprehension.

Some studies have reported twins "catch up" in speech and language development by 3–4 years of age, again with female twins ahead of male twins [37, 38, 40]. Although one study suggested twins continue to struggle with more complex speech sound combinations compared with their peers at the age of 6 years [40], while other evidence indicates language delays in twins are resolved by middle childhood [34, 35, 41].

28.5.3 Ongoing and Future Research

Although research has been conducted on the speech and language development of twins, it focuses on children aged from about 2 to 6 years. Research in progress continues to examine the effects of laser therapy to treat TTTS on speech and language [42]. However, future research should also seek to understand the long-term course of language development for twins and ramifications of language delay in early childhood with longitudinal study designs as well as test intervention paths [34, 37, 43].

28.6 Parental and Family Health

28.6.1 Background

Parents of multiples may experience higher rates of mental health problems compared with parents of singletons. Hay et al.'s La Trobe Twin Study found mothers of multiples reported having anxiety at three times the rate than mothers of singletons and "extreme" depression at five times the rate [44]. Fathers of multiples have been reported to experience twice the levels of anxiety and four times rate of depression [45]. Even at 5 years after birth, one study indicated a higher proportion of mothers of twins may experience depression compared with mothers of singletons [46].

28.6.2 What We Know from Existing Research

Many challenges are associated with being parents to multiples and include medical, financial, psychological, and social obstacles [47]. Financial concerns, marital problems, lack of space in the home, and the need for a larger car have all been correlated with anxiety and depression scores in mothers of newborn twins [44]. Poor sleep quality is also associated with worse depression and anxiety symptoms [48]. In addition, Hay et al. found higher postnatal depression in mothers of twins was mainly predicted by whether the twins came home from hospital after birth at the same time as the mother [44].

Furthermore, mothers of very preterm multiples who have suffered a bereavement of one of the multiples may be more vulnerable to psychological distress. One recent study found that compared with mothers who had not experienced a bereavement, those that had were 3.6 times (95% CI 1.05, 12.5) more likely to report increased anxiety symptoms and 3.6 times (95% CI 1.05, 12.3) more likely to report increased depressive symptoms when their very preterm child had reached 7 years of age [49]. Further, Bryan's work found mothers are faced with a number of challenges including simultaneously mourning one child and celebrating the other; differentiating between the deceased baby and the surviving baby; and coping with unsupportive friends, neighbours, and clinicians [50].

28.6.3 Future Research

Families of multiples, clinicians, and researchers from the Global Twins and Multiples Priority Setting Partnership prioritised postpartum depression as an area for future research: "What interventions prevent or minimise the impact of postpartum depression in parents/families of multiples (including twins)?" Wenze et al. have recently initiated investigations into perinatal mental health interventions for parents of multiples [48]. In this study, parents of multiples perceived the most challenging parenting periods to be birth to 3 months (56%) and pregnancy (almost 20%). During the parenting period that they perceived the most difficult, 26.1% of parents of younger multiples expressed interest for treatment for depression and 29.5% for anxiety. All participant sub-groups (mothers, partners, and parents of younger multiples) were most interested in individual, internet-delivered, and group therapy modes of treatment delivery. The researchers suggested e-Health interventions as promising given parents of multiples are interested in technology-based treatment modalities, are frequent users of technology, and face barriers to treatment such as lack of time, requiring childcare, financial strain, and confinement to bedrest. Future research will need to determine whether e-Health interventions can effectively prevent or minimise the impact of postpartum depression for parents of multiples.

28.6.4 Policy

The following questions related to postpartum depression were also considered important by the Global Twins and Multiples Priority Setting Partnership, but are more relevant to policy to support parents of young multiples. One concerned the impact of disrupted sleep on both mental and physical health: "How does long-term lack of sleep/continual sleep interruption impact the physical and mental health of parents or single parents with multiples?" Similarly, findings from the following question would provide evidence to supply and fund services to build protective factors for parents of multiples: "Does attending multiple specific antenatal classes improve parenting resilience and reduce postnatal depression for families?"

28.7 Conclusion

This chapter provides an overview of the research priorities considered most significant to families of twins and multiples, clinicians, and researchers for the future health of multiples and their families. These priorities were determined by the Global Twins and Multiples Priority Setting Partnership across five disciplines: antenatal care, intrapartum and postpartum care, neonatal and paediatric health, child psychiatry and development, and parent and family health. Following the review of existing research, further investigation is required in the following areas:

Antenatal Care

- The benefits of Aspirin in pre-eclampsia prevention in multiples
- The prediction and prevention of preterm deliveries

Intrapartum and Postpartum Care

- Long-term investigation of the development of physical and mental health issues in mothers
- A comparison between twin and multiple and singleton mothers postnatally to investigate the prevalence of medical comorbidities and limitations to quality of life

Neonatal and Paediatric Health

- The development of twin-specific infant growth charts specific to gestational age of delivery, as well as birthweight to assess normal growth trajectory after birth
- Methods to reduce neonatal unit admissions

Child Psychiatry and Development

- An investigation into the long-term course of language development in twins and the impacts of language delay in early childhood
- Testing intervention paths for language delay in twins

Parental and Family Health

- What interventions (including those online) can effectively prevent or minimise the impact of postpartum depression for parents of multiples

Research across this breadth of domains is imperative to improving the future health of twins, multiples, and their families. These priorities were developed through a multidisciplinary and collaborative effort between families, clinicians, and researchers and a continued partnership will be necessary to progress this work for the benefit of twins, multiples, their families, and communities worldwide.

28.7.1 Review Questions

1. What areas should future research focus on to benefit twins and multiples in:
   (a) Antenatal care
   (b) Postpartum care
   (c) Neonatal and paediatric health
   (d) Child psychiatry and development
   (e) Parental and family health
2. If speech and language delays in twins are usually considered mild, why should research continue to investigate this developmental concern?
3. At what age have speech and language delays been identified in twins? How large are these delays compared with children of single births?
4. Why is future research necessary to understand the speech and language developmental trajectories of twins?
5. Which developmental periods have been reported to be the most challenging for mothers of multiples, in terms of their impact on mental health?
6. Which policy areas are a priority for the mental and physical health of parents of multiples?
7. How can research support policy to benefit the mental health of parents?
8. What are the main causes of neonatal unit admissions in twins and multiples?
9. What is the main neonatal morbidity in twins after 34 weeks?
10. What are the benefits of using twin-specific growth charts during pregnancy?

28.7.2 Multiple-Choice Questions

1. Which group is most affected by speech and language delays?
   (a) Twins
   (b) Female twins
   (c) Male twins
   (d) Both (b) and (c)

Answer: (c)

2. At what developmental stage does existing evidence suggest language delays are resolved?
   (a) 3–4 years old
   (b) 6 years old
   (c) Middle childhood
   (d) Both (a) and (c)

Answer: (d)

3. What key speech and language areas should future research focus on?
   (a) Outcomes for twins 6 years and older
   (b) Consequences of language delay in early childhood
   (c) Intervention paths
   (d) All of the above

Answer: (d)

4. Which study design would be most appropriate to investigate the speech and language developmental trajectories of twins?
   (a) Randomised controlled trial
   (b) Longitudinal study
   (c) Cross-sectional study

Answer: (b)

5. What factors can contribute towards depression in young mothers of twins or multiples?
   (a) Financial concerns
   (b) Marital problems
   (c) Lack of space in the home
   (d) Poor sleep quality
   (e) Whether twins come home from hospital after birth at the same time as the mother
   (f) All of the above

Answer: (f)

6. What types of interventions look promising for the treatment of depression in parents of multiples?
   (a) Group therapy
   (b) Individual therapy
   (c) Internet-based therapy
   (d) All of the above

Answer: (c)

7. At what gestational age does growth begin to slow down for dichorionic twins?
   (a) 28 weeks
   (b) 30 weeks
   (c) 32 weeks
   (d) 34 weeks

8. What are the two main maternal complications in twin pregnancies?
   (a) Pre-eclampsia and gestational diabetes
   (b) Gestational diabetes and obstetric cholestasis
   (c) Antepartum haemorrhage and pre-eclampsia
   (d) Postpartum haemorrhage and pre-eclampsia

9. What can be offered to parents of triplet pregnancies to try and reduce the rate of miscarriage and very preterm delivery?
   (a) Progesterone suppository
   (b) Cervical cerclage
   (c) Selective fetal reduction
   (d) No intervention has been proven effective

References

1. The American College of Obstetricians and Gynecologists. Postpartum depression. The American College of Obstetricians and Gynecologists, The United States of America; 2019. https://www.acog.org/Patients/FAQs/Postpartum-Depression?IsMobileSet=false. Accessed November 2019.
2. Lam JR, Liu B, Bhate R, Fenwick N, Reed K, Duffy JMN, et al. Research priorities for the future health of multiples and their families: the global twins and multiples priority setting partnership. Ultrasound Obstet Gynecol. 2019;54(6):715–21. https://doi.org/10.1002/uog.20858.
3. Kilby MD, Baker PN, Critchley HO, Field DJ. Consensus views arising from the 50th Study Group: multiple pregnancy. In: Multiple pregnancy. London: RCOG Press; 2006. p. 283–6.
4. Sairam S, Costeloe K, Thilaganathan B. Prospective risk of stillbirth in multiple-gestation pregnancies: a population-based analysis. Obstet Gynecol. 2002;100(4):638–41. https://doi.org/10.1016/s0029-7844(02)02174-9.
5. Ehsanipoor RM, Haydon ML, Lyons Gaffaney C, Jolley JA, Petersen R, Lagrew DC, et al. Gestational age at cervical length measurement and preterm birth in twins. Ultrasound Obstet Gynecol. 2012;40(1):81–6. https://doi.org/10.1002/uog.10130.
6. Townsend R, Khalil A. Fetal growth restriction in twins. Best Pract Res Clin Obstet Gynaecol. 2018;49:79–88. https://doi.org/10.1016/j.bpobgyn.2018.02.004.
7. Hall JG. Twinning. Lancet. 2003;362(9385):735–43. https://doi.org/10.1016/s0140-6736(03)14237-7.
8. Pasquini L, Wimalasundera RC, Fisk NM. Management of other complications specific to monochorionic twin pregnancies. Best Pract Res Clin Obstet Gynaecol. 2004;18(4):577–99. https://doi.org/10.1016/j.bpobgyn.2004.04.011.
9. Santana DS, Cecatti JG, Surita FG, Silveira C, Costa ML, Souza JP, et al. Twin pregnancy and severe maternal outcomes: the World Health Organization multicountry survey on maternal and newborn health. Obstet Gynecol. 2016;127(4):631–41. https://doi.org/10.1097/aog.0000000000001338.

10. Peter C, Wenzlaff P, Kruempelmann J, Alzen G, Bueltmann E, Gruessner SE. Perinatal morbidity and early neonatal mortality in twin pregnancies. Open J Obstet Gynecol. 2013;3(1):12. https://doi.org/10.4236/ojog.2013.31017.
11. Russo FM, Pozzi E, Pelizzoni F, Todyrenchuk L, Bernasconi DP, Cozzolino S, et al. Stillbirths in singletons, dichorionic and monochorionic twins: a comparison of risks and causes. Eur J Obstet Gynecol Reprod Biol. 2013;170(1):131–6. https://doi.org/10.1016/j.ejogrb.2013.06.014.
12. National Institute for Health and Clinical Excellence. Twin and triplet pregnancy. NICE clinical guideline 137. London: National Institute for Health and Clinical Excellence; 2019.
13. Blickstein I. How and why are triplets disadvantaged compared to twins? Best Pract Res Clin Obstet Gynaecol. 2004;18(4):631–44. https://doi.org/10.1016/j.bpobgyn.2004.04.014.
14. Khalil A, Beune I, Hecher K, Wynia K, Ganzevoort W, Reed K, et al. Consensus definition and essential reporting parameters of selective fetal growth restriction in twin pregnancy: a Delphi procedure. Ultrasound Obstet Gynecol. 2019;53(1):47–54. https://doi.org/10.1002/uog.19013.
15. Stirrup OT, Khalil A, D'Antonio F, Thilaganathan B. Fetal growth reference ranges in twin pregnancy: analysis of the Southwest Thames Obstetric Research Collaborative (STORK) multiple pregnancy cohort. Ultrasound Obstet Gynecol. 2015;45(3):301–7. https://doi.org/10.1002/uog.14640.
16. Chaveeva P, Kosinski P, Puglia D, Poon LC, Nicolaides KH. Trichorionic and dichorionic triplet pregnancies at 10-14 weeks: outcome after embryo reduction compared to expectant management. Fetal Diagn Ther. 2013;34(4):199–205. https://doi.org/10.1159/000356170.
17. Morlando M, Ferrara L, D'Antonio F, Lawin-O'Brien A, Sankaran S, Pasupathy D, et al. Dichorionic triplet pregnancies: risk of miscarriage and severe preterm delivery with fetal reduction versus expectant management. Outcomes of a cohort study and systematic review. BJOG. 2015;122(8):1053–60. https://doi.org/10.1111/1471-0528.13348.
18. Khalil A, Rodgers M, Baschat A, Bhide A, Gratacos E, Hecher K, et al. ISUOG practice guidelines: role of ultrasound in twin pregnancy. Ultrasound Obstet Gynecol. 2016;47(2):247–63. https://doi.org/10.1002/uog.15821.
19. Curado J, D'Antonio F, Papageorghiou AT, Bhide A, Thilaganathan B, Khalil A. Perinatal mortality and morbidity in triplet pregnancy according to chorionicity: systematic review and meta-analysis. Ultrasound Obstet Gynecol. 2019;54(5):589–95. https://doi.org/10.1002/uog.20209.
20. Hutton EK, Hannah ME, Ross S, Joseph KS, Ohlsson A, Asztalos EV, et al. Maternal outcomes at 3 months after planned caesarean section versus planned vaginal birth for twin pregnancies in the Twin Birth Study: a randomised controlled trial. BJOG. 2015;122(12):1653–62. https://doi.org/10.1111/1471-0528.13597.
21. Hofmeyr GJ, Barrett JF, Crowther CA. Planned caesarean section for women with a twin pregnancy. Cochrane Database Syst Rev. 2015;(12):CD006553. https://doi.org/10.1002/14651858.CD006553.pub3.
22. Barrett JF, Hannah ME, Hutton EK, Willan AR, Allen AC, Armson BA, et al. A randomized trial of planned cesarean or vaginal delivery for twin pregnancy. N Engl J Med. 2013;369(14):1295–305. https://doi.org/10.1056/NEJMoa1214939.
23. Gielen M, Lindsey PJ, Derom C, Loos RJ, Souren NY, Paulussen AD, et al. Twin-specific intrauterine "growth" charts based on cross-sectional birthweight data. Twin Res Hum Genet. 2008;11(2):224–35. https://doi.org/10.1375/twin.11.2.224.
24. Min SJ, Luke B, Min L, Misiunas R, Nugent C, Van de Ven C, et al. Birth weight references for triplets. Am J Obstet Gynecol. 2004;191(3):809–14. https://doi.org/10.1016/j.ajog.2004.01.052.
25. Li Z, Umstad MP, Hilder L, Xu F, Sullivan EA. Australian national birthweight percentiles by sex and gestational age for twins, 2001–2010. BMC Pediatr. 2015;15(1):148. https://doi.org/10.1186/s12887-015-0464-y.
26. Elliott JP, Istwan NB, Collins A, Rhea D, Stanziano G. Indicated and non-indicated preterm delivery in twin gestations: impact on neonatal outcome and cost. J Perinatol. 2005;25(1):4–7. https://doi.org/10.1038/sj.jp.7211205.
27. Blickstein I, Jacques DL, Keith LG. Total and individual triplet birth weights as a function of gestational age. Am J Obstet Gynecol. 2002;186(6):1372–5. https://doi.org/10.1067/mob.2002.122400.
28. Cheong-See F, Schuit E, Arroyo-Manzano D, Khalil A, Barrett J, Joseph KS, et al. Prospective risk of stillbirth and neonatal complications in twin pregnancies: systematic review and meta-analysis. BMJ. 2016;354:i4353. https://doi.org/10.1136/bmj.i4353.
29. Luke B, Bigger HR, Leurgans S, Sietsema D. The cost of prematurity: a case-control study of twins vs singletons. Am J Public Health. 1996;86(6):809–14. https://doi.org/10.2105/ajph.86.6.809.
30. Costello-Harris VA, Segal NL. The unmet concerns of twins with special needs: diagnostic challenges and service recommendations. Community Pract. 2015;88(2):32–5.
31. Zeltzer J, Shand AW, Kelly P, Hopper JL, Scurrah KJ, Nassar N. Early birth is a key factor in educational disadvantage of twins: a data linkage study. Acta Paediatr. 2019;109(3):534–40. https://doi.org/10.1111/apa.14966.
32. Mogford-Bevan K. Twins and their language development. In: Sandbank A, editor. Twin and triplet psychology: a professional guide to working with multiples. London and New York: Routledge; 1999. p. 36–60.

33. Sutcliffe AG, Derom C. Follow-up of twins: health, behaviour, speech, language outcomes and implications for parents. Early Hum Dev. 2006;82(6):379–86. https://doi.org/10.1016/j.earlhumdev.2006.03.007.
34. Thorpe K. Twin children's language development. Early Hum Dev. 2006;82(6):387–95. https://doi.org/10.1016/j.earlhumdev.2006.03.012.
35. Mullers SM, McAuliffe FM, Kent E, Carroll S, Mone F, Breslin N, et al. Outcome following selective fetoscopic laser ablation for twin to twin transfusion syndrome: an 8 year national collaborative experience. Eur J Obstet Gynecol Reprod Biol. 2015;191:125–9. https://doi.org/10.1016/j.ejogrb.2015.05.019.
36. Rutter M, Thorpe K, Greenwood R, Northstone K, Golding J. Twins as a natural experiment to study the causes of mild language delay. I: Design; twin-singleton differences in language, and obstetric risks. J Child Psychol Psychiatry. 2003;44(3):326–41. https://doi.org/10.1111/1469-7610.00125.
37. Hay DA, Prior M, Collett S, Williams M. Speech and language development in preschool twins. Acta Genet Med Gemellol. 1987;36(2):213–23. https://doi.org/10.1017/S000156600000444X.
38. Mittler P. Biological and social aspects of language development in twins. Dev Med Child Neurol. 1970;12:741–57.
39. Koch H. Twins and twin relations. Chicago: University of Chicago Press; 1966.
40. Rice ML, Zubrick SR, Taylor CL, Hoffman L, Gayán J. Longitudinal study of language and speech of twins at 4 and 6 years: twinning effects decrease, zygosity effects disappear, and heritability increases. J Speech Lang Hear Res. 2018;61(1):79–93. https://doi.org/10.1044/2017_JSLHR-L-16-0366.
41. Davis E. The development of linguistic skills in twins, singletons with siblings and only children from age five to ten years, Monograph 14. Institute of Child Welfare, University of Minnesota. Westport: Greenwood Press; 1977.
42. Bolch C, Fahey M, Reddihough D, Williams K, Reid S, Guzys A, et al. Twin-to-twin transfusion syndrome neurodevelopmental follow-up study (neurodevelopmental outcomes for children whose twin-to-twin transfusion syndrome was treated with placental laser photocoagulation). BMC Pediatr. 2018;18(1):256. https://doi.org/10.1186/s12887-018-1230-8.
43. Culloty AM, O'Toole C, Gibbon FE. Longitudinal study of expressive language and speech of twins at 3 and 5 years: outgrowing a twinning effect. J Speech Lang Hear Res. 2019;62(7):2425–37. https://doi.org/10.1044/2019_jslhr-l-18-0333.
44. Hay DA, Gleeson C, Davies C, Lorden B, Mitchell D, Paton L. What information should the multiple birth family receive before, during and after the birth? Acta Genet Med Gemellol. 1990;39(2):259–69. https://doi.org/10.1017/s0001566000005481.
45. Twins Research Australia. Multiple perspectives: what support do multiple birth families need to live happy and healthy lives. Melbourne: TRA, The University of Melbourne; 2019.
46. Thorpe K, Golding J, MacGillivray I, Greenwood R. Comparison of prevalence of depression in mothers of twins and mothers of singletons. BMJ. 1991;302(6781):875–8. https://doi.org/10.1136/bmj.302.6781.875.
47. Scoats R, Denton J, Harvey M. One too many? Families with multiple births. Community Pract. 2019;91(10):28–31.
48. Wenze SJ, Battle CL. Perinatal mental health treatment needs, preferences, and barriers in parents of multiples. J Psychiatr Pract. 2018;24(3):158–68. https://doi.org/10.1097/pra.0000000000000299.
49. Treyvaud K, Aldana AC, Scratch SE, Ure AM, Pace CC, Doyle LW, et al. The influence of multiple birth and bereavement on maternal and family outcomes 2 and 7 years after very preterm birth. Early Hum Dev. 2016;100:1–5. https://doi.org/10.1016/j.earlhumdev.2016.04.005.
50. Bryan EM. The death of a newborn twin: how can support for parents be improved? Acta Genet Med Gemellol. 1986;35(1–2):115–8. https://doi.org/10.1017/s0001566000006322.

Key Reading

Lam JR, Liu B, Bhate R, Fenwick N, Reed K, Duffy JMN, et al. Research priorities for the future health of multiples and their families: The Global Twins and Multiples Priority Setting Partnership. Ultrasound Obstet Gynecol. 2019;54(6):715–21. https://doi.org/10.1002/uog.20858.

Scoats R, Denton J, Harvey M. One too many? Families with multiple births. Community Pract. 2019;91(10):28–31.

Twins Research Australia. Multiple perspectives: what support do multiple birth families need to live happy and healthy lives. Melbourne: TRA, The University of Melbourne; 2019.

Wenze SJ, Battle CL. Perinatal mental health treatment needs, preferences, and barriers in parents of multiples. J Psychiatr Pract. 2018;24(3):158–68. https://doi.org/10.1097/pra.0000000000000299.

Twin and Higher-Order Pregnancy – Patient Voice

Natasha Fenwick and Alyson Chorley

Contents

A. Khalil et al. (eds.), *Twin and Higher-order Pregnancies*,
https://doi.org/10.1007/978-3-030-47652-6_29

Trailer

The experience of a multiple-birth family is very different from that of a singleton family, from diagnosis throughout pregnancy, into the early years, and beyond. Beginning with a high-risk pregnancy, and increased chance of prematurity, baby loss or disability, parents may go on to face physical and mental health difficulties, relationship challenges, financial strain, social stigma, and difficult decisions around schooling and upbringing, as well as the practical challenges of having multiple children of the same age. It is vital that healthcare professionals can recognise these challenges and adapt their practice to best meet these families' needs.

Definitions

Health professional – midwife, sonographer, consultant, health visitor, paediatrician, or other professional involved in delivering care to multiple-birth families

Higher-order multiples – triplets, quadruplets, or more

Multiple pregnancy – a twin, triplet, or higher-order pregnancy

Multiples or multiple-birth children – referring to twins, triplets, or higher-order multiples

Parent – unless otherwise specified, parent refers to all parents in a family

Learning Objectives

- To understand the issues unique to a multiple pregnancy compared to a singleton pregnancy
- To understand what multiple-birth parents want and need from their antenatal and postnatal care and in the early days of parenthood
- To understand the complex issues surrounding baby loss in a multiple pregnancy
- To understand the experiences of parents facing a prenatal diagnosis or complicated pregnancy
- To understand the needs of multiple-birth families who conceive by assisted reproductive technology
- To understand the specific challenges faced by different types of multiple-birth families

29.1 Different from a Singleton Pregnancy

For parents expecting a multiple pregnancy, everything changes at diagnosis – their expectations of life with their new baby are suddenly replaced by the considerably more daunting task of raising two, three, or more [7, 19].

Having a pregnancy at higher risk of complications including anaemia, hyperemesis gravidarum, pre-eclampsia, gestational diabetes, obstetric cholestasis and postnatal illness, as well as some unique to multiple pregnancies, means that from the very beginning parents are likely to be anxious about their pregnancy and their future life with two or more babies [28].

Practically, antenatal care entails more appointments and closer monitoring, potentially requiring more time off work than a singleton pregnancy even before considering the increased risk of ill health and hospitalisation [15, 28].

Once babies are born, they are more likely to need neonatal care, parents can be split between babies with very different needs, and for many their parental leave will be spent waiting for their babies to come home [2, 28].

Yet the challenges do not end at discharge – rather, caring alone for two or more babies for the first time can be isolating and overwhelming for many parents, compounded by poor sleep, mental health difficulties, financial stresses, and increased challenges with getting out of the house [8, 32] (◘ Fig. 29.1).

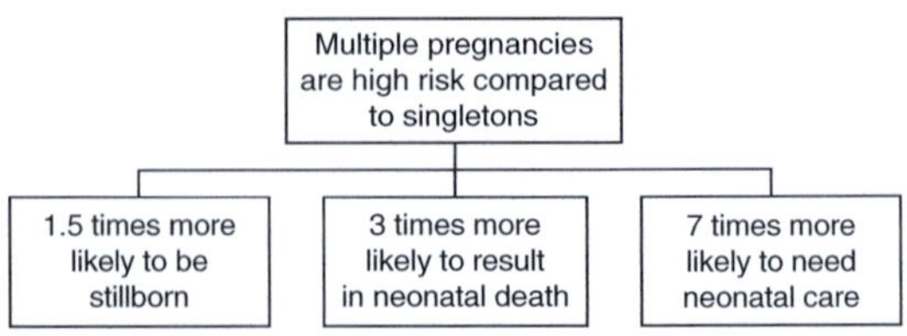

◘ **Fig. 29.1** Major risks of multiple pregnancy [27]

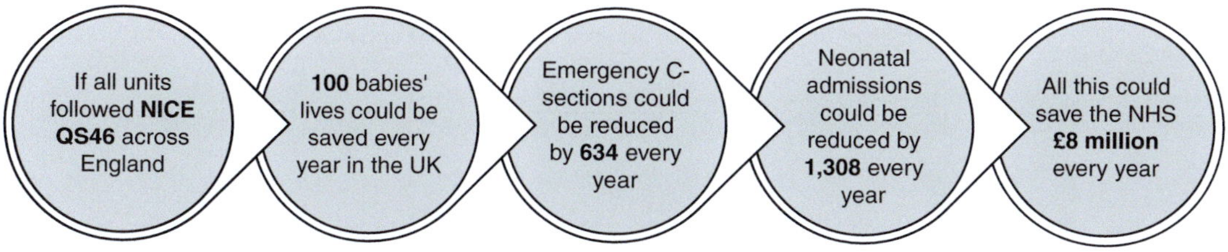

Fig. 29.2 Results of the Maternity Engagement programme to implement NICE QS46 [27]

This set of unique experiences requires health professionals who can offer support and reassurance throughout, adapting their skills and knowledge to the specific needs of these families.

29.2 Specific Guidelines for Multiple Pregnancies

Twin and higher-order multiple pregnancies must receive specialist care due to the high-risk nature of these pregnancies and the different patterns they follow. Several guidelines exist to help provide appropriate antenatal care for multiple pregnancies, including the NICE guideline for Twin and Triplet pregnancy NG137 [18] and quality standard QS46 [17], Green-Top guideline number 51 on the management of monochorionic twin pregnancy [13], and ISUOG Practice Guidelines on the role of ultrasound in twin pregnancy [12].

Since 2016, Twins Trust has supported maternity units to increase adherence to NICE QS46. Key elements of the standard include appointments with a multidisciplinary core team, a specialist care plan determined by chorionicity and amnionicity, and discussions about preterm birth, and mode and timing of delivery [17]. The project's pilot demonstrated that in 12 months, where all units increased adherence to NICE QS46, neonatal admissions and emergency Caesarean sections were reduced by 5.8% and 3.1%, respectively. Additionally, if all units across England followed NICE QS46, up to 100 stillbirths could be prevented every year in the United Kingdom, with 634 fewer emergency Caesarean sections and 1308 fewer neonatal admissions, making care safer and saving the NHS £8 million per year [27]. The benefits of implementing multiple-specific guidance are clear (Fig. 29.2).

Parents also value guideline implementation, with qualitative evidence indicating that being seen by a multidisciplinary core team, having an appropriate care plan, and being well prepared for preterm birth all improve the patient experience [30].

29.3 Antenatal Care

When parents reflect on their pregnancy and birth, the care received is a huge factor in how they feel about their experiences later on [8]. Although expecting a multiple birth is joyful and exciting, for many parents it can also be daunting, shocking, and worrying [19].

In 2019, Twins Trust conducted a survey of multiple-birth parents' experiences of antenatal care. This survey revealed that, overall, parents feel happy with the quality of their antenatal care – 70% would recommend the hospital where they gave birth, and 76% felt confident in the staff caring for them [30]. However, this leaves a large minority whose care could have been improved considerably.

Approximately 82% of expectant multiple-birth parents have chorionicity and amnionicity explained at the dating scan, leaving 18% who lack important information about their pregnancy and antenatal care from the start. Similarly, 72% of parents have an antenatal care plan which explains their appointments to them, but 16% report missing out on this vital information, and 12% are unsure if they received this [30].

Qualitative evidence shows that patients find high-quality, specialist antenatal care reassuring after being told their pregnancy is

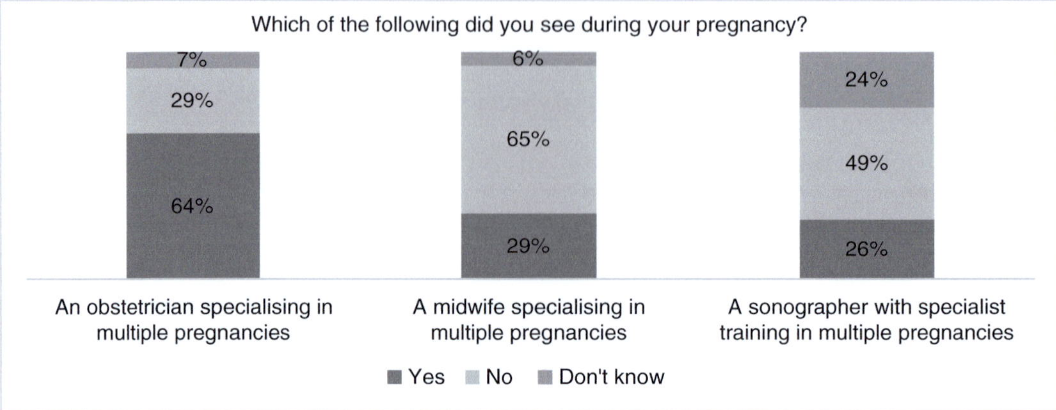

Fig. 29.3 Results of the BeCOME survey showing percentage of parents who accessed a multiple specialist during their pregnancy [30]

high risk [14, 30]. Patients may be familiar with the care they need and expect professionals to be able to provide this. They feel safe under the care of knowledgeable professionals who can answer questions and meet their specific health needs. Conversely, parents feel anxious when staff have little knowledge or experience of multiple pregnancies, and may do research to compensate, in effect becoming the expert on their care. Since up to 30% of parents have no access to a multiple-birth specialist (midwife, sonographer, or obstetrician) during their pregnancy [30], with a decrease in the percentage of pregnancies seen by a specialist obstetrician since 2015 [16], this leaves a large proportion lacking such reassurance (Fig. 29.3).

Continuity of carer is appreciated among parents, who speak positively of their experience where this occurs compared to those who see different staff at each appointment. This allows patients to make the most of appointments and build trust with professionals who understand their particular needs, rather than recounting their history each time. Sixty per cent of parents see the same obstetrician at each appointment, 52% see the same midwife, and 25% see the same sonographer [30]. There is clearly room for improvement in this aspect. When continuity of carer is not possible, this positive experience can also be provided through consistency of care, when different professionals are familiar with the patient's notes, have good communication between individuals and teams, and offer consistent advice [14].

One aspect that needs improvement is preparation for preterm birth. Parents feel very unprepared when their babies come early, despite 60% of twins being born before 37 weeks and 75% of triplets before 35 weeks of pregnancy [29]. It is vital to educate parents about the risks and signs of preterm birth early on and help them prepare for this possibility, even if there are no other indications of risk. This could include a visit to the neonatal unit or meeting the neonatal care team prior to birth – something only around 30% of parents report having the chance to experience [30].

The survey also showed that health professionals are likely to overestimate how often these aspects of care are provided so it is vital to be mindful of them when delivering multiple-specific care.

29.3.1 Complicated Pregnancies

If the revelation of twins or more is daunting, a prenatal diagnosis, such as twin-to-twin transfusion syndrome (TTTS), can be shocking and worrying, overwhelming the joy of pregnancy [7]. It is vital that parents receive counsel and information following a diagnosis, with signposting to resources they can access. Treatment decisions are difficult to make, and require sensitive and unbiased guidance [5, 7]. Treatment can be simultaneously promising and agonising, and this exhausting time does not end once treatment appears successful. This emotional rollercoaster is worsened by the unpredictable nature of some conditions, and the effect on mental health can be long lasting, particularly where babies experience long-term complications [35].

29.3.2 Baby Loss During Pregnancy

It can be difficult for everyone involved when single intrauterine demise, miscarriage, or stillbirth occur. For parents, the death of a baby is likely the most difficult event they will ever face. No matter the circumstances in which bereavement occurs, what happens when babies die can affect how parents reflect on their experience for the rest of their lives, so it is paramount they receive quality care.

Experiencing a bereavement whilst simultaneously carrying a surviving baby is a very difficult situation which brings complicated emotions. The presence of a surviving baby does not lessen the grief parents feel for babies that have died, even if they feel grateful or glad for their survivors [20]. Parents value being prepared for what their loss means for the rest of their pregnancy and birth, and may want to see the baby that has died as well as survivors at future scans, although every parent grieves differently so it is important to communicate openly about each individual's wishes [2, 25].

When all babies in a pregnancy die, care should be given sensitively – for example, giving birth in a general labour ward can be a painful reminder of the babies a family cannot take home. Equally, mothers may wish to recognise their parenthood by giving birth in the usual way with a midwife and spending time making memories with their babies, holding them and taking photographs [2, 21].

In any pregnancy where there is a bereavement, parents want professionals to know that there is no silver lining to grief [21]. Regardless of the number of babies, gestation, age of the parents or other factors, baby loss is a devastating situation and parents must be allowed to grieve. They would much rather talk about the babies who have died than be rushed through their grief or have their difficult circumstances become the "elephant in the room" [20]. Staff who feel unsure of how to approach bereaved parents can begin by asking their babies' names. Other ways to support parents include recognising future challenges, asking about or attending funerals, and discussing parents' wishes for memory making and burying their children.

Overwhelmingly, these parents want professionals to refer to their babies as babies, regardless of the circumstances of their death [21]. Using terms such as "late miscarriage" or "intrauterine demise" may be appropriate in certain circumstances, but when talking to parents (in person or in writing) this can sound dehumanising and trivialising.

Following a bereavement, accuracy and honesty are essential when talking about the pregnancy. Inaccuracies can appear unprofessional and uncaring, and for a parent remembering their babies, names, dates, multiplicity, and the circumstances of their pregnancy and loss are vital aspects [2]. Patients want professionals to be realistic with them about what to expect during pregnancy, birth and when meeting their babies, even when this is hard to hear, as it helps them understand through their shock what is going to happen [20, 21]. In circumstances where consulting a more senior member of staff before answering patients' questions is appropriate, they value honesty much more than being given wrong or vague information.

When transitioning to postnatal or neonatal care, staff need to be made aware of the bereavement, as poor communication between teams or failure to read patients' notes can lead to unnecessary distress [20]. To avoid this, staff must read the notes of every patient who comes into their care.

All grieving families need support, and as the first people to speak to those bereaved during pregnancy, health professionals are in a unique position to provide this [20]. Families value being directed to appropriate, accessible support. When planning support in the hospital and at home, staff should consider that each family member, including any siblings,

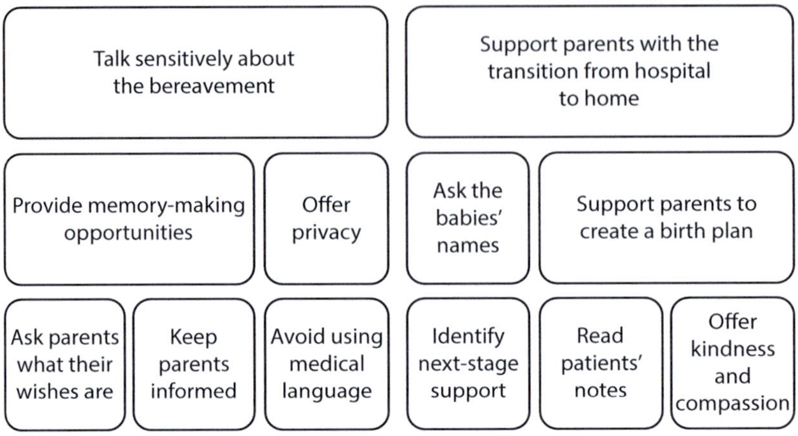

Fig. 29.4 Ways to support a multiple-birth family bereaved during pregnancy

may grieve differently, and need to be directed to both immediate and long-term support.

Above all, bereaved families value compassion, care, emotion, and kindness from staff [20, 21]. Those who exceed expectations to support families, ensure their needs and wishes are heard, and care for their babies like any other can make a truly devastating experience more bearable (Fig. 29.4).

29.3.3 Assisted Conception

Multiple pregnancy is a common effect of fertility treatment, although rates have decreased from around 24% in 2008 to around 10% in 2017 [10]. In fact, those who experience infertility may have a high desire for a multiple compared to a singleton pregnancy [3], often due to lack of knowledge of the risks and realities of parenting twins or more [23, 33]. Those who have been infertile or accessing ART for some time and who have no other children are more likely to desire an "instant family" through multiple pregnancy. However, this desire lessens once parents understand the associated difficulties [24].

Mothers of multiples conceived by ART are more likely to have poor mental health outcomes and be vulnerable to depression than mothers of ART singletons. Additionally, mothers of IVF multiples are less likely to enjoy parenthood than their singleton counterparts [24, 31]. The long journey to conceive and the life that such parents imagine afterwards can contrast starkly with the reality of struggling to meet the needs of two or more babies. These parents in particular need support postnatally.

Issues surrounding the method of conception can be sensitive, and parents may be reluctant to disclose such information. Even where families have not undergone assisted reproduction, they may experience judgement because of this misconception [22]. During antenatal care, mode of conception should only be discussed when medically relevant and should be asked in an unprejudiced way.

29.4 Postnatal Needs

Due to the high-risk nature of multiple pregnancies, it is reasonable that health professionals would focus on improving antenatal and intrapartum care. However, it is important to note that difficulties do not end at birth.

Many parents feel unprepared for the challenges that follow, and this is particularly true if their babies are premature. The BeCOME survey showed that 20% of parents feel preparation for postnatal care is poor or very poor, with 51% of health professionals agreeing that it could be improved [30]. The transition from specialist antenatal to routine postnatal care can be abrupt given that multiple-birth parents continue to have specific needs after birth, and there is a sense that these are not understood in this context. Parents may also have had complex or traumatic pregnancies and births and feel their postpartum needs are overlooked. This is compounded by high demand on staff attention in the postnatal ward.

Parents' satisfaction with neonatal care is high, and they feel confident in the neonatal staff, but transition between units and teamwork across the hospital are both concerns [30]. Parents' experiences of understanding and adjusting to the practices of the neonatal unit and participating in care of their babies are mixed, and it can take some time for these parents to feel like parents [11]. They value getting involved, as this helps them feel connected to their babies, supports bonding, and alleviates feelings of helplessness. However, logistical challenges such as caring for babies with different needs, in different wards or hospitals, establishing feeding with each baby and managing different feeding schedules, dividing their time and attention, and having a baby discharged before others, at the same time as recovering from birth can prove a barrier to effectively caring for and bonding with multiple babies [28]. Hospitals should provide flexible policies to parents of multiples to help relieve some of these pressures.

One area where parents struggle is feeding, and support is often inadequate or poorly signposted [20, 30]. Following the World Health Organisation advice of breastfeeding for at least 6 months [34] can be intimidating to a parent of two or more babies [4, 28]. Dishearteningly, parents who want to breastfeed are sometimes discouraged from doing so, or rarely babies are given formula without their consent. The situation becomes more complex when babies are very premature or split between wards or the family home. Parents value having their feeding goals considered so they can receive appropriate, high-quality support to achieve them, and feel empowered in choosing how to care for their babies.

Following discharge, both partners and birthmothers may experience social isolation, sleep deprivation, lack of confidence, and poor mental health [28, 33], and at all stages of life, parents of multiples undertake two or more times the care required by a singleton baby. Mothers of multiples experience more severe postpartum mental health difficulties and poorer mental health outcomes than mothers of singletons during the early years of parenthood [1, 35]. This is particularly true for those who experience difficult deliveries or whose babies experience postnatal complications, and can last for years. Even parents without a diagnosable mental health condition are likely to be exhausted. However, many parents report having no opportunity to discuss postnatal mental health with their healthcare providers and a larger proportion lack support at their time of need [32]. Parents of multiples should be monitored for mental health difficulties and signposted to support for mental health, sleep deprivation, financial strain, and other challenges (▫ Fig. 29.5).

In the community, there is little support from healthcare services [8], so it is invaluable to signpost families to external services that can support them long term. Leaving the house with more than one baby can be unfeasible, and check-ups, appointments, and support should be offered at the family home or online whenever possible to enable families to access services [32].

Families with two parents face high relationship stress after a multiple birth but also have more opportunities for both parents to care for the children, providing high levels of satisfaction and stability [6]. Where there is only one parent, relationship stress is relieved, but they may look to extended family, friends, peers, and services to help meet the needs of their children [9]. Nonetheless, these parents find parenthood a lonely experience and those in cultures that stigmatise lone parenthood can struggle to enjoy their new role. Although social support cannot replace a partner, families benefit from accessing support online, in the form of other parents of multiples, or at home [26].

29.5 The Multiple Experience

Although this chapter has focussed on the support needs, and therefore the challenges, of multiple-birth families, it is necessary to acknowledge that being part of a multiple-

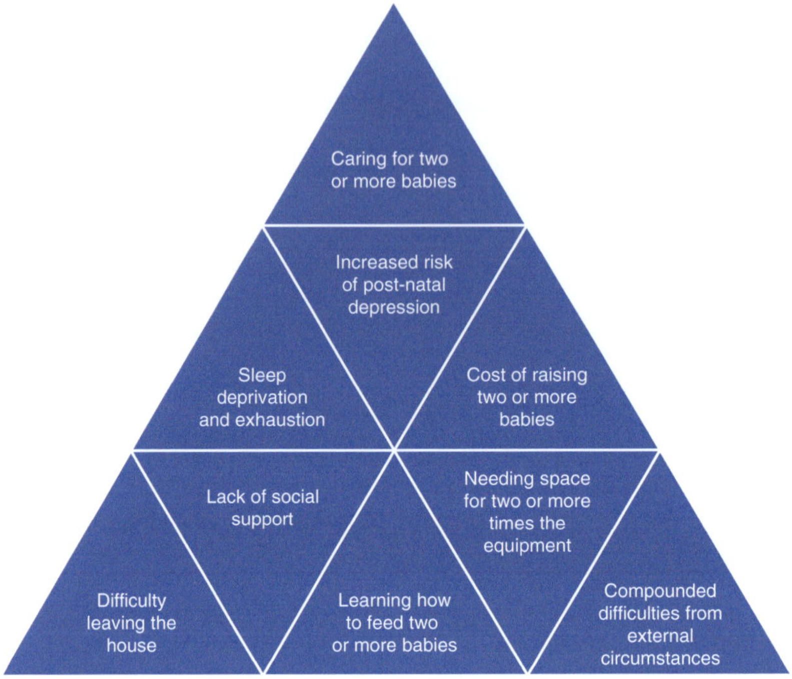

Fig. 29.5 Postnatal challenges faced by parents of twins and higher-order multiples

birth family can be deeply rewarding and satisfying. Multiples often describe having a special bond that is unique, and which provides strength and mutual affection throughout their lifetime. Multiple-birth children learn early on how to collaborate and cooperate, and parents also benefit from their child having a ready-made playmate. Twins and higher-order multiples, their parents, and their grandparents alike may all feel part of a special group of people who understand what it means to be part of a multiple-birth set or to raise multiples.

Patient Testimonials

TTTS Twins

Peter Etherington and wife Laura from Stamford, Lincolnshire, were surprised and thrilled to discover they were expecting twins. But during the 18-week scan, the couple were told that there was a clear size difference between the babies and that the smaller twin was unlikely to survive. They were devastated by this news.

"Unfortunately it seemed the sonographer hadn't been trained in scanning more complex twin pregnancies and gave us every impression the loss of one twin was imminent," said Peter.

Thankfully the consultant recognised that this was TTTS and immediately placed the couple under the care of Leicester Fetal Medicine Unit, where Stage 3 TTTS was confirmed.

The couple visited the Twins Trust website to find out all they could about TTTS and were urgently referred to Birmingham Women's Hospital where laser ablation was carried out and two litres of excess amniotic fluid drained.

The surgery was successful and the blood flow between the twins stabilised. The pregnancy continued under close observation and Laura gave birth via planned C-section at

34 weeks to Arthur (3 lbs 13) and Stanley (2 lbs 15).

The boys are doing well and the couple are both keen for more research to be carried out into TTTS.

Premature Twins

At 29 weeks, Rebecca Trede spontaneously went into labour.

One of the babies was breach so Rebecca agreed to a C-section – the safest route when the delivery team were struggling to pick up heartbeats. There were 22 people in the room helping to bring Gracie Ann (2 lbs 10) and Olivia Marie (2 lbs 15) safely into the world.

Being so tiny they were destined for neonatal care – but sadly not at the same hospital as Rebecca.

"I couldn't believe what had just happened. It was all so fast. The girls were transferred to Lister Hospital in Stevenage almost 60 miles from me in West Suffolk and I couldn't be taken there until the next day – but I just wanted my babies to be safe."

"Seeing them in the transfer incubators was so frightening, they were all wired up and looked so small and helpless. But I knew they would be just fine. They were in good hands."

Rebecca and Matt had not visited the neonatal unit before the birth, something she now regrets.

"Being a nurse, I wasn't particularly naïve but I didn't really think we would end up there because everything had been going so well, now I wish we'd taken that tour."

The journey into parenthood had begun, but Rebecca and Matt had to wait 6 days to hold their babies.

The girls stayed in neonatal care for 6 weeks with Rebecca expressing and feeding.

Five months later, Rebecca was offered a de-brief. It gave her the chance to ask important questions about the birth, why certain things happened and see it from the medical professionals' point of view.

Rebecca said, "This was invaluable. Nothing I did or didn't do made my babies come early. In a way it feels like because the answers weren't there I wouldn't get closure, but I did."

Twin Growth Charts

"Without the twin growth charts, my boys would have been born prematurely, their lives and health at risk. Because of research, they are healthy and happy!" Michelle, mum of identical twin boys.

Michelle Watson credits the twin growth charts, created by Professor Asma Khalil, consultant obstetrician at St George's Hospital, from Twins Trust funded research, with enabling her babies to be born healthy at 36 weeks.

"At my 28-week scan it was clear from the sonographer's demeanour that she was concerned," said Michelle.

"To date, all the growth scans had been uneventful, but this latest scan raised concerns that the abdominal circumferences of both twins, although increasing, had not increased enough according to the growth curve (on a singleton growth chart – widely used in scans)."

"The consultant felt the twins had stopped growing and so planned to deliver them much earlier and prescribed corticosteroids to bring on their lungs. He said we would be lucky if they got to 32 weeks and that there was no chance they would make 36 weeks, which is what the NICE guidance aims for."

"My gut instinct spurred me to seek a second opinion."

Michelle had read about twin growth charts on the Twins Trust website, and had asked her local hospital about them but they were still using the singleton growth charts to scan twins.

She then contacted Dr. Khalil who measured Michelle using the twin growth charts and was able to reassure her that the twins were, in fact, growing fine.

Michelle said, "From then on we transferred our care to the specialist twin team at St George's and our beautiful boys were safely delivered at just over 36 weeks."

"Without the twin growth charts, my boys would have been born prematurely, their lives and health at risk. Because of that research, they are healthy and happy!"

Currently only a handful of hospitals in the United Kingdom are using the twin growth charts which are free to use via Twins Trust.

References

1. Baptista J, Moutinho V, Mateus V. Being a mother of preterm multiples in the context of socioeconomic disadvantage: perceived stress and psychological symptoms. J Pediatr. 2017;94(5):491–7.
2. Bryan E. Loss in higher multiple pregnancy and multifetal pregnancy reduction. Twin Res. 2002;5(3):169–74.
3. Child TJ, Henderson AM, Tam SL. The desire for multiple pregnancy in male and female infertility patients. Hum Reprod. 2004;19(3):558–61.
4. Cinar ND, Alvur TM, Kose D, Nemut T. Breastfeeding twins: a qualitative study. J Health Popul Nutr. 2013;31(4):504–9.
5. Egan E, Reid K, O'Bien L, Erwin R, Umstad M. The outcome of twin pregnancies discordant for trisomy 21. Twin Res Hum Genet. 2013;17(1):38–44.
6. Ellison MA, Hall JE. Social stigma and compounded losses: quality-of-life issues for multiple-birth families. Fertil Steril. 2003;80(2):405–14.
7. Fischbein R, Meeker J, Saling J, Chyatte M, Nicholas L. Identifying families' shared disease experiences through a qualitative analysis of online twin-to-twin transfusion syndrome stories. BMC Pregnancy Childbirth. 2016;16:163–73.
8. Harvey M, Athi R, Denny E. Exploratory study on meeting the health and social care needs of mothers with twins. Community Pract. 2014;87(2):28–31.
9. Heinonen K. Describing being a single parent of multiples. Int J Caring Sci. 2019;12(3):1310–20.
10. Human Fertilisation and Embryology Authority. Fertility treatment 2017: trends and figures. London: HFEA; 2019.
11. Hutchinson SW, Spillet MA, Cronin M. Parent's experiences during their infant's transition from neonatal intensive care unit to home: a qualitative study. Qual Rep. 2012;17(12):1–20.
12. Khalil A, Rodgers M, Baschat A, Bhide A, Gratacos E, Hecher K, et al. ISUOG practice guidelines: role of ultrasound in twin pregnancy. Ultrasound Obstet Gynecol. 2016;47(2):247–63.
13. Kilby MD, Bricker L, on behalf of the Royal College of Obstetricians and Gynaecologists. Management of monochorionic twin pregnancy. BJOG. 2016;12(4):e1–e45.
14. Knox E, Martin W. Multiples clinic: a model for antenatal care. Semin Fetal Neonatal Med. 2010;15:357–61.
15. McAslan Fraser E, on behalf of Twins and Multiple Births Association. Multiple births parents' experience of maternity and paternity leave [Internet]. Guildford: Tamba; 2013. Available from: https://twinstrust.org/uploads/assets/f0eb962c-6967-459c-821bd38c01fcc215/MP-Leave-ReportLow-Res-Final.pdf.
16. National Childbirth Trust and Twins and Multiple Births Association. Maternity services and multiple births. Guildford: Tamba; 2015.
17. National Institute for Health and Care Excellence. Multiple pregnancy: twin and triplet pregnancies: quality standard [Internet]. London: NICE; 2019. Available from: http://nice.org.uk/guidance/qs46/resources/multiple-pregnancy-twin-and-triplet-pregnancies-pdf-2098670068933.
18. National Institute for Health and Care Excellence. Twin and triplet pregnancy: NICE guideline [Internet]. London: NICE; 2019. Available from: https://www.nice.org.uk/guidance/ng137/resources/twin-and-triplet-pregnancy-pdf-66141724389829.
19. Nys K, Colpin H, De Munter A, Vandemeulebroecker L. Feelings and the need for information and counselling of expectant parents of twins. Twin Res. 1998;1:142–9.
20. Pector E. How bereaved multiple-birth parents cope with hospitalization, homecoming, disposition for deceased, and attachment to survivors. J Perinatol. 2004;24(11):714–22.
21. Pector E. Views of bereaved multiple-birth parents on life support decisions, the dying process, and discussions surrounding death. J Perinatol. 2004;24(1):4–10.
22. Raj S, Morley R. "Are you asking me if we had sex to conceive?" To whom do parents of twins disclose mode of conception and what do they feel about being asked? Twin Res Hum Genet. 2007;10(6):886–91.
23. Ryan JL, Zhang SH, Dokras A, Syrop CH, Van Voorhis BJ. The desire of infertile patients for multiple births. Fertil Steril. 2004;81(3):500–4.
24. Sheard C, Cox S, Oates M, Ndukwe G, Glazebrook C. Impact of a multiple, IVF birth on post-partum mental health: a composite analysis. Hum Reprod. 2007;22(7):2058–65.

25. Swanson P, Kane R, Pearsall-Jones J, Swanson C, Croft M. How couples cope with the death of a twin or higher order multiple. Twin Res Hum Genet. 2009;12(4):392–402.
26. Twins and Multiple Births Association. Being a one parent family to twins, triplets and more. Aldershot: Tamba; 2015.
27. Twins and Multiple Births Association. NICE works: the final report. Aldershot: Tamba; 2019.
28. Twins Research Australia. Multiple perspectives: what support do multiple birth families need to live happy and healthy lives? Melbourne: TRA, The University of Melbourne; 2019.
29. Twins Trust. Birth plans [Internet]. Twinstrust.org. 2019 [cited 24 Oct 2019]. Available from: https://twinstrust.org/let-us-help/pregnancy-and-birth/preparing-for-birth/birth-plans.html.
30. Twins Trust. Better care of multiple pregnancies in the UK: an exploration. Aldershot: Twins Trust; 2020.
31. Van den Akker O, Postavaru GI, Purewal S. Maternal psychosocial consequences of twin and multiple births following assisted and natural conception: a meta-analysis. Reprod Biomed Online. 2016;33:1–14.
32. Wenze S, Battle C. Perinatal mental health treatment needs, preferences, and barriers in parents of multiples. J Psychiatr Pract. 2018;24(3):158–68.
33. Wenze S, Battle C, Tezanos K. Raising multiples: mental health of mothers and fathers in early parenthood. Arch Womens Ment Health. 2015;18:163–76.
34. World Health Organization. Breastfeeding [Internet]. World Health Organization; 2019 [cited 8 Nov 2019]. Available from: https://www.who.int/topics/breastfeeding/en/.
35. Ystrom E, Reichborn-Kjennerud T, Tambs K, Magnus P, Torgersen AM, Gustavson K. Multiple births and maternal mental health from pregnancy to 5 years after birth: a longitudinal population-based cohort study. Nor Epidemiol. 2014;24(1–2):203–8.

Key Reading

Fraser E, on behalf of Twins and Multiple Births Association. Bereavement support group booklet. Aldershot: Tamba; 2019.

Harvey M, Athi R, Denny E. Exploratory study on meeting the health and social care needs of mothers with twins. Community Pract. 2014;87(2):28–31.

Pector E, Green J, Ehrlers M, Ramsay Carr K, Brink Larsen S, Monaghan O, Damoiseau J, Wheeler M, Read B, Cuff J, Glahn A. Personal experiences of bereaved twins, parents of twins and their carers. Twin Res. 2002;5(3):236–44.

Sheard C, Cox S, Oates M, Ndukwe G, Glazebrook C. Impact of a multiple, IVF birth on post-partum mental health: a composite analysis. Hum Reprod. 2007;22(7):2058–65.

Twins and Multiple Births Association. NICE works. Aldershot: Tamba; 2019.

Twins Research Australia. Multiple perspectives: what support do multiple birth families need to live happy and healthy lives? Melbourne: TRA, The University of Melbourne; 2019.

Twins Trust. Better care of multiple pregnancies in the UK: an exploration (BeCOME). Aldershot: Twins Trust; 2020.

Wenze S, Battle C. Perinatal mental health treatment needs, preferences, and barriers in parents of multiples. J Psychiatr Pract. 2018;24(3):158–68.

Supplementary Information

A. Khalil et al. (eds.), *Twin and Higher-order Pregnancies*,
https://doi.org/10.1007/978-3-030-47652-6

Index

A

B

E

F

R

S

U

V

W

Z

MIX
Papier aus verantwortungsvollen Quellen
Paper from responsible sources
FSC® C105338

If you have any concerns about our products,
you can contact us on
ProductSafety@springernature.com

In case Publisher is established outside the EU,
the EU authorized representative is:
Springer Nature Customer Service Center GmbH
Europaplatz 3, 69115 Heidelberg, Germany

Printed by Libri Plureos GmbH
in Hamburg, Germany